Pediatric Oral and Maxillofacial Surgery

Pediatric Oral and Maxillofacial Surgery

Edited and with Contributions by

LEONARD B. KABAN, DMD, MD, FACS
Walter C. Guralnick Professor and Chairman
Department of Oral and Maxillofacial Surgery
Massachusetts General Hospital
Harvard School of Dental Medicine
Boston, Massachusetts

MARIA J. TROULIS, DDS, MSc
Assistant Professor
Director of Minimally Invasive Surgery Program
Department of Oral and Maxillofacial Surgery
Massachusetts General Hospital
Harvard School of Dental Medicine
Boston, Massachusetts

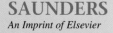
SAUNDERS
An Imprint of Elsevier

SAUNDERS
An Imprint of Elsevier

The Curtis Center
Independence Square West
Philadelphia, Pennsylvania 19106

PEDIATRIC ORAL AND MAXILLOFACIAL SURGERY   ISBN 0-7216-9691-0

NOTICE

Dentistry is an ever-changing field. Standard safety precautions must be followed, but as new research and clinical experience broaden our knowledge, changes in treatment and drug therapy may become necessary or appropriate. Readers are advised to check the most current product information provided by the manufacturer of each drug to be administered to verify the recommended dose, the method and duration of administration, and contraindications. It is the responsibility of the licensed prescriber, relying on experience and knowledge of the patient, to determine dosages and the best treatment for each individual patient. Neither the publisher nor the author assumes any liability for any injury and/or damage to persons or property arising from this publication.

International Standard Book Number 0-7216-9691-0

Publishing Director: Linda Duncan
Executive Editor: Penny Rudolph
Senior Developmental Editor: Jaime Pendill
Publishing Services Manager: Patricia Tannian
Project Manager: John Casey
Book Design Manager: Gail Morey Hudson
Cover Art and Medical Illustrations: Bill Winn

Printed in China

Last digit is the print number: 9   8   7   6   5   4   3   2

Contributors

JEAN E. ASHLAND, PHD, CCC-SLP
Speech and Language Pathologist
Research Associate
Department of Speech Language Pathology
Massachusetts General Hospital
Boston, Massachusetts

ARNULF BAUMANN, DMD, MD
AO-ASIF Research Fellow in Pediatric Oral and Maxillofacial
  Surgery
Massachusetts General Hospital
Boston, Massachusetts

MYRON L. BELFER, MD, MPA
Professor of Psychiatry, Department of Social Medicine
Harvard Medical School;
Senior Associate, Department of Psychiatry
Children's Hospital
Boston, Massachusetts

JEFFREY D. BENNETT, DMD
Associate Professor
Department of Oral and Maxillofacial Surgery
School of Dental Medicine, University of Connecticut
Farmington, Connecticut

MARJORIE A. CURRAN, MD
Instructor, Department of Pediatrics
Massachusetts General Hospital, Harvard Medical School
Boston, Massachusetts

JEFFREY B. DEMBO, DDS, MS
Professor of Oral and Maxillofacial Surgery
University of Kentucky College of Dentistry;
Professor, Department of Anesthesia
University of Kentucky College of Medicine
Lexington, Kentucky

THOMAS B. DODSON, DMD, MPH
Associate Professor and Director of Resident Training
Department of Oral and Maxillofacial Surgery
Massachusetts General Hospital
Harvard School of Dental Medicine
Boston, Massachusetts

ROLAND D. EAVEY, MD
Associate Professor
Department of Otology and Laryngology
Harvard Medical School;
Director of Pediatric Otolaryngology
Massachusetts Eye and Ear Infirmary
Boston, Massachusetts

MICHAEL T. LONGAKER, MD
Professor of Surgery, Director, Children's Surgical Research
Stanford University Medical Center
Stanford, California

JOHN B. MULLIKEN, MD
Professor of Surgery
Harvard Medical School;
Director, Craniofacial Centre
Children's Hospital
Boston, Massachusetts

ODED NAHLIELI, DMD
Professor and Chairman
Department of Oral and Maxillofacial Surgery
Barzilai Medical Center, Ashkelon, Israel

HOWARD L. NEEDLEMAN, DMD
Clinical Professor of Oral and Development Biology
Department of Dentistry, Children's Hospital
Harvard School of Dental Medicine
Boston, Massachusetts

ROBERT A. ORD, MD, DDS, FACS, FRCS, MS
Professor
Department of Oral and Maxillofacial Surgery
University of Maryland;
Professor
Greenebaum Cancer Center Oncology Program
Baltimore, Maryland

BONNIE L. PADWA, DMD, MD
Assistant Professor
Department of Oral and Maxillofacial Surgery
Children's Hospital, Harvard School of Dental Medicine
Boston, Massachusetts

JEFFRY R. SHAEFER, DMD
Instructor, Department of Oral and Maxillofacial Surgery
Massachusetts General Hospital
Harvard School of Dental Medicine
Boston, Massachusetts

ERIC S. SHANK, MD
Instructor, Department of Anesthesia
Massachusetts General Hospital, Harvard Medical School
Boston, Massachusetts

STEPHEN SHUSTERMAN, DMD
Associate Clinical Professor
Oral and Developmental Biology
Dentist-in-Chief, Children's Hospital
Harvard School of Dental Medicine
Boston, Massachusetts

JOAN M. STOLER, MD
Instructor
Department of Pediatrics, Genetics and Teratology Unit
Harvard Medical School, Massachusetts General Hospital
Boston, Massachusetts

KARIN VARGERVIK, DDS
Chair, Department of Growth and Development
Director, Center for Craniofacial Anomalies
University of California at San Francisco
San Francisco, California

W. BRADFORD WILLIAMS, BS
AO-ASIF Research Fellow
Pediatric Oral and Maxillofacial Surgery
Massachusetts General Hospital
Boston, Massachusetts

To **our pediatric patients**
who made this book possible and who
it has been our pleasure to serve

To **Barbara, Jody,** and **Jeff**
LBK

To **Eva Rodousakis-Troulis** and **Michael Aronoff**
MJT

Preface

This book is the offspring of *Pediatric Oral and Maxillofacial Surgery* published by W.B. Saunders in 1990. Our purpose was to provide a resource and reference for students, residents, fellows, and practitioners who perceived a deficiency in oral and maxillofacial surgery (OMFS) training with regard to general management of pediatric patients and specific management of pediatric OMFS problems.

OMFS remains an "anatomically regional" specialty, and the majority of practitioners therefore treat patients of all ages. Common problems (e.g., impacted and supernumerary teeth, intraoral soft tissue lesions, tongue-tie, to name a few) are familiar to most practitioners who treat children. In this text, we present our experience with these conditions for the reader to judge the techniques and to compare with his or her own methods. On the other hand, primary jaw tumors, malignant tumors, salivary gland pathology, vascular lesions, cleft lip and palate, microtia, and head and neck infections in children are less common. This volume is intended to be a reference for surgeons rarely encountering these conditions. Although other texts have been published with chapters on subjects related to pediatric OMFS, and an excellent text, *Craniomaxillofacial Surgery in Children and Young Adults* (W.B. Saunders, 2000) has been edited by Posnick, this book remains the only volume dealing specifically with pediatric oral and maxillofacial surgery.

In 1974, the senior editor was fortunate to be given the opportunity to develop an oral and maxillofacial surgery program at Boston Children's Hospital. This was largely the result of the wisdom and foresight of three Harvard professors and service chiefs: Walter C. Guralnick (Chief of OMFS, Massachusetts General Hospital), Joseph E. Murray (Chief of the Division of Plastic Surgery, Children's Hospital) and Judah Folkman (Surgeon-in-Chief, Children's Hospital). This commitment made it possible to develop one of the first OMFS services devoted to children in a children's hospital. We

are happy to observe that interest in pediatric OMFS has increased since the first edition of this text was published. The American Association of Oral and Maxillofacial Surgeons (AAOMS) now sponsors clinical interest groups in pediatric OMFS and cleft/craniofacial surgery. At the 85th Annual Meeting of the AAOMS (Orlando, Fla, September 2003) there was a major symposium on pediatric maxillofacial tumors, and there have been recent symposia on hemifacial microsomia, pediatric facial trauma, cleft management among other subjects. Interest in congenital craniomaxillofacial anomalies has grown, as has the membership and participation of oral and maxillofacial surgeons in the American Cleft Palate/Craniofacial Association.

The current edition of this project began in 1995. I had discussions with a series of W.B. Saunders editors to determine the exact form of this new edition. Some preferred changing the book to a surgical atlas. I was very much against this concept. I thought the strength of the first edition was its emphasis on principles rather than on technique. I finally came to an agreement with the current editor, Penny Rudolph. Penny and I seemed to have a similar vision of this book, its purpose and its strengths. Plans were finalized, and the author list established in 2000. This is a greatly expanded version of the first edition. The illustrations are in color, and chapters have been added on molecular genetics and syndrome identification, psychological preparation of pediatric patients for maxillofacial surgery, facial growth, deep sedation, salivary gland tumors, head and neck malignancy, microtia, and sequential management of patients with cleft lip and palate. Other chapters have been updated and expanded, (e.g., inflammatory salivary gland disease and orthognathic surgery in children and adolescents), with the addition of new contributors and more photographs and drawings.

The book remains very personal in that it reflects, for the most part, the senior editor's experiences over a 30-year period—10 years each at Boston Children's Hospital, University of California San Francisco, and

Massachusetts General Hospital. The original chapters written by the senior author on dentoalveolar surgery, intraoral soft tissue problems, jaw tumors in children, vascular anomalies, facial trauma, and congenital and acquired TMJ abnormalities have been updated and expanded with the help of Dr. Maria Troulis. This experience has been greatly enhanced by the invited contributions of my respected colleagues. Maria and I thank all of them for their scholarly manuscripts, and we greatly appreciate their timely submissions. Although the book may not cover every OMFS problem you will encounter in the pediatric age group, it is meant to give the reader the benefit of one group's broad experience. We hope it will stimulate your interest and help you build your own experience.

This book would not have been possible without my close collaborator, partner, and friend, Maria J. Troulis. We originally started this project with three editors; one dropped out and ultimately had no role in the project. Dr. Troulis has added her extraordinary organizational and creative skills to this book, and our colleagues, for the most part from other tertiary care institutions, have contributed unique expertise and materials. As the readers I am sure will appreciate, the art in this volume is of the highest quality. Dr. Troulis and I very much enjoyed working with Bill Winn, who created all the original drawings in this text. He is an extraordinarily talented artist and it has truly been a pleasure for us to work with him on this project.

We would like to acknowledge the help of our editor Penny Rudolph, who pushed this project along from the very beginning, and Jaime Pendill, who added a tremendous amount of energy and a lot of persistence to keep the production of the book on track. It was a pleasure working with Penny and Jaime, and I think we all felt like a close-knit team by the time the book was completed. We especially appreciate the last-minute help we received from Bonnie Padwa and John Mulliken, the authors of the chapter on management of cleft lip and palate.

Finally, we would like to especially acknowledge Jennifer Hancock, our administrative assistant, whose talent in organizing, formatting, putting together, and entering the references and communicating and working with all the contributors has been superb. Dr. Troulis and I truly enjoyed working with Jennifer on this project and we deeply appreciate her skill, dedication and hard work.

Leonard B. Kaban, DMD, MD
Boston
September 2003

Contents

Pediatric Oral and Maxillofacial Surgery

PART 1

GENERAL CARE OF THE PEDIATRIC SURGICAL PATIENT

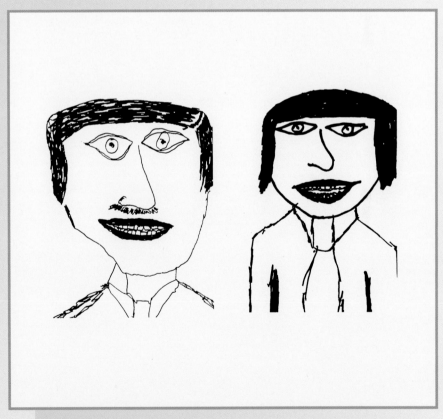

Self-portraits of a pediatric patient before *(left)* and after *(right)* surgery for hemi-facial microsomia

Preoperative Assessment of the Pediatric Patient

Marjorie A. Curran

The purpose of the preoperative assessment is to maximize patient safety and to anticipate potential medical problems during the perioperative period. Same-day admission decreases the length of hospital stay for the child but eliminates the comprehensive in-hospital preoperative evaluation. Therefore, it becomes necessary to determine if a child is a high-risk surgical or anesthetic candidate during a sometimes hurried outpatient visit.

Many of the issues to consider in pediatric patients may be similar to those in adults; however, some are unique to children and to specific age groups. As in all medical and surgical disciplines, it is critical to obtain a detailed and accurate history and physical examination. It is important for the specialist to alert the pediatrician about an upcoming elective operation to ensure that all the patient's medical conditions are well controlled. For example, a referral to the oral and maxillofacial surgeon may come from another specialist (e.g., orthodontist, orthopedic surgeon, or otolaryngologist) who may not be aware of or who might not mention a significant medical issue (e.g., heart murmur, diabetes, kidney disease). A healthy child with a negative medical history and normal physical examination findings does not require any preoperative laboratory studies for an elective operation with no expectation of significant blood loss. On the other hand, a premature infant with a history of lung disease and seizures may require multiple laboratory tests in preparation for even the simplest of operations.

GENERAL EVALUATION

The evaluation of any pediatric patient should begin with a detailed medical history that includes prenatal, birth, and maternal information, as well as a developmental screening evaluation. This history often is obtained from the referring pediatrician. The birth history provides important clues about a child's current health. Babies who are born significantly before term are at risk for multiple surgical or anesthetic complications. The parents should be asked the estimated gestational age at birth, the birth weight, Apgar score (Table 1-1) and, if applicable, issues that arose while in the neonatal intensive care unit. Specific attention should be paid to the duration of time the child was intubated, any intraventricular hemorrhages, history of feeding intolerance or necrotizing enterocolitis, and prolonged problems with apnea and bradycardia. Genetic abnormalities often are detected at birth and may have specific implications for management (see Chapter 2).

Maternal history including illnesses (e.g., gestational diabetes, hypertension), medications, or drug or alcohol

TABLE 1-1	Apgar Scores		
Score	0	1	2
Heart rate	Absent	Less than 100/minute	More than 100/minute
Respiratory effort	Absent	Slow, irregular	Good, crying
Muscle tone	Limp	Some flexion of extremities	Active motion
Reflex irritability (in response to nose catheter)	Absent	Grimace	Grimace and cough or sneeze
Color	Pale, blue	Acrocyanosis, pink body	No cyanosis Entirely pink

From Apgar V: *Curr Res Anesthesiol* 32:260, 1953.
Note: Each item is assessed and given a score of 0 to 2 at both 1 and 5 minutes postpartum. The total scores are the sum of the individual item scores at the respective times.

abuse must be documented. Children with prenatal infections (e.g., syphilis, rubella, cytomegalovirus, toxoplasmosis, or herpes) are usually small in size, of low birth weight, and at risk for developmental or congenital abnormalities. This is also true of children born to mothers who abused drugs or alcohol.

Developmental milestones always are evaluated and should be documented by the pediatrician. This sometimes is done on a formal basis using specific screening tools, such as the Denver Developmental Screening Test, but does not require all the apparatus suggested by the Denver test. Documentation of level of gross and fine motor activity (walking, crawling, pincer grasp) and language development (babbling, two words together) is adequate. The child's height, weight, and head circumference are measured periodically and compared with age-adjusted norms on growth charts (Figures 1-1 to 1-5). There should be appropriate support for the child's psychological needs during the perioperative period (see Chapter 3). Furthermore, children with suspected speech defects should have a formal speech evaluation before elective oral and maxillofacial procedures (see Chapter 5).

PREOPERATIVE LABORATORY TESTS

Preoperative laboratory tests generally are not required for healthy children undergoing elective oral surgical procedures. Any tests ordered should be individualized based on a child's history, physical examination, and the proposed procedure. A baseline hematocrit and hemoglobin is obtained if there is clinical evidence of anemia or if the scheduled procedure is likely to result in significant blood loss (bone graft, major reconstructive or orthognathic surgical cases).

Urinalysis is recommended only for children with a history of urinary tract infections or a family history of renal abnormalities. Urinalysis should also be obtained when the operation is anticipated to be of long duration or when a urine catheter will be used.

Coagulation studies such as bleeding time, platelet count, prothrombin time, and partial thromboplastin time are not routinely indicated for healthy children. During the preoperative evaluation, a bleeding history must be obtained. This should include episodes of spontaneous nosebleeds, prolonged bleeding after circumcision, unusual bruising history, hemarthrosis, and excessive bleeding during shedding of deciduous teeth or after dental extractions. A family history of specific bleeding disorders should also be obtained. Positive findings should prompt referral to a hematologist for evaluation and appropriate testing.

Electrolyte levels need not be evaluated in a healthy child with no history of kidney disease. Fluid replacement is sometimes required preoperatively and always required intraoperatively and during the early postoperative period. General guidelines for fluid requirements in healthy children are dependent on weight and age. Perioperative fluid replacement guidelines are described in detail in Chapter 8. For maintenance fluids in children, 5% dextrose in 0.25% normal saline (D5/0.25NS) is recommended for children under 5 years of age and D5/0.45NS for children over 5 years of age. Because children with immature kidneys do not preserve potassium, 20 to 40 mEq/L of potassium is added to the intravenous fluid. The rate of administration is dependent on the child's weight. The "4.2.1" rule for pediatric fluid replacement by weight is described in detail in Chapter 8. Children on potassium-wasting medications or with a history of renal failure should have electrolyte values monitored while receiving intravenous fluids and may have significantly different fluid requirements. Potassium should be added to intravenous fluids only with extreme caution for children with renal failure.

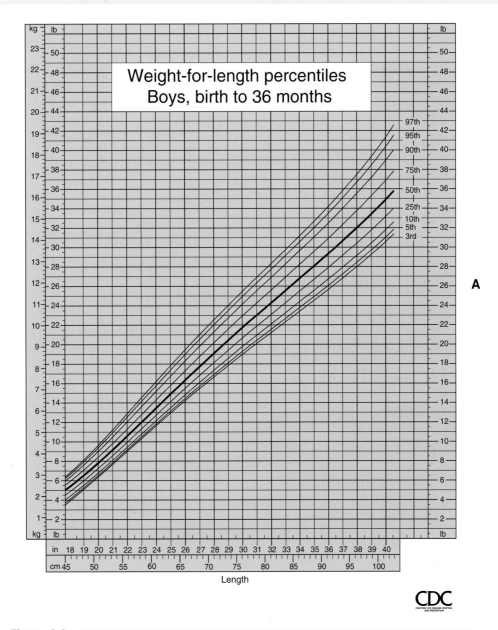

Figure 1-1

A, Weight-for-length percentiles for boys from birth to age 3. B, Head circumference-for-age percentiles for boys from birth to age 3. (From the National Center for Health Statistics in collaboration with the National Centers for Chronic Disease Prevention and Health Promotion, 2000 [modified 4/20/01].)

SPECIFIC CONSIDERATIONS

Premature Infant

Most infants are born an average of 40 weeks after conception (normal range is 38 to 42). This is known as the *gestational age* of the newborn. A premature infant is a baby born before 37 weeks of gestation. The earliest surviving infants are born at 23 weeks of gestational age. Babies born before 32 weeks of gestational age are at risk for a variety of medical problems such as bronchopulmonary dysplasia (BPD), apnea, intraventricular hemorrhages, sepsis, and necrotizing enterocolitis. Premature infants are at high risk for apnea after general anesthesia. Because there are no accurate screening tests to determine which infants will have apnea, any premature infant less than 60 weeks of postconceptual age should be monitored closely for the first 24 hours after an

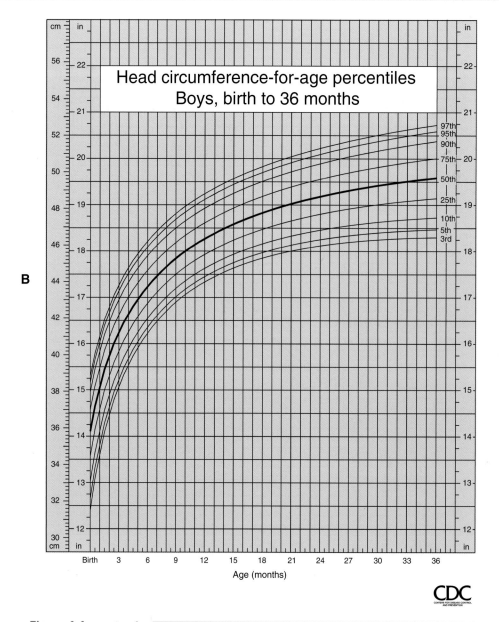

B

Figure 1-1—*continued*

operation.[1-3] Postconceptual age is determined by adding the child's gestational age at delivery to age at time of surgery. In other words, a 25-week "preemie" who has an operation 2 months after birth would be approximately 33 (25 + 8) postconceptual weeks of age and, therefore, at risk for apnea.

Bronchopulmonary Dysplasia. A premature infant with a history of endotracheal intubation during the neonatal period is at risk for development of BPD. This is thought to be caused by a combination of immature lung parenchyma with a decreased surfactant level. Exposure of these infants to positive pressure ventilation and oxygen results in ventilation/perfusion abnormalities. Children with BPD also have hyperreactive airways that place them at risk for pulmonary complications during the perioperative period. They are more susceptible to volume overload secondary to "leaky lung" and fluid accumulations in the lungs. Children with severe BPD may be dependent on diuretics, oxygen, or steroids, thus posing additional anesthetic risks. Consultation with a pediatric pulmonologist and anesthesiologist should be strongly considered in these cases.

Pulmonary development, with addition of alveoli, continues during the first few years of life, and BPD often improves (although the condition may persist for many years). Delay of nonurgent operations in these children may reduce the chances of perioperative pulmonary complications.

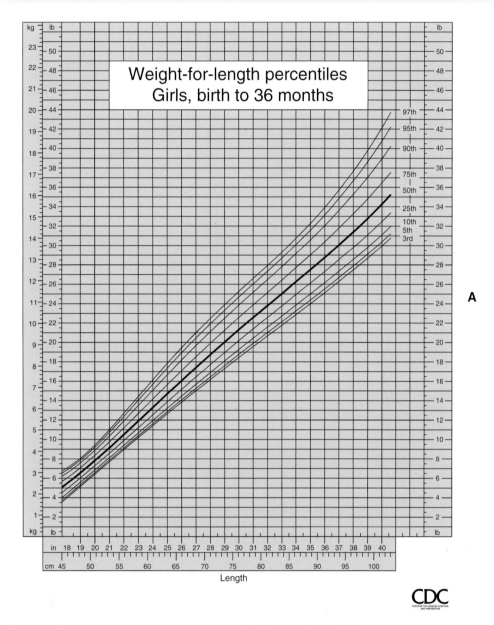

Figure 1-2

A, Weight-for-length percentiles for girls from birth to age 3. **B,** Head circumference-for-age percentiles for girls from birth to age 3. (From the National Center for Health Statistics in collaboration with the National Centers for Chronic Disease Prevention and Health Promotion, 2000 [modified 4/20/01].)

Intraventricular Hemorrhage. Intraventricular hemorrhage is a frequent complication of premature birth before 30 weeks of gestation. It is caused by bleeding from the subependymal germinal matrix into the ventricles and is believed to be a result of changes in cerebral blood flow and extreme sensitivity of the neonatal capillaries to hypoxic or ischemic injury. It is reported as grades I through IV, with grade IV being the most severe. Intraventricular hemorrhage can be unilateral or bilateral, and severe bleeding episodes may be fatal. Babies with a history of intraventricular hemorrhage are at increased risk for seizures, hydrocephalus, developmental delay, and cerebral palsy. They may have concurrent increased or decreased neuromuscular tone, which can lead to increased susceptibility to aspiration during the postoperative period.

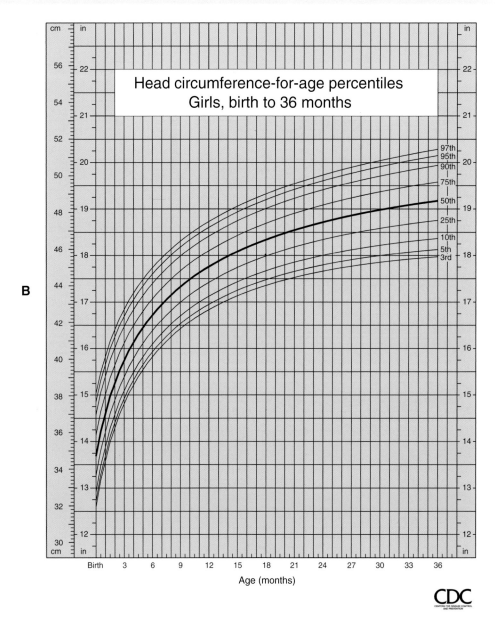

B

Head circumference-for-age percentiles
Girls, birth to 36 months

97th
95th
90th
75th
50th
25th
10th
5th
3rd

Age (months)

CDC
CENTERS FOR DISEASE CONTROL
AND PREVENTION

Figure 1-2—*continued*

Necrotizing Enterocolitis. Necrotizing entero-colitis is a serious gastrointestinal disease. It occurs most commonly in premature infants but also can occur in babies born at term. The etiology is unknown, but both ischemia and infectious causes are thought to play a role. Necrotizing enterocolitis is character-ized by mucosal or deeper necrosis in the terminal ileum, colon, or proximal small bowel. The infants may undergo resection of large segments of intestine, which can leave them with "short gut" syndrome, nutritional deficiencies, or dependence on parenteral nutrition. Dependence on parenteral nutrition can lead to cholestasis and liver failure, with concomitant bleed-ing diatheses. Special consideration to maximizing nutrition will lead to an improved ability to heal after surgery.

Genetic Disorders and Syndromes

Chromosomal abnormalities and syndromes usually are recognized during the newborn period; some may have particular importance for intraoperative manage-ment (see Chapter 2). Down's syndrome, or trisomy 21, places a child at risk for atlantoaxial instability during

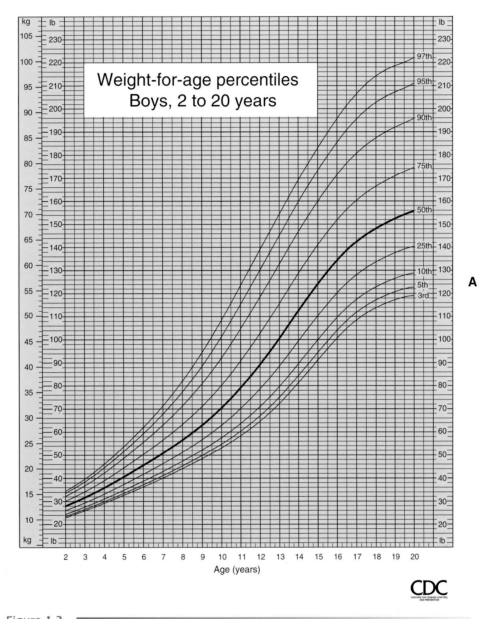

Weight-for-age percentiles
Boys, 2 to 20 years

Age (years)

CDC

Figure 1-3
A, Weight-for-age percentiles for boys, ages 2 to 20 years. **B,** Stature-for-age percentiles for boys, ages 2 to 20 years. (From the National Center for Health Statistics in collaboration with the National Centers for Chronic Disease Prevention and Health Promotion, 2000 [modified 4/20/01].)

endotracheal intubation. Atlantoaxial instability is caused by increased mobility of the cervical spine at the first and second vertebrae. Cervical flexion and extension radiographs are not good screening tools in children under 5 years of age, and many affected individuals will not exhibit any signs on physical examination.[4] Care must be taken when manipulating the neck during intubation so as not to cause subluxation, which may injure the spinal cord. In addition, approximately 40% of children with Down's syndrome have congenital heart disease that may complicate perioperative management.

Children with chondroplasia or other dwarfing conditions may also exhibit cervical spine abnormalities. Special positioning of the neck may be necessary during intubation.

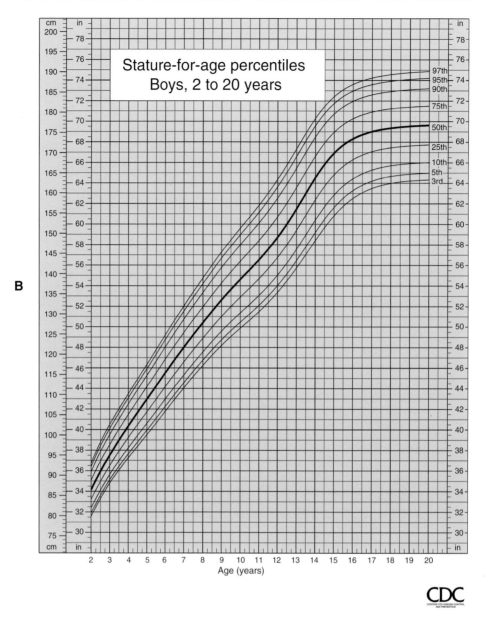

B

Stature-for-age percentiles
Boys, 2 to 20 years

Figure 1-3—*continued*

Craniofacial Anomalies

It should be recognized that infants and children with craniofacial anomalies are at risk for associated psychosocial problems (see Chapter 3) and anomalies of other systems such as the central nervous, cardiac, pulmonary, and renal systems (see Chapter 2). Preoperative testing and specialty consultations should be obtained. Respiratory difficulties (including airway obstruction) may be secondary to retrusive maxilla or mandible, choanal atresia, or macroglossia. Feeding issues and failure to thrive may be secondary to single anatomic defects (e.g., cleft lip and palate) or a combination of multiple craniofacial or other anomalies and neurologic deficits. Neurologic disorders such as increased intracranial pressure, hydrocephalus, or Chiari malformation may be present. Cervical spine anomalies, including intervertebral fusion, must be noted and are common in patients with hemifacial microsomia and craniosynostosis syndromes. Patients with nasal hypoplasia may have associated hypothyroidism.[5]

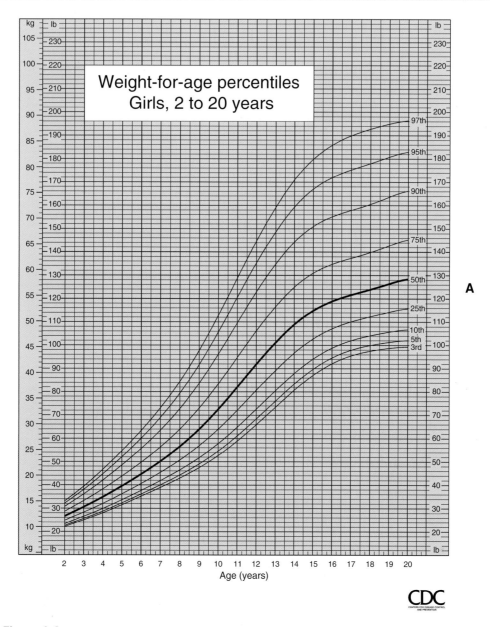

Figure 1-4 ▰▰▰▰▰▰▰▰▰▰▰▰▰▰▰▰▰▰▰▰▰▰▰▰▰▰▰▰▰▰

A, Weight-for-age percentiles for girls, ages 2 to 20 years. **B,** Stature-for-age percentiles for girls, ages 2 to 20 years. (From the National Centers for Health Statistics in collaboration with the National Centers for Chronic Disease Prevention and Health Promotion, 2000 [modified 4/20/01].)

Cardiovascular Disorders

Congenital heart disease, with an incidence of 1% of live births, is the most common type of birth defect. *If a history of heart murmur is elicited or if one is heard during the preoperative evaluation,* the child should be assessed for structural abnormalities such as ventricular septal defect or valvar abnormalities requiring endocarditis prophylaxis (Table 1-2). Patients with more complex congenital cardiac anomalies require specific evaluation and may require inotropic agents, calcium-channel blockers, anti-cholinesterase inhibitors, and other therapies during the perioperative period.[6] Children on these medications must be monitored carefully to prevent cardiac, pulmonary, and renal complications.

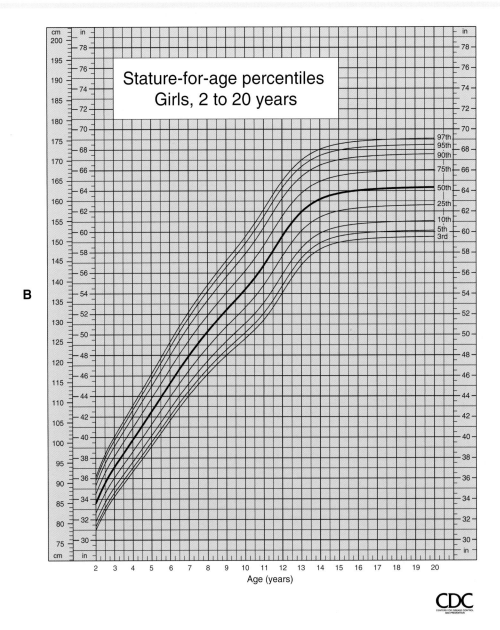

B

Stature-for-age percentiles
Girls, 2 to 20 years

Age (years)

CDC
CENTERS FOR DISEASE CONTROL
AND PREVENTION

Figure 1-4—*continued*

Preoperative laboratory tests including serum levels of electrolytes and medication, when applicable, should be obtained. Careful consideration must be paid to the patient's fluid volume status, and hours of preoperative oral intake restriction should be limited as much as possible (see Chapter 8). Specific therapies must be tailored to the individual patient.

Pulmonary Problems

The surgeon should concentrate on eliciting a history of asthma and any other underlying pulmonary problems such as cystic fibrosis.

Asthma. Asthma is the most common chronic illness in children, one of the most common causes for hospitalization, and a frequent cause of morbidity during the perioperative period. To facilitate management, it is useful to classify the severity of asthma based on clinical features of the illness. Patients who have symptoms fewer than 2 days per week and fewer than 2 nights per month are classified as having *mild intermittent asthma.* Those with symptoms more than 2 days per week but less than every day or more than 2 nights per month are considered to have *mild persistent asthma.* Children with *moderate persistent asthma* have daily symptoms and symptoms at night more than once

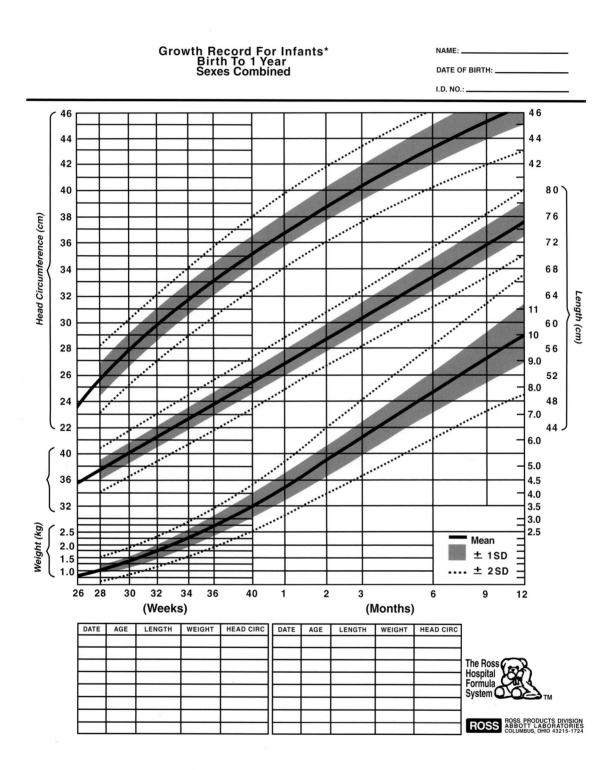

Growth Record For Infants*
Birth To 1 Year
Sexes Combined

NAME: _____

DATE OF BIRTH: _____

I.D. NO.: _____

Mean	—
± 1SD	▓
± 2SD	····

DATE	AGE	LENGTH	WEIGHT	HEAD CIRC		DATE	AGE	LENGTH	WEIGHT	HEAD CIRC

The Ross
Hospital
Formula
System™

ROSS ROSS PRODUCTS DIVISION
ABBOTT LABORATORIES
COLUMBUS, OHIO 43215-1724

Figure 1-5

Growth curves for premature infants. (Adapted from Babson SG, Benda GI: Growth graphs for the clinical assessment of infants of varying gestational age, *J Pediatr* 89:814-820, 1976.)

TABLE 1-2   American Heart Association Guidelines for Antibiotic Prophylaxis for Bacterial Endocarditis: Prophylactic Regimens for Dental, Oral, Respiratory Tract, or Esophageal Procedures

Situation	Agent	Regimen*
Standard general prophylaxis	Amoxicillin	Adults: 2.0 g; children: 50 mg/kg orally 1 hour before procedure
Unable to take oral medications	Ampicillin	Adults: 2.0 g intramuscularly (IM) or intravenously (IV); children: 50 mg/kg IM or IV within 30 minutes before procedure
Allergic to penicillin	Clindamycin	Adults: 600 mg; children: 20 mg/kg orally 1 hour before procedure
	OR Cephalexin[†] or cefadroxil[†]	Adults: 2.0 g; children: 50 mg/kg orally 1 hour before procedure
	OR Azithromycin or clarithromycin	Adults: 500 mg; children: 15 mg/kg orally 1 hour before procedure
Allergic to penicillin and unable to take oral medications	Clindamycin	Adults: 600 mg; children: 20 mg/kg IV within 30 minutes before procedure
	OR Cefazolin[†]	Adults: 1.0 g; children: 25 mg/kg IM or IV within 30 minutes before procedure

Reproduced with permission. Prevention of Bacterial Endocarditis. Copyright 1997, American Heart Association.
*Total children's dose should not exceed adult dose.
[†]Cephalosporins should not be used in individuals with immediate-type hypersensitivity reaction (urticaria, angioedema, or anaphylaxis) to penicillins.

per week. *Severe persistent asthma* is manifested by continual daily symptoms, as well as frequent nighttime symptoms.[7] In general, the more severe the clinical classification, the more complicated the medical management becomes and the greater the anesthetic and surgical risk.

Currently, there are four major categories of medications used to treat asthma (Table 1-3). First-line drugs are β-2 agonists. The short-acting agent is albuterol, which is used for flare-ups in patients with mild intermittent asthma. The longer acting β-2 agonists, salmeterol and formoterol, are used for patients with mild persistent asthma. Corticosteroids are used for patients with mild and moderate persistent asthma during exacerbations of symptoms and for children with severe asthma. Inhaled glucocorticoids have fewer side effects than oral steroids and may be used in mild persistent to severe asthma.

Oral steroids are reserved for severe asthmatics and acute exacerbations. Mast cell stabilizers such as cromolyn and nedocromil are helpful for allergy-induced asthma. Leukotriene inhibitors such as montelukast are used for moderate to severe asthma. The methylxanthine, theophylline, is now rarely used because of its many side effects and difficulties maintaining therapeutic levels. It should not be started as a new medication before a surgical procedure.

Children with asthma should be maintained on their baseline medications as they prepare for an operation. Patients who frequently use inhaled bronchodilators on an as-needed basis should use them on a regular schedule 24 hours before the operation. Children with moderate to severe asthma may require a course of oral steroids perioperatively for 2 to 3 days[3,7] (Table 1-4).

TABLE 1-3   Usual Dosages for Long-Term-Control Medications

Medication	Dosage Form	Adult Dose	Child Dose*
Inhaled Corticosteroids *(See Estimated Comparative Daily Dosages for Inhaled Corticosteroids.)*			
Systemic Corticosteroids *(Applies to all three corticosteroids.)*			
Methylprednisolone	2, 4, 8, 16, 32 mg tablets	■ 7.5–60 mg daily in a single dose in a.m. or qod as needed for control	■ 0.25–2 mg/kg daily in single dose in a.m. or qod as needed for control
Prednisolone	5 mg tablets, 5 mg/5 cc, 15 mg/5 cc	■ Short-course "burst" to achieve control: 40–60 mg per day as single or 2 divided doses for 3–10 days	■ Short-course "burst": 1–2 mg/kg/day, maximum 60 mg/day for 3–10 days
Prednisone	1, 2.5, 5, 10, 20, 50 mg tablets; 5 mg/cc, 5 mg/5 cc		
Long-Acting Inhaled Beta$_2$-Agonists *(Should not be used for symptom relief or for exacerbations. Use with inhaled corticosteroids.)*			
Salmeterol	MDI 21 mcg/puff	2 puffs q 12 hours	1–2 puffs q 12 hours
	DPI 50 mcg/blister	1 blister q 12 hours	1 blister q 12 hours
Formoterol	DPI 12 mcg/single-use capsule	1 capsule q 12 hours	1 capsule q 12 hours
Combined Medication			
Fluticasone/Salmeterol	DPI 100, 250, or 500 mcg/50 mcg	1 inhalation bid; dose depends on severity of asthma	1 inhalation bid; dose depends on severity of asthma
Cromolyn and Nedocromil			
Cromolyn	MDI 1 mg/puff	2–4 puffs tid-qid	1–2 puffs tid-qid
	Nebulizer 20 mg/ampule	1 ampule tid-qid	1 ampule tid-qid
Nedocromil	MDI 1.75 mg/puff	2–4 puffs bid-qid	1–2 puffs bid-qid
Leukotriene Modifiers			
Montelukast	4 or 5 mg chewable tablet 10 mg tablet	10 mg qhs	4 mg qhs (2–5 yrs) 5 mg qhs (6–14 yrs) 10 mg qhs (> 14 yrs)
Zafirlukast	10 or 20 mg tablet	40 mg daily (20 mg tablet bid)	20 mg daily (7–11 yrs) (10 mg tablet bid)
Zileuton	300 or 600 mg tablet	2,400 mg daily (give tablets qid)	
Methylxanthines *(Serum monitoring is important [serum concentration of 5–15 mcg/mL at steady state]).*			
Theophylline	Liquids, sustained-release tablets, and capsules	Starting dose 10 mg/kg/day up to 300 mg max; usual max 800 mg/day	Starting dose 10 mg/kg/day; usual max: ■ < 1 year of age: 0.2 (age in weeks) + 5 = mg/kg/day ■ ≥ 1 year of age: 16 mg/kg/day

From National Asthma Education and Prevention Program: Guidelines for the diagnosis and management of asthma—update on selected topics 2002, NIH Pub No 02-5075, July 2002.
*Children ≤ 12 years of age.

TABLE 1-4   **Estimated Comparative Daily Dosages for Inhaled Corticosteroids**

| Drug | Low Daily Dose | | Medium Daily Dose | | Medium Daily Dose | |
	Adult	Child*	Adult	Child*	Adult	Child*
Beclomethasone CFC 42 or 84 mcg/puff	168–504 mcg	84–336 mcg	504–840 mcg	336–672 mcg	> 840 mcg	> 672 mcg
Beclomethasone HFA 40 or 80 mcg/puff	80–240 mcg	80–160 mcg	240–480 mcg	160–320 mcg	> 480 mcg	> 320 mcg
Budesonide DPI 200 mcg/inhalation	200–600 mcg	200–400 mcg	600–1,200 mcg	400–800 mcg	> 1,200 mcg	> 800 mcg
Inhalation suspension for nebulization (child dose)		0.5 mg		1.0 mg		2.0 mg
Flunisolide 250 mcg/puff	500–1,000 mcg	500–750 mcg	1,000–2,000 mcg	1,000–1,250 mcg	> 2,000 mcg	> 1,250 mcg
Fluticasone MDI: 44, 110, or 220 mcg/puff	88–264 mcg	88–176 mcg	264–660 mcg	176–440 mcg	> 660 mcg	> 440 mcg
DPI: 50, 100, or 250 mcg/ inhalation	100–300 mcg	100–200 mcg	300–600 mcg	200–400 mcg	> 600 mcg	> 400 mcg
Triamcinolone acetonide 100 mcg/puff	400–1,000 mcg	400–800 mcg	1,000–2,000 mcg	800–1,200 mcg	> 2,000 mcg	> 1,200 mcg

From National Asthma Education and Prevention Program: Guidelines for the diagnosis and management of asthma—update on selected topics 2002, NIH Pub No 02-5075, July 2002.
*Children ≤ 12 years of age.

Children with asthma often will have episodes of bronchospasm postoperatively, and albuterol via nebulizer is the first line of treatment. Children under 5 years should be given 1.25 mg (0.25 ml of the standard 0.5% solution) with 3 ml of saline; children over 5 years should receive 2.5 mg (0.5 ml of the 0.5% solution). These treatments can be repeated as often as necessary.

Cystic Fibrosis. Children with cystic fibrosis have abnormally thick pulmonary secretions and chronic pulmonary infections. This puts them at risk for complications arising from general anesthesia and endotracheal intubation. Many patients with cystic fibrosis require preoperative "clean out" with intravenous antibiotics and vigorous chest physiotherapy for up to 10 days before surgery. This improves pulmonary function in preparation for a general anesthetic. Preoperative evaluation of patients with cystic fibrosis should include pulmonary function tests, liver function tests, complete blood count, and blood glucose value. If the patient has an arterial carbon dioxide concentration ($Paco_2$) of greater than 50 mm Hg, forced expiratory volume after 1 second/forced vital capacity (FEV1/FVC) ratios of less than 60%, or vital capacity less than 50%, elective operations under general anesthesia should be avoided because of the high risk of intraoperative and postoperative complications.[8] Older children with cystic fibrosis often develop diabetes. Blood sugar levels must be documented preoperatively and managed carefully during the postoperative period.

Gastrointestinal Disorders

Overall nutrition and any special dietary requirements should be assessed preoperatively. Patients with metabolic disorders such as maple syrup urine disease or phenylketonuria will require special formula. Simple adjustments such as notation of cow's milk allergy and procurement of soy formula must be done. Because adequate nutrition is essential for healing after an operation, the surgeon must ensure that the child will have access to proper caloric intake. There are many high-calorie (30 cal/oz) formulas available for nutritional supplementation. Most infants require between 85 and 150 cal/kg/day to grow well and will require additional calories to recover from an operation. Nasogastric feeding or intravenous supplementation with parenteral nutrition may be necessary in children who are particularly cachectic.

Special precautions may be needed for children who have a history of reflux; antireflux medications should be continued as soon as appropriate. Liver failure can cause clotting disorders or inability to metabolize anesthetic agents, leading to morbidity. Long-term malnutrition often will result in vitamin K deficiency with inhibition of the clotting mechanism. Patients with a history of liver failure or longstanding malnutrition should be evaluated for coagulation abnormalities. Liver function tests should also be obtained in these cases and special care given to administration of any medications that are metabolized in the liver. It should be remembered that acetaminophen, which often is given for postoperative pain relief, is metabolized in this fashion.

Renal Disease

Children with renal disease require careful evaluation of renal function and electrolytes preoperatively. Complete blood count, total protein (albumin-to-globulin ratio), and calcium and phosphate levels should also be documented. Such patients may require special restriction or supplementation of intravenous fluids, beyond what was discussed above. Fluid requirements should be addressed on a case-by-case basis. Patients with renal failure may have calcium and phosphate imbalances that may prolong healing times when bony structures are involved. Patients with end-stage renal disease may require dialysis to achieve a nonuremic and nonacidotic status to allow for appropriate healing. Consultation with a nephrologist is recommended. There must be careful consideration of medications used during and after surgery, because many medications are metabolized in the kidney, and half-life prolongation and renal toxicity may occur.

Hematologic Diseases

Patients with a history of sickle cell disease, hemophilia, or anemia require more specific interventions.

Sickle cell disease (SCD) places patients at risk for pain crisis, acute chest syndrome, renal infarction, and stroke whenever there is relative hypoxia or dehydration. In addition, patients with sickle cell disease are at increased risk for infection after an operation. Current recommendation for patients with SCD-SS and SCD-S β-thalassemia is transfusion to achieve a hemoglobin level of 10 g/dl. This should occur before all but the lowest risk procedures. Tonsillectomy and adenoidectomy should not be considered low-risk procedures, because children with sickle cell disease who are unable to take oral fluids are at increased jeopardy if they become dehydrated.[9]

Patients with factor VIII deficiency, factor IX deficiency, and von Willebrand's disease require specific clotting products before an operation. Consultation with the child's hematologist is recommended. General recommendations for patients with hemophilia are outlined in Box 1-1.[10] Local measures for achieving hemostasis have recently been introduced which have improved management for oral surgery for patients with hemophilia. Best results include factor infusion along with epsilon-aminocaproic acid (EACA), vasopressin (DDAVP), and a local agent such as Avitene (CR Bard, Murray Hill, NJ) or topical thrombin, applied directly to the wound.[10]

BOX 1-1	Guidelines for Managing Hemophiliac Patients Who Require Surgery

Before Surgical Procedure

Complete coagulation workup

Screen for inhibitor(s)

Calculate needs and stockpile therapeutic material in hospital

Survival study for recovery and half-life of therapeutic material

Nonorthopedic Surgical Procedures

Give dose calculated to bring patient's plasma level to 100%, 1 hour before procedure (50 IU/kg)

Maintain plasma level above 60% for 4 days

Maintain plasma level above 20% for the subsequent 4 days or until all drains and sutures are removed

Assay daily before dose

Orthopedic Surgical Procedures

Give dose calculated to bring patient's plasma level to 100%, 1 hour before procedure (50 IU/kg)

Maintain plasma level above 80% for 4 days

Assay daily before dose

Maintain plasma level above 40% for the subsequent 4 days

If patient is casted, discontinue replacement until rehabilitation program is begun

If not casted, maintain above 20% for ambulation

For rehabilitation program, maintain above 10% for 3 weeks

Dental Procedures

Give Amicar (EACA) 50 mg/kg 4 hours before surgery or Cyclokapron 10 mg/kg

Give factor replacement dose calculated to bring patient's plasma level to 100%, 1 hour before procedure

Continue Amicar 50 mg/kg tid for 7 days (adults, 2 g tid for 7 days)

Repeat one dose of replacement therapy in 3 days if procedure is extensive

---

Routine screening for anemia is not necessary in healthy children with normal physical examination findings. Patients with chronic illnesses and premature infants should be screened.

Neurologic Disorders

Seizure Disorders. Children with seizure disorders should be maintained on their usual anticonvulsant therapy. Before the surgical procedure, anticonvulsant levels, a baseline complete blood count, and liver function tests should be obtained. If the patient will be unable to take oral anticonvulsive agents postoperatively, the neurologist should be consulted for parenteral alternatives.

Neuromuscular Disorders. Certain patients with neuromuscular disorders are at increased risk from anesthetic agents. Neuromuscular blocking agents can cause prolonged muscle weakness in patients with myasthenia gravis. Duchenne's muscular dystrophy and other myopathies may increase a patient's risk of developing malignant hyperthermia. In infants with Duchenne's muscular dystrophy, succinylcholine can cause hyperkalemia leading to cardiac arrest. Patients with myotonic dystrophy can have prolonged respiratory depression after sedative or narcotic administration.

Malignant Hyperthermia. Malignant hyperthermia is inherited as an autosomal dominant trait with variable expression. Affected children have a 1 in 15,000 risk for malignant hyperthermia during anesthetic administration. The surgeon and pediatrician should elicit a familial history of an "anesthetic complication" or "reaction to an anesthetic" by any family member (including parents, aunts, uncles, and cousins). Because this is a rare but potentially fatal disorder, any positive family history should be followed up by a referral to the anesthesiologist for specific preoperative evaluation.

Clinically, malignant hyperthermia is characterized by a very rapid rise in body temperature, tachycardia, cardiac arrhythmias, hypercapnia, acidosis, muscular rigidity, and rhabdomyolysis. In children known to have had malignant hyperthermia, the anesthesiologist must be consulted in advance so that the appropriate anesthetic agents are chosen and perioperative management with dantrolene planned. A prophylactic regimen includes preoperative treatment with oral dantrolene, 4 to 8 mg/kg/day for 2 days. The last dose is administered 2 hours before administration of anesthesia.

Developmental Delay. It is important to document any history of developmental delay preoperatively. A child with significant impairments will respond inappropriately (relative to chronologic age) to the surgical experience. It is important for the medical staff to know this when the child wakes up from anesthesia. In most cases, it is helpful to allow the parents to be present in the recovery room when the child awakens. A child who has motor delay and doesn't sit or stand will clearly have the same issues postoperatively. Once again, this is important information for the nurses and physicians in the recovery room.

Endocrinologic Disorders

Diabetes Mellitus. Patients with insulin-dependent diabetes mellitus must have special adjustments made in their insulin dosage and dietary intake during the perioperative period. The aim is to prevent hyperglycemia, hypoglycemia, and ketosis. Both the stress of the operation and the anesthesia can lead to increased production of catecholamines, growth hormone, corticosteroids, and glucagons, which cause hyperglycemia. Administration of insulin should be carried out with the goal of keeping blood sugar less than 200 mg/dl while preventing hypoglycemia. One approach to perioperative management for surgical procedures is to give 30% to 50% of the patient's usual intermediate insulin dose subcutaneously on the morning of the operation. A sliding scale of regular insulin every 4 to 6 hours (0.05 to 0.1 U/kg) is started postoperatively and maintained until oral intake is adequate. Insulin can also be given intravenously, if preferred. In a patient receiving a 5% dextrose infusion, 0.05 to 0.1 U/kg/hr of regular insulin generally will be required to maintain the appropriate blood glucose level.[11]

Congenital Adrenal Hyperplasia. Children with congenital adrenal hyperplasia require daily corticosteroid and mineralocorticoid replacement. The glucocorticoid most often used is hydrocortisone and the dosage is tailored to the individual patient. A range of 6 to 15 mg/m²/day given orally in two divided doses (bid) is usually required. Fludrocortisone acetate 0.05 to 0.2 mg, given once daily, is the mineralocorticoid of choice. Stress-dose glucocorticoids are required before an operation. This is triple the usual dosage. Intravenous hydrocortisone can be given as 2.0 mg/m²/day in divided doses (q8h). If intravenous hydrocortisone is not readily available, equivalents of methylprednisolone or dexamethasone can be used. Because very high doses of glucocorticoids will have mineralocorticoid effects, no additional mineralocorticoids are necessary when stress doses of glucocorticoids are being given. Electrolytes should be monitored closely during surgery, because inadequate stress steroids will result in salt wasting and hyponatremia. Preoperatively, maintenance steroid doses must be documented carefully, as well as any extra sodium requirement.

Patients receiving long-term steroid therapy have suppression of the adrenal axis and may need stress-dose steroids during the perioperative period. Replacement therapy can be given as hydrocortisone 2.0 mg/kg/day divided every 8 hours.

Pregnancy Testing

Because it is difficult to be sure that an adolescent is telling the truth about sexual activity, the safest approach is to obtain a pregnancy test on all girls who have started their menses. If there is an institutional policy to this effect, it will avoid any conflict with unwilling parents who may be unaware of their child's activities. Testing the urine for human chorionic gonadotropin is fast and accurate.

Psychosocial Issues

Family support systems can be very stressed by a sick child. The economic hardship of paying for travel to and from the hospital, as well as lodging if the family comes from a distance, can adversely affect parents' abilities to care for their child. Maximizing social service support can allow the parents to spend time at the hospital and become comfortable in how to care for their child when it is time for discharge. Age-appropriate explanations for what is going to happen on the day of surgery will help to relieve the child's fears (see Chapter 3).

CONCLUSION

The preoperative evaluation provides a complete assessment of the patient, thereby enabling the surgical team to be prepared for any issues that may arise from pre-existing medical conditions or perioperative problems. The focused approach described in this chapter minimizes unnecessary testing while allowing the surgeon to collect adequate information to ensure patient safety. A thorough evaluation results in better surgical and anesthesia planning and promotes the best in patient care.

REFERENCES

1. Steward DJ: Preterm infants are more prone to complications following minor surgery than are term infants, *Anesthesiology* 56:304-306, 1982.
2. Liu LM, Cote CJ, Goudsouzian NG, et al: Life-threatening apnea in infants recovering from anesthesia, *Anesthesiology* 59:506-510, 1983.
3. Fisher QA, Feldman MA, Wilson MD: Pediatric responsibilities for preoperative evaluation, *Pediatrics* 125(5 Pt 1):675-685, 1994.
4. American Academy of Pediatrics Committee on Sports Medicine and Fitness: Atlantoaxial instability in Down syndrome: subject review, *Pediatrics* 96(1 Pt 1):151-154, 1995.
5. Gorlin RJ, Cohen, Hennekam RCM: Johnson Bizzard syndrome. In Gorlin RJ, Cohen MM, Hennekem RCM, editors: *Syndromes of the head and neck*, ed 4, Oxford, 2001, Oxford University Press.
6. Dajani AS, Taubert KA, Wilson W, et al: Prevention of bacterial endocarditis: recommendations by the American Heart Association, *JAMA* 277:1794, 1997.
7. National Asthma Education and Prevention Program: Guidelines for the diagnosis and management of asthma—update on selected topics 2002, NIH Pub No 02-5075, July 2002.
8. Taussig LM, Landau LI, Marks, MI: Respiratory system. In Taussig LM, editor: *Cystic fibrosis*, New York, 1984, Thieme-Stratton.
9. The management of sickle cell disease, revised June 2002, ed 4, NIH Pub No 02-2117, Chapter 24: Anesthesia and surgery, pp 149-151, 2002.
10. Hilgartner MA, Pochedly C: *Hemophilia in the child and adult*, ed 3, New York, 1989, Raven Press.
11. Ingelfinger JR, Wald ER, Polin RA: *Current pediatric therapy*, ed 16, Philadelphia, 1999, WB Saunders.

CHAPTER 2

Molecular Genetics and Syndrome Recognition for the Clinician

Joan M. Stoler

MOLECULAR GENETICS

Why is knowledge of genetics important? During the past century, physicians have made great strides in treating infectious diseases and lowering associated morbidity and mortality. Advances have also been made in the management of medical conditions such as hypertension, diabetes, and heart disease. There have been significant improvements in surgical management of disease, such as transplantation and repair of congenital and acquired facial deformities. In some ways, the last frontier is the field of genetics. Understanding the role of genes in the pathogenesis of anatomic and physio-logic abnormalities will aid in the diagnosis and the development of rational treatments. Twenty percent of infant deaths and 18% to 30% of pediatric hospitalizations[1,2] in advanced countries are due to congenital defects.[3] Understanding the etiology of such disorders and devising new methods of prevention and treatment would be of enormous benefit.

"New Genetics"

There has been an explosion in genetic knowledge during the past decade. The identification of specific genes responsible for many diseases has become a reality. In some cases, such identification has led to a better understanding of the pathophysiology of a disorder and, hopefully, genetic diagnosis will result in targeted treatment in the future. The identity and the role of genes responsible for various disorders inherited in the classic mendelian patterns (autosomal recessive, autosomal dominant, X-linked) have been documented. Similarly, genes responsible for multifactorial or complex inherited disorders have also been discovered. Congenital diseases that traditionally have been labeled *multifactorial*, such as cleft lip and palate, may represent abnormalities in multiple genes. Some of these genes may confer susceptibility to exogenous influences, thereby leading to the development of the disorder. Acquired conditions such as cancer, coronary artery disease, and hypertension may similarly have a specific genetic basis.

Human Genome Project

As a result of the Human Genome Project, the human genome map was published in February 2001.[4,5] The project has provided a valuable guide for researchers trying to discover pathologic changes in genes. This roadmap consists of markers (normal variants such as single nucleotide polymorphisms) which can be used to trace familial patterns to determine genetic linkage. The sequence of a particular gene from individuals affected with a congenital or acquired abnormality can be compared with the known mapped sequence of the gene. There are fewer genes than originally thought—roughly 26,500 to 39,000.[6] Only 1.1% of the genome actually codes for active portions of genes. Furthermore, genes are not located evenly on the 23 chromosome pairs. For example, chromosomes 17, 19, and 22 contain significantly more genes than chromosomes 4,13,18, and X.[6] Furthermore, some genes have multiple functions. The goal now is to identify the functions of these genes and their protein products. This will allow geneticists, scientists, and clinicians to understand a disease process when a specific protein or its function is altered.

Short Primer on Molecular Genetics

Genes are the basic unit of heredity and are composed of molecules of deoxyribonucleic acid (DNA). They are located on chromosomes, which are the physical structures transmitted in the sperm and ovum. From the Human Genome Project, it is known that most of the DNA on chromosomes does not code for specific genes. The genes themselves are composed of various compartments and regulatory elements needed for the machinery of transcription. Exons and introns are two examples of such elements. Exons contain the exact sequence needed to make a protein. A gene is transcribed into messenger RNA (mRNA) in the nucleus of the cell. The mRNA then leaves the nucleus for the cytoplasm. It contains the exact sequence for making the protein but lacks the intron components of the gene. The introns are removed after transcription of the RNA through a precise process called *splicing*. The mRNA is then translated into the respective protein (Figure 2-1). Mistakes affecting the production, composition, and activity of the protein may occur at various levels, from a single base pair change to duplication or deletion of whole genes, parts of chromosomes, and whole chromosomes.

BIRTH DEFECTS

Birth defects are a common cause of morbidity and mortality, with an incidence in newborns ranging from 1% to 4% depending on the population analyzed.[7] The method and period of ascertainment and the definition

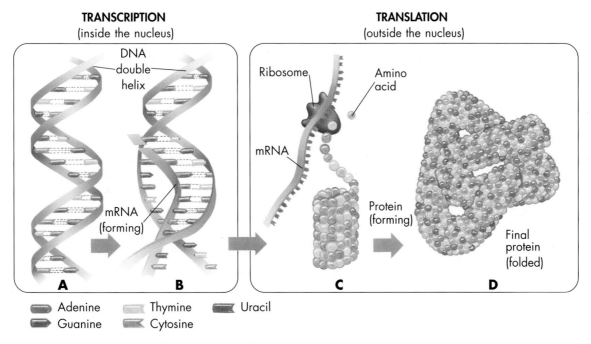

TRANSCRIPTION
(inside the nucleus)

TRANSLATION
(outside the nucleus)

DNA double helix

mRNA (forming)

Ribosome

Amino acid

mRNA

Protein (forming)

Final protein (folded)

A **B** **C** **D**

- Adenine
- Guanine
- Thymine
- Cytosine
- Uracil

Figure 2-1

Schematic representation of transcription and translation. **A,** The DNA molecule contains a sequence of base pairs (gene) that represents a sequence of amino acids. **B,** During transcription, the DNA recipe is "transcribed" as messenger RNA that forms (mRNA) in the nucleus. The forming mRNA is represented by the orange ribbon. **C,** The mRNA (orange ribbon) is "translated" into the proper sequence of coiled amino acids outside of the nucleus on the ribosome. **D,** To form the final complex protein molecule, the coiled amino acid strand coils again. (From Thibodeau GA, Patton KT: *The human body in health and disease*, ed 3, St. Louis, 2002, Mosby.)

of a malformation also affect the reported incidence. With age, the rate of diagnosis rises, doubling by 1 year of age and tripling by school age.[8] It is known that low birth weight, twinning, and consanguinity are all associated with an increased frequency of birth defects.[9,10] In addition, male sex is associated with an increased frequency of many, but not all, malformations.[11] The etiologies of birth defects are classified as chromosomal disorders, single gene disorders, genetic disorders resulting from teratogens, and multifactorial disorders (combinations of genes and environmental factors).

Chromosomal Disorders

Abnormalities in chromosome number and structure result in significant pathology. A normal karyotype consists of 46 chromosomes, divided into 23 pairs: 22 autosomal and 1 sex chromosome pair (2 X's or one X and Y). Normally, an individual receives one copy of each chromosome from each parent. Abnormal division of a chromosome pair (nondisjunction) can occur during maternal meiosis or during mitosis (after fertilization). Mosaicism, defined as populations of cells with differing chromosome constitutions, (e.g., some cells may have a normal chromosome number and others may have an extra chromosome), may occur as a result of abnormal division during mitosis. Theoretically, an extra copy of any chromosome pair (trisomies) can occur, but most of these affected fetuses abort spontaneously. Only a few trisomies are compatible with a liveborn infant: trisomy 21 (Down syndrome) (Figure 2-2), trisomy 13, trisomy 18 (Figure 2-3),

47,XXY (Klinefelter syndrome), 47,XXX, and 47,XYY. These usually are associated with advanced maternal age, and the features differ according to the chromosome involved.

Monosomy (one missing chromosome) has been reported only for the sex chromosomes, because fetuses with other monosomies are nonviable. Turner syndrome (45,X) has a high in utero mortality rate but some fetuses do survive (Figure 2-4). In general, 45,X is not associated with advanced maternal age. The X chromosome, in most cases (80%), is of maternal origin, indicating that the paternal copy was lost.[12]

Structural chromosomal abnormalities, such as deletions, duplications, and rearrangements (translocations, inversions), also occur. Deletions and duplications may be visible microscopically (seen with the usual method of performing a karyotype) or at a submicroscopic level using specialized cytogenetic techniques, such as FISH (fluorescent in situ hybridization).

A very common deletion is located on the long arm of chromosome 22 (22q11). This results in velocardiofacial syndrome and DiGeorge sequence (absent thymus and parathyroid glands, micrognathia, and heart abnormalities). The features are varied and include cleft palate, Pierre Robin sequence or velopharyngeal insufficiency in the absence of a cleft, conotruncal heart defects, learning disabilities, psychiatric problems, DiGeorge sequence, and a characteristic facial appearance (Figure 2-5).

Duplications of parts or regions of chromosomes result in different phenotypes. Cat's-eye syndrome is caused by tetrasomy (four copies) of chromosome 22

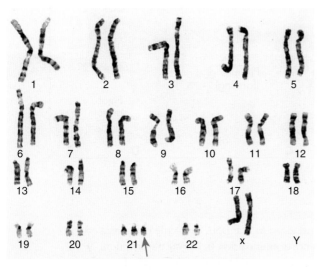

Figure 2-2

Karyotype of newborn female (two copies of X and no Y chromosome) with Down syndrome (trisomy 21). Note the extra copy of chromosome 21 *(arrow)*.

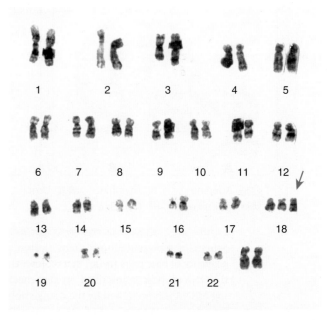

Figure 2-3

Karyotype of a newborn female who has trisomy 18 *(arrow)*.

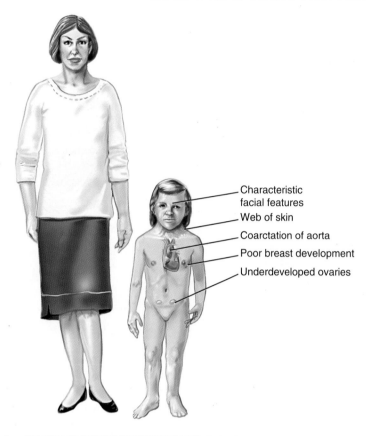

Figure 2-4

Turner syndrome (45,X) is a monosomy chromosomal disorder (one sex chromosome is missing). This drawing shows some of the clinical features of Turner syndrome: short stature and webbed neck.

material, with two copies present as an additional small chromosome pair. The clinical features include coloboma of the iris, anal atresia with fistula, down-slanting palpebral fissures, ear abnormalities including tags and pits, heart and kidney malformations, and mild mental impairment (Figure 2-6).

Single Gene Disorders

Single gene disorders are caused by one abnormal gene and are inherited in the traditional mendelian patterns: autosomal dominant, autosomal recessive, X-linked recessive, and X-linked dominant. Mutations in the responsible gene result in abnormal quantity or function of the protein. There may be a single point mutation (changing one nucleotide for another), insertion of one or more nucleotides, deletion of one or more nucleotides, expansion of a portion of a gene, or other rearrangements within the gene. Depending upon the site of mutation, the coded protein may not be produced at all or its stability may be altered. The configuration of the protein may be changed, resulting in alteration of

the protein's activity (higher or lower activity). Point mutations that do not affect protein function are not pathogenic.

Autosomal dominant disorders are the result of one abnormal copy of a gene on any of the 22 non–sex chromosome pairs. All children of an individual with an autosomal dominant disorder have a 50% chance of inheriting the abnormal gene and exhibiting the phenotype (Figures 2-7 and 2-8). In many cases, there is no family history of the disorder and it may represent a new mutation in the affected individual. Therefore, the absence of a positive family history does not exclude an autosomal dominant disorder. Typically, autosomal dominant disorders involve structural proteins or receptors. There may be phenotypic variability within families, with different degrees of expression (variable expressivity). For example, a very mildly affected parent may have a child who is more severely affected. Treacher Collins syndrome is a common craniofacial disorder with variable expressivity (Figure 2-9). The mechanism of this phenomenon is not well understood. However, in some disorders (such as myotonic dystrophy) there

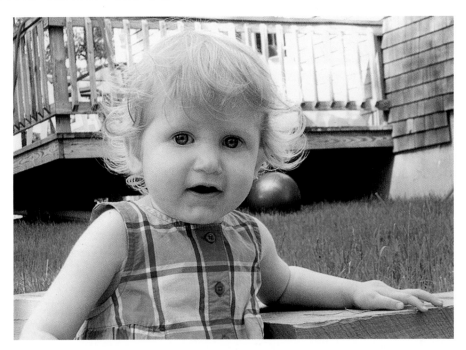

Figure 2-5

Photograph of 3-year-old girl with velocardiofacial/DiGeorge syndrome. The characteristic features of this syndrome include rectangular-shaped nose, low-set ears, micrognathia (mild in this patient), and long-tapered fingers (left hand in this patient). Patients also have cleft palate, velopharyngeal insufficiency, thymic aplasia, and cardiac anomalies.

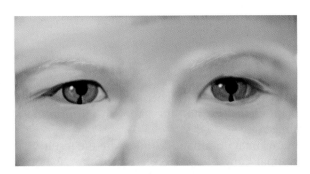

Figure 2-6

Drawing of the characteristic coloboma of the iris seen in cat's-eye syndrome. The genetic basis for this syndrome is four copies of chromosome 22. Other clinical features include anal atresia, downslanting palpebral fissures and ear abnormalities (tags and pits), and heart and kidney malformations.

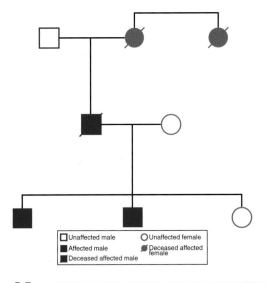

Unaffected male	Unaffected female
Affected male	Deceased affected female
Deceased affected male	

Figure 2-7

Autosomal dominant pedigree. Pedigrees reflect phenotypic data from several generations.

may be an expansion of part of the gene, which affects function in subsequent generations.

An autosomal recessive condition is the result of two copies of the abnormal gene, one inherited from each parent. The parents each have one normal and one abnormal copy and are, therefore, asymptomatic carriers. A carrier couple has a 25% risk of having an affected male or female child in each pregnancy (Figure 2-10).

Typically, autosomal recessive conditions involve synthesis of enzymatic proteins. These enzyme deficiencies result in inborn errors of metabolism, as well as malformation syndromes. For example, Smith-Lemli-Opitz syndrome, which consists of microcephaly, cleft palate, a characteristic facial appearance, cardiac defects,

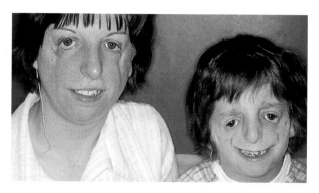

Figure 2-8

Mother *(left)* and daughter *(right)* with Treacher Collins syndrome (autosomal dominant *TCOF1* gene). Offspring of a parent with an autosomal dominant disorder have a 50% chance of inheriting the abnormal gene. (Photograph courtesy Dr. L.B. Kaban.)

ambiguous genitalia in the male, postaxial polydactyly and syndactyly of toes, and growth and mental retardation, is due to an abnormality in cholesterol metabolism.[13]

X-linked disorders, as the name implies, are due to abnormal genes located on the X chromosome. In general, males with X-linked disorders are more symptomatic than females. A female who has one copy of an X-linked recessive gene may have only mild or no signs, while the male expresses the full condition. This differential expression is due to X inactivation. One of the X chromosomes in the female becomes inactivated early in development. In contrast, a female with an X-linked dominant disorder is symptomatic, although less so than males. Some X-linked dominant disorders, such as Rett syndrome and incontinentia pigmenti, are lethal in males. With X-linked inheritance, male-to-male transmission is not possible, because a male receives the X chromosome from the mother. Each son of a carrier mother has a 50% chance of inheriting the abnormal gene. Each daughter has a 50% chance of inheriting the abnormal gene (carrier) and a 50% chance of inheriting the normal gene (Figure 2-11). The Y chromosome is passed from father to son only. Therefore, a male with an X-linked disorder who can reproduce will pass on the abnormal X chromosome to each of his daughters, and they will be carriers. None of his sons will inherit the abnormal gene. The affected male can have affected grandsons (via the daughter), but not sons. Hemophilia is a classic example of X-linked inheritance.

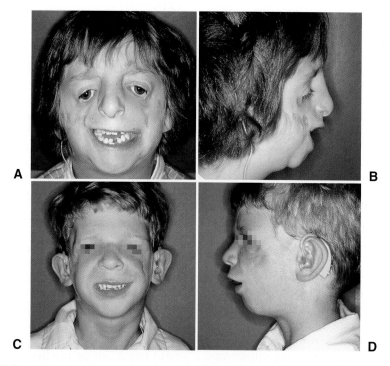

Figure 2-9

Treacher Collins syndrome is an autosomal dominant disorder of variable expressivity. Frontal **(A)** and lateral **(B)** photographs of a girl with severe involvement of the orbits, eyelids, midfacial soft tissue, mandible, and ears. Frontal **(C)** and lateral **(D)** photographs of a boy with moderate orbital and periorbital soft tissue involvement and mild ear and mandibular deformities. (Photograph courtesy Dr. L.B. Kaban.)

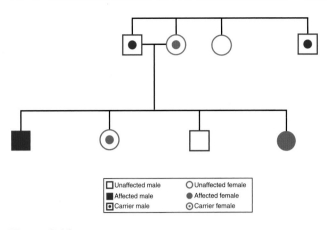

Figure 2-10

Autosomal recessive pedigree. The parents each have one normal and one abnormal copy of a gene and are asymptomatic carriers. A carrier couple has a 25% risk of producing an affected child, male or female (at each pregnancy).

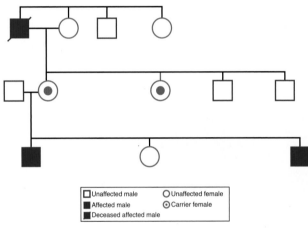

Figure 2-11

X-linked pedigree.

Nontraditionally Inherited Disorders

Mitochondrial Inheritance. Mitochondria are the energy organelles of human cells and contain their own DNA. Mitochondrial DNA can be inherited in two ways: (1) from genes which are encoded in the nucleus (as part of the nuclear genome) or (2) from genes which are located in the mitochondria themselves (the mitochondrial genome). Abnormalities inherited from the nuclear genome follow the usual mendelian modes of inheritance. Abnormalities of genes located in the mitochondrial genome follow a maternal pattern of inheritance. This is because the mitochondrial genome is produced by mitochondria present in the cytoplasm of the oocyte. Very few mitochondria are derived from DNA in the sperm. (Figures 2-12 and 2-13). A woman may have mutations in a small number of mitochondria, produc-

ing a variable proportion of mitochondria with mutant DNA in her oocytes. The degree of phenotypic expression from these mutant mitochondria depends upon the proportion of mutant and normal mitochondria in the fertilized egg.

Multifactorial Inheritance. Some conditions do not exhibit the traditional mendelian inheritance patterns. In these disorders, it is thought that multiple genes or significant environmental interactions are responsible.

Imprinting. Some gene functions are dependent upon whether the gene is inherited paternally or maternally. Such genes may be active only if inherited from the mother and others only if inherited from the father.

SYNDROME RECOGNITION FOR THE CLINICIAN

As genes are identified and assigned to specific disorders, DNA-based diagnostic testing is becoming a realistic possibility for a variety of conditions. However, there is often a lag time between identification of a gene and clinical correlation. The explosion of genetic information and the rapid rate of identification of new genes has made it unrealistic for someone who is not a geneticist to remain current and completely informed. Consultation with the clinical geneticist is, therefore, imperative.

A syndrome is defined as "a pattern of malformations that occur together from a single cause."[14] A major role of the clinical geneticist is to determine whether a child with a particular anomaly has a syndrome or whether the anomaly is an isolated finding. This helps to determine testing options, prognosis, medical problems to anticipate, possible treatments, and recurrence risks for other family members.

The geneticist obtains a careful and detailed medical and family history. The patient and, in some cases, other family members undergo a physical examination, laboratory evaluation, and follow-up counseling and management.

Review of Medical History

Details regarding the pregnancy, delivery, newborn period, and childhood should be obtained from the parents. A particularly important issue is the maternal drug history during pregnancy, because certain medications are known to be teratogenic. For example, warfarin taken during the first trimester is associated with significant nasal hypoplasia (Figure 2-14). It should be determined whether any prenatal testing, such as chorionic villus sampling, amniocentesis, or ultrasonography, was done. This is important to determine what information was available prenatally and whether any untoward complications occurred from the

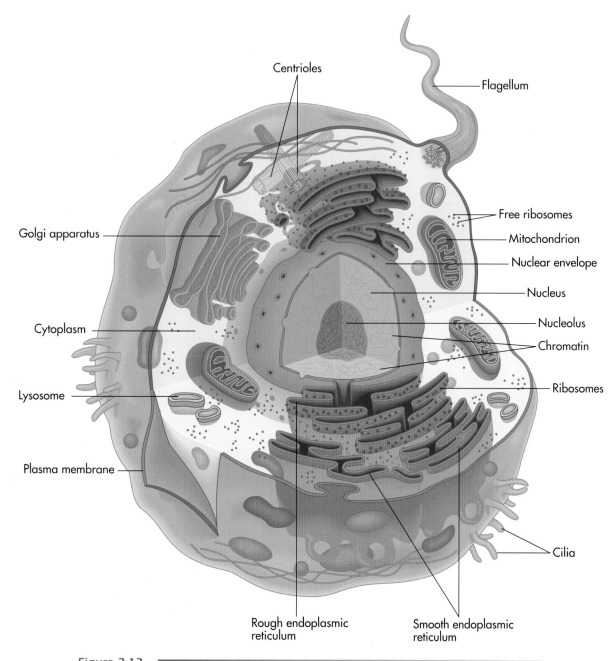

Centrioles

Flagellum

Golgi apparatus

Free ribosomes

Mitochondrion

Nuclear envelope

Nucleus

Cytoplasm

Nucleolus

Chromatin

Lysosome

Ribosomes

Plasma membrane

Cilia

Rough endoplasmic reticulum

Smooth endoplasmic reticulum

Figure 2-12

Schematic representation of a cell. Note the presence of the nucleus and mitochondria. The mitochondria (energy organelles) contain their own DNA. The components of the mitochondria are encoded in genes located in the nucleus or in the mitochondria. (From Thibodeau GA, Patton KT: *The human body in health and disease*, ed 3, St. Louis, 2002, Mosby.)

procedure. For example, chorionic villus sampling has been implicated in the etiology of transverse limb and several other vascular disruption defects (gastroschisis, intestinal atresia, and clubfoot).[7,15] Obstetric issues such as bleeding, trauma, intrauterine growth retardation, oligohydramnios or polyhydramnios, or decreased fetal movements are also important. A child with a malformation and intrauterine growth retardation may be more likely to have an underlying syndromic etiology for the defect. Decreased fetal movements may indicate an underlying neurologic or neuromuscular problem. The type of delivery, complications during delivery, birth parameters, and the baby's feeding history should be recorded. An infant with a cleft palate and a small head should be evaluated for an underlying disorder of multiple systems.

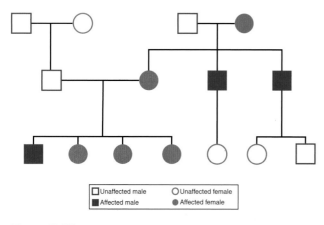

Figure 2-13

Mitochondral inheritance pedigree. Abnormalities of the mitochondrial genome follow a maternal pattern of inheritance.

Any developmental or cognitive difficulties should be noted. Growth history, with examination of growth curves (appropriate to gender and ethnic background, if available), is essential. Hospitalizations, operations, and frequent illnesses must be documented. Episodic illnesses may lead the clinician to pursue a metabolic etiology. Previous laboratory data should be reviewed.

Family History

This should include details about other siblings, parents, grandparents, and cousins. Specific questions are asked about recurrent miscarriages, stillbirths, neonatal deaths, and family members with birth defects and mental retardation. The family's ethnic background should be noted, because certain conditions are more common in specific ethnic groups. Consanguinity must be determined, because this increases the risk of birth defects and the chance of rare autosomal recessive disorders.

Several key points are important when analyzing a family history.

1. A negative family history does not eliminate the possibility of a genetic disorder. The disorder may be autosomal recessive and multigenerational involvement would not be expected, or the disorder could be secondary to a new autosomal dominant mutation.
2. An attempt should be made to identify other high-risk family members and to determine if they have any physical resemblance to the affected child. Based on variable expressivity, previously unrecognized affected relatives may be discovered.
3. For male children, the presence of similarly affected males on the maternal side suggests X-linked inheritance. However, the absence of any other affected males does not eliminate the possibility of X-linked inheritance with the mother as the carrier.

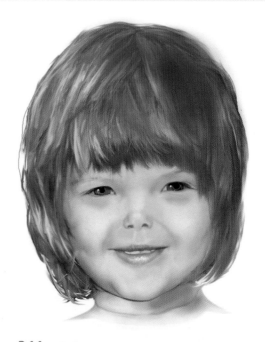

Figure 2-14

Representation of a girl with nasal hypoplasia (vertically short and flat nasal bridge secondary to hypoplasia of the nasal bones) secondary to maternal Coumadin ingestion during the first trimester of pregnancy.

Physical Examination

The physical examination is detail oriented and comprehensive, and specific features may also be assessed in the parents. Careful measurements of height or length, weight, and head circumference are done and are plotted on appropriate growth curves. If a disorder of growth or the skeleton is suspected, arm span and upper and lower segments are measured. Major and minor anomalies and normal variants are noted. Minor anomalies may not be of significance, but they may provide clues to the diagnosis. Specific details about the examination are listed in Table 2-1.

In cases of facial dysmorphism, the individual is compared with other family members at the same age to assess for familial resemblance. The presence of certain anomalies may serve as clues to the diagnosis. These anomalies may be minor themselves, but they are highly correlated with a specific diagnosis. For example, pits (depressions in the skin) in various locations are often clues to the diagnosis. Lower lip pits are associated with van der Woude syndrome, an autosomal dominant disorder consisting of cleft palate and lip pits. Pits and creases on the back of the external ear should make one think of Beckwith Wiedemann, an overgrowth syndrome. Palmar pits are associated with nevoid basal cell carcinoma syndrome. The presence of more than one malformation or a malformation in

TABLE 2-1	Components of a Genetic Physical Examination
System	**Feature Assessed**
General	Size, body proportions, general appearance
Skin and hair	Pigmentation, hair distribution, and texture, and any lesions or birthmarks are noted
	Comparison is made to the pigmentation of family members
Head size and shape	Asymmetry, sutural synostosis, microcephaly, macrocephaly
Eyes	Slant, size, placement, morphology of irides
	Measure palpebral fissures and inner canthal, outer canthal, interpupillary distances
Ears	Shape, size, location, ear lobe creases, ear pits, tags, morphology
Nose	Shape, configuration of nasal bridge, root, columella, nares
Mouth	Vermilion, shape, dentition, palate, uvula
Philtrum	Length, groove
Chin	Size, position
Neck	Webbing, masses, sinuses, pits, thyroid
Chest	Heart auscultation, symmetry, pectus excavatum, pectus carinatum, placement of nipples
Abdomen	Hepatosplenomegaly, masses, scars
Extremities	Size, symmetry, configuration of hands, feet, nails, creases
	Range of motion of distal and proximal joints, pes planus, pes cavus, syndactyly
Back	Curvature, lesions
Neurologic	Developmental status, cranial nerves, motor tone, motor strength, gait, cerebellar function, reflexes

association with a minor anomaly may be clues to a specific diagnosis.

The clinical geneticist should recognize the pattern of anomalies seen in various disorders. This is based on the geneticist's personal experience, review of the literature, or use of various databases such as POSSUM, the London dysmorphology database, and OMIM (Online Mendelian Inheritance in Man). Another strategy is for the geneticist to concentrate on the most unusual feature and to determine what conditions are associated with it. In addition, the geneticist must be highly aware of the variable expressivity of certain disorders and be open to exploring new possibilities.

Laboratory and Testing Methods

After the geneticist has formulated a differential diagnosis or suspects a specific diagnosis, laboratory testing is performed.

In the case of a specific genetic disorder, it must be determined if the problem is at the chromosomal level or if it is a single gene disorder. In chromosomal disorders, there is a deletion or duplication of a particular chromosome or chromosomal segment. If the disorder is suspected to be submicroscopic, special techniques such as FISH are used to detect the abnormality.

If the condition is a single gene disorder, then the clinician must determine if the responsible gene has been identified, whether pathogenic mutations are known, and whether testing is available. Clinical testing is not available for all identified genes.

A karyotype involves cell culture. Cells are harvested, fixed, and stained for mitoses. The specimen is then examined under the microscope (Figure 2-15). A karyotype can be performed on white blood cells from a peripheral blood sample, fibroblasts from skin, and epithelial cells from a buccal smear. The FISH technique requires additional steps to hybridize fluorescent-labeled DNA probes to specific areas on the gene (Figures 2-16 and 2-17).

When the disease is caused by a specific number of mutations which can be identified, analysis can be done using direct sequencing, restriction enzymes, or hybridization techniques for the specific mutations (Figures 2-18 and 2-19).

If the family has a unique mutation, analysis can be accomplished by direct sequencing of the gene and analyzing each base pair. This is very labor intensive and expensive and is not possible for every gene. An alternative is indirect or linkage testing.

Linkage testing involves tracking the gene in a family by using normal variations either around or within the gene (Figure 2-20). These variants do not cause disease and differ among individuals. However, they allow differentiation between the two chromosomes containing the gene in question. Linkage analysis does not test the actual gene for possible disease-causing mutations. It requires that one be confident of the diagnosis and of the identity of the gene causing the disorder. Samples

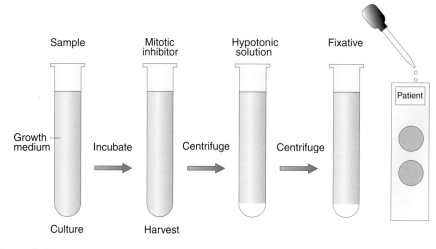

Figure 2-15

Chromosome processing. Cells are harvested, fixed, and stained for mitoses and examined under a microscope.

from multiple affected and unaffected family members are required. Interpretation of linkage studies is also limited, because members of a chromosome pair can exchange material (recombination).

Both DNA methods have limitations. When using direct testing, the expected detection rate for the disorder must be known. If the test detects only 70% of possible pathogenic mutations, then a negative test result does not completely eliminate the disorder in question. Linkage testing is predominantly useful when the diagnosis is known and for estimating the probability that an individual has inherited the chromosome containing the abnormal gene.

These tests help confirm a clinical diagnosis and help guide the geneticist in management of the patient and family. Furthermore, location of a specific mutation facilitates prenatal diagnosis and identification of at-risk family members.

There are some concerns about genetic testing. DNA analysis of presymptomatic individuals may have adverse effects on their insurability and employment. Some states have enacted laws to prevent such discrimination. However, there is no uniform policy on a national level.

Testing individuals for a late-onset disease for which there is no treatment is controversial. While testing for some autosomal dominant disorders, other family members with the disease may be identified against their wishes. For example, a man seeks testing for an adult-onset autosomal dominant disorder, which his grandfather had. His own parent has not shown signs of the disorder and has not been tested. If the man's test

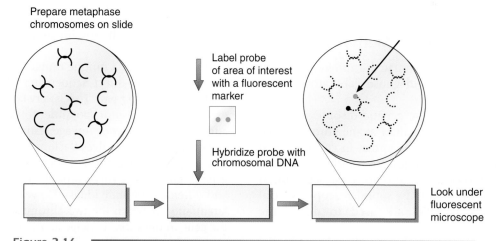

Figure 2-16

In the FISH (fluorescent in situ hybridization) technique, extra steps are taken to hybridize fluorescent-labeled DNA probes to specific areas of the chromosome.

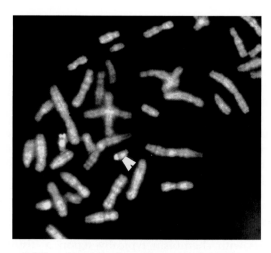

Figure 2-17 ▰▰▰

Photograph of a FISH processed karyotype showing deletion of 22q11.2. One of the fluorescent probes indicates that it is chromosome 22, the other is a specific probe for the region of interest (in this case, 22q11.2). The arrowhead shows the missing area on one of the no. 22 chromosomes.

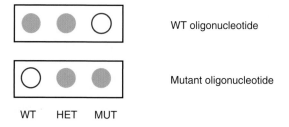

Figure 2-18 ▰▰▰

Mutational analysis using oligonucleotide probes. A oligonucleotide is a small piece of DNA that includes the base pairs of interest. The wildtype (WT, normal) probe is an exact match for the normal gene. The mutant probe is an exact match for the mutant (abnormal) gene. The WT sample does not hybridize with the mutant probe (represented by the open circle). The mutant sample will hybridize only with the mutant probe (solid circle). A carrier sample will hybridize with both. *WT*, Wildtype; *HET*, heterozygote or carrier; *MUT*, affected individual.

result is positive, then the parent can also be assumed to have the disease. The parent may not wish to know this, which poses an ethical dilemma. Geneticists try to counsel their patients extensively about these issues prior to testing. Such counseling should be part of the decision-making process.

When an unknown disorder exists, screening tests are available. A karyotype may be ordered if one or more of the following are present: (1) a particular pattern of anomalies, (2) an unrecognized pattern of multiple congenital anomalies, (3) ambiguous genitalia, (4) developmental

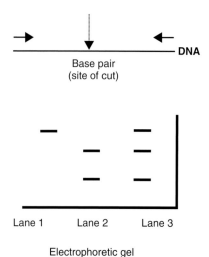

Electrophoretic gel

Figure 2-19 ▰▰▰

Schematic of restriction enzyme digest test. Restriction enzymes cut pieces of DNA *(line)* at specific points. A change in a base pair *(vertical arrow)* can change the enzyme's ability to cut the DNA. The pieces of DNA vary in size depending on whether there was a change in a base pair (mutation). The lower part of the schematic is a gel. Lane 1 shows an intact piece of DNA (mutant—the enzyme did not cut it). Lane 2 shows normal DNA that was cut by the enzyme. Lane 3 reflects a carrier: there is cut DNA (normal) and uncut DNA (mutant).

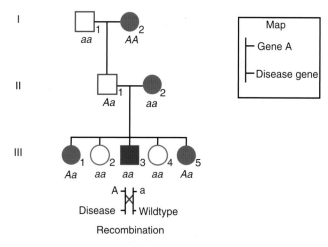

Figure 2-20 ▰▰▰

Schematic representation of linkage testing. Linkage testing involves tracking the gene in a family by using normal variations either around or within the gene. The pattern of these variations is then correlated with the abnormal phenotype. This technique is limited by the possibility of recombination between chromosomes during meiosis. In this pedigree the "A" variation cosegregates with the disease (i.e., affected individuals are II-1, III-1 and III-5). However, individual III-3 is "aa" and is affected due to recombination.

delay with major or minor anomalies, (5) presence of two single gene disorders in the same individual.

A geneticist may order a subtelomeric deletion FISH study for a child with unexplained mental retardation and a normal karyotype. This study looks for deletions at the ends of chromosomes and has detected abnormalities in about 7% of individuals with unexplained moderate to severe mental retardation.[16]

Metabolic studies such as analysis of amino acids, organic acids, and lysosomal enzymes are ordered in certain circumstances. This testing is based on the signs and symptoms, such as episodic illnesses, food avoidance, cyclic nature of the symptoms, and regression and deterioration of mental state.

COMMON SYNDROMES WITH FACIAL DEFORMITY

Branchio-Oto-Renal Dysplasia

The clinical features of branchio-oto-renal (BOR) syndrome include sensorineural, conductive, or mixed hearing loss, cup-shaped pinnae (lop ear), preauricular pits, Mondini's malformation (hypoplasia of cochlear apex), bilateral branchial cleft fistulae or cysts, high arched palate, cleft palate, bifid uvula, and various renal anomalies. Renal anomalies may include renal dysplasia or aplasia, abnormalities of the collecting system, and polycystic kidneys.[17] This diagnosis should be considered whenever deafness, malformed pinnae, preauricular pits, and branchial clefts are present with or without a cleft palate.

The kidney abnormalities may be unrecognized, especially if renal evaluation has not yet been carried out. If there are affected family members, the diagnosis can be made with the presence of only two findings (hearing loss, preauricular pits or tags, lop-ear deformity, branchial fistula, or renal anomalies). If there are no affected family members, three findings are necessary to make the diagnosis. Other diagnoses to consider include cat's eye syndrome, branchio-otic syndrome (which does not include renal abnormalities and deafness is variable), and BOR-Duane-hydrocephalus contiguous gene syndrome (which has the additional features of Duane anomaly and hydrocephalus).

BOR syndrome is an autosomal dominant disorder with variable expressivity. Accordingly, each child of an affected individual has a 50% chance of inheriting the abnormal gene and exhibiting the phenotype, although expression may vary. In approximately 40% to 45% of families with BOR syndrome, there is a mutation in the *EYA1* gene (eyes absent-1 gene) located at the chromosomal locus 8q13.3.[18] Over 35 different mutations have been reported, including small insertions, deletions, and missense and nonsense mutations.[19] *EYA1* testing is available clinically. However, one must interpret the results of such testing with caution, because 55% to 60% of families with BOR syndrome appear to have a different abnormal gene.[20,21] Unless one knows that the *EYA1* gene is the responsible gene in that family, a negative *EYA1* gene test result does not eliminate the possibility of this diagnosis.

Renal evaluation must be done in affected individuals because of the potential severity of the renal disease. In addition, the family should be counseled about the possibility of significant renal abnormalities in subsequent affected family members.

Cherubism

Patients with cherubism typically report a history of progressive swelling of the lower face during early childhood, which eventually tilts the eyes upward, giving the "cherubic" appearance (Figure 2-21). The swelling is due to fibro-osseous tissue containing multinucleated giant cells. Radiographs show multilocular radiolucencies in the mandible, maxilla, and ribs. The lesions may occupy a large portion of the ramus and body of the mandible and the zygomatic–maxillary complex. Generally the swelling recedes after puberty.[22,23] This condition may have a significant impact on facial appearance. It causes concern on the part of the parents, pediatricians, and dentists regarding adverse effects on tooth eruption and the possibility of root resorption and pathologic fracture of the jaw. There may also be secondary complications with swallowing, speech, and vision. The diagnosis is based on the clinical features and should be distinguished from Caffey's disease, which has a different radiologic appearance and has more involvement of the skeleton.[24]

Cherubism is an autosomal dominant disorder with abnormalities in the *SH3BP2* gene located on chromosome 4p16.3. Point mutations causing amino acid substitutions have been described.[25] The protein normally produced by this gene affects the bone cell's responses to incoming signals; these mutations may result in gain of function.

Most cases are due to new dominant mutations. Therefore, the absence of a positive family history does not rule out the possibility of this diagnosis. Cherubism also is characterized by incomplete penetrance, with some gene carriers not exhibiting any signs of the disorder.[25]

Nevoid Basal Cell Carcinoma Syndrome

The clinical features of this syndrome include numerous basal cell carcinomas, epidermal cysts, odontogenic keratocysts, palmar and plantar pits, various tumors or hamartomas, skeletal abnormalities of the ribs and vertebrae, macrocephaly, cleft lip, and cleft palate[26,27]

A

B

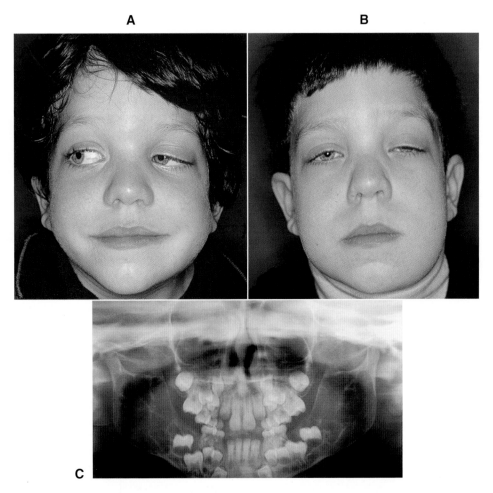

C

Figure 2-21

Frontal photograph of a boy with cherubism at age 5 years **(A)** and at age 12 years **(B)**. Note the progressive swelling of the cheeks and lower face. **C,** Panoramic radiograph shows the large multilocular radiolucencies that occupy the body and ramus of the mandible. (Photograph courtesy Dr. L.B. Kaban.)

(Figure 2-22). The criteria to make the diagnosis of nevoid basal cell carcinoma syndrome (NBCCS) include two major or one major and two minor features.[28]

The major features include (1) two or more basal cell carcinomas or one tumor in patients under 20 years of age, (2) odontogenic keratocyst, (3) palmar pits, (4) calcification of falx cerebri, (5) bifid, fused, or splayed ribs, and (6) an affected first-degree relative.

Minor criteria include (1) macrocephaly, adjusted for height, (2) frontal bossing, cleft lip or palate or both, hypertelorism, (3) Sprengel deformity, pectus, syndactyly, (4) bridging of sella turcica, hemivertebrae, flame-shaped radiolucencies, (5) ovarian fibroma, and (6) medulloblastoma.

NBCCS is an autosomal dominant disorder with complete penetrance but with variable expressivity. The gene is called PTCH and is located at chromosome 9q22.3. Mutations occur throughout the gene and there is no apparent correlation between the specific mutation and the physical effects.[29,30] Thirty-five to fifty percent of the cases are due to new mutations and there is an effect of increasing paternal age.[31]

PTCH is a tumor suppressor gene and is a cell cycle regulator.[32] The developmental effects are seen when only one mutation is present, accounting for the autosomal dominant inheritance pattern.[33] With tumor suppressor genes, unregulated cell growth occurs when both copies of the gene are not working. For people who have inherited an abnormal tumor suppressor gene, the likelihood of a "second hit" (a change in the remaining gene somewhere in the body) is very high. This leads to unregulated cell growth in that tissue. In the tumors that

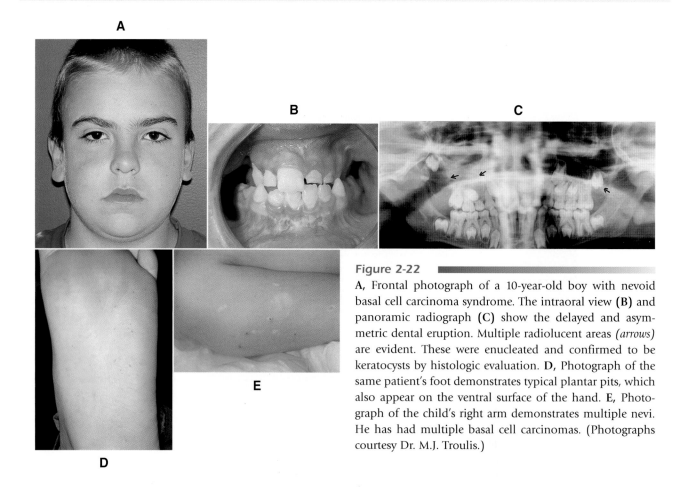

Figure 2-22

A, Frontal photograph of a 10-year-old boy with nevoid basal cell carcinoma syndrome. The intraoral view (**B**) and panoramic radiograph (**C**) show the delayed and asymmetric dental eruption. Multiple radiolucent areas *(arrows)* are evident. These were enucleated and confirmed to be keratocysts by histologic evaluation. **D,** Photograph of the same patient's foot demonstrates typical plantar pits, which also appear on the ventral surface of the hand. **E,** Photograph of the child's right arm demonstrates multiple nevi. He has had multiple basal cell carcinomas. (Photographs courtesy Dr. M.J. Troulis.)

develop in NBCCS, there does appear to be an abnormality of the other gene of the pair. This is presumed to be responsible for the change in cell growth.[34,35]

Genetic testing is available for correlation with clinical findings. Such testing detects the genetic abnormality in approximately 60% of clinical cases. Indications for genetic testing include confirmation of the clinical diagnosis in patients with the classic features, confirmation of NBCCS in a child with medulloblastoma and in individuals less than 20 years of age with a basal cell carcinoma, and insufficient associated clinical findings. It can also be used for prenatal diagnosis and identification of at-risk family members who may appear to be asymptomatic.

The risk to other family members depends on whether the mutation in the affected person is inherited or has arisen de novo. Each child of an affected individual has a 50% chance of inheriting the abnormal gene and of expressing the disorder to some extent. If there is no family history of the disorder and the parents of the affected individual have been examined extensively for mild expression, then the recurrence risk is low.

However, one has to factor in the possibility of gonadal mosaicism: one of the parents carries the mutation only in the gonads.

Pierre Robin Sequence

The clinical features include micrognathia, glossoptosis, and cleft palate (Figure 2-23). This constellation of features is considered to be descriptive and not etiologic. This sequence is associated with various syndromes (Table 2-2) and the geneticist should evaluate the child for these other conditions. This involves a detail-oriented history and physical examination, as outlined previously.

The genetics, counseling about recurrence risks, testing, and prognosis depend on the nature of the definitive diagnosis; hence the importance of searching for the underlying condition. About 65% of patients with Pierre Robin sequence have associated syndromes. The most common syndromes are Stickler syndrome, in about 35% of cases; velocardiofacial syndrome, 11%; fetal alcohol syndrome, 10%; and other syndromes, 10%.[36-39] As seen in Table 2-2, the inheritance patterns

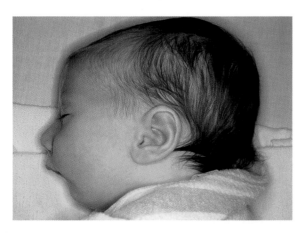

Figure 2-23
Lateral photograph of an infant shows the typical micrognathia of Pierre Robin sequence. (Photograph courtesy Dr. L.B. Kaban.)

may differ by condition. This results in different implications for the family and a different treatment plan and prognosis for the patient.

CONCLUSION

The field of genetics is expanding dramatically, with new developments occurring almost daily. The impact of genetic knowledge on medicine will continue to grow and will result in a new understanding of the pathogenesis of many different diseases. This new information should lead to better and more rational treatments. The role of the clinical geneticist is to evaluate patients for various disorders with the goal of obtaining specific diagnoses. Having a specific disorder can provide accurate recurrence counseling for the family, prognosis, guidance for what medical problems may arise, and, in some cases, appropriate treatment.

TABLE 2-2   Conditions with Pierre Robin Sequence[36-43]

Classification	Condition	Inheritance; Gene
Single gene disorders	Stickler syndrome	AD; *COL2A1, COL11A1, COL11A2*
	Marshall syndrome	AD; *COL11A1*
	Weissenbacher-Zweymuller syndrome	AD; *COL11A2*
	Otospondylomegaepiphyseal dysplasia	AD; *COL11A2*
	Congenital myotonic dystrophy	AD; *DMPK expansion*
	Spondyloepiphyseal dysplasia, congenita	AD; *COL2A1*
	Treacher Collins syndrome	AD; *TCOF1*
	Van der Woude syndrome	AD
	Cerebrocostomandibular syndrome	AD
	Toriello-Carey syndrome (corpus callosum, agenesis of, with facial anomalies and Robin sequence)	AR
	Carey-Fineman-Ziter syndrome (myopathy, congenital nonprogressive with Moebius and Robin sequences)	AR
	Arthrogryposis multiplex congenita with whistling face	AR
	Otopalatodigital syndrome type I	X-linked dominant
	Catel-Manzke syndrome	X-linked
	Osteopathia striata with cranial sclerosis	X-linked dominant
Chromosomal	Velocardiofacial syndrome	AD; 22q11 deletion
	Miller-Dieker lissencephaly syndrome	17p13.3 deletion
	Other duplication, deletion syndromes	—
Teratogenic	Fetal alcohol syndrome	—
	Fetal anticonvulsant syndrome	—
Disruption	Amniotic band sequence	—
Unknown	CHARGE association	—
	Oculo-auriculo-vertebral syndrome	—

AD, Autosomal dominant; *AR,* autosomal recessive; *CHARGE,* coloboma, heart defects, atresia of the choanae, retardation of growth and development, genital and urinary abnormalities, and ear abnormalities with or without hearing loss.

REFERENCES

1. Soltan HC, Craven JL: The extent of genetic disease in human populations, *CMAJ* 124:427-442, 1981.
2. Weatherall DJ: The frequency and clinical spectrum of genetic diseases. In Weatherall DJ, editor: *The new genetics and clinical practice*, New York, 1991, Oxford University Press.
3. Shepard TH, Fantel AG, Fitzsimmons J: Congenital defect rates among spontaneous abortuses: twenty years of monitoring, *Teratology* 39:325-331, 1989.
4. Venter J, Adams MD, Meyers EW, et al: The sequence of the human genome, *Science* 291:1304-1351, 2001.
5. International Human Genome Sequencing Consortium: Initial sequencing and analysis of the human genome, *Nature* 409:860-921, 2001.
6. Alberts MJ: Genetics update: impact of the human genome projects and identification of a stroke gene, *Stroke* 32:1239-1241, 2001.
7. Stoler JM: Prevalence and etiology of birth defects. In McCormick MC, Siegel JE, editors: *Prenatal care: effectiveness and implementation*, Cambridge, UK, 1999, Cambridge University Press.
8. Graham J: Congenital anomalies. In Levine MD, Carey WB, Crocker AC, editors: *Developmental-behavioral pediatrics*, Philadelphia, 1992, WB Saunders.
9. Mili F, Edmonds LD, Khoury MJ, McClearn AB: Prevalence of birth defects among low-birth-weight infants. A population study, *Am J Dis Child* 145:1313-1318, 1991.
10. Schinzel AA, Smith DW, Miller JR: Monozygotic twinning and structural defects, *Pediatrics* 96:921-930, 1979.
11. Carter CO: Genetics of common single malformations, *Br Med Bull* 32:21-26, 1976.
12. May KM, Jacobs PA, Lee M, et al: The parental origin of the extra X chromosome in 47,XXX females, *Am J Hum Genet* 46:754-761, 1990.
13. Irons M, Elias ER, Salen G: Defective cholesterol biosynthesis in Smith-Lemli-Opitz syndrome, *Lancet* 341:1414, 1993.
14. Jones KL: *Smith's recognizable patterns of human malformation*, Philadelphia, 1997, WB Saunders.
15. Matroiacovo P, Cavalcanti DP: Limb-reduction defects and chorion villus sampling, *Lancet* 337:1091, 1991.
16. Knight, SJ, Regan R, Nicod A: Subtle chromosomal rearrangements in children with unexplained mental retardation, *Lancet*, 354:1676-1681, 1999.
17. Chen A, Francis M, Ni L, et al: Phenotypic manifestations of branchio-oto-renal syndrome, *Am J Med Genet* 58:365-370, 1995.
18. Vincent C, Kalatzis V, Abdelhak S, et al: BOR and BO syndromes are allelic defects of *EYA1*, *Eur J Hum Genet* 5:242-246, 1997.
19. Abdelhak S, Kalatzis V, Heilig R, et al: A human homologue of the *Drosophila* eyes absent gene underlies branchio-oto-renal (BOR) syndrome and identifies a novel gene family, *Nat Genet* 15:157-164, 1997.
20. Rickard S, Boxer M, Trompeter M, Bitner-Glindzicz M: Importance of clinical evaluation and molecular testing in the branchio-oto-renal (BOR) syndrome and overlapping phenotypes, *J Med Genet* 37:623-627, 2000.
21. Stratakis CA, Lin JP, Rennert OM: Description of a large kindred with autosomal dominant inheritance of branchial arch anomalies, hearing loss, and ear pits, and exclusion of the branchio-oto-renal (BOR) syndrome gene locus (chromosome 8q13.3), *Am J Med Genet* 79:209-214, 1998.
22. Timosca GC: Cherubism: regression of the lesions and spontaneous bone regeneration, *Rev Stomatol Chir Maxillofac* 97:172-177, 1996.
23. Von Wowern N: Cherubism: a 36-year long-term follow-up of 2 generations in different families and review of the literature, *Oral Surg Oral Med Oral Pathol* 90:765-772, 2000.
24. Emmery L, Timmermans J, Christens F, Fryns JP: Familial infantile cortical hyperostosis, *Eur J Pediatr* 141:56-58, 1983.
25. Ueki Y, Tiziani V, Santanna C, et al: Mutations in the gene encoding c-Abl-binding protein SH3BP2 cause cherubism, *Nat Genet* 28:125, 2001.
26. Gorlin RJ: Nevoid basal-cell carcinoma syndrome, *Medicine* 66:98-113, 1987.
27. Evans DG, Ladusans EJ, Rimmer S: Complications of the naevoid basal cell carcinoma syndrome: results of a population based study, *J Med Genet* 30:460-464, 1993.
28. Kimonis VE, Goldstein AM, Pastakia B, et al: Clinical manifestations in 105 persons with nevoid basal cell carcinoma syndrome, *Am J Med Genet* 69:299-308, 1997.
29. Hahn H, Wicking C, Zaphiropoulous PG, et al: Mutations of the human homology of *Drosophila* patched in the nevoid basal cell carcinoma syndrome, *Cell* 85:841-851, 1996.
30. Wicking C, Shanley S, Smith I, et al: Most germ-line mutations in the nevoid basal cell carcinoma syndrome lead to a premature termination of the PATCHED protein, and no genotype-phenotype correlations are evident, *Am J Hum Genet* 60:21-26, 1997.
31. Jones KL, Smith DW, Harvey MA, et al: Older paternal age and fresh gene mutation: data on additional disorders, *Pediatrics* 86:84-88, 1975.
32. Johnson RL, Rothman AI, Zie J, et al: Human homolog of patched, a candidate gene for the basal cell nevus syndrome, *Science* 272:1668-1671, 1996.
33. Gailani MR, Bale SJ, Leffel SJ, et al: Developmental defects in Gorlin syndrome related to a putative tumor suppressor gene on chromosome 9, *Cell* 39:111-117, 1992.
34. Levanat S, Gorlin RJ, Fallet S, et al: A two-hit model for developmental defects in Gorlin syndrome, *Nat Genet* 12:85-87, 1996.
35. Shilo BZ: Tumor suppressors: dispatches from patched, *Nature* 382:115-116, 1996.
36. Shprintzen RJ: Pierre Robin, micrognathia and airway obstruction: the dependency of treatment on accurate diagnosis, *Int Anesthesiol Clin* 26:64, 1988.
37. van den Elzen AP, Semmekrot BA, Bongers EM, et al: Diagnosis and treatment of the Pierre Robin sequence: results of a retrospective clinical study and review of the literature, *Eur J Pediatr* 160:47-53, 2001.
38. Witt PD, Myckatyn T, Marsh JL, et al: Need for velopharyngeal management following palatoplasty: an outcome analysis of syndromic and nonsyndromic patients with Robin sequence, *Plast Reconstr Surg* 99:1522-1529, 1997.
39. Holder-Espinasse M, Abadie V, Cormier-Daire V, et al: Pierre Robin sequence: a series of 117 consecutive cases, *Pediatrics* 139:588-590, 2001.
40. Denion E, Capon M, Martinot V, et al: Neonatal permanent jaw constriction because of oral synechiae and Pierre Robin sequence in a child with van der Woude syndrome, *Cleft Palate Craniofac J* 39:115-119, 2001.
41. Aboura A, Coulombe-Hermiane A, Audebert F, et al: De novo interstitial direct duplication 1(q23.11q31.1) in a fetus with Pierre Robin sequence and camptodactyly, *Am J Med Genet* 108:153-159, 2002.
42. Morin G, Gekas J, Naepels P, et al: Cerebro-costo-mandibular syndrome in a father and female fetus: early prenatal ultrasonographic diagnosis and autosomal dominant transmission, *Prenat Diagn* 21:890-893, 2001.
43. Cohen MM Jr: Robin sequences and complexes: causal heterogeneity and pathogenic/phenotypic variability, *Am J Med Genet* 84:311-315, 1999.

CHAPTER 3

Psychological Preparation of the Child Undergoing a Maxillofacial Surgical Procedure

Myron L. Belfer

CHAPTER OUTLINE

Appropriate preoperative psychological preparation of the child and his or her family for a maxillofacial surgical procedure is essential for a successful outcome. Objective results may be overshadowed by failure of the patient and, often more importantly, the family to have an appreciation of the process and outcomes to be expected from the operation. In the case of an adverse outcome, adequate preparation may facilitate positive management of complications and disappointment. In this chapter we address basic considerations in the psychological preparation of the child and family for an operation. In addition, special attention is devoted to preparation of the "difficult patient" and the family with complex issues, such as separation or divorce, psychological illness, and history of surgical failure. The basic approach and concerns raised apply to both in-hospital and ambulatory surgery.

PSYCHOLOGICAL DEVELOPMENT

It is not possible to work with children and families without some basic understanding of psychological development.[1] Knowing what the child is capable of understanding, and the child's capacity to participate in the decision-making process and other aspects of surgical planning and postoperative care, is crucial to achieving a positive outcome. Likewise, helping parents to focus on realistic expectations and understanding the dynamics between child and parent, between parents, and among parents and the surgeon are crucial to having the parents as allies throughout the course of treatment and follow-up.

To evaluate a child based only on chronologic age, without an appreciation of developmental stage, will result in a failure to understand cognitive abilities and emotional conflicts that may need to be considered. Goin and Goin[2] provide a succinct review of body image development in children and adolescents in relation to overall development. For the maxillofacial surgeon, understanding the patient's developmental level is of particular importance, because many children have major or subtle cognitive delays associated with facial deformity or the presence of a syndrome. In addition, the expected socialization and cognitive development of a child may be delayed or distorted because of parental sheltering or overprotection. The developmental distortions conceived by parents can be in the direction of immaturity or in the attribution of precocious abilities to the child. Thus, understanding the child's socialization and cognitive development, preferably from more than one source, is crucial to appreciating the pediatric patient's preoperative and postoperative adaptive potential.

It is important to assess the developmental level of the child both independently and with input from the parents. This is not as complex a process as it might seem. A framework of observations, questions, and potential sources of information is provided in Table 3-1. These sources of information usually are accessed easily during

TABLE 3-1   Developmental Assessment

Age	Observation (Problem Concern)	Question/Observation	Source of Additional Information
3 - 5	Interaction with parents	Lack of relatedness, hyperactivity	Parents: Is this typical?
	Lack of speech	What is this . . . ?	Speech and hearing evaluation
5 - 7	Muteness	What do you like to do?	Parents: Is this typical?
	Apparent cognitive delay	Tell me about your school.	School report
	General concern	Do you have a best friend?	
7 - 10	Socialization	Do you have a best friend?	
		What things do you like to do?	
	Cognitive delay	What do you do in school?	School report
		What is your favorite subject?	
	Anxiety	Do you know about having an operation?	
		What do you think about having an operation to . . . ?	
10 - 13	Socialization	Do you have a best friend?	
	Anxiety	What do you think about having surgery?	
		What do you want the operation to do for you?	
	Cognitive delay	How are you able to do in school?	School report
		Do you need help in school?	
13 - 18	Socialization	What things do you like to do?	
		Do you have a best friend?	
		Do you think that an operation will help you with being with people?	
	Anxiety	Are you worried about the surgery?	Psychological report
		Have you ever spoken with someone about worries you have? Are you now speaking with someone? Does this help you?	
	Cognitive delay	Are you able to keep up with your schoolwork?	School report
		Do you get help in school?	

the preoperative period. Independent assessment by a specialist is indicated when the surgeon has concerns or when the answers to the questions do not seem reassuring.

With the preverbal patient it is not possible to obtain a statement of expectations. One can ask if the verbal child wishes something could be different or changed. This often can be done at a very early age. At earlier ages, and with limited cognitive function at any age, the focus of desired change is likely to be on some functional problem, such as difficulty chewing, or drooling.

Parents may state that the child has no appreciation of the facial deformity, but without talking about deformity per se, a simple question often can elicit that the child wants his ears made smaller, to be able to chew more easily, or something of that nature. Making the parent aware of the child's knowledge of a problem and the desire for change, even if crudely stated, can be of great help in overcoming parental ambivalence about pursuing surgical correction. If a complication occurs, this knowledge is an important factor in preventing the parent from engaging in self-blame for allowing the child to have an operation. Such guilt can seriously complicate the surgeon's relationship with the family in the event of an adverse outcome.

A relatively easy, well-documented technique for assessing a child's self-perception as different is the draw-a-person exercise.[3] This technique involves asking the child to draw a picture of a person, then to draw a self-portrait, and finally to draw one of the whole family. This simple task may provide the surgeon with a great deal of useful information and takes very little time. From the picture it is possible to make an assessment of cognitive function relative to age and an assessment of how the child perceives self in relation to the family. It is also possible, with some frequency, to determine whether the child has an internalized idea of his/her deformity. The draw-a-person test can be done in the waiting room and can be supervised by an assistant (Figure 3-1).

It is essential to understand the psychological defense of denial when evaluating a child for maxillofacial surgery.[4] To what extent is the patient or the parent denying the impact of the deformity, the life-threatening nature of some underlying or chronic illness, or the degree to which the child is ostracized? For example, the child who has been treated with high-dose radiation for a malignancy may have parents who wish to mask or deny the ongoing threat to the patient's overall health. In other cases, parents may be seeking correction for a

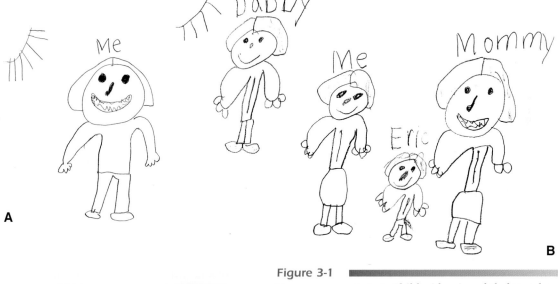

Figure 3-1

Draw-a-person test. **A,** Child with microphthalmos draws herself with eyes that are darkened and, therefore, more prominent relative to her other facial features. **B,** Same child draws herself and family, again with her eyes relatively more prominent. These drawings reveal the child's internalization of her deformity. **C,** Child with hemifacial microsomia draws himself with facial asymmetry corresponding to his deformity. **D,** Six months postoperatively, the child has integrated his new facial appearance and draws himself with the head symmetric and in more normal proportion to the rest of his body.

maxillofacial deformity as part of an overall attempt to deny the patient's underlying cognitive deficit. In this situation, without clarification regarding the potential effect of an operation on cognitive functioning and socialization, the stage may be set for disappointment.

In these cases and others, such denial is not an absolute contraindication to an operation, but it requires assessment and an attempt to better understand it in relation to the request for a procedure. For instance, the parents of the child with Down syndrome may actually be in touch with the child's deficits but seek, in a first interview, to mask their concerns for fear that they will present themselves as negative. It is possible to assess denial without so disturbing the defense, when it is pathologic, that one gets into difficulty with the parent or child.

The patient with temporomandibular joint (TMJ) dysfunction, particularly if accompanied by pain, requires a more in-depth psychological assessment.[5] Objective anatomic findings often do not correspond to expressed pain and functional deficit. During the postoperative period, objective surgical correction may not yield an expected resolution of discomfort and pain. It is necessary to evaluate aspects of family dynamics and depression as possibly significant contributing factors to the TMJ dysfunction clinical picture.

INITIAL EVALUATION OF CHILD AND PARENTS

Referral

The surgeon's relationship with the family and child actually begins before the first appointment, with the referral process and the referring person. The referring doctor, patient, friend, or other health care provider may convey a set of expectations. The patient and family may also have predetermined ideas about treatment from a brochure or other materials they have read. It is often difficult to know precisely what expectations have been transmitted to the family but, without fail, one must find out what they are at the outset. Regardless of the laudatory nature of the referrer, *do not promise more than you can deliver*.

Often, the maxillofacial surgeon is seen as having special powers. Newspaper and television accounts of the accomplishments of maxillofacial surgeons now routinely raise expectations for virtually flawless outcomes. To support this expectation is to lay the groundwork for later problems. It is better to have a grateful, nonlitigious patient and family than one who thinks you are "God." Most referrals to maxillofacial surgeons come through pediatricians, pediatric dentists, other physicians and dentists, or former patients. The latter are usually the most supportive if they are making a referral. Counterintuitively, the professional referral often

must be viewed with the greatest caution. It is essential that you understand precisely what the referral source told the patient, what expectations have been held out, and to what degree the referrer will maintain responsibility for the patient and later care.

It is important to have all relevant information from the referral source and to have access to the materials that parents can provide before the initial appointment. Too often, the patient is sent with no referral letter, information, or records, and the parents expect that you have received these materials. In complex cases, it is essential to go over the history with the parents to verify the information you have received.

A particular point that is often overlooked, but that may have consequences, is the mental status of the child. With complex deformities such as velocardiofacial syndrome there may be an accompanying psychological problem of some significance, such as schizophrenia or bipolar disorder. If this is not noted prior to the operation, bizarre behavior or responses during the postoperative period may be attributed to hospitalization or the impact of anesthesia, and not rightly seen as a preexisting condition. Acute psychiatric intervention may seem inappropriate, or families may feel that they can attribute the postoperative psychological problem specifically to the surgical procedure. This may lead to protracted and difficult discussions.

For patients with TMJ dysfunction, the history is critically important to understand the etiology of the problem. Although parafunctional habits and trauma are to be questioned, possible psychological contributants must be ascertained.[5] A history of loss, such as the death of a parent, can be a trigger or reinforcer of TMJ pain and dysfunction. Other psychological factors may be physical or sexual abuse, stress leading to bruxism, attention seeking, or identification with a similar parental complaint. A relatively simple screen for depression in younger children[6] is illustrated in Figure 3-2. For older children and adolescents, it is sufficient simply to ask the following: (1) Have you felt sad at any time in the recent past? (2) Do you feel as if you have lost something? (3) Have you lost someone important to you? (4) Are you worried about something that has happened or might happen you? A positive answer to any of these questions is sufficient to warrant a more in-depth psychological evaluation, as is a positive response to the screening test for younger children.

First Interview

Let the parents and patient do the talking. This does not mean that the surgeon should not interact or show affect. Rather, the surgeon should not start prematurely to describe what can and cannot be done for the patient until the expectations of all concerned have been

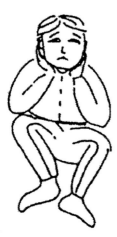

Figure 3-2

Sadness assessment. A child is shown this picture of a "sad person" and asked questions: Do you get like him? How much? Do you feel sad the way he does? Do people tell you that you look sad? How much? What about crying? How much does it happen to you? (From Ernst M, Cookus BA, Moravec BC: *J Am Acad Child Adolesc Psychiatry* 39:94-99, 2000.)

articulated. If any of the "red flag" circumstances described below (absent parent, multiple prior referrals, previous dissatisfaction) are apparent, they should be noted and discussed.

Remember, regardless of the important role of ancillary personnel (administrative, dental assistants, nurses), the surgeon is the key person in relation to the patient and family and the only person seen to have authority. However, the concerns of other staff should be considered based on their observations of the family in the waiting room, during routine workup procedures, making appointments, or in their verbal interaction. Nurses, dental assistants, or administrative staff may learn or observe something that might not be divulged in an interview.

The patient and family usually are seen together at the first visit. The surgeon should address all and ask each if they have questions.

In some cases, the surgeon may want to see the parents alone, at a separate appointment, before seeing the child. This strategy is useful for a particularly difficult or complex problem and avoids a rushed interview with all parties during a scheduled office visit. With adolescents, the surgeon should meet first with the patient. This generally establishes a more trusting relationship with the teenager.

Trust your instincts. If you feel uncomfortable with the parents or patient, do not dismiss the feeling. Explore this reaction with yourself and discuss it with colleagues who have also seen the patient and family. If it is not

evident what the reasons are (litigious attitude, overly directive parents, threat, unreasonable expectations, or inability to grasp the possible procedure), then say how pleased you were to meet the patient and family but that you do not think that you would be the best person to perform the operation. Refer the patient back to the referring doctor. Explain the situation and suggest other surgeons so that you do not risk losing a referral source. Do not be persuaded to engage in a situation with which you are not comfortable. *Note:* this is quite different from taking on a complicated family situation or complex operative procedure that may require ancillary support for the family and patient, but where you feel you have a basic understanding with the family and potentially a good relationship.

Try to come away from the first interview with a clear understanding of expectations, the family's view of the child, an understanding of what the family knows or does not know about the procedure, and their response to the possibility of a less than perfect outcome. The surgeon should also have a subjective feeling of comfort with the family and patient.[4] It is very important to understand and to document views divergent from the parents' regarding expected outcomes and desire for the operation. Discrepant views can come back to haunt the surgeon during the postoperative period if there are complications or a negative outcome.

Campis[7] found that maternal adjustment and maternal perceptions of the mother-child relationship were more potent predictors of children's emotional adjustment than either medical severity or maternal social support. Without needing to probe in depth, it is possible to ascertain how the parents and, in particular the mother, feel about their relationship with their child and to what extent they are able to communicate. For instance, asking, "Please tell me how easy it is for you to talk with your child about things, including this proposed surgery" is sufficient to get useful information. When a problem exists, the answer will be clearly truncated or elaborated beyond a reasonable expectation. In the case of a perceived problem, it is then possible to ask if the family has or plans to seek help to deal with the issue.

The use of nursing, social work, or other ancillary staff associated with the hospital or the maxillofacial practice is very important. Nursing staff often can provide a vital link with the child and family. However, they should not be asked to triage problems that might have broader significance for the patient, such as to treat an infection without the surgeon's direct involvement or to answer a technical question when the surgeon's answer might differ from a standard answer. Nursing staff can and should be supportive and should reinforce messages and directions that the patient or family may not have understood.

APPROACH TO THE CHILD
Explaining the Procedure

Once is never enough; pictures help (but are not necessarily the definitive answer). Despite the accompanying administrative difficulties in this era of managed care, second preoperative visits represent a good investment on the part of the surgeon and patient. Even more visits are desirable for complex cases. The additional contact helps patients gain a better appreciation of the operation and familiarity with the surgeon. It helps the surgeon to gain a better rapport with the patient and family and to further assess potential problems.

When there is an expectation for significant improvement in appearance, it is important to point out to the parents and patient that they should not expect an immediate acknowledgment of improvement no matter how great the change. Everyone involved must recognize that it takes time for the patient to integrate and to internalize a changed sense of self and a corresponding acknowledgment of an improved body image. This may take months, and the interim may be accompanied by regressive behaviors suggesting that the patient is testing out the new image with those nearby.[8]

First Conversation

Do not start by talking to the child about the proposed procedure. Ask about a favorite hobby, the doll they are carrying, or any other neutral topic. Then, ask if they know why they have come to see you. Have they been to the hospital (office) before? What would they like you to do? The child may not answer these questions, but it is important to ask. There is no need to pressure for an answer, but state that you hope the child may tell you later about what they have thought of in response to your questions.

Concept of Time and Use of a Calendar

In preparing a pediatric patient for an operation, it is not uncommon to be misunderstood, because children do not have a well-formed sense of time. For instance, to say to a child that "braces" will come off in 6 weeks has little concrete meaning. It is more helpful to indicate the time with the use of a calendar, or to target the time to some holiday or other event familiar to the child. This will aid greatly the appreciation of the time frame for the operation and the postoperative recovery. Supporting this understanding of time can reduce postoperative difficulties with compliance.

During the preoperative visits, it may be helpful to provide the family with a calendar on which key dates are indicated. Anxiety around the upcoming operation often leads parents to misinterpret or to misunderstand the time frames that may have been stated clearly. A particularly important part of this calendar exercise is to avoid negotiations about the often pressured concern on the part of children as to when they can go swimming, return to sports, or otherwise engage in normal activities.

Use of Hospital Surgical Preoperative Programs

Hospital, in particular pediatric hospital, preoperative programs are now almost universally sophisticated and useful to both parents and children.[9-11] Even parents who say that they have been through preoperative programs should be encouraged to participate again if there has been a span of years between operations. New information is always helpful to avoid confusion or misunderstandings during the hospital stay. Some programs offer ongoing contact through child life specialists, and this service should be utilized.

Anesthesia

This is, perhaps, the most difficult aspect of the overall surgical experience for both the parents and patient. It is important to understand that subjecting a child to general anesthesia is, for some parents, tantamount to killing their child. Therefore, the fears or anxieties associated with anesthesia may outweigh the concerns regarding the operation itself. This fear may not be made explicit by the anxious parent. It is important for the surgeon to be as precise as possible about the way in which the anesthesia will be administered. It is also essential that the surgeon and the anesthesiologist indicate the same procedures. In this regard, it is important that the anesthesiologist be fully informed about the operation so as not to venture an opinion at odds with that of the responsible surgeon. When explaining the anesthesia, there is an opportunity to inquire about the parents' experience with anesthesia and surgery. There is a high correlation between a negative parental experience and a negative reaction by the child to the experience of surgery or anesthesia induction. A possibly emotional scene at the time of induction or movement to the operating room can be avoided if these risks are appreciated. In such cases, it is important to help parents to avoid sharing their experiences with the child. Sometimes it is beneficial to insist that the parents not be present during the induction. In addition, the use of behavioral techniques to ease the anesthesia induction process can result in a far less traumatic experience for all involved.

A second aspect of the anesthesia that may be traumatic, for both parents and the patient, is the necessity for postoperative intubation. If this is a possibility, it should be explained prior to the operation. The family should be informed that the child may require assistance in maintaining an airway and, therefore, the endotracheal tube or other airway device may be kept for a time after the operation. The resultant temporary loss of voice or throat irritation should be explained.

ASKING THE DIFFICULT QUESTIONS

As an example of needing to ask difficult questions, consider the full evaluation of the pediatric patient with TMJ dysfunction and facial pain. Questions need to be asked that may be difficult for the surgeon, the patient, and the family. However, failure to ask these questions may result in an unfavorable outcome. The risk inherent in asking difficult questions is outweighed by the potential benefit to the patient. Typical questions follow: (1) Can you think of a loss around the time the TMJ pain was first noticed? (2) What response (from your parents, other family members, friends, and teachers) do you get when you complain of TMJ pain or dysfunction? (3) Have you felt sad or depressed? (4) Over what? (5) Have you ever felt that someone has done something to you they should not have? (6) Please explain. (7) Can you think of anything good that has come from your TMJ problem? With congenital deformities the questions are usually not focused on such charged emotional issues but could involve asking if one parent or the other has a family member with a similar deformity.

PROCEDURES REQUIRING SPECIAL CONSIDERATION
Distraction Osteogenesis

This modern, minimally invasive technique, while enthusiastically embraced by surgeons, can be seen by parents and the child as bordering on torture. The balance between media reports of sensational outcomes accomplished by essentially noninvasive means, and the reality of the means to accomplish these outcomes, is difficult for some parents and children to grasp. It is essential to explain in detail the goals of distraction osteogenesis, not just the outcome, and to be very clear with parents about the details of the process and how long it will take. It is also essential to be clear with both parents and the child about the details of the distraction procedure for which they will be responsible, such as who will turn the screws and when, and how much pain will need to be tolerated. Potential complications such as pin loosening, device failure, and requirement for additional procedures to correct the vector of distraction or to adjust the result also need to be discussed.

Maxillomandibular or Intermaxillary Fixation

It is not adequate to describe intermaxillary fixation or maxillomandibular fixation as being analogous to having braces. Immobilization of the jaws almost universally leads to a concern with choking, inability to breathe, and inability to talk. These concerns must be acknowledged. In all cases the safety procedures associated with use of maxillomandibular fixation should be explained and the tools provided to release the fixation.

External Devices

External fixation or distraction osteogenesis devices require compliance on the part of the child. In these cases, the likelihood of the child being the subject of teasing in school or being barraged by questions requires careful preoperative explanation directly with the child. The child should be part of the decision to use such devices.

Grafts

Although the language may be common and the concept well known, it is remarkable how often parents and patients fail to hear that "taking bone" or "making a graft" actually means that the surgeon will have to make an incision and remove bone from the hip or elsewhere. During the postoperative phase, pain associated with the donor site and the additional scar may become more of a focus of concern than the primary operation itself. It is best to avoid this situation by asking if the parents and child understand this and note this recognition in the chart. It is also helpful to point to the part of the anatomy from which the bone will be taken and state explicitly that there will be a scar and pain associated with this procedure.

HOSPITALIZATION

During the hospitalization, it is essential that families and children know how to get in touch with the surgeon. Most complications with families and patients arise not from problems with the operation, but from poor communication. How do you wish to be contacted? Is there a nurse working with you who can be reached? Who is in charge of the patient on the ward? Who is the resident in charge on the service? These questions should be answered clearly for the family.

A uniquely important part of the hospitalization is the first postoperative visit of the parents to the recovery room, intensive care unit, or regular nursing unit. It is a danger sign if one or the other parent is unable or unwilling to come to the recovery room. This may indicate lack of mutual support or an inability to accept the child or may predict difficulty in postoperative care and adjustment.

Nursing staff, familiar with the operation, can be helpful in accompanying parents to the recovery room during the postoperative period. Parents should not go to the recovery room without being accompanied by someone from the surgical team or from the clinic nursing staff or, in rare instances, by the psychiatric or social service consultant who worked with the child and family prior to the surgery.

When complications arise or when the nursing service thinks it is necessary to get a psychological consultation, it is best to remember "sooner rather than later." Reasons for thinking about a psychiatric consultation are non-compliance or changes in mental status noted by parents or ward staff, even the most vague expressions of suicidal ideation, unremitting anxiety, disproportionate complaints of pain, and extreme expressions of dissatisfaction with the surgical outcome. Likewise, if the nursing staff suggests a psychological consultation, find out why and get it regardless of the reason.

That a consultation will be requested needs to be conveyed to the parents as well as the child. The responsible consultant should speak with you or a designated member of the surgical team before seeing the patient, should be familiar with the procedure and underlying disorder of the patient, and should be available to give you rapid and precise feedback. All psychological consultations need to be documented in the record, as would any other consultation; more delicate material can be communicated in a less formal manner, if necessary. There is always a question about the most appropriate way in which a therapeutic intervention can be carried out during the course of hospitalization. In general, it is not possible to carry out a definitive psychological intervention given the time constraints of today's environment, but the establishment of a therapeutic alliance and an intervention to alleviate the acute problem should be possible. The consultant implementing a therapeutic intervention has a responsibility to provide the linkage to a community provider upon discharge, if indicated. The patient, the family, and the surgeon should not be left with this responsibility.

ACUTE COMPLICATIONS

It is inevitable that at some time during the course of a surgical career there will be an intraoperative or post-operative catastrophe resulting in a death, disability, or other serious complication. These situations, while often anticipated in the informed consent, can be devastating to the surgeon, the family, the operative team, and the surviving patient. The worst possible response is to deny the event or to attempt to withdraw from involvement and to seek the protection of the hospital. The best practice is to be immediately forthcoming with the family, to be involved with the family (and patient) in their grief, and to work with the family to either preserve the memory of their child or to optimize the recovery of the patient. This does not mean that one should admit guilt, for often this is not the issue and may not be the case, nor should you try to seek an immediate settlement in an attempt to put the incident past you. It is important to be in touch with the hospital authorities and your insurance carrier, and not to abdicate your physician-patient-family relationship. Parents and patients will interpret withdrawal as a sign of guilt, and involvement as at least a sign of caring and desire for restitution.

There is no need to invoke the involvement of the psychological support services as a first step, but it is helpful to offer grief counseling or coping services as provided by the hospital. You may wish some psychological support for yourself or members of your team, and these should be sought at the earliest possible time. It is not a sign of weakness to avail yourself of some psychological help, but rather can be seen as a way to be supportive to members of your team and an effort for you to return to full functioning as soon as possible. Failure to recognize the psychological toll on yourself can lead to unwarranted negative interactions with others, depression, withdrawal, and other disruptions in your normal life.

POSTSURGERY ISSUES
Meeting Again with the Child and Parents

The role of the surgeon does not end with the operation, and surgeons should recognize the postoperative phase of their relationship with the patient as crucial to a successful outcome. Although meeting with the parents and child following a procedure is not mandatory, it is the best practice. To leave the postoperative visit to nursing or resident staff without a final contact with you does not complete the contract with the parent and child. Because the longer term consequences of any procedure may be uncertain, the ability to meet face to face with parent and child offers the opportunity to discuss the overall experience, review any issues directly, and leave the family with a sense of closure. If there are to be multiple procedures, it is good at this meeting to indicate the longer term course of action to avoid uncertainties that may lead to dissatisfaction. *Remember:* a child does not integrate a changed physical image immediately postoperatively no matter how satisfactory the outcome, and this internalization of changed, positive self-image is likely to occur over a period of months after the surgery. It may be important to reiterate this observation to the patient and family postoperatively.[8]

Dealing with Negative Psychological Reactions

Negative psychological consequences may occur post-operatively. The following comments are meant to put in perspective what may be seen initially as an untoward reaction. In reality such a reaction may consist of expected psychological responses that can be dealt with easily. *Remember:* a surgical procedure is a traumatic event, no matter how good the outcome. The apparent smoothness of the postoperative course in medical terms should not lead you to assume that there may not be a more conflicted psychological outcome.

After an operation both the patient and family will be anxious. Expressions of anxiety are to be expected, and the surgeon's failure to recognize such concerns is perhaps a problem because it represents a lack of engagement. Reassurance is the appropriate response. Any attempt to minimize or negate the anxiety usually will lead to more anxiety or the undesirable consequence of the family seeking information or reassurance from others. The responsible surgeon should be the key person during this postoperative period.

Acute psychological responses during the early postoperative period are rare and often secondary to anesthesia effects, such as may be seen with ketamine. The anesthesiologist should be involved if this is suspected and appropriate treatment provided. Psychiatric consultation should be requested sooner rather than later to assess the child's mental status if there are concerns. Unlike consultation for long-term problems, this can be introduced to the parents as a routine measure.

Offering Ongoing Contact

The surgical event and postoperative period may precipitate psychological problems. The procedure may have failed to meet the patient's or parent's expectations despite a satisfactory anatomic result, or there may be an emergence of conflict in the family or a disruption in school. The surgeon, although not directly responsible for any of these events, can be seen by the parent or child as linked to them. Offering ongoing contact, rather than fleeing from the distress, is probably the best way to manage the situation. There is, of course, a difference between offering ongoing contact and providing a therapeutic intervention in a situation with which a surgeon may have no professional experience. In these cases, the surgeon should make an appropriate referral. In rare instances, the surgical experience is one of the best experiences of caring a patient or parent has had. This may lead to an almost magical dependence on the surgeon for support long after the operation has been performed and the patient is well. Telephone calls, unexpected visits to the clinic, notes, or gifts may be signs of this type of response. Do not be overly flattered by these responses, but try to put the relationship with the patient and parent in a professional perspective. To encourage this type of dependence is to come to regret its long-term consequences when disappointment ensues or complexities emerge.

Use of the Psychological Referral Postoperatively

Some psychological problems cannot be anticipated. If a need for psychological or psychiatric consultation following a surgical procedure arises, it is best that the surgeon stay in control of this postoperative referral process. First, the surgeon can and should know the person to whom the patient is being referred. If not, the danger that the consultant may offer advice at odds with that of the referring surgeon could pose problems. Although the issue is psychological in nature, it is particularly important for the consultant to be familiar with the surgical procedures to be discussed, the time course for the usual recovery, the expected outcomes, and some of the history of the family with the surgeon, institutions, and procedures. The consultant must realize a responsibility to you as the attending referring surgeon and should not communicate solely through the chart. You should be responsible for making the effort to understand the consultation results and incorporate the guidance that you and the consultant deem appropriate.

DIFFICULT SITUATIONS WITH PATIENTS
Separated and Divorced Parents

It is not uncommon to have pediatric patients whose parents are separated or divorced. In some instances, the child has been the source of marital stress leading to the separation and divorce. In other cases, the child's deformity has been the excuse for the parental behaviors leading to the divorce.

Resolving family conflicts is not the job of the surgeon. However, understanding how the conflicts might contribute to behaviors of the child and the parents is important. Parental conflict over the decision to have an operation, disagreements about desired outcomes, negative concerns about the parent who cares for the child (on the part of the other parent), or blaming one parent for passing on the undesirable gene can influence the nature of the discussion about surgery.

It is incumbent upon the surgeon to obtain a clear statement from both parents about the desire and need for the operation and an agreement on the treatment plan. In reality, this will not always be possible. Therefore, it is important to note clearly in the record the legally designated guardian for the child. This is the person who ordinarily has the right to make decisions. Assuming that both the child and the guardian are in agreement about the operation, it is safe to proceed. However, it is best not to get into a situation in which the relationship with one parent precludes discussion with the other parent. Should there be an adverse outcome, the parental conflict can precipitate litigation. It cannot be emphasized enough that the surgeon should be clear about the identity of the legal guardian of the child after the presurgical interviews.

Child with Negative Prior Experience

It is not uncommon for children with complex maxillofacial deformities to have more than one surgical procedure. The surgeon always should make inquiries as to past experiences. In the process, clarify how the currently contemplated procedure will be similar to or different from past procedures. Parents' experiences with surgery and their fears in relation to the experience are often relevant. Be aware that parental fears are transmitted to the child.

"You Can Do What No One Else Has Been Able To Do"

"I heard how great you are, doctor. I am sure you can make my daughter look like all the other children." Beware of heightened expectations. "You can do what no else can do." This is invariably a trap. Work at keeping expectations realistic. If expectations are set too high or if they are totally unrealistic, postoperative psychological and adjustment problems often occur. It is far better for the family and the child to feel that they have achieved a better outcome than they could have hoped for than to be disappointed. The surgeon should not minimize the necessary skills or be too pessimistic about outcome but should not seek to reinforce "God-like" perceptions on the part of the family.

Absent Mother or Father

Experience over many years indicates that a danger signal for psychological complications and dissatisfaction is the absence of one parent from any part of the operative planning or the operation itself. An example is a father who brings the child for evaluation appointments and consistently says that the mother is too busy or burdened to attend. A second common scenario is the father who is a reluctant participant and who does not come to the hospital for the surgery or who is not present at the time the child is brought to the recovery room. These circumstances may reflect symptoms of some element of family dysfunction; in rarer instances, it is evidence of frank family psychopathology. When all goes smoothly, these issues may not surface, but if there are complications, the absence of either parent can greatly complicate decision making, leave the child feeling abandoned, and decrease the capacity for all to cope.

Additional Medical Condition(s) with Life-Threatening Dimensions

Congenital facial abnormalities often are accompanied by less visible physical abnormalities, some of which may be life-threatening. An example is velocardiofacial syndrome with severe cardiac complications. In these cases, it is important to make sure that the nonmaxillofacial aspects of the syndrome are being cared for in a responsible manner. The surgeon should not assume the care of a problem beyond the area of expertise.

It is important to differentiate specifically, for the parents, nonmaxillofacial aspects of the syndrome. If there are nonmaxillofacial complications during the perioperative period, another physician or caregiver might criticize the decision to undertake an "elective" procedure when the child suffered from a co-existing "more serious" and life-threatening problem. The parents may then ask: "Why did the surgeon agree to do that operation, knowing that my child suffered from . . . ?" If there are cardiac, neurologic, urologic, or other known physical ailments, it is incumbent on the surgeon to make sure that appropriate preoperative clearances appear in the medical record and are discussed with the family.

"My Child Is Special"

Sometimes, in an effort to be reassuring or supportive of the young child with a facial deformity, parents will describe their child as "special." This may or not become an internalized perception. This label can have varying meanings but, when internalized, the perception of the parent can quickly and firmly guide parental and child behavior. Unfortunately, this is usually a maladaptive way of supporting the child, particularly in social situations. It is a given that any child is special to his or her parents. However, the world does not view children with facial deformities as special, but rather as different. By labeling the child *special*, the parent does not help the child to develop a set of coping skills. This does not undermine the notion that a focus on the development of skills that may compensate for functional deficits is important. For example, some parents have the child develop skill in drawing when he or she is not articulate because of cleft palate.

The label of *special* becomes particularly difficult when there is an element of cognitive delay. The disconnect between the label and the way the child will be treated creates conflict and often serves to distance both the child and parents from potential helpers and friends. In some circumstances, the internalized "specialness" on the part of the child or adolescent can result in deviant behavior.

Effort To Put the Child at Risk

A most troublesome but, thankfully, rare situation occurs when a parent has adopted a child with a congenital or traumatic injury and then finds that there is a need for corrective surgery (Case Report 3-1). In addition, the parent may desire the corrective surgery to allow the child to enter the mainstream. In some circumstances the desired cosmetic result is truly not worth the operative risk. When there is no predictable functional gain from the proposed operation, and yet the parent strongly desires the child to undergo the operation rather than coming to grips with the child's deformity, one has to consider that the parent has unresolved feelings about the adoption of this "defective" child. In these circumstances, careful assessment may reveal that the parent would just as soon be rid of the child. The surgeon must evaluate the potential risk versus gain from the operation when there may be a very strong request on the part of the parent for potentially life-threatening, nonessential treatment. Acquiescence in this circumstance is counter to the best interests of the child, whose welfare must always be first.

Child with Known Preexisting Psychological Problems

Mental illness or psychological disturbance, such as attention deficit hyperactivity disorder, is not an absolute contraindication to maxillofacial surgical procedures. However, it is important to elicit any history of existing psychological problems. In some special situations, such as patients with TMJ dysfunction and facial pain, it is critical to get a precise history that may be psychologically relevant to the complaint and course.[5] In these children, the frequency of depression as an etiologic factor warrants careful scrutiny. It is most important to

know about the disorder prior to the surgery and to make arrangements for continued active treatment postoperatively. The need for documentation is critical, because some parents will attribute behavioral change to the operation and others will attribute a worsening of a preexisting condition to the operation. The latter may be the case, but it is more difficult to understand without a thorough baseline evaluation. This diagnostic workup may simply involve obtaining available records, contacting a treating clinician, or a referral to a specialist. Transient adjustment reactions may be expected but are usually self-limited or resolved with minimal psychological support, as opposed to the regressions seen with more serious emotional disturbance.

When there is a mental health clinician involved with the patient, it is important to have direct contact with that person. This will help the surgeon to gauge the clinical status of the patient and the ongoing treatment and to secure the services of the provider to cover the patient before, during, and after the surgery if necessary. It is important to inform the mental health provider about the procedure and the type of support that may be required perioperatively. The surgeon can be most helpful in facilitating the psychological preparation of the patient by explaining accurately to the mental health consultant the nature of the procedure and the areas that may need to be addressed.

Child with Developmental Delay

Cognitive delay is associated with several craniomaxillofacial syndromes. In cases of Apert, Crouzon, trisomy, and other syndromes, care must be taken to make an accurate assessment of cognitive function. This assessment is needed to gauge the capacity of the individual to comprehend the procedure, to comply, and to prioritize outcomes. For instance, many patients with limited cognitive ability will focus on functional outcomes such as chewing rather than on improved appearance. Preoperative documentation of cognitive function is also

---

CASE REPORT 3-1

HK, a 5-year-old Asian girl, was brought by her single, older, adoptive mother for correction of a webbed neck without any other associated malformation or apparent cognitive deficit. The child, from the time of adoption, evidenced hyperactivity which resulted in the mother having to appear at school for many appointments. HK's behavior required intervention. At home, HK did not respond to the mother as she would have wished. The surgical evaluation suggested that HK's webbing was not as significant as viewed by the mother and that the likely surgical outcome and intraoperative risk did not warrant

the procedure. When this message was conveyed to the mother, she expressed disappointment and during the following years requested the operation several more times. Consultations with other surgeons resulted in the same recommendation. Psychological evaluation of mother, in the context of the overall evaluation of the child, indicated that she was profoundly disappointed in HK. The child did not provide her with the gratification she sought and significantly limited her lifestyle. The consultant's concern was that the mother deliberately was seeking to put the patient at risk.

important in the assessment and determination of the etiology of any postoperative changes. In many young people an element of psychological regression can be seen postoperatively, that is, more immature behavior but not a loss of cognitive function.

DIFFICULT SITUATIONS WITH COLLEAGUES
Differing Views on the Approach to the Child Heard by the Family

It is enormously helpful, especially in training settings, to have a group discussion of a patient's condition and options for the surgical approach to the problem. Unfortunately, the dialogue in such situations can sometimes wrongfully convey to the patient and family uncertainty about the ultimate approach, or cast unintended negative aspersions on the operating surgeon's acumen. These latter outcomes are to be avoided. If the setting where patients are reviewed has too little organization and too great a propensity to stimulate discussions that a lay person might not understand, then the surgeon should consider having the broader discussion in some type of office case review or rounds and keep the more public meeting limited to an opportunity to view the patient.

The Team

It is common to have a "maxillofacial team," and that is generally considered a strength.[12] The team can offer support to the surgeon, the patient, and the family. However, it must be remembered that a team needs an identifiable leader and the leader must orchestrate the team function and procedures. It is not sufficient to identify to a parent "the team" and then leave the parent and patient to figure out what may be a complex set of interrelationships. This complexity can lead to confusion and dysfunction that contributes to an unsatisfactory result, even when the surgical outcome, itself, is quite satisfactory. It is helpful to have some written document explaining the role of the team and its members. *Remember:* there is no collective responsibility for an operation. The surgeon is always the responsible person.

Coverage

You can expect that patients and families will want or need you at the most inopportune times. It is essential to arrange for knowledgeable and available coverage. "I could not get hold of the doctor" is a prelude to many negative outcomes and greatly increases the surgeon's liability. It is important to know who is covering for you and inform them of what they can expect in relation to particular patients. It is very disconcerting to parents to hear from the covering physician that they know nothing

about a procedure or that if they had done the operation they would have done it differently. Therefore, know and inform your covering surgeon or resident, and make sure that person will be an ally.

House Officer Versus Staff

"Who is going to do my child's operation?" The answer must be truthful. There is no reason to assume that operative records will be privileged communication. Informed in the proper way, most families will understand the role of the attending surgeon and the participation of trainees. If they do not, then the surgeon must consider what approach will be taken in performing the operation. It is not sufficient to say that the institution is a training institution.

Hospital Billing Versus Professional Billing

The surgical outcome may have been just what was expected, but the parents may complain bitterly that the experience was bad. Often this feeling comes from confusion over billing, repeat billing, or inaccurate billing. This scenario is increasingly frequent because of the complex relationships between surgeons and hospitals, hospitals and third party payers, and surgeons and third party payers. The degree to which this confusion can lead to permanent dissatisfaction and litigation cannot be underestimated. When the outcome is less satisfactory than the family expected, receiving a bill perceived to be unjust will only fuel litigious responses. The surgeon should recognize this as an important issue, and the support office staff should be trained to help patients and their families with these conflicts. Otherwise, the family will feels abandoned and this issue will fuel considerable discontent.

UNFAVORABLE OUTCOME

The term *unfavorable outcome* is used by Goldwyn[13,14] to describe a myriad of outcomes viewed by the patient, family, and surgeon as unfavorable. The term and its implication are considered in the chapter on preparation, because to some extent, short of surgical error, a great deal of the grief associated with unfavorable outcomes can be anticipated and dealt with during the preparation of the patient for surgery.[15] When there is adequate preparation that anticipates a possible unfavorable outcome, then the surgeon is in a better position to work with the patient and family to ameliorate disappointment, anger, and litigation.

When the family presents the concern that the outcome is not what they wanted or expected, it does no good to be defensive. It is important to listen to the family. In this process, the surgeon should hear from all involved members of the family: father, mother, child, siblings, and any other accompanying party. It may become clear that the patient is satisfied but a parent is not, or vice versa. The surgeon should help the family understand if the result that is considered "unfavorable" is likely to change or improve over time, if there has been some miscommunication, or if after surgery the family has modified its expectations. The latter instance illustrates the importance of documentation and discussion of expectations during the preoperative phase.

How should the surgeon respond when the result is objectively as good or better than one could have expected but the patient or family remains unhappy? It is important to ascertain, as noted above, who is disappointed. However, in this case a more sophisticated psychological assessment is required. If it is the patient who remains unhappy in the case of a good anatomic result, then some other psychological issues should be considered. For instance, rarely there may be a persistent somatic delusion. This may not have been as evident when there was an objective deformity but becomes all too clear when surgery has improved the individual's physical appearance. In other instances, the dissatisfaction comes not from anyone in the room but emanates from comments made by others. In this case, it is important to try to help the family to put these comments in context.

What happens when there has been an intraoperative mistake? First, one needs to document carefully and precisely what happened and the circumstances. There is no such thing as medical record confidentiality today. It is best, at the earliest possible moment and preferably prior to the error being discovered by the parents or patient, for you to consult the legal department of your facility and then meet with the parents or guardian and patient under circumstances dictated by the legal staff. Be direct, do not blame anyone other than yourself (if this is the case), indicate what the longer term consequences may be, suggest corrective action if possible, and offer your apology. By all means do not try to avoid interaction with the family, but interact in accord with the policies of your institution. Parents and the patient will feel supported if you demonstrate your concern and forthrightness.

CONCLUSION

The vast majority of maxillofacial operations go forward in a most benign way with excellent patient and family satisfaction. Over the years, preoperative preparation for children and families has become the standard. In this chapter we reviewed issues and techniques that will be of use, either as a reminder or for enhancing one's approaches.

REFERENCES

1. Campis LK, Pillemer FG, DeMaso DR: Psychological consideration in the pediatric surgical patient. In Kaban LB, editor: *Pediatric oral and maxillofacial surgery*, Philadelphia, 1990, WB Saunders.
2. Goin JM, Goin MK: *Changing the body: psychological effects of plastic surgery*, Baltimore, 1981, Williams & Wilkins.
3. DiLeo JH: *Children's drawings as diagnostic aids*, New York, 1973, Brunner/Mazel.
4. Macgregor FC: *After plastic surgery: adaptation and adjustment*, New York, 1979, Praeger.
5. Belfer ML, Kaban LB: Temporomandibular joint dysfunction with facial pain in children, *Pediatrics* 69:564-567, 1982.
6. Ernst M, Boojus BA, Moravec BC: Pictorial instrument for children and adolescents (PICA-III-R), *J Am Acad Child Adolesc Psychiatry* 39:94-99, 2000.
7. Campis LK, DeMaso DR, Twente AW: The role of maternal factors in the adaptation of children with craniofacial disfigurement, *Cleft Palate Craniofac J* 32:55-61, 1995.
8. Belfer ML, Harrison AM, Murray JE: Body image and the process of reconstructive surgery, *Am J Dis Child* 133:532-535, 1979.
9. Meng AL: Parents' and children's reactions toward impending hospitalization for surgery, *Matern Child Nurs J* 9:83-98, 1980.
10. Elkins PO, Roberts MC: Psychological preparation for pediatric hospitalization, *Clin Psychol Rev* 3:275-295, 1983.
11. O'Connor-Von S: Preparing children for surgery—an integrative research review, *AORN J* 71:334-343, 2000.
12. Murray JE, Mulliken JB, Kaban LB, Belfer M: Twenty year experience in maxillocraniofacial surgery, *Ann Surg* 190:320-331, 1979.
13. Goldwyn RM, editor: *The unfavorable result in plastic surgery*, Boston, 1984, Little, Brown.
14. Whitaker LA: Problems and complications in craniofacial surgery. In Goldwyn RM, editor: *The unfavorable result in plastic surgery*, Boston, 1984, Little, Brown.
15. Padwa BL, Evans CA, Pillemer FC: Psychosocial adjustment in children with hemifacial microsomia and other craniofacial deformities, *Cleft Palate Craniofac J* 28:354-359, 1991.

Practical Considerations in Facial Growth

Karin Vargervik

Any operation for a pediatric patient, whether it is emergency treatment for trauma, reconstruction after tumor resection, or correction of a birth defect, may have adverse effects on growth. Therefore, knowledge about wound healing and normal growth patterns and the timing of slow and accelerated growth periods should be a pre-requisite for anyone planning or executing surgical procedures in children. This guides the clinician to design and carry out interventions with the least potential for adverse consequences on facial growth.

GENERAL OBSERVATIONS ON GROWTH DATA

Most studies on growth of craniofacial structures are based on longitudinal cephalometric radiographs. Many cross-sectional studies have also been conducted. Measurements are linear or angular and changes are assessed in time intervals. They may be recorded and displayed as velocity curves, changes in given time intervals, or as distance curves, actual measurements at given ages. Cephalometric x-ray units produce a film with an average of 9% magnification. Errors may result from: (1) inaccuracies in head position, (2) variations in landmark location, and (3) inaccuracies in measuring lines and angles. This third source of errors has been reduced significantly by current digitizing technology. The sum of errors should be within 1 mm for linear and 1 degree for angular measurements in order to yield reliable growth information.

During childhood, most craniofacial structures grow at a slow rate, often within the measurement error during 1-year intervals. The exceptions are vertical changes of the alveolar processes and length increases of the mandible where readily measurable changes take place, even during short intervals.

DIMENSIONAL AND PROPORTIONAL GROWTH CHANGES IN THE CRANIOFACIAL SKELETON

Cranium and the Cranial Base

The size of the cranium is determined by growth of the brain. The length and width of the cranium have reached 60% to 65% of adult size at birth and this is also the case for orbital size. The optic nerve and eye are extensions of the brain and follow brain growth rather than growth of the facial skeleton. The internal volume of the skull reaches its full size by age 4 to 5 years. The external dimensions increase as the skull bones thicken and muscle attachment areas develop.

The cranial base has reached 55% of total length at birth and continues to grow, particularly at the sphenoccipital synchondrosis, which remains open until skeletal maturity is achieved. Growth in width of the cranial base occurs at sutures and is determined by the shape of the growing brain. A distinction usually is made between a narrow, elongated, dolichocephalic head shape with a cephalic index (maximum breath of the skull divided by its length and multiplied by 100) of 75 or less, and a broad, brachycephalic skull with a cephalic index of 80 or greater. The flexion and length of the cranial base are determinants for the relative vertical and horizontal positions of the maxilla and mandible.[1] The width of the anterior cranial fossa is also one of the determinants for the width of the nose and the palate.

Upper face width usually is measured as the bizygomatic distance. It is, on average, 60% of adult size at birth and increases by 31%, or 32 mm, from age 2 to early adulthood in males and by 26%, or 27 mm, in females.[2] There is great variation among individuals in actual measurements.

Maxilla

The maxilla occupies the space between the zygomatic bones laterally, the nasal structures medially, and the orbits superiorly. During growth, sutures divide the frontal bone, nose, and maxilla in the midline, allowing increase in width. This occurs along with the more dramatic increase in vertical development that takes place in the face. It is interesting to note that the position of the zygomas is not dependent upon the maxilla. For example, in circumstances in which the maxilla has been resected as treatment for a tumor, the zygomatic bones do not exhibit any growth abnormality. Similarly, when the lateral segments of the maxilla have collapsed medially, as a consequence of a cleft condition, the adjustments occur on the maxillary side of the zygomaticomaxillary suture.[3]

Posture of the mandible and tongue are also factors that play important roles in maxillary development, in the sagittal, transverse, and vertical planes. If the tongue is not resting in the palate, as it normally should, the typical adaptation is a narrow maxilla with increased vertical height and sagittal length. This results in clockwise (backward) rotation of the mandible with a class II malocclusion, often with an anterior open bite, proclined maxillary incisors, and retroclined mandibular incisors.[4]

The depth of the face, which also indicates the sagittal position of the maxilla, can be measured from the anterior nasal spine to the most anterior point on the condyles. The average dimension in whites is 80 mm at age 4 years. This dimension increases on an average of 1.25 mm per year during growth. Face height can be measured as the distance from nasion to gnathion, demonstrating an average increase of 1.7 mm per year during the growth period. The facial profile commonly is described by the angle of convexity, measuring the relative prominence of the forehead, the midface, and the chin (Figure 4-1). This angle increases an average of 1 degree per year, mostly as a consequence of mandibular growth and chin projection.[5]

According to data from the Burlington Growth Study, the maxillary unit length, as measured from condylion to the anterior nasal spine, grows an average of 1.5 mm per year, slightly less in females than in males[4,5] (Tables 4-1 and 4-2).

Mandible

Based on animal experiments and clinical studies, it is now generally assumed that the mandible is carried forward during growth by its suspension system of muscles and ligaments. Condylar growth occurs as an adaptation rather than as a driving force. Nevertheless, some endocrine effect on mandibular growth must be assumed, because the length increase of the mandible

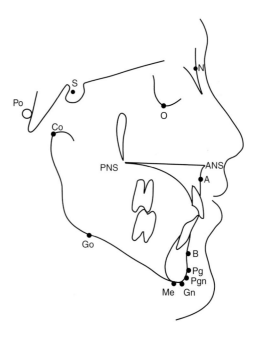

Figure 4-1

Tracing of lateral head film with commonly used landmarks and the angle of convexity between Pg-ANS and ANS-N. (Redrawn from Ousterhout DK, editor: *Aesthetic contouring of the craniofacial skeleton*, New York, 1991, Little, Brown.)

TABLE 4-1 Growth Changes in a Random Group of Boys Observed on Standard Cephalometric Profile X-Rays (Magnification 9%)

| Age (yr) | No. | LENGTH (mm) | | | Standard Deviation |
		Minimum	Mean Value	Maximum	
Temporomandibular Point (TM)* – Anterior Nasal Spine (ANS)†				**(1a)**	
6	118	76	82	90	3.19
9	102	80	87	97	3.43
12	96	85	92	101	3.73
14	66	88	96	108	4.52
16	72	93	100	111	4.17

| Age (yr) | No. | LENGTH (mm) | | | Standard Deviation |
		Minimum	Mean Value	Maximum	
Temporomandibular Point (TM) – Prognathion (pgn)			**(2a)**		
6	118	90	99	108	3.85
9	102	98	107	117	4.40
12	96	102	114	127	4.90
14	66	107	121	137	6.05
16	72	116	127	139	5.25

| Age (yr) | No. | LENGTH (mm) | | | Standard Deviation |
		Minimum	Mean Value	Maximum	
The Lower Face Height: Anterior Nasal Spine (ANS) – Gnathion (gn)				**(3a)**	
6	118	52	59	72	3.55
9	102	53	62	74	4.25
12	96	53	64	76	4.62
14	66	56	68	82	5.23
16	72	57	71	86	5.73

| Age (yr) | No. | LENGTH (mm) | | | Standard Deviation |
		Minimum	Mean Value	Maximum	
Difference between (TM – PGN) and (TM – ANS)			**(2a – 1a)**		
6	118	10	17	27	
9	102	13	20	28	
12	96	12	22	30	
14	66	14	25	38	
16	72	17	27	39	

*Temporomandibular point: A point in the articular fossa on the line from prognathion through the condyle that indicates the maximum length of the mandible.
†Anterior nasal spine: A point on the lower curvature of the spine where the vertical thickness is 3 mm.

TABLE 4-2   Growth Changes in a Random Group of Girls Observed on Standard Cephalometric Profile X-Rays (Magnification 9%)

Age (yr)	No.	LENGTH (mm) Minimum	LENGTH (mm) Mean Value	LENGTH (mm) Maximum	Standard Deviation
Temporomandibular Point (TM)* – Anterior Nasal Spine (ANS)† (1b)					
6	88	73	80	89	2.96
9	79	78	85	93	3.43
12	71	80	90	102	4.07
14	49	81	92	104	3.69
16	53	86	93	105	3.45

Age (yr)	No.	LENGTH (mm) Minimum	LENGTH (mm) Mean Value	LENGTH (mm) Maximum	Standard Deviation
Temporomandibular Point (TM) – Prognathion (pgn) (2b)					
6	88	88	97	105	3.55
9	79	94	105	113	3.88
12	71	102	113	124	5.20
14	49	104	117	128	4.60
16	53	109	119	128	4.44

Age (yr)	No.	LENGTH (mm) Minimum	LENGTH (mm) Mean Value	LENGTH (mm) Maximum	Standard Deviation
The Lower Face Height: Anterior Nasal Spine (ANS) – Gnathion (gn) (3b)					
6	88	49	57	65	3.22
9	79	50	60	70	3.62
12	71	53	62	74	4.36
14	49	54	64	72	4.39
16	53	55	65	74	4.67

Age (yr)	No.	LENGTH (mm) Minimum	LENGTH (mm) Mean Value	LENGTH (mm) Maximum	Standard Deviation
Difference between (TM – PGN) and (TM – ANS) (2b – 1b)					
6	88	10	17	24	
9	79	13	20	28	
12	71	16	23	36	
14	49	18	26	39	
16	53	19	26	39	

*Temporomandibular point: A point in the articular fossa on the line from prognathion through the condyle that indicates the maximum length of the mandible.
†Anterior nasal spine: A point on the lower curvature of the spine where the vertical thickness is 3 mm.

so closely follows the length increase of long bones, presumed to be hormonally controlled. It has been observed also that, although growth of the mandible can occur in the absence of a condyle, the growth is usually less than normal. A crucial element in mandibular growth is the lateral pterygoid muscle. If this muscle is missing, mandibular length will be impacted severely as is seen in individuals with hemifacial microsomia (HFM). Restriction of movement, such as can be seen in ankylosis following trauma, will also result in severe growth impairment.

The normal mandible is often the very last bony structure to stop growing. According to data from the Burlington Growth Study, mandibular length measured from condylion to prognathian increases by an average of 2.5 mm per year, slightly less for females than for males. The advancement of the chin that this growth produces is determined by the vertical development of the face which, in turn, is determined by the dentoalveolar development in both jaws[4,5] (see Tables 4-1 and 4-2).

Spatial Relationships Between the Jaws

Many cephalometric analyses have been developed since Broadbent published his first work on the cephalostat and the value of oriented head films in assessing growth and planning treatment for malocclusions in 1931.[6] There are many different measurement techniques for head film analysis, which indicates that no single one has been accepted as superior to the others. One reason for the many approaches is that different analyses have been developed for different purposes. Several of the most frequently used analyses are available as software packages for personal computers (Downs, Steiner, Ricketts, Bjork, McNamara).[7-9] Most analyses use similar landmarks, planes, angles, and reference lines. Databanks have been developed for normative data that can be accessed and used as controls for various study samples. The largest and most commonly used databanks are the Bolton Standards, the Michigan Standards, and the Burlington Orthodontic Research Centre Standards.

Most analyses and software programs have been developed for the lateral cephalogram. When asymmetries are present, other views, such as posteroanterior, right and left oblique, and submental vertex, are needed. Three-dimensional computed tomographic data are also helpful for complex deformities.

In the following paragraphs, some easy-to-use methods for assessing position, size, and relationship of the maxilla and mandible are presented. Commonly used landmarks are shown in Figure 4-1, lines and planes in Figure 4-2.[10]

Methods of relating the maxillary–mandibular complex to the forehead represented by nasion are shown in Figures 4-3 and 4-4. Harvold developed a simple but

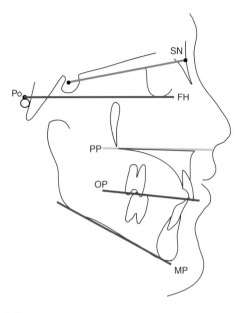

Figure 4-2

Tracing of lateral head film with commonly used reference lines and planes. *SN*, Sella nasion line; *FH*, Frankfort horizontal; *PP*, palatal plane; *OP*, occlusal plane; *MP*, mandibular plane. (Redrawn from Ousterhout DK, editor: *Aesthetic contouring of the cranio-facial skeleton*, New York, 1991, Little, Brown.)

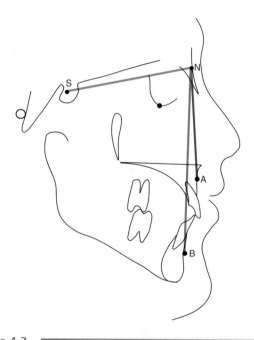

Figure 4-3

The angles SNA and SNB are used to assess the relative prominence of the upper and lower anterior alveolar processes to the forehead and to each other. (Redrawn from Ousterhout DK, editor: *Aesthetic contouring of the cranio-facial skeleton*, New York, 1991, Little, Brown.)

practical method to relate the maxilla and mandible to each other, taking into account both the sagittal and vertical relationships. The Harvold triangle is presented in Figure 4-5. The length and height dimensions of this triangle are projected on the midsagittal plane. The center is at condylion, with one radiant extending to the anterior nasal spine and the other to prognathian. These two distances, as well as the distance between the anterior nasal spine and menton, are measured in millimeters and commonly are referred to as *maxillary* and *mandibular unit lengths* and *anterior face height*, respectively. For this triangle the point on the lower contour of the anterior nasal spine, where the thickness of the spine is 3 mm, is used for the horizontal measurement. The corresponding point on the superior surface is used for the vertical measurement. The measured maxillary and mandibular unit lengths and lower face height are used to relate the jaws to each other and to compare with data from a random sample of serial radiographs of male and female subjects from the Burlington Orthodontic Research Centre (see Tables 4-1 and 4-2). This databank was obtained by taking standard cephalometric lateral head films of a random group of boys and girls at ages 6, 9, 12, 14, and 16.

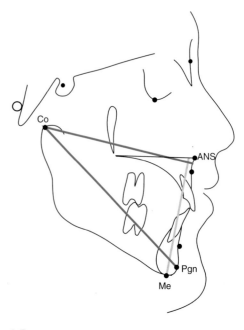

Figure 4-5

The Harvold triangle relates the two jaws to each other both in the sagittal and vertical planes. (Redrawn from Ousterhout DK, editor: *Aesthetic contouring of the craniofacial skeleton*, New York, 1991, Little, Brown.)

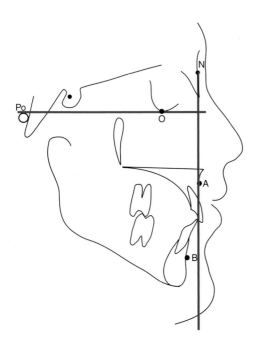

Figure 4-4

The position of the lower face relative to the upper skeleton can also be measured by the distance of point *A* and point *B* from a perpendicular to the Frankfurt horizontal, drawn through nasion. (Redrawn from Ousterhout DK, editor: *Aesthetic contouring of the craniofacial skeleton*, New York, 1991, Little, Brown.)

The unit length difference between the jaws is a significant indicator of how the jaws are matched in size. Difference toward either end of the sample range show unfavorable matching and may indicate a need for jaw surgery in order to achieve good occlusion and well-balanced facial proportions. The vertical dimension must be taken into account, as well. Dentoalveolar compensations may mask skeletal disproportions and must be considered in treatment planning.

With regard to growth changes and predicting the effects of growth after surgical interventions, it is important to keep in mind that the two jaws grow forward at different rates. The mandibular unit length increases a yearly average of 1 mm more than the maxilla. At the same time, the lower anterior face height increases by 1 mm per year on an average. The eruption path of the teeth in the maxilla is as much forward as it is downward, at about 55 degrees to a line drawn from condylion to the anterior nasal spine (Figure 4-6). The mandibular teeth erupt at about right angles to the lower border of the mandible (Figure 4-7). This means that influencing vertical development also influences sagittal relationships among the upper and lower jaws and teeth (Figure 4-8). Tongue size and posture, mandibular posture, thumb and finger sucking, and other habits all influence the shape and relationship of the dental arches.

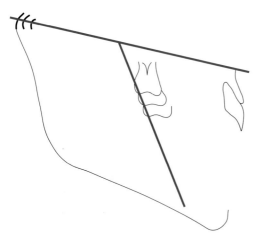

Figure 4-6
The path of eruption of maxillary molars relative to a line drawn from condylion to the anterior nasal spine, approximately 55 degrees.

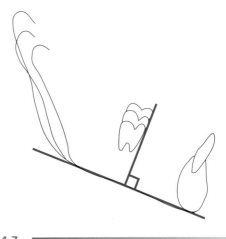

Figure 4-7
The path of eruption of mandibular molars relative to the mandibular plane, approximately 90 degrees.

General Rules for Timing of Surgical Procedures of the Jaws

Mandibular deficiencies: can be approached early if needed.

Mandibular excess: intervention should be postponed until end of growth.

Maxillary deficiency: intervention should be postponed until end of mandibular growth.

Maxillary excess: impaction can be done after eruption of permanent teeth, at 12 to 14 years, if indicated.

GROWTH CONSIDERATIONS IN MANAGEMENT OF MANDIBULAR MALFORMATIONS

Hemifacial Microsomia

HFM is the second most common congenital cranio-facial anomaly after cleft lip and palate. The most frequently quoted incidence estimate is 1 in 5,600 live births.[11] Often referred to as *oculo-auriculo-vertebral* spectrum, this birth defect represents very heterogeneous phenotypes. In the mildest form the only clinical manifestation may be ear tags, with or without malformed ears. The most severe cases may have malformed ears, temporal bone involvement including missing glenoid fossa, missing both condylar and coronoid processes, rudimentary muscles, and facial nerve involvement. Descriptions, management protocols, and outcomes have been described in several publications.[12-14]

In this condition, the very structures that are necessary for normal mandibular growth are affected and growth impairment is always present, but varying in degree according to primary tissue deficiencies. Typically, both the bony elements and the soft tissues develop less on the affected side, resulting in facial asymmetry with midline deviations and canting of the nasal floor and of the occlusal and mandibular planes (Figure 4-9, *A*).

Surgical intervention usually is indicated when the facial asymmetry is outside of normal variation (Figure 4-9, *B*). Two important questions must be answered

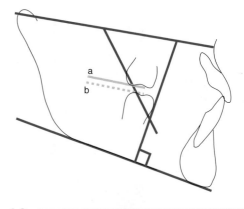

Figure 4-8
The relative vertical position of the upper and lower molars will determine their sagittal relationship. At level *a*, the molar relationship will be class I; at level *b*, class II. Treatment intervention during growth with headgear or functional appliance can change a class l molar relationship to class II by holding back maxillary vertical development.

before proceeding with any surgical procedure. When, relative to growth, is surgical reconstruction most beneficial for the patient's final outcome and what type of procedure will give the best long-term result?

In a treatment outcome study on 25 individuals with HFM, it was found that in 15 of them in which the surgical correction was done after completion of growth, the symmetry that was obtained remained stable because there was no growth recorded on either side of the mandible. In the 10 individuals in whom the surgical correction was done while they were still growing, the contralateral side continued to grow at what seemed to be a normal rate, while the surgically lengthened side increased in most of them, but less than the contralateral side and not at all in 3 of the 10. Three of these individuals required a second surgical procedure. In examining the records, it was found that those who had growth on the reconstructed side had been cooperating with functional appliance wear as instructed.[15]

Use of costochondral grafts, in patients with absence of the ramus-condyle unit, has been reported.[12,16] The preferred method to lengthen the mandible in less severe forms of HFM is distraction. Some remnant of the mandibular ramus must be present for this technique to be used. If the proximal extension does not have a condyle with cartilage, it is likely that the top of this structure will remodel and shorten as it is pushed against the temporal bone during the distraction phase. This must be taken into account when the amount of needed distraction is calculated. It is not likely that growth expectations after mandibular lengthening by distraction would be different from what we have learned to expect from previous techniques.[17]

Timing of Surgical Procedures. If adequate growth in length of a reconstructed mandibular ramus could be expected to occur routinely, early reconstruction would be preferable. This would provide for the best environment for soft tissue development and growth of the maxilla on the affected side and would be beneficial for the overall development of the child. If early reconstruction frequently results in recurrence of asymmetry and a second lengthening procedure, the benefits and disadvantages of this approach must be evaluated carefully and discussed with the patient and parents. At this time it is not possible to predict with reasonable certainty that a reconstructed mandibular ramus will keep up with the growth of the other side.[18] Because of congenital absence of factors that contribute to mandibular growth, compliance with appliance wear during the remaining growth period is essential. Soft tissue procedures, such as augmentations, should not be done until the skeletal framework has been corrected, usually at the end of the growth period.

Mandibulofacial Dysostosis and Nager's Syndrome

In addition to being bilateral, these syndromes often are associated with severe restrictions in jaw movements. In general, the structural abnormalities and disproportions seen at birth or early infancy tend to become more marked during growth. Midline structures such as the

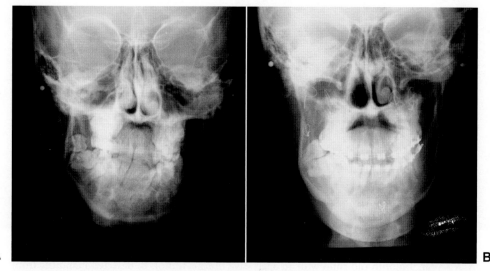

Figure 4-9

A, Posteroanterior radiograph of child with hemifacial microsomia, demonstrating canting of nasal, occlusal, and mandibular planes and deviation of both maxillary and mandibular structures to the right of the face midline. **B,** After orthodontic dental arch coordination, surgical repositioning of both maxilla and mandible, including an asymmetric genioplasty, was done.

nose and maxilla continue to grow forward, while the lateral facial structures, primarily the zygomatic arch, remain hypoplastic or missing. The mandible remains abnormal in shape, with restriction in growth corresponding to the degree of joint abnormality and restrictions in mobility. In cases of severe restrictions, no growth of the mandible will occur and intervention should take place as early as possible. Several procedures are most often necessary, and spontaneous growth in length of the mandible is not expected. If jaw movements are not restricted, the same considerations apply as have been detailed for HFM.[13]

Timing of Surgical Procedures. The first priority for surgical intervention in which mandibular movements are severely restricted is mobilization of the mandible. This may have to be done in infancy and may require more than one procedure. Later reconstructive procedures should be guided by the same principles described for HFM.

After Trauma or Tumor Resection

Timing of Surgical Procedures. Reconstruction of the mandible in a normal neuromuscular system is very likely to result in near-normal morphology and in subsequent normal growth (Figure 4-10). The necessary surgical reconstructive procedures generally are done either immediately following trauma or resections or as soon after initial healing as possible.

GROWTH CONSIDERATIONS IN MANAGEMENT OF MIDFACE MALFORMATIONS
Cleft Lip and Palate

Surgical restoration of soft tissue continuity of the lip and palate results in approximation of the maxillary segments regardless of surgical technique. The degree of maxillary width reduction depends on several factors, including surgical technique, the surgeon's skill, scar

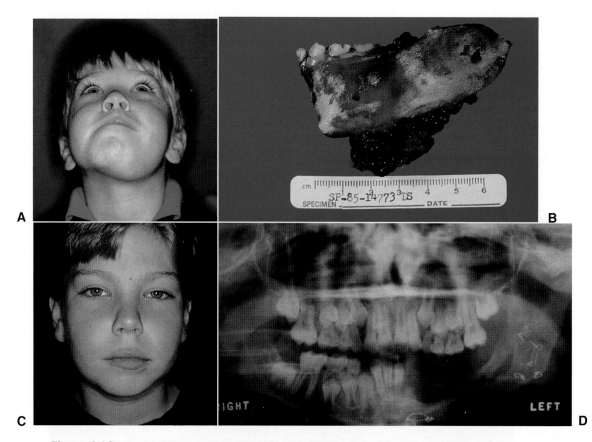

Figure 4-10

A, A 3-year, 9-month-old child with an aggressive fibrous tumor. **B,** Resected mandible from lateral incisor anteriorly to the ascending ramus posteriorly. The mandible was reconstructed using costochondral grafts. **C,** Same child 5½ years later with excellent facial symmetry. **D,** The reconstructed mandibular ramus 5 years after tumor removal and reconstruction. The reconstructed side has kept up with the growth of the contralateral side. (Courtesy Dr. L.B. Kaban.)

formation, degree of tissue deficiency, and timing of procedures. Different treatment scenarios have been devised to manipulate the position of the maxillary segments preoperatively and to control their position postoperatively. Data are not yet available to demonstrate definitively the efficacy or usefulness of such treatment.

When continuity of the lip has been restored, the pressure from the lip will mold the alveolar process and the anterior teeth will be retroclined as they erupt. An anterior crossbite and crossbite of the cuspid on the cleft side in unilateral clefts are common findings. The permanent incisors will often erupt into crossbite, as well. The position of the anterior nasal spine is usually normal in the 6-year-old or 7-year-old child[19] (Figure 4-11).

Leaving the alveolar defect unrepaired allows easy expansion of the maxilla to regain full width before alveolar bone grafting is done, usually at some time between 8 and 10 years of age. Whether alveolar bone grafting interferes with growth is still being debated, but even if it does not, it is an advantage to be able to readily expand the maxilla by moving the segments apart, which is possible only before bony continuity has been established. Expansion of the maxilla and normalization of tongue position in the palate are important prerequisites for subsequent normal growth during the preadolescent and adolescent growth periods.

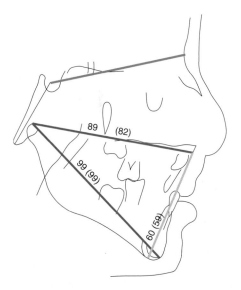

Figure 4-11
Tracing of a 5-year-old child with repaired cleft lip and palate. The position of the midface and anterior nasal spine is normal, but the incisors are retroclined, as is usually seen in repaired clefts before orthodontic treatment has started. This is orthodontically correctable.

Assessing relative jaw relationship in both sagittal and vertical dimensions is easily done by using the Harvold triangle described earlier. If jaw size proportions are outside of normal range, jaw surgery becomes necessary (Figure 4-12, *A*). Usually it is the maxilla that is underdeveloped and must be advanced (Figure 4-12, *B*). If the mandible is large, two-jaw surgery may be indicated but should not be done until growth is completed.

Timing of Surgical Procedures. The cleft palate team with which the individual surgeon works generally will have a standard protocol for timing of surgical repair of the lip, palate, and alveolus by bone grafting and for final surgical revisions of the lip and nose. If orthognathic surgery is needed, this is done after orthodontic preparation and usually after completion of growth.[20]

Trauma to the Midface

Trauma to the midface, particularly damage to the nose and ethmoid plate, may result in reduced forward and downward growth of the midface.[21] Timing and type of surgical intervention will depend on age at injury and the severity of growth inhibition (Figure 4-13).

Timing of Surgical Procedures. The most reliable and consistent treatment outcome is achieved when the surgical reconstruction is done after orthodontic preparation and at completion of growth.

Maxillary Vertical Excess

Excessive downward and forward development of the maxilla is seen often in class II malocclusions. This may be the result of low posture of the mandible and tongue caused by airway obstruction. Because the etiologic factors usually have disappeared by the time the youngster comes for treatment, surgical corrections are expected to be stable when combined with appropriate orthodontic management.

Timing of Surgical Procedures. Surgical impaction can be done after eruption of the permanent teeth before growth is completed, if the causative functional problems have been alleviated.

Craniosynostosis Syndromes

One of the characteristic findings in craniosynostosis syndromes is an underdeveloped and retropositioned maxilla (Figure 4-14, *A*). This causes difficulties in infancy for breathing, feeding, eustachian tube function, and later for mastication, as well. Visual acuity and corneal injury may also be problems. In addition to the functional impairments, the strikingly dysmorphic appearance may also have detrimental psychological effects.

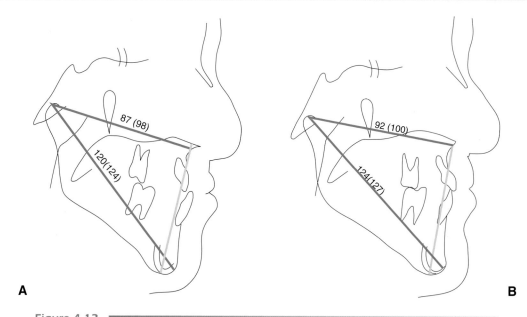

A

B

Figure 4-12
A, Tracing of a 15-year-old boy with repaired cleft lip and palate who had a retruded and hypoplastic maxilla. **B,** At age 19, after orthodontic treatment and maxillary advancement surgery, the maxilla is still retruded, but the occlusion is class I.

Surgical interventions to release prematurely closed cranial sutures and normalize skull shape are done routinely during the first months of life. The fused sutures that inhibit downward and forward development of the facial structures are not easily accessible and, even if approached, their surgical release would not result in correction, because there is no force for expansion and bone growth equivalent to that of the growing brain.

The desire to improve both essential functions and esthetics have moved craniofacial teams to attempt midface correction at earlier and earlier ages, even as early as infancy. It generally is recognized that the post-surgical position of the midface will remain stable, but subsequent growth at osteotomy sites or "sutures" will not take place, thus leaving these midface structures behind as the rest of the face, particularly the mandible, continues to grow. The midface again becomes deficient and in need of further surgical advancement procedures.

If functional impairments such as severe airway problems do not necessitate very early advancement, the ideal timing for a Le Fort III type midface advancement would be at an age when the upper portion, such as the infraorbital region, has reached its adult position, thus avoiding a second procedure in that area. The maxilla would then be advanced later, after orthodontic preparation and after most of mandibular growth has taken place.

We conducted a study on longitudinal growth changes in the infraorbital region, at orbitale on a control group of nonaffected children, and found little change in the position of the infraorbital rim after 8 years of age.[22] This area grows primarily with the expansion of the optic nerve and the eye, which follow the growth pattern of the brain more closely than that of the facial skeleton. A study of the position of orbitale and changes in position of this cephalometric landmark was also done on individuals with craniosynostosis syndrome.[23] The results showed that the infraorbital area was very retruded in these individuals compared with the controls and that also in this group there was minimal growth change from 8.5 to 11.5 yeas of age. As a result of these studies, our preferred age for the Le Fort III advancement, whether done by distraction or the conventional immediate advancement, is now between 8 and 10 years. The corrected position of the midface is expected to remain stable, without growth, but also without relapse[24,25] (Figure 4-14, *B*).

Timing of Surgical Procedures. If the midface advancement is done during early childhood, before 7 to 8 years of age, the expectation must be that a second Le Fort III procedure will become necessary.

If, however, the advancement is done after age 8 or 9, it is expected that the infraorbital area will be in an acceptable position for the adult face, and the lower maxilla can be advanced by a Le Fort I procedure after orthodontic treatment, toward the end of the growth period.

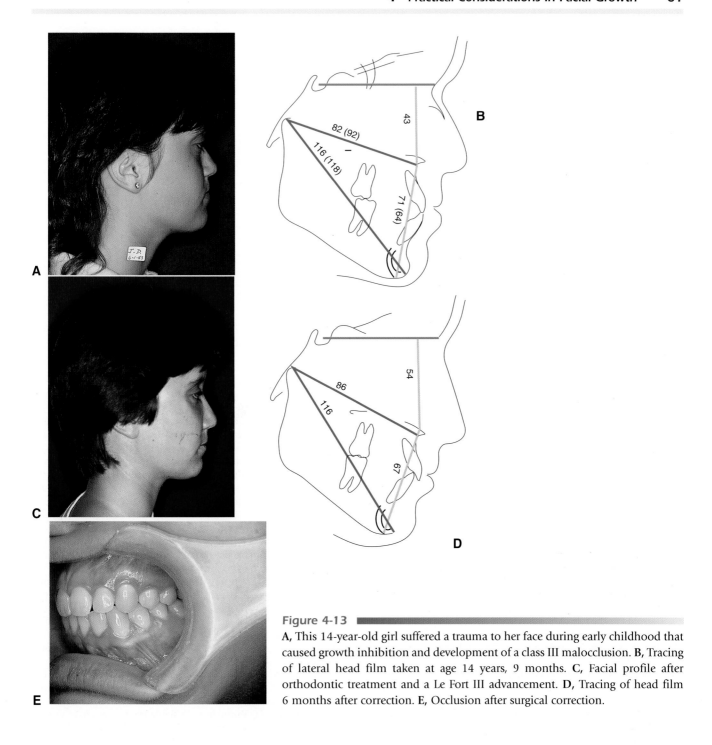

Figure 4-13

A, This 14-year-old girl suffered a trauma to her face during early childhood that caused growth inhibition and development of a class III malocclusion. **B,** Tracing of lateral head film taken at age 14 years, 9 months. **C,** Facial profile after orthodontic treatment and a Le Fort III advancement. **D,** Tracing of head film 6 months after correction. **E,** Occlusion after surgical correction.

It is important to recognize that a second midface advancement is not only a psychological burden but is also a much more difficult surgical undertaking than the first one, regardless of age.

CONCLUSION

In this chapter we have reviewed the dimensional and proportional growth changes that occur in the craniofacial skeleton with time. Any clinician who treats craniomax-

illofacial deformities in growing children must understand these principles and changes in order to develop a rational treatment plan. Mandibular deficiencies and vertical maxillary excess may be corrected prior to the completion of growth. Under certain circumstances, patients with HFM, Treacher Collins syndrome, and posttraumatic defects will also benefit from early correction. Treatment of mandibular excess conditions, maxillary deficiency, and midface deficiency associated with craniosynostosis is most stable when carried out

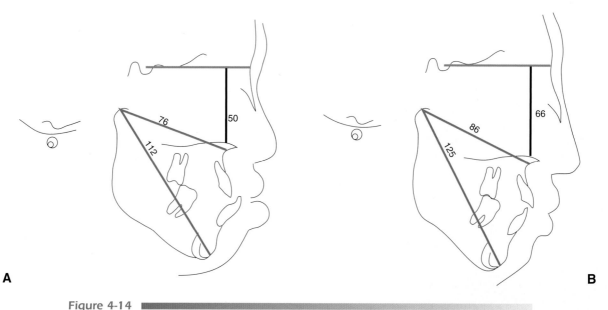

Figure 4-14

A, Tracing of lateral head film of a 14-year-old boy with Crouzon syndrome. **B,** After Le Fort III advancement and orthodontic treatment.

after completion of growth. However, in the case of severe deformity, the surgeon and family may choose early correction for psychosocial benefits, to protect the eyes, and to improve the functional airway.

REFERENCES

1. Enlow DH, Hans MG: *Essentials of facial growth,* Philadelphia, 1996, WB Saunders.
2. Meredith HV: Selected anatomic variables. In Lipsitt LP, Spiker CC, editors: *Advances in child development and behavior,* New York, 1965, Academic Press.
3. Chierici G, Harvold EP, Vargervik K: Morphologic experiments in facial asymmetry, *Am J Phys Anthropol* 38:291, 1973.
4. Harvold EP: The role of function in the etiology and treatment of malocclusion, *Am J Orthod* 54:883, 1968.
5. Harvold EP: *The activator in interceptive orthodontics,* St Louis, 1974, Mosby.
6. Broadbent BH: A new technique and its application to orthodontics, *Angle Orthod* 1:45, 1931; reprinted in *Angle Orthod,* vol 51, 1981.
7. Broadbent BH, Broadbent BH, Golden WH: *Bolton standards of dentofacial development growth,* St Louis, 1975, Mosby.
8. McNamara JA: A method of cephalometric evaluation, *Am J Orthod* 86:449, 1984.
9. Bjork A, Skieller V: Normal and abnormal growth of the mandible. A synthesis of longitudinal cephalometric implant studies over a period of 25 years, *Eur J Orthod* 5:1, 1983.
10. Vargervik K: Cephalometry in assessment of craniofacial form and proportions. In Ousterhout DK, editor: *Aesthetic contouring of the craniofacial skeleton,* Boston, 1991, Little, Brown.
11. Gorlin RJ, Cohen MM Jr, Hennekamp RCM, editors: *Syndromes of the head and neck,* ed 4, New York, 2001, Oxford University Press.
12. Kaban LB, Moses ML, Mulliken JB: Correction of hemifacial microsomia in the growing child, *Cleft Palate J* 23(suppl):50, 1986.
13. Vargervik K: Congenital and developmental temporomandibular disorders. In Fonseca RJ, editor: *Oral and maxillofacial surgery,* vol 4, *Temporomandibular disorders,* Philadelphia, 2000, WB Saunders.
14. Vargervik K, Ousterhout DK: Factors affecting long-term results in hemifacial microsomia, *Cleft Palate J* 23(suppl):53, 1986.
15. Vargervik K, Hoffman WY, Kaban LB: Comprehensive surgical and orthodontic management of hemifacial microsomia. In Vig K, Turvey T, Fonseca RJ, editors: *Principles and management of facial clefts and craniosynostosis,* Philadelphia, 1996, WB Saunders.
16. Kaban LB, Padwa BL, Mulliken JB: Surgical correction of mandibular hypoplasia in hemifacial microsomia: the case for treatment in early childhood, *J Oral Maxillofac Surg* 56:628-638, 1998.
17. Vargervik K, Hoffman WY: Mandibular distraction: factors in timing of the procedure. In Samchukov ML, Cope J, Cherkasin AM, editors: *Craniofacial distraction osteogenesis,* St Louis, 2000, Mosby.
18. Peltomaki T: Growth of the costochondral graft in the rat temporomandibular joint, *J Maxillofac Surg* 50:851, 1992.
19. Vargervik K: Orthodontic management of unilateral cleft lip and palate, *Cleft Palate J* 18:359, 1981.
20. Vargervik K, Ferrari C: Embryogenesis and management of the cleft patient. In Fonseca RJ, editor: *Oral and maxillofacial surgery,* Philadelphia, 2000, WB Saunders.
21. Ousterhout DK, Vargervik K: Pediatric trauma: resultant growth changes. In Habal MB, Ariyan S, editors: *Facial fractures,* Philadelphia, 1989, BC Decker.
22. Horowitz SI, Baumrind S, Vargervik K, Ben Bassat Y: Growth displacement of orbitale in normal subject between 8.5 and 15.5 years, *J Dent Res* 78:A125, 1999 (abstract).
23. Lee YP, Baumrind S, Vargervik K: Orbital growth in craniosynostosis, *Annual Program ACPA,* May 18-21, 1994, Toronto (abstract).
24. Ousterhout DK, Clark S, Vargervik K: Stability of midface position following Le Fort III advancement, *Cleft Palate J* 23:91, 1986.
25. Bu B, Kaban LB, Vargervik K: Effects of Le Fort III osteotomies on mandibular growth in patients with Crouzon and Apert syndromes, *J Oral Maxillofac Surg* 47:666, 1989.

CHAPTER 5

Speech Disorders Associated with Dentofacial Anomalies

Jean E. Ashland

The position of the teeth and the occlusion can influence the quality of speech production.[1] The neuromuscular and respiratory systems also play a key role in the quality and coordination needed for functional speech. They influence the accuracy of movement of the oral musculature and the coordination of respiration and phonation to achieve adequate control of the air stream during articulation. This is a dynamic and sequential process. Age and expected developmental milestones for speech sounds must also be considered when attempting to determine the influence of dentition and occlusion on speech performance.[1] Seventy percent of speech is learned by age 2 and 90% by age 4[2,3,5] (Box 5-1).

Speech sound production can be differentiated by anatomy or place of articulation and manner of production or degree of airflow obstruction between the articulators (Box 5-2). It is important to note that "90% of all consonants are made in the anterior portion of the oral cavity."[1] Thus, the maxilla often provides a boundary for the tongue. One of the groups of phonemes more vulnerable to misarticulations are sibilants /s, z, sh, ch, zh, dg [soft "g"]/,[3] especially the /s/ sound.[4] Production for sibilants involves sustained, partially obstructed airflow. The continuant feature of these sounds requires greater fine motor control than the complementary manner of production called *stops* or *plosives*. Plosive sounds are produced by complete obstruction of airflow followed by a release of the air stream. The complexity of sibilant sound production also contributes to the later age at which they are acquired when compared with plosives.

BOX 5-1	Milestones for Speech Development

p, m, b, h, n, w, b (90% by age 3 years)
k, g, d, t, ng, f, y (90% by age 4 years)
r, l, s; sh, ch, z; j, v; th; dj, zh (6-8 years)
Speech intelligibility: 70% age 2 years; 80% age 3 years; 90% age 4 years

Adapted from Sander EK: *J Speech Hear Disord* 37:55-63, 1972; Templin MC: Certain language skills in children, Institute of Child Welfare Monograph 26, Minneapolis, 1957, University of Minnesota Press.

| BOX 5-2 | **Speech Production Classification by Placement and Manner** |

Placement
Labials (p, b, m)
Labial and lingual-dental (f, v, th)
Lingual alveolar (t, d, n, l)
Palatal (sh, zh, ch, dj)
Velar (k, g, ng)

Manner
Continuants (h)
Plosives (p, b, t, d, k, g)
Sibilants (s, z)

Adapted from Singh SS, Singh KS: *Phonetics principles and practices,* Baltimore, 1976, University Park Press.

Oral and maxillofacial surgeons contending with anomalies of dental occlusion and skeletal jaw relationships often work in tandem with speech pathologists to ascertain the nature of existing or potential speech problems. If speech difficulties, such as problems with pronunciation or nasal resonance, are present, the speech pathologist can assist with differential diagnosis regarding contributions from dentofacial anomalies, delays in speech development, or neurophysiologic factors. Sometimes the speech pathologist may provide preoperative and postoperative speech evaluations to assess alterations in velopharyngeal structural relationships and potential vocal resonance changes (e.g., hypernasality).

SPEECH AND DENTAL ANOMALIES

There are numerous discrepancies with respect to the impact of skeletal malocclusion or malpositioned teeth and speech production. Early studies were vague about links between dental occlusion and misarticulations. Early reports had incomplete information with regard to the type of malocclusion or speech problem and reported that 20% to 80% of individuals with malocclusion had articulation difficulties.[4,6-8] The most common dental problems associated with speech difficulties included class III malocclusion, class II (divisions 1 and 2) malocclusion, open bite, and cleft palate.[9-13]

Lubit[4] recommended a variety of other factors to consider with dental anomalies and speech such as age, articulation score, palate width, palate height, type of occlusion, presence of an overbite or overjet, and upper anterior spacing. This multifactorial approach to speech and occlusion did not yield a causal relationship between the two, although /s/ productions improved after correction of the occlusion and with closure of diastemas. No

relationship was found between the palate vault height or width and the articulation. Johnson and Sandy[10] added that although the relationship was inconclusive, the severity of speech problems increased with greater severity of dental anomalies. Sounds acquired later are more vulnerable to misarticulation with dental anomalies given the greater physical complexity required for their production (e.g., sibilants).[7,10,14] Recently, Marcheson[13] described malocclusions and facial shape with respect to impact on facial tone (e.g., lip muscle tone) and subsequent speech production patterns. For example, individuals with a long face shape tend to have low facial tone and to be mouth breathers. The lower third of the face is longer and can create more difficulty achieving lip closure for labial sounds, because the tongue is more distant from the palate. A short face results in reduced intraoral vertical dimension and restricted space for the tongue to adequately move superiorly for precise production of /s/ and /z/.

Open Bite

The most common misarticulations with an anterior open bite are distortions of lingual alveolar sounds /s, z, t/ as the tongue glides between the arches and the air stream is altered against the anterior teeth.[11] Bilabial /b, p, m/ or labial dental sounds /f, v/ can also be difficult if the severity of the open bite compromises upper lip or upper teeth closure with the bottom lip. Laine[7] added that an open bite results in contraction of the hyoglossus muscle and that this can interfere with central grooving of the tongue needed for sibilant production.

Cross Bite

A cross bite occlusion can allow lateral air escape over the tongue resulting in distortion of sibilants /s, z/ sounds. Marcheson explains this phenomenon by inward and downward growth of the maxilla on the "working side." Consequently, the palatal vault space becomes crowded and provides less space for accurate tongue placement. This pattern can be seen in myofunctional swallow cases with forward motion of the tongue during swallowing. Farret and colleagues[12] examined 113 individuals with malocclusion aged 9 to 14 years and found that those with anterior cross bite were able to compensate with the lower lip to direct the air stream anteriorly.

Class III Malocclusion: Mandibular Prognathism

Mandibular prognathism interferes with production of many speech sound groups. Lip closure is difficult and can disrupt accurate production of bilabials /p, b, m/ sounds. Likewise, distortions of sibilants /s, z/ result from interdental placement of the tongue. In addition, anterior tongue placement alters the relationship of the tongue to the alveolar ridge, contributing to the distortion of sibilants.[10-12] Marcheson[13] adds that the tongue generally is positioned between the arches, and this can make the tongue seem larger.

Missing and Malpositioned Teeth

Generally children adapt to missing or malpositioned teeth with respect to speech production, especially when the occlusion is normal. However, the greater the severity of dental crowding and missing or malpositioned teeth, the more difficult it is to compensate to maintain a normal speech pattern.[10] Missing upper central incisors most frequently affect speech.[11] The speech sounds most vulnerable are lingual alveolar sibilants /s, z/. This is especially true if the child tends to carry the tongue more anteriorly at rest, such as with nasal congestion or enlarged tonsils. Thus, when the barrier of the upper teeth is missing, the tongue slides forward during articulation, resulting in distortion of /s, z/. Supernumerary teeth that appear within the palatal vault can compromise lingual-palatal tongue placement in severe cases.

Other Dentofacial Anomalies

Ankyloglossia. In a small percentage of patients, a short frenulum results in impaired speech production.[15,16] When the tongue range of motion is restricted sufficiently (e.g., the tongue cannot protrude past the lower teeth) to alter speech, lingual alveolar speech sounds generally are the first sound group to be affected. The child may compensate by using the midblade of the tongue to achieve these sounds with sufficient acoustic accuracy. In more severe cases, deviant compensatory speech patterns may be observed, such as pharyngeal fricatives (i.e., producing /s/ with the tongue base against the posterior pharynx) and glottal stops (i.e., occluding air at the glottis as a sound substitution). Feeding in young infants also can be disrupted if the lingual motion is restricted sufficiently to limit range of motion needed for sucking. Some breast-feeding mothers and lactation specialists have reported that the baby's ability to latch onto the breast has been compromised by a short lingual frenulum.[17] Surgical intervention (frenotomy or frenuloplasty) can be helpful in the more severe cases when speech or feeding function is disrupted. However, surgical intervention continues to be controversial across disciplines (oral and maxillofacial surgeons, otolaryngologists, pediatricians, speech pathologists, and lactation consultants), with pediatricians recommending surgery less frequently.[17]

Myofunctional Disorder. Myofunctional disorder, or tongue thrust, refers to a deviant swallowing pattern

in which the tongue moves anteriorly during the swallow, often with the tongue protruding between the incisors. This pattern can be seen in young children who suck their thumbs, creating an overjet and open bite. Typically when digit sucking is identified and stopped at a young age, the occlusal pattern self-corrects. However, the latter is not always the case. Dahan and colleagues[18] added that reduced oral perception, especially reduced sensory perception of the tongue tip, may be another factor contributing to myofunctional problems. Mouth breathing is sometimes a feature of a myofunctional swallowing pattern and is also associated with a narrow palatal vault.[19] During mouth breathing and myofunctional swallowing, the resting pattern of the tongue also tends to be more anterior and this contributes to a more constant pressure of the tongue against the upper incisors. Marcheson[13] contends that the tongue serves as one source to help shape the dental arch. Subsequently, a more anterior tongue position with an elevated dorsum and downward tongue tip position can contribute to reduced mandibular growth and simultaneously foster anterior growth of the maxilla, resulting in a class II malocclusion pattern. If the tongue is resting completely in the floor of the mouth, forward growth of the mandible can result in prognathism.[13] Other common occlusal patterns seen with a myofunctional swallow pattern include a cross bite. Speech productions frequently are characterized by distortion of sibilant sounds /s, z/. Normalizing the swallow pattern, including lingual strength and endurance activities, can facilitate improvement in speech production for sibilants.[20] In addition, Gross and colleagues[19] contended that establishing appropriate tongue placement in tandem with use of fixed appliances for correcting orthodontic issues may enhance outcomes of the orthodontic treatment.

Cleft Palate and Velopharyngeal Insufficiency. Approximately 20% of children with cleft palate repair demonstrate subsequent speech problems.[21] Common factors contributing to speech difficulties include dentoalveolar structural changes, craniofacial dysmorphism, and vocal tract anomalies that contribute to changes in dental occlusion. Breathing and phonation patterns necessary to support speech production are also abnormal.[14,22] The greater the severity of palatal clefting (e.g., bilateral cleft lip and palate versus unilateral), the more frequently speech errors are noted, especially with production of pressure sounds and lingual-alveolar consonants /s, r, l/.[23] Likewise, Pulkkinen and colleagues[24] found a greater frequency of surgical intervention (pharyngeal flap) for children with cleft palate compared with unilateral cleft palate. Furthermore, both groups showed a good recovery from velopharyngeal insufficiency (VPI) and hypernasality symptoms by age 8 years. Early examination of prespeech development provides preliminary views of future speech outcomes. Lohmander-Agerskov and colleagues[25] examined pre-speech development in children with cleft palate and cleft lip and palate. They reported more anterior speech sounds with cleft palate only, whereas there were greater posterior speech sound productions with cleft lip and palate anomalies. Thus, speech development patterns in the babbling stage, before cleft repair, appear to set the stage for error patterns that develop with the onset of words. Kummer and colleagues[26] documented /s, z, sh, ch, j/ as the most frequently occurring speech errors in 8 subjects with cleft compared with 8 subjects without cleft before Le Fort I osteotomy. The rationale provided for this pattern was that all of these sounds require maxillary and mandibular incisor contact for accurate production.

ASSESSMENT OF SPEECH PROBLEMS
Differential Diagnosis

Differential diagnosis of speech errors in patients with dentofacial anomalies includes developmental, structural, and neurologic factors. Developmental errors often occur with predictable, consistent patterns, such as omissions or sound substitutions secondary to late acquisition of certain sounds. For example, children aged 2 to 3 years may substitute /t/ for /k/ (tat/cat) or omit endings of words. It must be determined, based on the age of the child, whether developmental speech errors are deviant or within age-expected limits. Sound distortions, compensatory speech patterns (e.g., pharyngeal fricative), and incorrect placement of the articulators are observed more frequently with structural deviations of the speech mechanism. Vallino and Tompson[27] outlined a classification system for speech errors identified in patients with malocclusion: *frontal distortion I* (tongue through teeth); *frontal distortion II* (tongue posterior with flat body: air scattered); *dentalization* (tongue tip to the teeth); *lateralization* (lateral air escape), *whistling* (high frequency sound from air between palate and tongue), *mandibular movement* (mandible anterior or shifts laterally); and *labiodentalization* (lower lip contacts maxillary incisors).

In addition to misarticulations, the soft palate can be insufficient in length, resulting in hypernasality secondary to VPI. When VPI is present, consonant production can be affected adversely, impeding the ability to achieve adequate intraoral pressure for pressure /p, b/ or fricative /s, z/ sounds.[28] In contrast, neuromuscular abnormalities that impact speech production generally manifest with alterations in strength, precision, or timing of oral movements. Slurred or imprecise articulation patterns may be demonstrated. These may be accompanied by hypernasality secondary to weak or uncoordinated velar movements that compromise velopharyngeal closure. VPI can also have a learned or behavioral component, and a child can develop a compensatory speech pattern before palate repair (e.g., glottal substitutions). Persistent use of compensatory patterns after palate repair can give a false impression of VPI[22] (e.g., valving at the level of the glottis instead of the palate so that air escapes nasally). A number of possible speech and resonance errors can occur depending on the underlying etiology (Table 5-1).

Speech Assessment

Assessment of speech requires a multifaceted approach. The speech language pathologist (SLP) assesses oral motor function and structure related to speech production using a motor speech examination. This yields information about strength, precision, coordination, and speed of the oral musculature for speech. In addition, orofacial symmetry, palate shape, and a general examination of dental occlusion provide information regarding potential anatomic patterns and orofacial anomalies that may affect speech.[1] Formal tests of articulation are used and if VPI is suspected, there are articulation tests that contain targets of specific sound groups more vulnerable to error with impaired velopharyngeal closure (e.g., Bzoch Error Pattern Diagnostic Test[29]; Templin-Darley Articulation Test[30]). Potential speech errors when VPI is present may include difficulty with plosives and nonsibilant fricatives. Posterior lingual sounds /k, g/ are distorted more than tongue tip sounds /t, d/. There are more misarticulations with voiceless versus voiced sounds, and weak consonants are produced due to decreased intraoral pressure.[28] If resonance abnormalities are present in addition to speech errors, assessment for VPI is indicated. The severity of VPI is determined by the degree of speech and resonance compromise: hypernasality, compensatory speech patterns, reduction of intraoral pressure for speech, changes in vocal loudness or quality, audible or inaudible nasal air emissions, and facial grimacing during speech.

Resonance Assessment: Screening

An initial speech screening for VPI may include a mirror test, as well as use of a nasometer (nasal pressure plate to measure nasal air flow) to determine the degree of nasal air emission during speech. VPI rating scales frequently are used before and after speech therapy or surgery (e.g., Bzoch Perceptual Instrument[29]). Such scales generally rate the velopharyngeal mechanism as intact, borderline, or incompetent based on degree of nasality, nasal air leak, compensatory speech errors, intraoral pressure, and vocal loudness during speech production. Borderline cases generally can be addressed first with speech intervention; however, in cases of an incompetent mechanism, mechanical or surgical intervention is needed.

TABLE 5-1 Differential Diagnosis of Speech and Resonance Problems

	Sound omission/ substitutions	Distortions	Hypernasality	Hyponasality
Developmental				
Speech delay	x (e.g., /w/l, f/th, b/v/)	x /s, z, sh/		
Hearing loss	x	x		
Frequent ear infections	x	x		
Structural				
Cleft palate	x (deviant articulation placement)	x	x	
Submucous cleft		x (sibilants)	x	
Dental malocclusion (moderate to severe cases)				
Class II	x (changes articulation placement)	x (sibilants)		
Class III	x (lingual dental errors)	x (sibilants)		
Open bite	x (bilabial errors)			
Cross bite		x (sibilants)		
Short soft palate	X		x	
Maxillary or mandibular advancement		x	x (infrequent, often transient)	
Neurological				
Brain tumor				
Cerebellar or brain stem	x	x	x	
Weak palate (hypotonia)	x		x	
Cerebral palsy	x	x		
Speech apraxia	x		x	
Other				
Ankyloglossia (severe)	x			
Myofunctional swallow (tongue thrust)		x		
Allergies with congestion				x
Adenoid hypertrophy				x
Tonsillar hypertrophy (severe)			x	
Persistent compensatory speech pattern (glottal stop)			x	
Shallow depth of hypopharynx			x	
Fast rate of speech or reduced jaw excursion			x	

Sibilants: /s, z, sh, f/ ; *lingual alveolars:* /t, d, n, l/ ; *lingual dental:* /th/ ; *bilabials:* /p, b, m/ ; *glottal stop:* glottal sound for a plosive /p, b/.

Resonance Assessment: Instrumentation

Videofluoroscopy and nasoendoscopy can provide a dynamic view of the velopharyngeal mechanism to determine the movement patterns of the velum and pharynx during production of specific speech sound groups (e.g., plosives: /p, b/; fricatives, affricates, and sibilants: /s, z, sh, f/; liquids: /l, r/. These examinations assist with surgical planning, as well as potential use of a palate prosthesis as an alternative to surgery (e.g., speech bulb, palate lift) (Figure 5-1). Videofluoroscopy provides lateral, anteroposterior, and coronal views of the velopharyngeal mechanism. This yields specific information regarding velar stretch and thickening, relationship of velar height and the hard palate during phonation, and symmetry and range of lateral pharyngeal wall motion (Figure 5-2).[28] Limitations include radiation exposure, patient cooperation, and restrictions in viewing the actual site of velopharyngeal closure.[31] Other measures of the velopharyngeal mechanism include cephalometrics, magnetic resonance imaging (MRI), and functional MRI (fMRI). Cephalometric radiographs provide a two-dimensional static radiographic image of the anatomy (Figure 5-3). Measurements of pharyngeal depth, velum length, and adenoid size can be made from such images. fMRI images offer brief, simulated "virtual endoscopy" segments of dynamic speech samples in three dimensions. Limitations to fMRI techniques include cost, machine noise, and the effect of gravity in supine position; its efficacy has not been established.[31] fMRI technology is evolving to use rapid scan techniques that will allow longer speech segments to be viewed; currently segments of ~1.3 seconds are possible.[32] MRI technology has the potential to provide new insights regarding velopharyngeal dynamics for speech.

Myofunctional Assessment

Assessment for tongue thrust includes a general speech evaluation and a swallowing screening. Observing the child during drinking and eating with controlled bolus sizes allows the clinician to determine the presence of a reverse swallow pattern. The examiner asks the child to hold a small amount of water intraorally and then swallow while the clinician pulls down on the child's lower lip to expose the teeth. If the tongue protrudes interdentally past the incisors, this is an indication of a possible myofunctional problem. Other potential signs of a myofunctional swallow pattern include food crumbs remaining on the tongue after swallowing, a cross bite, distorted sibilant speech sounds, anterior resting position of tongue, and a narrow maxillary arch.[13,19] There are training programs for speech language pathologists to be certified to provide myofunctional therapy.

ORTHOGNATHIC SURGERY AND SPEECH PERFORMANCE
Cleft Palate Repair: Palatoplasty

The general consensus today for palate closure is that delayed hard palate closure (e.g., after 12 months of age) often results in greater articulation and resonance problems while not yielding much advantage in maxillofacial growth.[33,34] Approximately 20% of children develop speech problems, including VPI,[35] after palatoplasty. Primary approaches to palate repair include Veau-Wardill-Kilner "push-back," Furlow double-opposing Z plasty, and Von Langenbeck.[35] Examining speech outcomes is influenced by multiple factors including cleft severity, age of child, surgeon's experience, and study designs to examine the surgical outcomes. Witt and Marsh[35] concluded from a retrospective review of 25 years that the surgical approach used was not the primary factor affecting the outcome of speech, but rather the timing and staging of the repair and the severity of the cleft.

Maxillary and Mandibular Advancement

Resonance Outcomes. Multiple factors can impact speech and resonance outcomes when there is manipulation of the maxillary or mandibular arches: the presence of a cleft repair, type of speech errors before surgery, degree of dentofacial dysmorphology, and pre-morbid hypernasality.[22,26,36,37] When the maxilla is moved anteriorly, such as in a Le Fort procedure, the system tries to compensate. Therefore, there might be increased velar stretch secondary to greater velopharyngeal depth, mild changes in nasal resonance or nasal air emission, or reduced velar height related to superior movement of the maxilla.[26,38] Kummer and colleagues[26] reported that subjects without cleft palate were the least vulnerable to resonance changes after a Le Fort I procedure, followed by subjects with cleft palate alone and cleft lip/palate with normal resonance before surgery. Witzel[37] reported similar findings and added that subjects with borderline or incompetent velopharyngeal function before surgery were the most vulnerable for VPI following movement of the maxilla. Palatal scarring from prior surgeries can

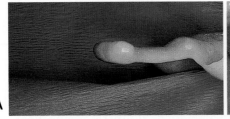 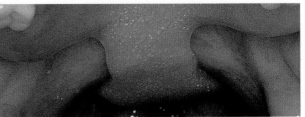

Figure 5-1

Palatal lift appliance. **A,** A palatal lift extension on a maxillary prosthesis. **B,** Intraoral view of appliance "lifting" soft palate. (Courtesy Dr. M. Jackson.)

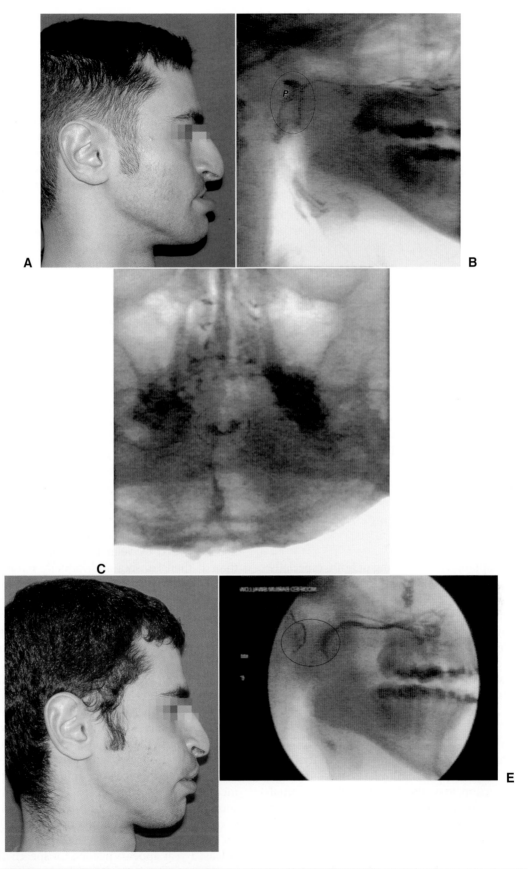

Figure 5-2

A 28-year-old patient with bilateral complete cleft lip and palate. **A,** Lateral photograph depicts severe maxillary retrognathia and lack of nasal support. **B,** Static lateral view captured from the patient's videofluoroscopy demonstrates limited maximal palatal excursion and incomplete velar closure even in the presence of a large Passavant's ridge *(P)*. **C,** Static anteroposterior view captured from videofluoroscopy shows the maximal lateral wall excursion, which is again limited in this patient. **D,** Lateral photograph after completion of maxillary advancement using semi-buried (transmucosal) Le Fort I distraction devices. **E,** Static lateral view a few months after maxillary advancement shows large increase in the velopharyngeal gap compared with **B.**

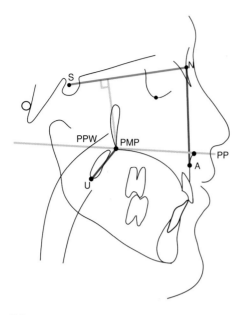

Figure 5-3

Cephalometric landmarks commonly include *S*, sella; *N*, nasion; *A*, A-point; *PPW*, posterior pharyngeal wall along the palatal plane; and *U*, uvula. The palatal plane *(PP)* is the most important plane. The posterior maxillary point *(PMP)* is determined by the intersection of the PP and a perpendicular line drawn through the pterygomaxillary fissure. Pharyngeal depth is the distance between PMP and PPW. Velar or soft palate length is the distance from PMP to U.

result in less adaptability or tethering or both, especially with more extensive operations. Sabry, Marsh, and Marty-Grimes[39] reported a low risk for postoperative velopharyngeal dysfunction (VPD) in 12 subjects with prior pharyngeal flaps or sphincter pharyngoplasty with controlled VPD. Six of 12 patients had preoperative bubbling on nasoendoscopy. The maxillary advancement for these individuals ranged from 7 to 12 mm, with a vertical impaction of 5 mm. Only 2 of the 6 subjects with abnormal findings (bubbling) developed postoperative VPD. However, it is important to note that delayed relapse in speech production for sibilants has been reported 1 year postoperatively for individuals with class III malocclusion.[40] Similarly, patients with maxillary distraction may also be vulnerable to initial changes in speech and resonance with changes in maxillary height. However, Guyette and colleagues[43] found that speech and resonance normalized over time after distraction.

Speech Outcomes. Mandibular and maxillary advancements provide correction of craniofacial deformities[41] and improve breathing, occlusion, and speech.[42] The gradual nature of tissue stretching with distraction

techniques reduces the potential negative outcomes on speech by allowing time for adaptation.[41,43] In cases of maxillary advancement to normalize occlusion, there can be positive effects on speech, especially in individuals without clefts. Vallino[44] described 34 subjects with class II and III malocclusion, with and without an open bite. Distortion of sibilants was the primary speech error. Postoperatively, 30 of 34 had improved speech, with a reduction of a mean of 16 errors to a mean of 3 errors. The greatest improvement was noted with open bite occlusal patterns. Changes also have been reported with respect to place of articulation. Wakumoto and colleagues[45] found that the tongue placement was improved and acoustic changes were maintained 6 months postoperatively.

Physician Screening for Speech

When considering the impact of orthognathic surgery, speech and resonance outcomes can be weighted more heavily in patients with a history of previous cleft palate repair, a baseline speech disorder, or abnormal resonance balance related to craniofacial dysmorphology or neurologic issues. The degree of maxillary or mandibular displacement certainly plays a major role in functional outcomes such as speech performance. Ko and colleagues[46] refer to the *need ratio* that includes the intersection of the palatal plane and posterior pharyngeal wall. The need ratio can be calculated using a cephalogram with the velum at rest during occlusion to predict postoperative VPD (Figure 5-4): pharyngeal depth divided by velar length. If need ratio is greater than 1, then Fonseca and Zeitler[47] report an increased likelihood of postoperative VPD. However, Park and colleagues[48] caution against the use of cephalometric measures in isolation to predict VPD, because other factors such as palate length, mobility, and strength also influence function during speech. Varying degrees of resonance change have been documented with increasing the pharyngeal depth with maxillary advancement. Ko and colleagues[46] reported 14% of patients (3 of 21) had a decline in hypernasality with an average of 8.9 mm of maxillary advancement. Patients with preoperative pharyngeal flaps did not have postoperative changes in nasality. Cedar and colleagues[49] also reported mild changes in resonance with midface maxillary advancement (mean 14 mm) for 5 of 11 patients. However, spontaneous resonance improvement was documented over the first year with no reported surgical intervention for velopharyngeal closure. Postoperative follow-up of at least 1 year appears needed for speech and resonance outcomes to account for spontaneous recovery or degree of compensation to orthognathic changes. Preoperative speech evaluations by a speech pathologist can assist with discerning any cause-and-effect relationship between speech difficulties and dentofacial anomalies, as well as establishing baseline resonance balance (Box 5-3). The scale outlines the impact of dentofacial anomalies on speech and resonance performance. When nasal air leak and abnormal speech compensatory patterns are observed, this is a strong indicator of VPD. The screening tool yields a rating score of velopharyngeal function that includes the presence of articulation errors, facial grimacing, nasal air emissions, and abnormal nasal resonance. A score of 2 or greater indicates the need for a speech evaluation. As the severity of VPD increases, additional testing is indicated, such as instrumental evaluation of the velopharyngeal mechanism. Speech and language pathologists, such as those on a cleft palate team, frequently use velopharyngeal rating scales as one means of speech and resonance evaluation (e.g., Perceptual Rating Scale[29]).

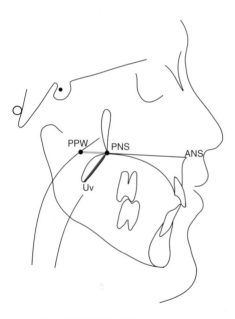

Need ratio = PPW–PNS/PNS –Uv

Figure 5-4

The lateral cephalogram can be used to calculate the need ratio that predicts the risk of velopharyngeal insufficiency after a maxillary advancement. *PPW,* Posterior pharyngeal wall (intersection of PP and PPW); *PNS,* posterior nasal spine; *ANS,* anterior nasal spine; and *Uv,* tip of uvula, are identified. The pharyngeal depth is the distance (in millimeters) between PPW and PMP, and the velar or soft palate length is the distance (in millimeters) from Uv to PMP. These measurements are then inserted into the equation. If the need ratio is greater than 1, there is an increased likelihood of postoperative velopharyngeal insufficiency after the maxillary advancement. (Adapted from Ko EW, Figueroa AA, Guyette TW, et al: *J Craniofac Surg* 10(4):321-322, 1999.)

BOX 5-3	*Physician Velopharyngeal Insufficiency Screening*

Articulation

Developmental speech errors (e.g., wabbit/rabbit, top/stop, da/dog)	0
Weak consonant production (related to nasal air leak)	1
Abnormal or compensatory speech errors (e.g., glottal stop, nasal snorts, pharyngeal)	1
Fricatives (e.g., using the back of the tongue against the pharynx to make an /s/)	1

Facial Grimace (e.g., pinching or wrinkling at the nasal root during speech)

Absent or mild	0
Moderate or severe	1

Nasal Air Emissions (audible, or visible on mirror)

Nasal air emission: audible or inaudible	1
Nasal turbulence	1

Nasal Resonance

Hyponasal	0
Mild hypernasality	1
Moderate-severe hypernasality	2

Total Score

Other Risk Factors on Patient Examination

Short-appearing palate; bifid uvula
Reduced pharyngeal contraction on phonation
Asymmetric palate or palatal weakness on phonation
Abnormal muscle tone; developmental delays

Referral Guideline

0-1 No referral indicated
2-3 Speech evaluation and referral to ear, nose, and throat specialist
4+ Speech evaluation and velopharyngeal insufficiency study or nasoendoscopy; referral to ear, nose, and throat specialist

---

Adapted from Bzoch K: *Communication disorders related to cleft lip and palate,* ed 4, Austin, Tex, 1997, PRO-ED.

Other risk factors for VPD include craniofacial anomalies such as Apert, Crouzon, Treacher Collins, Moebius, fetal alcohol syndrome (FAS), Stickler, oto-facial-digital, and velocardio-facial syndromes.[50]

Intraoral Prostheses: Speech Outcomes

An alternative to operative anatomic correction for VPD is the use of an oral prosthesis. Such devices include obturators or speech bulbs, as well as palate lifts, the former to compensate for lack of tissue and the latter for impaired palate movement related to weakness or degenerative problems.[28] Other prostheses include a premaxillary positioning appliance for complete bilateral cleft lip and palate, a nasal conformer, and an articulation development prosthesis (to assist with articulation development while awaiting palate repair).[51] Hardin-Jones and colleagues[52] reported no observable changes in prespeech sound development with young infants fitted at 6 months with anterior palate obturators. They attributed this to the open posterior palate that inhibited pressure sound production. Compliance is the most significant factor, especially for young children. Success with a speech bulb requires strong motivation by the child and family, and the best success is often with adolescents or adults. Turner and Williams[53] suggest the use of fluoroscopy or nasoendoscopy in tandem with a prosthodontist and speech pathologist to assess need, design, and effectiveness of an oral prosthesis. Sometimes a combined lift and obturator may be warranted if there is both velar weakness and a short palate. A new design for a palate lift combined with a palate bar has been reported to have improved stability. Ueda and colleagues[54] constructed a palate bar that acts as a fulcrum against the palate and reduces dislodgement of the prosthesis from palatal force.[51]

Once a speech bulb or lift is placed, speech treatment may still be needed to establish optimal speech patterns. Habitual patterns of speech may not change with a mechanical alteration of the mechanism, and the patient may need to learn new patterns. Speech bulbs are contraindicated with phoneme-specific errors for which speech treatment should be considered. One possible benefit of a speech bulb or a hybrid bulb plus a lift is to enhance function of the levator palatine muscle. This potentially enhances the reserve capacity, allowing greater muscle activity while reducing muscle fatigue during speech.[55,56] This concept continues to be investigated, with inconsistent findings.[57]

GUIDELINES FOR REFERRAL

The decision-making process to guide the maxillofacial surgeon for making referrals to the speech pathologist is multifaceted (see Box 5-3). Consideration should be given to the child's age, speech development, degree of dentofacial anomaly, psychosocial impact of speech compromise, and surgical procedures planned. In general, when an operation is planned, a preoperative speech screening to gather baseline data on speech performance, resonance, and oral motor function is indicated. This is especially true when there are baseline speech or voice problems or potential for sufficient structural change postoperatively that could alter speech. The speech pathologist can also provide insight regarding any confounding factors such as developmental issues, neuro-development, and dentition that may be impacting speech abilities.[1] In cases of cleft palate, the speech pathologist generally is involved throughout the process of surgical repairs to facilitate optimal feeding, speech, and voice performance.

CONCLUSION

Problems with speech cause some patients to seek treatment for malocclusion or dentofacial skeletal deformities. The ability to specify a cause-and-effect relationship is variable because of confounding factors. However, there are certain risk factors and craniofacial relationships for the oral and maxillofacial surgeon to consider when determining functional outcomes, including speech performance:

- The greater number of dental anomalies increases the potential impact on speech performance. Not all individuals with dental anomalies have speech problems.
- Class III malocclusions are more likely to be associated with speech difficulties than those in class II. However, in extreme cases class II and open bite problems can impact speech.
- Successful surgical correction of class III malocclusion can result in improved speech.
- Velopharyngeal function postoperatively in Le Fort and distraction cases will depend on the degree of maxillary advancement and preexisting speech and voice status.
- Individuals with cleft palate repair have less ability to compensate after maxillary advancement secondary to scarring and palate length.
- The presence of neuromuscular deficits increases the risk of hypernasality after orthognathic surgery.
- Hypernasality issues are generally first addressed with speech treatment before consideration for surgical intervention. In cases of severe VPI, speech treatment will not likely correct the problem.
- fMRI has the potential to offer new insights regarding velopharyngeal function and dysfunction.

REFERENCES

1. LeBlanc EM, Cisneros GJ: The dynamics of speech and orthodontic management in cleft lip and palate. In Shprintzen RJ, Bardach J, editors: *Cleft palate speech management: a multidisciplinary approach,* New York, 1995, Mosby.

2. Sander EK: When are speech sounds learned? *J Speech Hear Disord* 37:55-63, 1972.

3. Singh SS, Singh KS: *Phonetics principles and practices,* Baltimore, 1976, University Park Press.

4. Lubit EC: The relationship of malocclusion and faulty speech articulation, *J Oral Med* 22(2):57-55, 1967.

5. Templin MC: Certain language skills in children. In *Institute of child welfare monograph,* ed 26, Minneapolis, 1957, University of Minnesota Press.

6. Snow K: Articulation proficiency in relation to certain dental abnormalities, *J Speech Hear Dis* 26:209-212, 1961.

7. Laine T, Jaroma M, Linnasalo A: Articulatory disorders in speech as related to position of the incisors, *Eur J Orthod* 7:260-266, 1985.

8. Hale ST, Kellum GD, Bishop FW: Prevalence of oral muscle and speech differences in orthodontic patients, *Int J Orofacial Myology* 14:6-10, 1988.

9. Campbell R, Dock M: Dental anomalies associated with cleft lip and palate. In Kummer AW, editor: *Cleft palate and craniofacial anomalies: the effects on speech and resonance,* San Diego, 2001, Singular Publishing.

10. Johnson NCL, Sandy JR: Tooth position and speech—is there a relationship? *Angle Orthod* 69(4):306-310, 1999.

11. Kent K, Schaaf NG: The effects of dental abnormalities on speech production, *Quintessence Int* 12:1353-1362, 1982.

12. Farret MMB, Jurach EM, Brandao L, et al: Relationship between malocclusion and fonoarticulatory disorders, *Int J Orofacial Myology* 24:20-26, 1998.

13. Marcheson IQ: The speech pathology treatment with alterations of the stomatognathic system, *Int J Orofacial Myology* 26:5-12, 2000.

14. Laine T: Malocclusion traits and articulatory components of speech, *Eur J Orthod* 14(4):302-309, 1992.

15. Fletcher SG, Meldrum JR: Lingual function and relative length of the lingual frenum, *J Speech Hear Res* 2:382-390, 1968.

16. Willging JP, Kummer AW: Facial and oral anomalies: effects on speech and resonance. In Kummer AW, editor: *Cleft palate and craniofacial anomalies: the effects on speech and resonance,* San Diego, 2001, Singular Publishing.

17. Messner AH, Lalakea ML: Anklyoglossia: controversies in management, *Int J Pediatr Otorhinolaryngol* 54:123-131, 2000.

18. Dahan JS, LeLong O, Celant S, Leysen V: Oral perception in tongue thrust and other oral habits, *Am J Orthod Dentofacial Orthop* 118(4):385-391, 2000.

19. Gross AM, Kellum GD, Hale ST, et al: Myofunctional and dentofacial relationships in second grade children, *Angle Orthod* 60(4):247-253, 1990.

20. Gommerman SL, Hodge MM: Effects of oral myofunctional therapy on swallowing and sibilant production, *Int J Orofacial Myology* 21:9-22, 1995.

21. Witt PD, D'Antonio LL: Velopharyngeal insufficiency and secondary palatal management: a new look at an old problem, *Clin Plast Surg* 20:707-721, 1993.

22. Pulkkinen J, Haapanen ML, Laitinen J, et al: Associations between velopharyngeal function and dental consonant misarticulations in children with cleft lip and palate, *Br J Plast Surg* 54:290-293, 2001.

23. Laitinen J, Haapanen ML, Paaso M, et al: Occurrence of dental consonant misarticulations in different cleft types, *Folia Phoniatr Logop* 50:92-100, 1998.

24. Pulkkinen J, Haapanen ML, Paaso M, et al: Velopharyngeal function from the age of three to eight years in cleft palate patients, *Folia Phoniatr Logop* 53:93-98, 2001.

25. Lohmander-Agerskov A, Soderpalm E, Friede H, et al: Pre-speech in children with cleft lip and palate or cleft lip only: phonetic analysis related to morphologic and functional factors, *Cleft Palate Craniofac J* 31(4):271-279, 1994.

26. Kummer AW, Strife JL, Grau WH, et al: The effects of LeFort I osteotomy with maxillary movement on articulation, resonance, and velopharyngeal function, *Cleft Palate J* 26(3):193-199, 1989.

27. Vallino LD, Tompson B: Perceptual characteristics of consonant errors associated with malocclusion, *J Oral Maxillofac Surg* 51:850-856, 1993.

28. Shprintzen RJ, Bardach J, editors: *Cleft palate speech management: a multidisciplinary approach,* New York, 1995, Mosby.

29. Bzoch KR: Perceptual assessment instrument. In *Communicative disorders related to cleft lip and palate,* ed 4, Austin, 1997, Pro-ed.

30. Templin MC, Darley F: *Screening and diagnostic tests of articulation,* Iowa City, Iowa, 1960, Bureau of Educational Research and Service Extension Division, State University of Iowa.

31. Witt PD, Marsh JL, McFarland EG, Riski JE: The evolution of velopharyngeal imaging, *Ann Plast Surg* 45:665-673, 2000.

32. Ettema SL, Kuehn DP, Perlman AL, Alperin N: Magnetic resonance imaging of the levator veli palatini muscle during speech, *Cleft Palate Craniofac J* 39(2):130-144, 2002.

33. Rohrich RJ, Rowsell AR, Johns DF, et al: Timing of hard palatal closure: critical long-term analysis, *Plast Reconstr Surg* 98(2):236-246, 1996.

34. Rohrich RJ, Love J, Byrd SH, Johns DF: Optimal timing of cleft palate closure, *Plast Reconstr Surg* 106(2):413-422, 2000.

35. Witt PD, Marsh JL: Advances in assessing outcomes of surgical repair of cleft lip and cleft palate, *Plas Reconstr Surg* 100(7):1907-1917, 1997.

36. Corcoran J: Orthognathic surgery for craniofacial differences. In Kummer AW, editor: *Cleft palate and craniofacial anomalies: the effects on speech and resonance,* San Diego, 2001, Singular Publishing.

37. Witzel MA: Commentary, *Cleft Palate J* 26(3):199-201, 1989.

38. Jaques B, Herzog G, Muller A, et al: Indications for combined orthodontic and surgical (orthognathic) treatments of dentofacial deformities in cleft lip and palate patients and their impact on velopharyngeal function, *Folia Phoniatr Logop* 49:181-193, 1997.

39. Sabry MZ, Marsh JL, Marty-Grimes L: The effect of surgical maxillary advancement on velopharyngeal function in previously managed velopharyngeal dysfunction patients. Poster session: Annual American Cleft Palate Association Meeting, Seattle, May 2002.

40. Lee ASY, Whitehall TL, Ciocca V, Samman N: Acoustic and perceptual analysis of the sibilant /s/ before and after orthognathic surgery, *J Oral Maxillofac Surg* 60:372-373, 2002.

41. Mofid MM, Manson NP, Bradley CR, et al: Craniofacial distraction osteogenesis: a review of 3278 cases, *Plas Reconstr Surg* 108(5):1103-1114, 2001.

42. Van Slyke PA, Figueroa AA, Polley JW: Pre and postoperative speech assessment for maxillary distraction. Seminar: Annual American Cleft Palate Association Meeting, Seattle, May 2002.

43. Guyette TW, Polly JW, Figueroa AA, Cohen MN: Mandibular distraction osteogenesis: effects on articulation and velopharyngeal function, *J Craniofac Surg* 7(3):186-191, 1996.

44. Vallino LD: Speech, velopharyngeal function, and hearing before and after orthognathic surgery, *J Oral Maxillofac Surg* 48:1274-1281, 1990.

45. Wakumoto M, Isaacson KG, Friel S, et al: Preliminary study of articulatory reorganization of fricative consonants following osteotomy, *Folia Phoniatr Logop* 48:275-289, 1996.

46. Ko EW, Figueroa AA, Guyette TW, et al: Velopharyngeal changes after maxillary advancement in cleft patients with distraction osteogenesis using a rigid external distraction device: a 1-year cephalometric follow-up, *J Craniofac Surg* 10(4):321-322, 1999.

47. Fonseca RJ, Zeitler DL: Management of dentofacial deformities in the cleft palate patient. In Bell WH, editor: *Surgical correction of dentofacial deformities: new concepts,* Philadelphia, 1980, WB Saunders.

48. Park S, Omori M, Kato K, et al: Cephalometric analysis in submucous cleft palate: comparison of cephalometric data obtained from submucous cleft palate patients with velopharyngeal competence and incompetence, *Cleft Palate Craniofac J* 39(1):105-109, 2002.

49. Cedars MG, Linck DL, Chin M, Toth BA: Advancement of the midface using distraction techniques, *Plast Resconstr Surg* 103(2):429-441, 1999.

50. Shprintzen RJ: *Syndrome identification for speech-language pathology,* San Diego, 2000, Singular Publishing.

51. Reisberg DJ: Dental and prosthodontic care for patients with cleft or craniofacial conditions, *Cleft Palate Craniofac J* 37:534-537, 2000.

52. Hardin-Jones MA, Chapman KL, Wright J, et al: The impact of early palatal obturation on consonant development in babies with unrepaired cleft palate, *Cleft Palate Craniofac J* 39(2):157-163, 2002.

53. Turner GE, Williams WN: Fluoroscopy and nasoendoscopy in designing palatal lift protheses, *J Prosthetic Dent* 66:63-71, 1991.

54. Ueda N, Sato YS, Senoo Y, et al: New design of a palatal lift prosthesis combined with a palatal bar, *Cleft Palate Craniofac J* 39(1):12-17, 2002.

55. Tachimura T, Nohara K, Wada T: Effect of placement of a speech appliance on levator veli palatini muscle activity during speech, *Cleft Palate Craniofac J* 37(5):478-482, 2000.

56. Tachimura T, Nohara K, Fujita Y, Wada T: Change in levator veli muscle activity for patients with cleft palate association with placement of a speech-aid prosthesis, *Cleft Palate Craniofac J* 39(5):503-508, 2002.

57. Witt PD, Rozelle AA, Marsh JL, et al: Do palatal lift prostheses stimulate velopharyngeal neuromuscular activity? *Cleft Palate Craniofac J* 32(6):469-475, 1995.

CHAPTER 6

Behavior Management and Conscious Sedation of Pediatric Patients in the Oral Surgery Office

Stephen Shusterman and Howard L. Needleman

BEHAVIOR MANAGEMENT

Behavior management of pediatric patients prior to and during oral surgery procedures is a challenge. Children may experience pain or anxiety, both of which mediate fear. Because children are likely to require more of the surgeon's time, attention, and management skills than routine adult patients, it may be tempting to use general anesthesia frequently or exclusively as an adjunct to office surgical procedures. The actual procedure, however, may be relatively minor, the referral may have been made with the understanding that it could be accomplished with local anesthesia, and the parents may not want to submit their child to the risk of general anesthesia. Behavior management in the office is, therefore, an important part of pediatric surgical care.

Developmental Influences on the Dental Experience

A surgeon's expectations for the behavior of pediatric patients should be based on some understanding of psychological and emotional development.

The surgeon should speak directly to the child, as well as to the parent. Language skills develop early and increase with age. By the age of 2 years, children may have a vocabulary of from 12 to 1000 words.[1] By the age of 3 years, most have a sizable vocabulary and are capable of speaking in short phrases or sentences. For young children, therefore, verbal descriptions should consist of simple words and phrases that do not elicit unpleasant thoughts or fears. For example, a local anesthetic solution may be called "sleepy drops" that will leave the lips feeling "fat and fuzzy." Nitrous oxide may be "magic air" that will give the patient a "floating feeling." Extraction of a tooth involves "wiggling, pushing, turning, and crunchy noises."

Avoid fear-provoking words and phrases or conversation that leaves the child feeling small or intimidated. By telling children that an action "won't hurt," we may actually be alerting them to the possibility that it might hurt. Similarly, by describing a procedure in "little" terms, such as "I'm going to put my little mirror in your little mouth . . . ." we simply emphasize the helplessness of the small child in a big world.

Unpleasant stimuli are inherent to dentistry.[2] It is critical in patient management, however, to speak in terms that minimize the impact of those stimuli. At the same time, we must alert a child to the sensations and sounds that will be experienced.

School, preschool, and day-care programs introduce structure to the child's day. They create exposure to group activities, separate the child from parents, and introduce the concept that solid accomplishment brings praise and reward. Some young children may not have had these opportunities and are, therefore, suspicious of new situations. They fear strange people, noises, and surroundings and, therefore, usually benefit from the presence of a parent in the operatory. Although preschool may begin the socialization process, fear of the unknown usually peaks between 40 and 47 months of age. Frank[3] pointed out that the presence of the mother in the operatory during this period is beneficial to the child. However, this overriding concept may require modification in the setting of a surgical procedure, no matter how minor. The surgeon must weigh the possibility that the parent will be queasy and perhaps have a syncopal episode at the sight of blood. This will compromise the experience and care of the child and endanger the parent.

Between the ages of 4 and 5, children are capable of greater understanding and may become more assertive or stubborn. These children may question, stall, and attempt to manipulate and control a particular situation. Experiences in kindergarten and grammar school reduce the child's dependence on parents, introduce other authority figures, present the opportunity for group interactions, and teach the child to cope with fear.

The home environment shapes a child's response to minor surgical procedures. When both parents work and spend more time away from home, the child is exposed to social interactions sooner (baby-sitters, day-care programs). Because of this, some children may appear to develop social and psychologic maturation earlier while, in fact, they become more dependent on parents when they are available. For example, they may "cling" to parents in the presence of strangers. Similarly, some ethnic groups foster independence in their children, while others may be indulgent and overprotective. These children may become overly dependent on parents or extended families.

Systemic disease and mental and physical impairment also influence the child's capacity to understand and respond. For example, cerebral palsy may leave a child with hemiparesis or paraplegia and resultant athetoid or spastic movements. Many of these children have normal intelligence and are frustrated by their inability to cooperate. Systemic diseases such as diabetes, congenital heart disease, hematologic disorders, and rheumatoid arthritis may expose the child to constant medical care and unpleasant experiences. Any additional intervention, such as an oral surgical procedure, may be more than the child can tolerate.

Appointment Timing and Length

Appointments for children should be made as early in the day as possible. Pediatric patients are usually more alert, responsive, and cooperative in the morning and there will be more time before the hour of sleep to monitor recovery. After-school appointments should be reserved for older children. School time may be more critical for these patients, and they are more capable of cooperative behavior after a long workday.

Length of appointment is also considered an important management tool by some practitioners. While many pediatric dentists feel that shorter appointments enhance patient cooperation, others feel that longer appointments allow more treatment to be accomplished.[5] The resultant reduction in total number of visits is important to some children and their parents. In a survey of pediatric dentists in Washington, less than half (35%) preferred shorter appointments.[4] The oral surgeon performs both long and short surgical procedures. Primary teeth may be removed simply and quickly but, on other occasions, such as the removal of unerupted permanent teeth or supernumerary teeth, more lengthy appointments are necessary. The length of an oral surgery visit can be controlled only by electing to do procedures in a single quadrant at a particular sitting. With proper behavior management, long procedures may be completed successfully with the child's cooperation.

Office Environment

The office waiting room should be a comfortable and reasonably warm environment for the child, with age-appropriate reading material, toys, and other paraphernalia to keep the child busy. Sturdy, safe toys, with large parts and no sharp edges or points, are selected for the waiting room. Waiting time should be kept to a minimum to control apprehension, which increases with time spent in the reception area. An effort should be made to separate the waiting child from those recovering or leaving. Confrontations between entering patients and those who might be exiting with gauze in their mouths or tears in their eyes are counterproductive. Once inside the operatory, the mood should have a calming effect. The dental chair should cradle the child without being so large as to make approach and visibility difficult.

Patient Contact

When approaching the child to render treatment, surgeons must be straightforward and direct. A review of the medical history with a parent is necessary, but surgeons should introduce themselves directly to the child. After entering the operatory, the introduction may include a handshake with the child to establish, through personal contact, a sense of caring. The surgeon should crouch or kneel at the child's level. Parents who remain in the operatory are asked not to interrupt the conversation or cling to the patient. Parents who act as interpreters, when both doctor and patient speak the same language, are doing more harm than good. When the surgeon asks a child to "open wide," it is unnecessary and disconcerting for the parent to echo from aside, "open your mouth for the doctor."

We must clarify the parent's role as passive if we are to maintain the child's attention. The oral surgeon should explain the procedure to the child in understandable terms using the "tell-show-do" method. Tell the child what will be done, show what will be used and how, and then begin the procedure.

For example, after obtaining anesthesia, the surgeon might explain, "I am going to remove your tooth by pushing on it (demonstrate by pushing the child's arm) and turning it (turn the arm), and wiggling it. You will hear crunchy noises but nothing will bother you." Everything should be explained directly to the patient, maintaining eye contact at all times. Do not become bogged down in lengthy questions and answers that may be used by the child to avoid the procedure.

MANAGEMENT TECHNIQUES

With an understanding of the psychosocial development of the child and the array of behavioral guidance techniques, treatment of children safely and comfortably with local anesthesia becomes the modality of choice.

INJECTION TECHNIQUES

Before an injection, a topical anesthetic with a pleasant taste and odor, such as EMLA (lidocaine and prilocaine; AstraZeneca, Wilmington, Del.) or Benzo-Jel (Henry Schein, Melville, NY), should be applied to the mucosa and left in place long enough to induce surface anesthesia (approximately 1 minute). Disposable syringes with preattached fine needles are preferable to the traditional stainless syringe, which is more threatening and likely to attract the child's attention. Twenty-seven gauge needles are large enough to permit aspiration of blood and to allow a comfortable injection for mandibular blocks, whereas 30-gauge needles are adequate for infiltrative injections. The mucosa should be stretched tight, and the solution warmed and injected slowly in advance of the needle to minimize discomfort. During the injection, eye contact and constant supportive conversation should be maintained. Adequate amounts of anesthetic solution should be used but care must be taken not to exceed the toxic levels for lidocaine in children (approximately 4 mg/kg)[6,7] (Table 6-1).

Children easily tolerate infiltration anesthesia; however, mandibular block injections, resulting in anesthesia of the lip, may be disturbing. Pediatric patients should be alerted to avoid testing or chewing the lip. Bilateral mandibular nerve blocks generally are avoided by pediatric dentists. Some children may panic after developing

TABLE 6-1	Maximum Recommended Doses of Commonly Used Local Anesthetics*									
	LIDOCAINE 2% WITH/WITHOUT VASOCONSTRICTOR		MEPIVACAINE 2% OR 3%			PRILOCAINE 4% WITH/WITHOUT VASOCONSTRICTOR		ARTICAINE 4% WITH VASOCONSTRICTOR			
	2.0 MG/LB, 300 MG MAX.		2.0 MG/LB, 300 MG MAX.			2.7 MG/LB, 400 MG MAX.		ADULT 3.2 MG/LB, 500 MG MAX.		CHILD 2.3 MG/LB, 500 MG MAX.	
Patient Weight (lb)	mg	No. of Cartridges	mg	No. of Cartridges (2%)	(3%)	mg	No. of Cartridges	mg	No. of Cartridges	mg	No. of Cartridges
20	40	1.1	40	1.1	0.8	54	0.75	64	0.9	46	0.6
40	80	2.2	80	2.2	1.5	108	1.5	128	1.8	92	1.3
60	120	3.3	120	3.3	2.0	162	2.25	192	2.7	138	1.9
80	160	4.4	160	4.4	3.0	216	3.0	256	3.6	184	2.5
100	200	5.5†	200	5.5	3.5	270	3.75	320	4.4	230	3.0
120	240	6.5	240	6.5	4.0	324	4.5	384	5.33		
140	280	7.5	280	7.5	5.0	378	5.0	448	6.2		
160	300	8.0	300	8.0	5.5	400	5.5	500	7.0		
180	300	8.0	300	8.0	5.5	400	5.5	500	7.0		
200	300	8.0	300	8.0	5.5	400	5.5	500	7.0		

*Doses indicated are for normal healthy patients. Drug doses should be decreased for debilitated or elderly patients.
†0.2 mg epinephrine dose is limiting factor for 1:50,000 epinephrine.

the sensation of not being able to swallow or talk, while others may not be capable of resisting the temptation to test or chew the area postoperatively. These fears may be exaggerated when bilateral blocks anesthetize the entire lower lip and anterior portion of the tongue.

Management of Aversive Behavior

Not all pediatric patients are capable of complete cooperation. Some may cry or refuse to enter the operatory. In most cases, crying is a normal expression of fear, the result of being in a threatening situation. Brown and Smith[8] pointed out that developing a sense of security in the patient is the best way to modify fear and reduce anxiety. The child's attention must be gained before one can begin to develop that security. A firm, steady, but gentle approach, including a comprehensible description of the upcoming procedure, is usually adequate to gain a child's attention.

Thrashing, sobbing, or clinging to a parent may make it impossible to prepare for and, thus, perform a procedure. Rather than attempt to wrestle the child from a parent's arms, the surgeon should ask the parent to place the child in the chair. The chair is then moved to a comfortable reclining or semi-reclining position. This makes it more difficult for a child to sit up and attempt to leave. The parent must then move out of the patient's vision, allowing the surgeon to capture the child's attention. The parent may demonstrate a continuing presence and support by holding a hand or otherwise maintaining contact.

If a pediatric patient is combative, physical restraint may be necessary to prevent injury to the child or nearby equipment. Before resorting to physical restraint, an explanation must be given to the parent. It should be emphasized that the child will be handled gently and not injured. An assistant should be present; reassuring conversation directed toward the child is continued.

The use of a restraint for office oral surgery procedures is rarely indicated. In the case of an emergency procedure, however, when the patient has eaten within the past 6 to 8 hours, there is no choice. A very minor elective procedure, such as extraction of a loose tooth, may not warrant general anesthesia or deep sedation.

Restraining techniques include holding the patient's arms and legs, and the use of Velcro ties, straps, or commercial nylon wraps. The Papoose Board (Olympic Medical, www.olymed.com) and the Rainbow Stabilizing System (Specialized Care, www.specializedcare.com), while usually accomplishing the purpose, are frightening and uncomfortable and should be used only as a last resort. These devices should be used more commonly in the emergency room for suturing and debriding small wounds or during conscious sedation procedures. If a long or complicated procedure is necessary, the wounds

should be dressed and the child treated under general anesthesia.

Another method of controlling obstreperous behavior is the so-called *hand-over-mouth exercise (HOME)*. With this approach, the surgeon's hand is placed over the child's mouth to muffle sound. At the same time, the child is told that the hand will be taken away[9] when he or she becomes quiet. The same phrase should be repeated firmly, close to the child's ear, such as "when you are quiet and listen to me, I'll take my hand away." The purpose of this technique is to gain the child's attention for an explanation of the procedure to follow. The HOME approach has *no* role in the management of children who are too young to comprehend or who are developmentally delayed.

In a 1971 survey by the Association of Pedodontic Diplomates, 75% of the respondents reported that there were occasions when HOME should be used.[10] Today, HOME with airway restriction (HOMAR) is not considered an acceptable management tool, and the use of HOME is declining; 80% of all pediatric dentists do not use HOMAR, and 34% no longer use HOME.[11,12] If chosen, it should be used selectively to gain attention and prevent persistent avoidance responses. In theory, the child exposed to HOME learns that (1) the disruptive avoidance response will not succeed, and (2) the anxiety-provoking stimuli are actually far less noxious than imagined. The choice of HOME must be preceded by a full explanation to the parents and can be used only after obtaining their informed consent.

CONSCIOUS SEDATION

When behavior management techniques are insufficient to manage a pediatric patient, the use of conscious sedation should be considered. Conscious sedation is "a controlled, pharmacologically induced, minimally depressed level of consciousness that retains the patient's ability to maintain a patent airway independently and continuously and respond appropriately to physical stimulation and/or verbal command." The drugs, dosages, and techniques used should carry a margin of safety that is unlikely to render the child noninteractive and nonarousable."[13] The American Academy of Pediatric Dentistry divides conscious sedation into three distinct levels: level 1, mild sedation or anxiolysis; level 2, interactive; and level 3, noninteractive to arousable with mild-to-moderate stimulus.[13] This continuum, particularly in pediatric patients, may result in different states of consciousness that may or may not be predictable in every instance.[14] Table 6-2 describes the goals, responsiveness, personnel, and monitoring equipment associated with each of these levels, as well as those for deep sedation and general anesthesia. It is important to distinguish these levels of conscious sedation from that

TABLE 6-2 Template of Definitions and Characteristics for Levels of Sedation and General Anesthesia

	Conscious Sedation			Deep Sedation	General Anesthesia
Functional level of sedation	Mild sedation (anxiolysis)	Interactive	Noninteractive/arousable with mild/moderate stimulus	Noninteractive/nonarousable except with intense stimulus	General anesthesia
Goal	Level 1: Decrease anxiety; facilitate coping skills	Level 2: Decrease or eliminate anxiety; facilitate coping skills	Level 3: Decrease or eliminate anxiety; facilitate coping skills; promote noninteraction sleep	Level 4: Eliminate anxiety; coping skills overridden	Level 5: Eliminate cognitive, sensory and skeletal motor activity; some autonomic activity depressed
Responsiveness	Uninterrupted interactive ability; totally awake	Minimally depressed level of consciousness; eyes open or temporarily closed; responds appropriately to verbal commands	Moderately depressed level of consciousness; mimics physiologic sleep (vital signs not different from those of sleep); eyes closed most of time; may or may not respond to verbal prompts alone; responds to mild/moderate stimuli, e.g., repeated trapezius pinching or needle insertion in oral tissues elicits reflex withdrawal and appropriate verbalization (complaint, moan, crying); airway only occasionally may require readjustment via chin thrust	Deeply depressed level of consciousness; sleeplike state, but vital signs may be depressed slightly compared with physiologic sleep; eyes closed; does not respond to verbal prompts alone; reflex withdrawal with no verbalization when intense stimulus occurs, e.g., repeated, prolonged and intense pinching of the trapezius; airway expected to require constant monitoring and frequent management	Unconscious and unresponsive to surgical stimuli; partial or complete loss of protective reflexes, including the airway; does not respond purposefully to physical stimulus and verbal command
Personnel	2	2	2	3	3
Monitoring equipment	Clinical observation*	PO; precordial stethoscope recommended†	PO, precordial, BP; capno desirable†	PO and capno, ECG; precordial, BP; defibrillator required	PO, capno, precordial, BP; ECG, temperature, and defibrillator required
Monitoring information	None	HR, RR, O₂ before; during (q15min); after, as needed	HR, RR, O₂, BP cuff; CO₂ if available before; during (q10min); after until stable or discharge criteria met	HR, RR, O₂ and CO₂, BP cuff, ECG; before; during (q5min); after until stable or discharge criteria met	HR, RR, O₂, CO₂, BP; ECG, temperature before; during (q5min minimum); after until stable or discharge criteria met

Monitors: *HR*, heart rate; *RR*, respiratory rate; *PO*, pulse oximetry; *capno*, capnography; *BP*, blood pressure cuff; *ECG*, electrocardiography.
*Clinical observation should accompany any level of sedation and general anesthesia.
†"Recommended" and "desirable" should be interpreted not as a necessity, but as an adjunct in assessing patient status.

of deep sedation (level 4), which is defined as "a controlled, pharmacologically induced state of depressed consciousness from which the patient is not easily aroused and which may be accompanied by a partial loss of protective reflexes, including the ability to maintain a patent airway independently or respond purposefully to physical stimulation or verbal command."[13] Nitrous oxide and oxygen sedation, with or without oral premedication, have a broader range of safety and are easier to control than parenteral techniques.

Conscious sedation is particularly advantageous in pediatric patients. It reduces stress for both the surgeon and the child, and respiratory depression is less likely than with the use of deep sedation. Conscious sedation also produces some degree of mood alteration, amnesia, and analgesia.

Because the patient is conscious during the procedure, it is imperative that the operator continuously employ the behavior management techniques previously introduced. This allows for smooth induction, even maintenance, and smooth emergence from the sedated state. Conscious sedation is indicated for the anxious, frightened child who is capable of cooperating when anxiety levels are reduced. If the child is too uncooperative to allow induction with the drug, alternative approaches, such as deep sedation or general anesthesia, must be used.

General Considerations

The drugs and techniques used for conscious sedation in children must have a large margin of safety to avoid unintended loss of consciousness and other complications.[14] Pediatric patients who are deeply sedated may quickly develop respiratory depression and obstruction because their airways are smaller than that of an adult and they have a more variable response to drugs than do adults. Another consideration in pediatric patients is the sensitivity of the respiratory mucosa and airway smooth muscle to blood and secretions. Children may develop laryngospasm or bronchospasm in response to minimal stimulation of the airway. Only children who fit ASA (American Society of Anesthesiologists) class I or II should be considered candidates for conscious sedation in the office setting.

Indications for conscious sedation in pediatric oral surgery patients include the following: (1) age: younger than 4 years, (2) behavior: separation anxiety, short attention span, inability to understand simple commands or follow directions, (3) special needs: language barrier or learning disability, (4) extent of the procedure: less than 45 minutes and requires less than the maximal dosage of local anesthesia, and (5) noxious, extensive, or difficult procedure.

A minimum of two individuals (an operator and an assistant trained to monitor the appropriate physiologic parameters) is necessary for the administration and maintenance of sedation and monitoring of the patient. A third person should be available to circulate and assist in managing any adverse reactions.

Proper monitoring during conscious sedation is of the utmost importance.[15] Except for the very lightly sedated patient (level: anxiolysis, i.e., those sedated with nitrous oxide alone), the heart and respiratory rates should be monitored continuously with a precordial stethoscope and pulse oximetry.[16] When level 3 (noninteractive to arousable with mild-to-moderate stimulus) conscious sedation is anticipated, blood pressure and expired carbon dioxide levels[17] should be monitored. This enables the operator to detect early changes in cardiopulmonary parameters that could indicate serious life-threatening adverse reactions including drug toxicity, hypersensitivity reaction, airway obstruction, other medical complications, or administration mishaps. Normal values for vital signs of the pediatric patient are shown in Tables 6-3 to 6-5.[18,19]

The most commonly used and safest agent for pediatric sedation is nitrous oxide. The inhalation route by which it is administered allows a rapid, pleasant induction and emergence, and the operator may titrate dosage easily. A major disadvantage, however, is that patient cooperation is required to induce and maintain sedation. Children under 3 years of age and those who are extremely apprehensive generally do not allow the introduction of a nasal hood. These patients require enteral sedation preoperatively.

The combination of preoperative enteral sedation and intraoperative nitrous oxide may be used for managing difficult pediatric patients. Preoperative enteral sedation offers a number of advantages: (1) the pain and anxiety of the parenteral route is avoided, (2) a familiar person

TABLE 6-3	**Heart Rate per Minute**		
Age	Lower Limits	Normal Value	Upper Limits
Newborn	70	120	170
1–11 months	80	110	160
2 years	80	110	130
4 years	80	100	120
6 years	75	100	115
8 years	70	90	110
10 years	70	90	110

From Smith R: *Anesthesia for infants and children,* ed 4, St Louis, 1980, Mosby.

TABLE 6-4 Normal Blood Pressure for Various Ages

Ages	Mean Systolic ± 2 SD	Mean Diastolic ± 2 SD
Newborn	80 ± 16	46 ± 16
6 months–1 year	89 ± 29	60 ± 10
1 year	96 ± 30	66 ± 25
2 years	99 ± 25	64 ± 25
3 years	100 ± 25	67 ± 23
4 years	99 ± 20	65 ± 20
5–6 years	94 ± 14	55 ± 9
6–7 years	100 ± 15	56 ± 8
7–8 years	102 ± 15	56 ± 8
8–9 years	105 ± 16	57 ± 9
9–10 years	107 ± 16	57 ± 9
10–11 years	111 ± 17	58 ± 10
11–12 years	113 ± 18	59 ± 10
12–13 years	115 ± 19	59 ± 10
13–14 years	118 ± 19	60 ± 10

From Smith R: *Anesthesia for infants and children*, ed 4, St Louis, 1980, Mosby.

TABLE 6-6 Drugs Used in Pediatric Sedation

Drug	Dose
Oral Agents Administered Alone	
Chloral hydrate	50–70 mg/kg
Hydroxyzine	1.0–1.5* mg/kg
Promethazine	1.0 mg/kg
Diazepam	0.2–0.6 mg/kg
Oral Agents Administered in Combination	
Chloral hydrate	55 mg/kg
and	
Hydroxyzine	1.0 mg/kg
Meperidine	1.0–1.5 mg/kg
and	
Promethazine	1.0 mg/kg
Intravenous Drugs (Healthy, Euvolemic Patients)	
Meperidine	0.5–1.0 mg/kg
Diazepam	0.1–0.2 mg/kg
Midazolam	0.01–0.03 mg/kg
Pentobarbital	0.5–1.0 mg/kg

*Maximum of 50 mg when given in conjunction with narcotics.

can administer the medication in a nonthreatening environment, and (3) it is less likely to produce deep sedation than the parenteral route. The disadvantages are: (1) administration and absorption are not predictable due to lack of compliance or variable gastric or rectal absorption, (2) sedation may last beyond the required time, because the drugs have a long duration of action, (3) sedation is difficult to reverse, and (4) the dosage and effect cannot be finely titrated. In spite of these disadvantages, surveys indicate that oral administration is the route most commonly used by pediatric dentists.[20,21]

TABLE 6-5 Respiratory Rates per Minute of Normal Children, Sleeping and Awake

Age	SLEEPING		AWAKE		Mean Difference Between Sleeping and Awake
	Mean	Range	Mean	Range	
6–12 months	27	22–31	64	58–75	37
1–2 years	19	17–23	35	30–40	16
2–4 years	19	16–25	31	23–42	12
4–6 years	18	14–23	26	19–36	8
6–8 years	17	13–23	23	15–30	6
8–10 years	18	14–23	21	15–31	3
10–12 years	16	13–19	21	15–28	5
12–14 years	16	15–18	22	18–26	6

From Khatri IM, Freis ED: *J Appl Physiol* 22:867, 1967.

The recommended dosages of sedative drugs for adults are not directly applicable to children. Pediatric patients often require a higher dosage per unit of body weight because of such factors as surface area, organ size, cardiac rate and output, basal metabolic rate, distribution in tissue compartments, and glomerular filtration rate. In addition, manufacturers' recommended dosages usually are calculated for sedation of a cooperative individual. Such recommended dosages serve only as a starting baseline for managing the highly anxious, uncooperative pediatric patient. Therefore, many of the dosages recommended in this section may exceed the manufacturer's maximal recommendation. These dosages are based both on clinical experience and numerous studies reporting on the use of sedative drugs in children (Table 6-7).[22] In addition, these drugs often are used in combination, which may improve the efficacy of the particular agent versus when it is used alone (Table 6-8).[22]

If a child refuses to take a drug by mouth, the parenteral (intramuscular) route can be used with various sedative combinations such as hydroxyzine or promethazine with meperidine. This route is more reliable than the oral route because (1) latency is standard, (2) it does not depend on patient cooperation, (3) the uptake is less variable, and (4) the operator can better titrate the drug.

Most oral and maxillofacial surgeons do not use physical restraints for elective procedures but reserve them for emergency procedures, usually in the hospital emergency room. However, during the sedation session, most clinicians find the use of physical restraints such as the Papoose Board (Olympic Medical, www.olymed.com) or the Rainbow Stabilizing System (Specialized Care, www.specializedcare.com) helpful. The device restricts patient movement but should not impair respiration or the surgeon's ability to observe chest excursions. Many children "fight" the feeling of sedation, thereby diminishing the effectiveness of the drugs. With restraints, the child is forced to be still, which allows the onset and increases the success rate of sedation.

Sedation Techniques

Inhalation Route: Nitrous Oxide. Nitrous oxide inhalation results in a euphoric state and analgesia.[23,24] In addition, it alters the perception of time. Surgical procedures may proceed without the fidgeting associated with the short attention span of many young children. The sedative effect of nitrous oxide via nasal hood, in concentrations equal to or less than 60%, is not accompanied by any significant cardiopulmonary changes in pediatric patients. In studies that show a decrease in pulse rate and blood pressure, such decreases may have been produced by the relaxation response rather than a direct effect of the drug.[25]

TABLE 6-7 Drugs Commonly Used for Sedation and Analgesia in Pediatric Dentistry	
Agents	**Route and Dosage**
Antihistamines	
Diphenhydramine	PO: 1.25 mg/kg
Hydroxyzine	PO: 1-2 mg/kg
	IM: 0.6 mg/kg
Barbiturates	
Pentobarbital	PO: 2 mg/kg
Benzodiazepines	
Diazepam	PO: 0.3-0.5 mg/kg
	IV: 0.2 mg/kg
Midazolam	PO: 0.3-0.7 mg/kg
	IM: 0.04-0.1 mg/kg
Dissociative Agents	
Ketamine	IV: 1-2 mg/kg (loading dose)
	IM: 3 mg/kg
	PO: 6-8 mg/kg
Local Anesthetic Agents	
Lidocaine	2% with 1:100,000 epinephrine (maximum: 4 mg/kg)
Neuroleptic Agents	
Chlorpromazine	PO or IM: 0.25-0.5 mg/kg
	pr: 0.5-1.0 mg/kg
	IV: 0.5-2.0 mg
Promethazine	PO: 1-2 mg/kg
	IM: 1 mg/kg
Nitrous Oxide	
Nitrous oxide	40-60% N_2O/O_2
Opioids	
Fentanyl	IV: 1-4 mcg/kg
Meperidine	PO: 1-3 mg/kg
	IM: 1.0-1.5 mg/kg
	IV: 1-2 mg/kg
Sedative/Hypnotic Agents	
Chloral hydrate	PO: 50-55 mg/kg (maximum: 1 g)

Modified from Pham-Cheng A, Needleman HL: Sedation and analgesia in dental office practice. In Krauss B, Brustowicz RM, editors: *Pediatric procedural sedation and analgesia*, Philadelphia, 1999, Lippincott Williams & Wilkins.

Potential adverse reactions to nitrous oxide include (1) hypoxia, either due to mechanical failure or physiologic diffusion, (2) pressure/volume effects in air spaces

TABLE 6-8   Indications for Common Drug Combinations Used in Pediatric Dental Practice

Procedures	Combinations	Route and Dosage
Age: <3 years **Treatment:** <30 minutes **Behavior:** moderately difficult to approach **Weight:** <20 kg	Chloral hydrate Hydroxyzine	po or pr: 55 mg/kg po: 2 mg/kg
Age: >2 years **Treatment:** <30 minutes **Behavior:** difficult to approach	Meperidine Promethazine	IM: 1.1 mg/kg IM: 1.1 mg/kg
Age: >3 years **Treatment:** 30-60 minutes **Behavior:** moderate to very difficult, disruptive **Weight:** >20 kg	Chloral hydrate Meperidine Hydroxyzine	po: 30-50 mg/kg po: 1 mg/kg po: 25 mg
Age: >6 years **Treatment:** <30 minutes **Behavior:** moderate anxiety, special needs (e.g., cerebral palsy)	Diazepam Fentanyl	po: 0.25 mg/kg sl: 4 mcg/kg 1 hr after diazepam

From Pham-Cheng A, Needleman HL: Sedation and analgesia in dental office practice. In Krauss B, Brustowicz RM, editors: *Pediatric procedural sedation and analgesia*, Philadelphia, 1999, Lippincott Williams & Wilkins.
sl, Sublingual.

such as the middle ear, (3) psychotic reactions, (4) depressed bone marrow after prolonged use, (5) possible decrease in protective reflexes, and (6) nausea and vomiting.[26]

Technique. It is helpful to give the parents written preoperative instructions to take home. This will minimize needless appointment failures and potentially minimize intraoperative complications. It is not necessary for a child to have nothing by mouth prior to nitrous oxide analgesia. However, the preceding meal should consist of clear liquids. The operatory should be quiet, to prevent distraction and to enhance the sedative state. The tell-show-do method is essential in helping to allay the child's anxiety and to gain cooperation for placement of the nasal hood. It is often helpful to give the child the nasal hood to take home prior to the surgical visit to practice nasal breathing and to allow desensitization to the placement of the hood. Flavored nasal hoods make it easier and more pleasant for the child to practice and accept the procedure. These hoods (PIP+ Nasal Hoods, Accu-Tron, www.accutron-inc.com) are available in various sizes and flavors. Many children are unable to understand the command "breathe through your nose." Therefore, the instruction to "smell" the particular scent is important to ensure proper inhalation of the nitrous oxide–oxygen mixture. Terms such as "magic air" are also useful.

Demonstration of the nasal hood by placing one on the surgeon's own nose and showing the child how to make the reservoir bag move is helpful. If the child is resistant, the mask can be placed in front of the nose and mouth and the percentage of nitrous oxide raised to 70% or more. On occasion, it may be necessary to force the mask over the nose or mouth of a resistant child to establish initial sedation.[27] If this is unsuccessful, additional sedative medications may be needed at a subsequent session (see Enteral and Parenteral Agents and Techniques).

It is important to explain the associated effects of nitrous oxide in positive terms such as a "tingling or bubbling of the fingers, toes, and limbs" and a "floating, warm feeling." If the child does not expect these sensations, he or she may become fearful and agitated. A level of 50% to 60% nitrous oxide should be used for 2 to 3 minutes prior to administering local anesthesia or performing any painful procedure. Sufficient sedation is established when the child's eyes fixate and extraneous movements cease. After the injection is completed, lower levels such as 40% nitrous oxide can be used for maintenance during the procedure.

For children under 8 years of age, a total flow of 6 liters per minute of the nitrous oxide–oxygen mixture is sufficient for the minute respiratory volume requirement. Nasal respiration should be monitored to ensure maintenance of adequate sedation. It is not uncommon for a child to fall asleep during the procedure when adequately sedated and if the procedure is performed around his or her nap time.

When the procedure is completed, the patient is placed on 100% oxygen for 2 to 3 minutes to minimize the effect of diffusion hypoxia and to adequately scavenge the residual exhaled nitrous oxide. Within 3 to 5 minutes after cessation of sedation, the patient's behavior and affect are usually back to normal. The child should satisfy the discharge criteria in Box 6-1 before being released. In addition, the parent is advised to monitor the patient closely over the next few hours, because the child may be so relaxed that falling is possible.

Enteral and Parenteral Agents and Techniques. The administration of sedative drugs must be preceded by an evaluation of the patent's preoperative oral intake. The following guidelines must be followed in order to ensure optimal absorption and to prevent aspiration: (1) no milk or solids for 6 hours for children 6 to 36 months old and 6 to 8 hours for children 36 months or older, and (2) clear liquids up to 3 hours before the procedure for children ages 6 months and older.[13] Depending on the drug used, a waiting period of between 30 and 60 minutes is required to achieve a maximal sedative effect. According to a recent study,[28] waiting a sufficient amount of time between administration of the sedative drug and the local anesthetic may be a critical variable for a successful sedation outcome. The child and parent should rest in a quiet room and trained office personnel should assist in monitoring the patient. If the child is not somnolent after the initial waiting period, induction with 50% nitrous oxide is recommended. If the child then fails to cooperate, the procedure may have to be abandoned. A reappointment is scheduled for the procedure with alternative enteral medications, deep parenteral sedation, or general anesthesia.

The combination of enteral medication and nitrous oxide inhalation may result in deep sedation, depending on the drugs used, their dosages, and the patient's drug sensitivity. The operator should, therefore, be prepared to monitor the patient appropriately. While it is not the intention to produce deep sedation with the drugs discussed in this section, the possibility always exists.

The technique for a deep muscular injection is similar to that for adults. The preferred sites of injection for children are the anterior aspect of the thigh and the upper outer quadrant of the buttocks. The preferred needle size is 22 gauge (1½ inch long) or 23 gauge (1 inch long) for smaller children. Most sedative agents administered by this route are effective 20 to 40 minutes after injection.

The drugs listed in Table 6-7 occasionally are used alone, but more often they are used in combination to complement each other's sedative effect and to decrease adverse reactions (Table 6-8). No one drug or combination of drugs is clearly superior to others; therefore, clinicians must base their choice of sedatives on their training, clinical experience, and new information in the medical and dental literature.[29]

CONCLUSION

The public has become increasingly aware of the inherent risks involved in the office use of deep sedation and general anesthesia in children. This has made parents more inclined to request that procedures be done with local anesthesia and conscious sedation. Most states now have regulations for the use of sedation, which all practitioners must follow. Some states require separate licensure or certification for the use of deep sedation and general anesthesia in the office setting. The potential for producing unintended deep sedation or general anesthesia with conscious sedation in any given individual must be considered. The morbidity and mortality reported for deep sedation in pediatric patients are a direct result of overmedication.[30,31] Local anesthetics are central nervous system depressants and potentially toxic. When excessive amounts of local anesthetics, narcotics, and other drugs are used in combination, serious morbidity and mortality can occur. It is important to keep the total dosage of local anesthesia below toxic levels (see Table 6-1) and not to exceed the recommended dosages for the sedative drugs discussed in this chapter (see Table 6-7). A recent report indicates that there may be a gender difference in responses to sedative agents, with boys having more successful sedations than girls.[32]

The surgeon should be aware of the psychologic and physiologic differences between adults and children. Emergency equipment must be readily available in the operatory, including a positive pressure oxygen delivery system that can accommodate children of all ages and sizes. The recovery area must also have equipment to monitor children, and emergency drugs with pediatric dosages should be available. The staff must be trained to manage any pediatric emergency situation.

BOX 6-1	Discharge Criteria

Cardiovascular function satisfactory and stable
Airway patency uncompromised and satisfactory
Patient easily arousable and protective reflexes intact
State of hydration adequate
Patient can talk, if applicable
Patient can sit unaided, if applicable
Patient can ambulate, if applicable, with minimal assistance
For the child who is very young or disabled and incapable of the usually expected responses, the presedation level of responsiveness or the level as close as possible for that child should be achieved
Responsible individual available

The surgeon should consider carefully which behavior or sedation modality to use for a specific oral surgical procedure. The factors to be considered in making this decision include: (1) length of the procedure, (2) difficulty and potential pain associated with the procedure and, most importantly, (3) age and level of anticipated cooperation of the child. When the planned procedure is long and difficult and the anticipated cooperation is poor, the operator should consider moving from behavior modification techniques and conscious sedation to deeper sedation and general anesthesia. When the exact extent and difficulty of a procedure is unknown, the operator should use a level of sedation that will allow the operation to be completed with optimal results. This may necessitate using a deeper level of sedation than originally anticipated. With experience gained from performing many procedures on children, the surgeon will become more confident in selecting the appropriate management technique.

REFERENCES

1. Gesell AL: *The first five years of life: a guide to the study of the pre-school child,* New York, 1940, Harper Brothers.
2. Wright FAC, Lucas JO, McMurray NE: Dental anxiety in five-to-nine–year-old children, *J Pedod* 4:99-115, 1980.
3. Frankl SN, Shiere FR, Fogels HR: Should the parent remain with the child in the dental operatory? *J Dent Child* 29:150, 1962.
4. Levy RL, Domoto PK: Current techniques for behavior management: a survey, *Pediatr Dent* 1(3):160-164, 1979.
5. Taylor MH, Peterson DS: Effect of length and number of appointments on children's behavior in a dental setting, *J Dent Child* 50(5):353-357, 1983.
6. Moore PA, Mickey E, Hargreaves J, et al: Sedation in pediatric dentistry: a practical assessment procedure, *J Am Dent Assoc* 109:564-569, 1984.
7. Moore PA: Pediatric sedation and anesthesia: monitoring and management considerations. In Dionne RA, Laskin DM, editors: *Anesthesia and sedation in the dental office,* New York, 1986, Elsevier.
8. Brown JP, Smith IT: Childhood fear and anxiety states in relation to dental treatment, *Aust Dent J* 24:256-259, 1979.
9. Craig W: Hand over mouth technique, *J Dent Child* 38:387-398, 1971.
10. Association of Pedodontic Diplomates: Survey of attitudes and practices in behavior management, *Pediatr Dent* 3(3):246-250, 1981.
11. Davis MJ, Rombom HM: Survey of the utilization of and rationale for hand-over-mouth (HOM) and restraint in postdoctoral pedodontic education, *Pediatr Dent* 1(2):87-90, 1979.
12. Nathan JE: Management of the difficult child: survey of pediatric dentists' use of restraints, sedation, and general anesthesia. Data presented at Conference on Behavior Management for the Pediatric Dental Patient, sponsored by the American Academy of Pediatric Dentistry, Iowa City, Iowa, Sept 30, 1988.
13. Guidelines for the elective use of conscious sedation, deep sedation, and general anesthesia in pediatric patients, *Pediatr Dent* 7:334-337, 1985.
14. Krippaehne JA, Montgomery MT: Morbidity and mortality form psychosedation and general anesthesia in the dental office, *J Oral Maxillofac Surg* 50:691-698, 1992.
15. Wilson S: Review of monitors and monitoring during sedation with emphasis on clinical applications, *Pediatr Dent* 17:413-418, 1995.
16. Grandy SR: The use of pulse oximetry in dentistry, *J Am Dent Assoc* 126:1274-1278, 1995.
17. Primosch RE, Buzzi IM, Jerrell G: Monitoring pediatric dental patients with nasal mask capnography, *Pediatr Dent* 22:120-124, 2000.
18. Smith R: *Anesthesia for infants and children,* ed 4, St Louis, 1980, Mosby.
19. Khatri IM: Hemodynamic changes during sleep, *J Appl Physiol* 22:867, 1967.
20. Wilson S: A survey of the American Academy of Pediatric Dentistry membership: nitrous oxide and sedation, *Pediatr Dent* 18:287-293, 1996
21. Houpt M: Project USAP the use of sedative agents in pediatric dentistry: 1991 update, *Pediatr Dent* 15:36-40, 1993.
22. Pham-Cheng, A, Needleman HL: Sedation and analgesia in dental office practice. In Krauss B, Brustowicz RM, editors: *Pediatric procedural sedation and analgesia,* Philadelphia, 1999, Lippincott Williams & Wilkins.
23. Berger DE, Allen G, Everett GB: An assessment of the analgesic effect of nitrous oxide in the primary dentition, *J Dent Child* 39:265-268, 1972.
24. Zuniga JR, Knigge KK, Joseph SA: Central 13-endorphin release and recovery after exposure to nitrous oxide in rats, *J Oral Maxillofac Surg* 44:714-718, 1986.
25. Aspes T: The effect of nitrous oxide sedation on the blood pressure of pediatric dental patients, *J Dent Child* 42:364-366, 1975.
26. Duncan GH, Moore P: Nitrous oxide and the dental patient: a review of adverse reactions, *J Am Dent Assoc* 108:213-218, 1984.
27. Wald C: Methods of introducing nitrous oxide to the handicapped or difficult child, *J Am Analg Soc* 15:11-18, 1977.
28. Leelataweedwud P, Vann WF: Adverse events and outcomes of conscious sedation for pediatric patients. Study of an oral sedation regimen, *J Am Dent Assoc* 132:1531-1539, 2001.
29. Nathan J: Dosage selection for pediatric oral conscious sedation: a practical approach, *J Southeast Soc Pediatr Dent* 5:26-27, 1999.
30. Goodson JM, Moore PA: Life-threatening reactions after pediatric sedation: an assessment of narcotic, local anesthetic and antiemetic drug interaction, *J Am Dent Assoc* 107:239-245, 1983.
31. Moore P: Adverse drug interactions in dental practice: interactions associated with local anesthetics, sedatives and anxiolytics, *J Am Dent Assoc* 130:541-556, 1999.
32. Needleman HL, Joshi A, Griffith DG: Conscious sedation of pediatric dental patients using chloral hydrate, hydroxyzine and nitrous oxide—a retrospective study of 382 sedations, *Pediatr Dent* 17:424-431, 1995.

CHAPTER **7**

Deep Sedation for Pediatric Patients

Jeffrey D. Bennett and Jeffrey B. Dembo

CHAPTER OUTLINE

Anesthetic management of the pediatric patient in the oral surgery office varies considerably from that of the adult patient. There are anatomic and physiologic differences that the surgeon must consider. The pharmacokinetics and pharmacodynamics of most medications differ by age and weight. Finally, psychological development of children and their ability to cope with the stress of the surgical experience varies with age and the stage of development. Selection of the anesthetic technique and medications for each child should be dictated by an understanding of these parameters.

ANATOMIC AND PHYSIOLOGIC CONSIDERATIONS IN THE NONINTUBATED CHILD

The scope and complexity of oral and maxillofacial surgery (OMFS) procedures performed in the outpatient setting has been increasing with improvements in technique and with pressure from third party payers.

The unique and challenging nature of anesthetic management in the oral surgery office setting relates to the performance of intraoral procedures in anesthetized, nonintubated patients. The surgical site within the oral cavity is in close proximity to the pharynx, which renders the pediatric patient especially susceptible to airway obstruction and airway irritation. These factors may cause a significant degree of hypoxia.[1,2] Decreased minute ventilation and airway tone secondary to sedative medication also may contribute to hypoxia.

Anatomic differences between the pediatric and adult airway increase the risk of obstruction in the nonintubated child. Between the ages of 4 and 10, lymphoid hypertrophy occurs with enlargement of the tonsils and adenoids. The young child has a tongue that is large relative to the size of the oral cavity. The tongue is positioned higher in the oral cavity and impinges on the palate because of the more rostrally positioned larynx. Lymphoid hypertrophy, relative macroglossia, and rostral positioning of the tongue in the child all contribute to the potential for airway obstruction.

The trachea and bronchi of a child are more compliant than that of an adult. These airways are susceptible to collapse with an increase in negative inspiratory pressure. Such an increase in transluminal pressure may be seen when the child is crying or attempting to compensate for upper airway obstruction. Throughout all branches of the airway, the diameter is relatively smaller in a child. Because airway resistance is inversely proportional to the radius of the lumen to the fourth power, any narrowing secondary to secretions, edema, or bronchospasm has a more profound adverse effect on air exchange in the pediatric patient than in the adult.

Anatomic differences in the pediatric patient diminish the efficacy of ventilation. In the adult, each rib has a caudal slant, whereas in children ribs are more horizontally angled relative to the vertebral column.[3] The accessory muscles of respiration are less developed in the child. These factors result in less efficient thoracic expansion and a greater dependence on diaphragmatic breathing. Upper airway obstruction in the sedated young child can result in paradoxic chest wall movement. Inward movement of the chest opposes the expansile downward movement of the diaphragm. Greater energy is therefore required for breathing, which may lead to fatigue and subsequent hypoxia.

Exchange of gas takes place within the alveoli, which are smaller and fewer in the child. The alveoli increase in number until approximately 8 years of age and continue to increase in size until growth is completed. The number of alveoli may increase more than 10-fold from infancy to adulthood, with a resultant increase in surface area by a multiple of 60.[4-6]

Functional residual capacity (FRC) is the volume of gas in the lung after a normal expiration. The pediatric patient has a diminished FRC expressed on a basis of weight[7] (Table 7-1). For the pediatric patient, who has a higher metabolic demand and greater oxygen consumption, the decreased FRC (which provides oxygen reserve) results in a more rapid desaturation of hemoglobin during periods of respiratory depression.[8-10] In one model calculation comparing children with adults, an apneic period of 41 seconds in the pediatric patient would result in an arterial oxyhemoglobin saturation of 85%. A similar reduction would take an 84-second apneic period in an adult.[11] Closing volume, the lung volume at which dependent airways begin to close, is greater in the pediatric patient. This results in increased dead space ventilation and more rapid development of hypoxemia.

Perfusion is dependent on cardiac output and peripheral resistance. Cardiac output is dependent on heart rate and stroke volume. The pediatric heart is less compliant than that of the adult and has less ability to alter stroke volume. Adequate cardiac output is, therefore, dependent on an adequate heart rate. This is important, because some sedative agents may produce a significant decrease in heart rate.

The myocardium is innervated by both the sympathetic and parasympathetic systems. The parasympathetic system has a greater influence on the myocardium in children versus adults. In one retrospective study, the incidence of bradycardia during anesthesia was reported to be age related, and the greatest effect appeared to occur in patients less than 3 to 4 years of age.[12] There was an approximate threefold increase in the incidence of bradycardia in 2- to 3-year-old children when compared with the 3- to 4-year-old group. Blood pressure is the product of cardiac output and peripheral resistance, and children have less ability to alter peripheral resistance. A bradycardia that results in decreased cardiac output also results in a decrease in blood pressure, because the child cannot compensate by increasing peripheral resistance.

PREOPERATIVE EVALUATION OF THE PATIENT

Psychological Assessment

The perioperative period can be very stressful for a child. The child is confronted with an unfamiliar environment, unfamiliar people, apprehension about the unknown, and loss of control. The child faces the fear of separation from the parents, the threat of needles, the perception of impending pain, and the fear of mutilation. Younger children frequently cannot verbalize their concerns. Behavioral manifestation of perioperative anxiety may vary from hyperventilation, trembling, crying, and agitation to physical resistance. Children younger than the age of 6 frequently cannot comprehend the need for the procedure or that it is for their benefit. Children older than 6 years of age or those who have participated in social programs may be better able to comprehend the situation and communicate their concerns.[13] If possible, allow older children to participate in the choice of anesthetic management. Introduce them to the various routes of induction, such as intravenous, intramuscular, oral, or a mask. Adolescents may be more mature and capable of comprehending the planned surgery and anesthetic management. Emotionally, they are seeking independence and self-control. However, they are not adults and they may exhibit a multitude of behaviors with rapid mood changes. A paradoxical reaction to sedation, in which the adolescent appears to become agitated after the administration of anxiolytic medication, may necessitate a deeper level of anesthesia than what originally may have been planned.

TABLE 7-1	Normal Respiratory Functions			
	3 Years	5 Years	12 Years	Adult
Tidal volume (ml)	112	270	480	575
Minute ventilation (L/min)	2.46	5.5	6.2	6.4
Vital capacity (ml)	870	1160	3100	4000
Functional residual capacity (ml)	490	680	1970	3000

Modified from O'Rourke PP, Crone RK: The respiratory system. In Gregory GA, editor: *Pediatric anesthesia*, ed 2, New York, 1989, Churchill Livingstone.

The presence of parents during administration of the sedative agent may reduce the stress of the procedure and improve the child's cooperation. However, parents may also be anxious and this can worsen the child's anxiety.[14] Clear, simple, and succinct explanations to both parents and children may minimize adverse behavior. The explanation must be appropriate for the age of the child. For example, telling young children that they are "to be put to sleep" may recall for them what happened to the family pet. Children must also know what will be done when they are sedated and what to expect when they awaken.

Preoperative Fasting

Anesthetic medications have the potential to blunt protective airway reflexes and increase the risk for pulmonary aspiration of gastric contents. This has been reported to be as high as 10 per 10,000 pediatric patients.[15-17] Preoperative fasting guidelines have been established to minimize the risk of aspiration. However, requiring a pediatric patient to fast for an extended period will cause irritability and discomfort and may increase the incidence of hypotension secondary to dehydration.

The patient who has recently ingested food is at risk for both particulate and fluid aspiration, and a 6- to 8-hour fast from solids is recommended to minimize this risk. However, over the past decade there have been numerous reports challenging guidelines for consumption of clear liquids.[18-22]

The risk of aspiration pneumonitis (Mendelson's syndrome) is dependent on both the quantity and acidity of the aspirate. In 1974, published data indicated that the critical volume was more than 0.4 ml/kg and the critical pH less than 2.5.[23] In a subsequent study, it was reported that a volume of 0.8 ml/kg would be necessary to cause aspiration pneumonitis.[24]

Gastric emptying time for clear liquids is approximately 15 minutes. After a 1-hour fast, 80% of consumed clear liquid should be emptied from the stomach. Residual gastric volume after consumption of unlimited amounts of clear liquids has been assessed from 2 to 8 hours prior to surgery. These studies demonstrated that individuals who consumed unlimited volumes of clear liquids up to 2 to 3 hours prior to surgery had gastric residual volumes and pH similar to those who fasted for the more traditional 6 to 8 hours. Therefore, the current recommendation for a healthy, ASA (American Society of Anesthesiologists) class I or II, pediatric patient who will undergo elective surgery is to have no solids by mouth for 6 to 8 hours preoperatively. The child, however, may consume clear liquids up to 2 to 3 hours prior to surgery. Children who are scheduled in the afternoon may have a light breakfast at least 6 hours prior to the operation.

Upper Respiratory Tract Infections

Upper respiratory tract infections (URIs) may produce pathophysiologic changes in the upper and lower airways. Changes include diminished diffusion capacity, increased closing volumes, increased secretions, and airway hyperactivity.[25-27] URIs also have been demonstrated to cause respiratory muscle weakness that can persist for up to 12 days.[28] Increased hyperactivity with associated bronchoconstriction, increased closing volume compounded by an increased oxygen uptake (secondary to the inflammatory response of the infection), and a decreased FRC (that normally occurs with general anesthesia) all increase the risk of hypoxemia during sedation.[29]

URIs are common in pediatric patients. Reports of children arriving for surgery with symptoms of a URI or having had a recent infection are as high as 22.3% and 45.8%, respectively.[30] It is important for the surgeon to distinguish between allergic rhinitis, which is not a contraindication for anesthesia, and a mild URI. While there is no controversy as to whether or not a child with a severe URI (symptoms including a productive cough, fever, and mucopurulent discharge) should be anesthetized, it is unclear as to whether a child with a mild URI can be safely anesthetized or sedated.

There have been numerous reports on the incidence of adverse perioperative respiratory events in patients with a URI. There is an increased incidence of laryngospasm, bronchospasm, and a higher rate of oxygen desaturation.[31-37] Oxygen desaturation has been reported both intraoperatively and postoperatively. (The latter indicates the need for postoperative monitoring.) Other adverse events included increased secretions, breath holding, and severe cough. Children undergoing endotracheal anesthesia have an increased incidence of adverse respiratory events when compared with those anesthetized by face mask or laryngeal mask airway. The increased risk of adverse respiratory events persists for up to 4 to 6 weeks after the URI. Despite this increased incidence of adverse respiratory events, most are not associated with severe morbidity.

It is important to appreciate that traditional office-based ambulatory anesthesia in OMFS is dependent on spontaneous ventilation in the nonintubated patient. Tait and Knight[38] documented no increase in adverse respiratory events in patients who had mask ventilation for myringotomies. While the patient undergoing OMFS may not be intubated, surgery involving the airway has been shown to increase the risk of adverse respiratory events. Although intraoral surgery is not truly airway surgery, it encroaches on the airway and may contribute to airway irritability. The nonintubated OMFS patient is susceptible to periods of hypoventilation and apnea while receiving supplemental oxygen. In conclusion, the patient who arrives for elective surgery with an allergic rhinitis or a mild URI that is not of acute onset may be safely sedated in the office. If the patient has a significant URI, the procedure should be rescheduled. Traditional guidelines suggest that the procedure should be rescheduled 4 to 6 weeks later if the patient is to be intubated. Many healthy children have three to eight URIs per year.[39] If surgery is canceled, it may be difficult to find an opportunity to reschedule it when the child is without symptoms within this 4- to 6-week period. Considering the above knowledge, a period of 2 weeks is probably acceptable for the short office-based minor dentoalveolar procedure in which the patient is not intubated.

DEEP SEDATION TECHNIQUES

It is generally agreed that managing the anxious, uncomfortable, and uncooperative pediatric patient in the office is one of the more challenging tasks for the oral surgeon. The primary goals should be to (1) reduce anxiety, (2) establish cooperation, (3) ensure comfort, (4) produce amnesia, (5) achieve analgesia, and (6) ensure hemodynamic stability. While the goals of sedation are similar for both the child and the adult, reducing anxiety in the child may not establish cooperation. The child may require a greater depth of sedation to achieve cooperation and to facilitate completion of the planned surgical procedure.

Sedation should be accomplished in a nonthreatening manner. Some children exhibit an intense fear of needles. Therefore, establishing intravenous access may be impossible. The surgeon must be familiar with alternative techniques that will allow for a safe, satisfactory induction and recovery from anesthesia. Each child must be considered individually to select both the most appropriate drug and route of administration. The following factors should be considered when developing the anesthetic plan: (1) age of the patient, (2) level of anxiety and ability to cooperate with medical and dental staff, (3) medical history of the patient, (4) patient's prior surgical or anesthetic experience, (5) infringement of the procedure on the airway, and (6) duration of procedure. The selected technique ideally should be painless, accepted by the patient and parents, rapid in onset, appropriate in duration with rapid recovery, and have minimal side effects and a broad margin of safety (Table 7-2).

The benefit of sedation is minimized if administration of the sedative agent is associated with pain or unpleasant memories. The anesthetic must provide an environment in which the procedure can be completed. In certain situations a moderate degree of movement may be acceptable, whereas in other situations no movement is acceptable.

Routes of Administration

Sedative medication can be administered by oral, intranasal, transmucosal, rectal, intramuscular, inhalational, and intravenous routes. The intravenous route results in the most rapid onset, rapid offset, and most predictable effect. The disadvantage in children is the initial requirement of intravenous access. A percentage of pediatric patients will not cooperate with intravenous catheter insertion. Many children report the needle puncture from either intravenous placement or intramuscular injection as the most unpleasant part of the surgical experience.

The inhalational route of induction with a potent anesthetic agent also provides rapid onset, rapid offset, and a predictable effect. The advantage of this technique, similar to that of the intravenous route, is the availability of short-acting agents. This also allows the effect of the anesthetic to be terminated rapidly at the end of the procedure.

The traditional inhalation induction is accomplished by administering oxygen or a mixture of oxygen (minimum concentration of 30%) and nitrous oxide, using a full face mask. The potent vapor agent is increased gradually every few breaths until the induction is complete. For brief procedures (e.g., extraction of a deciduous tooth), the face mask can be removed, the procedure performed, the face mask reapplied, and the patient allowed to awaken breathing 100% oxygen. Administration of a vapor agent using a traditional dental nasal hood provides a significantly diluted concentration of anesthetic agent and potentially results in excessive environmental pollution. Therefore, for longer cases, once a general anesthetic depth is achieved intravenous access should be established.

The vasodilatory effects of the inhalation agent may optimize conditions for establishing intravenous access. Once intravenous access is established, fluids and maintenance intravenous anesthetic agents can be administered. An intravenous line provides the ability to administer intravenous agents for a prolonged surgery, as well as to administer medication to manage a potential adverse event, if either becomes necessary.

There are a few disadvantages to the inhalation technique. The vapor agent has a scent that may be objectionable to some. The odor may be minimized by applying a more pleasant scent to the mask and by reminding the child to breath through the nose.[40] The technique is also dependent on the child accepting a face mask. If physical restraint is necessary, an alternative technique should be considered.

The intramuscular route approximates the rapidity and predictability of onset of intravenous administration. Its primary disadvantage is the discomfort associated with the injection. Four anatomic regions are used for intramuscular administration of drugs (deltoid, vastus

TABLE 7-2   Anesthetic Management of Pediatric Patients

Agent	Technique	Depth of Sedation	Advantages	Complications	Monitoring
Nitrous oxide/ oxygen sedation (nitrous oxide 30%-70%)	Can be administered via a nasal hood or full face mask. The advantage of the full face mask is the achievement of a greater percentage of inhaled nitrous oxide. The mask is removed only for injection of local anesthetic and the brief surgical procedure.	Anxiolysis and sedation. A small percentage of individuals become profoundly sedated from higher concentrations of nitrous oxide.	In a young child maximal effect for very brief procedures is achieved with a full face mask. Administration of N2O 70% with oxygen 30% via a nasal hood is effective for a mildly anxious adolescent presenting for extraction of premolars.	Concentrations higher than 50% have increasing emetic effects. However, when used as a sole agent, it does not require dietary restrictions. Potentiates the sedative effects of other anesthetic agents.	As a sole agent no monitoring is required. In conjunction with other agents, pulse oximetry should be used.
Oral midazolam	Recommended dose is 0.5 mg/kg, up to a maximum 20 mg dose. The drug should be administered in the office.	Anxiolysis and sedation. The onset of effect occurs in about 20 minutes. Working time lasts for about 20 minutes.	Oral midazolam provides a greater anesthetic depth than nitrous oxide. It can provide adequate anxiolysis and sedation for a brief procedure (15 minutes) in a mildly anxious child. A more profound anesthetic depth can be achieved with the co-administration of nitrous oxide. Oral midazolam can also be administered as a premedicant before establishing intravenous access.	Relaxation of upper airway musculature can result in airway obstruction. Airway reflexes can be compromised, and the patient should be npo.	Pulse oximetry should be used from the time the drug is administered until the patient is considered stable for discharge.
Oral ketamine	Recommended dose is 6-10 mg/kg. Its primary advantage is when inhalation and intramuscular techniques are	Ketamine establishes a cataleptic state that is different from both sedation and general anesthesia. As a sole	Onset of sedation is achieved in about 20 minutes. A 6 mg/kg dose provides a mean working period of about	The sympathetic effect of ketamine may potentially cause tachycardia and hypertension. Postoperatively it may be	Pulse oximetry should be used to follow both oxygen saturation and heart rate. Blood pressure.

TABLE 7-2   Anesthetic Management of Pediatric Patients—cont'd

Agent	Technique	Depth of Sedation	Advantages	Complications	Monitoring
	not options in gaining control of the patient.	agent administered orally in lower doses that will facilitate early discharge, it may not be as effective as midazolam. Its primary advantage (alone or with midazolam) is its ability to "immobilize" the patient.	30-40 minutes. Mean recovery time is about 60 minutes. However, recovery is variable and may last a few hours. Higher doses that provide longer working times may have excessively long recovery periods. For an older, stronger, or mentally impaired patient in which the patient will not allow other routes of induction, oral ketamine establishes a dissociative state.	associated with hallucinations, as well as nausea and vomiting. Unlike other anesthetic agents it maintains airway patency and airway reflexes as well as FRC. Increased salivation.	
Intramuscular ketamine	Recommended dose is 2-5 mg/kg with or without midazolam 0.05 mg/kg. An antisial-agogue is frequently co-administered. Glycopyrrolate is advantageous in that it produces less tachycardia. If intravenous access is to be established, consideration should be given to administering the antisialagogue intravenously, which will achieve a more rapid effect.	The lower dose establishes a dissociative sedative/analgesic state, compared with a dissociative anesthetic state established after the administration of the higher dose.	Onset occurs within 3-5 minutes. The technique is advantageous for an uncooperative child in whom a mask induction is not an option. A dose of 2 mg/kg sedates the patient but requires the practitioner to tolerate some movement and vocalization. Recovery, however, is more predictable, with the ability to discharge the patient in about 60 minutes from time of injection.	The technique requires an injection. The injection is only mildly uncomfortable, and induction follows rapidly.	Pulse oximetry, blood pressure, and ECG.

continued

TABLE 7-2   Anesthetic Management of Pediatric Patients—cont'd

Agent	Technique	Depth of Sedation	Advantages	Complications	Monitoring
Sevoflurane	MAC: 2.05	Induction can be achieved by incrementally increasing the percentage of sevoflurane administered or by administering 8%. The administration of N2O with sevoflurane does not alter MAC of sevoflurane to the degree that occurs with the co-administration of nitrous oxide with halothane.	Provides rapid induction. After the patient is asleep, a redistribution of the drug may result in a lightening of the anesthetic depth. This may occur if the percentage of sevoflurane administered is too rapidly decreased. Establishing intravenous access is recommended after induction. For all but brief procedures, anesthetic maintenance should be with intravenous drugs.	Excessive force is necessary to restrain an individual who is uncooperative. This creates more of a problem in an older child. Loss of airway in a patient who is anesthetized without intravenous access. Maintenance of an excessively high dose results in myocardial depression.	Pulse oximetry, blood pressure, and ECG.

lateralis, gluteus maximus muscles, and ventrogluteal area). These sites are preferred because they have minimal numbers of both nerves and large blood vessels, and adequate bulk to accommodate the volume of injected drug. The rapidity of absorption and onset of action of the drug is dependent upon the perfusion of the muscle.

Oral administration is considered by many to be the least threatening, because children (including mentally impaired and autistic patients) are familiar with taking medications orally. However, this technique has significant limitations. In one study of children 20 to 48 months of age, one third of patients required medication to be administered into the back of the throat with a needle-free syringe.[41] An oral sedative agent also can be used as a premedication to help establish intravenous access or prior to inducing deep sedation by a different route (e.g., inhalation or intramuscular). The limited volume of fluid administered with oral medication is not associated with an increased risk for aspiration pneumonitis.[42]

The primary disadvantage of oral sedation is the slow onset, variable response, and prolonged recovery. An oral sedative should not be given to a young child in a car seat prior to arrival in the office. The respiratory depressant effect of the medication, combined with the positioning of the unattended child in the car, can result in unrecognized upper airway obstruction or respiratory impairment, with resultant death or significant neurologic impairment.[43] Injecting a sedative agent into the back of the throat with a needle-free syringe also has been associated with adverse consequences. It has been theorized that the drug intended for orogastric administration can be aspirated by a crying child, with bronchial absorption resulting in an excessive plasma level of the drug.

Intranasal administration of a medication may result in a rapid rise in the plasma level of the drug. The nasal mucosa is relatively thin and has an abundance of capillaries and an extensive surface area. Once the drug is absorbed through the nasal mucosa, it avoids first-pass hepatic degradation. Furthermore, the nasal mucosa provides a direct connection to the central nervous system through the cribriform plate. Medication may be absorbed through the cribriform plate directly into the central nervous system through the capillary beds, the olfactory neurons, or directly into the cerebrospinal fluid.[44] Intranasal administration provides a more rapid onset than either oral or rectal administration.[45] However, this route of administration may be less effective in an individual with a URI or allergic rhinitis.[46]

The intranasal route initially was proposed for pediatric sedation because some felt that it would be less traumatic than the alternatives. However, the intranasal route frequently is not well accepted by children because a portion of the volume is often swallowed, thus producing the same unpleasant taste as oral administration. Midazolam, the most common, intranasally administered medication, has an acidic pH resulting in nasal mucosal irritation.

Transmucosal administration has also been considered, although this requires cooperation of the patient to keep the drug in contact with the oral mucosa. This route produces rapid onset due to the rich mucosal blood supply. The medication may be administered as a solution placed sublingually or as a lozenge. The lozenge should be held against the buccal mucosa because this promotes better absorption than is achieved from under the tongue.[47] Currently, the only commercially available lozenge with an acceptable flavor is fentanyl citrate.

The rectal route has been used for the administration of antiemetics, antipyretics, and analgesics to both adults and pediatric patients. Many sedative drugs administered either intravenously or orally can be administered rectally. Rectal administration may also be used in the management of emergencies. For example, rectal administration of diazepam is an acceptable alternative route for the treatment of seizures.

The absorption of a drug that is administered per rectum is affected by several factors including the venous drainage of the rectum, exact location of agent deposition, and type of agent (solution, suppository). Stool within the rectal vault and expulsion of drug result in delayed or decreased absorption. An uncooperative child may close the anal sphincter tightly during the administration process.

Pharmacologic Agents: Ketamine

Ketamine is a unique pharmacologic agent that produces a dissociation between the thalamoneocortical and limbic systems. This dissociation interrupts the brain from interpreting visual, auditory, or painful stimuli.[48] A state that resembles catalepsy is induced, in which the patient may appear awake but is noncommunicative. The eyes are open, with a blank nystagmic stare and with intact corneal and light reflexes.[49] Increased skeletal muscle tone may result in nonpurposeful skeletal muscle movement. Ketamine produces amnesia and intense analgesia, which is mediated partially by ketamine binding to the μ-opioid receptors.[50] The analgesic effects of ketamine are present at subanesthetic plasma levels and persist into the postoperative period, potentially decreasing the need for postoperative analgesia.

Ketamine may stimulate dreams and hallucinations. These have been described as "out-of-body" experiences, sensation of floating, and delirium.[51] They may occur as a misinterpretation of the visual and auditory stimuli. The incidence is zero to 10% in children.[52,53] Co-administration of a benzodiazepine decreases the incidence of emergence phenomenon.

Ketamine has several advantageous respiratory effects. In the usual clinical dosages, respiratory impairment is rare. Upper airway muscle tone, which frequently is decreased by other anesthetic agents, is preserved, minimizing the risk of upper airway obstruction.[54] In contrast to most other agents, FRC is also preserved.[55] This maintains pulmonary oxygen reserve and minimizes the potential for ventilation-perfusion abnormalities that result in hypoxia. Although respiratory depression can occur with the administration of ketamine,[56] slow intravenous infusion over 30 to 60 seconds, using dosages between 0.5 to 1.0 mg/kg, should minimize this complication.

The pharyngeal and laryngeal protective airway reflexes are better maintained with ketamine than with most other anesthetic agents. Preservation of these reflexes allows patients to maintain the ability to swallow and cough. This provides protection against, but does not totally eliminate the possibility of, pulmonary aspiration.[57,58] On the other hand, ketamine stimulates salivary and tracheobronchial secretions and may predispose the patient to laryngospasm.[59,60] Ketamine produces sympathetic stimulation and is considered beneficial in the management of the asthmatic patient. It has been shown to relax bronchial smooth muscle and cause bronchial dilation.[61,62] The cardiovascular effects of this sympathetic stimulation are an increase in blood pressure and heart rate. However, children generally manifest minimal changes in blood pressure with more pronounced changes in heart rate.

Ketamine can be administered intravenously, intramuscularly, orally, intranasally, and rectally. When administered by the intramuscular route, onset occurs within 3 to 5 minutes. One investigation prospectively assessed pediatric patients requiring sedation for procedures in the emergency department. A dose of 4 mg/kg ketamine used in conjunction with local anesthesia was effective for 93.5% of the children. The working time achieved from a 4 mg/kg dose can last from 15 to 30 minutes.[63] A disadvantage of intramuscular ketamine is that recovery is variable and can be quite long.

Benzodiazepines are at times administered along with ketamine. The premise for the co-administration of a benzodiazepine is to reduce the amount of ketamine required, reduce the incidence of ketamine-induced hallucinations, attenuate the cardiovascular effects of ketamine, and provide more amnesia.[64-66]

Co-administration of a benzodiazepine and ketamine may prolong recovery.[67] In a prospective investigation ketamine 3 mg/kg with midazolam 0.5 mg/kg was administered to pediatric patients requiring sedation for minor surgical procedures in the emergency department.[68] Thirty percent of the pediatric patients who received this dosing regimen manifested "intermittent crying or fighting." Of these patients, however, only 14% required additional medication to establish a satisfactory anesthetic state.

The level of sedation and immobilization is dependent on the planned procedure. While the intent is to provide an atraumatic experience for the child, a dissociative sedative and analgesic state, rather than a dissociative anesthetic state, may be acceptable for a brief dentoalveolar procedure. The intent is to modify the patient's perception of the procedure. In this situation the patient will not be profoundly sedated, and the practitioner will have to tolerate some movement and possibly some vocalization. Ketamine 2 to 3 mg/kg given intramuscularly should provide this desirable behavioral sedative depth. It has been reported that ketamine 3 mg/kg given intramuscularly was successful 99% of the time in allowing a minor procedure to be completed.[69] The lower dosage of 2 mg/kg is advantageous in that recovery from injection to discharge approximates 60 minutes. If a satisfactory sedative depth is not achieved, additional intramuscular ketamine can be administered. Alternatively, for many children the low-dose intramuscular ketamine achieves a depth of sedation that allows the placement of an intravenous line. The depth of sedation can then be modified using intravenous medications. In one study it was reported that 31% of children resisted intravenous placement with a dosage of 3 mg/kg.[70]

When intravenous access is established, incremental doses of ketamine, 5 to 10 mg, can be administered to the sedated patient. Onset occurs within 30 to 60 seconds. Duration of sedation is from 10 to 15 minutes. A dose of ketamine 0.5 to 1.0 mg/kg administered over 60 seconds will establish dissociation in the patient who has not been premedicated.

An anticholinergic agent (e.g., glycopyrrolate or atropine) frequently is administered with ketamine to decrease hypersalivation. Tachycardia and postoperative psychomimetic effects are problems associated with ketamine, and atropine combined with ketamine does produce a significantly higher heart rate when compared with ketamine and glycopyrrolate. However, the incidence of adverse emergence phenomenon was found to be similar with either glycopyrrolate or atropine.[71,72] Both drugs can be mixed in the same syringe with ketamine for an intramuscular injection.

Ketamine can also be administered orally.[73] Bioavailability is approximately 17% following oral administration, compared with 93% after intramuscular administration.[74,75] Onset of sedation occurs in approximately 20 minutes. While dosages reported have ranged from 3 to 10 mg/kg, a more consistent effect is achieved with dosages larger than 6 mg/kg.[76] The mean sedation time achieved after orally administered ketamine 6 mg/kg is 30 to 40 minutes. The combination of oral midazolam and ketamine also has been described. This drug combination may provide effective sedation when oral midazolam alone has been ineffective. One study that demonstrated a greater efficacy with this combination used ketamine 4 mg/kg with midazolam 0.4 mg/kg.[77] The reported dosing regimens have varied from ketamine 4 to 10 mg/kg with midazolam 0.25 to 0.5 mg/kg.

Situations may occur in the management of a mentally impaired patient, autistic patient, or an older child in which an intravenous line cannot be inserted, an intramuscular injection cannot be administered without harm to the patient or the healthcare provider, or the patient will not accept a face mask. Oral ketamine alone or combined with oral midazolam will establish a cataleptic state facilitating treatment of the combative patient.[78,79] When administering the medication, it may be advantageous for you or the child's escort to drink a similar-appearing liquid to reassure the child.

Pharmacologic Agents: Midazolam

Midazolam is a water-soluble, short-acting benzodiazepine. As a class, the benzodiazepines provide anxiolysis, sedation, and amnesia. Midazolam can be administered intravenously, intramuscularly, orally, sublingually, intranasally, or rectally. Because of its water solubility, in contrast to diazepam, intramuscular injection of midazolam is pain free and absorption is predictable.

Oral midazolam is probably the most widely used premedication in children. The recommended dosage is 0.5 to 1.0 mg/kg, with a maximum of 20 mg. Seventy to eighty percent of patients who receive midazolam 0.5 mg/kg will achieve anxiolysis. The anesthetic depth may be potentiated by the administration of nitrous oxide. The combined administration of 40% nitrous oxide with midazolam 0.5 mg/kg produces deep sedation in 12% of patients.[80]

Midazolam causes loss of airway muscle tone. Although airway obstruction is not common with dosages of 0.5 to 1.0 mg/kg, airway obstruction has been reported after 0.5 mg/kg of oral midazolam.[81] The incidence of airway obstruction may increase with the administration of nitrous oxide. In one study there was a 56% incidence of upper airway obstruction in children with enlarged tonsils with the combined administration of 50% nitrous oxide and 0.5 mg/kg of oral midazolam.[82] With mechanical or positional maintenance of airway patency, however, oral midazolam dosages of 0.5 to 0.75 mg/kg generally do not result in a change in oxygen saturation, heart rate, or blood pressure.[83]

The onset of effect of oral midazolam is within 20 minutes and sedation lasts for 20 to 40 minutes. Patients generally can be discharged within 60 to 90 minutes from the time of administration of the drug.

Midazolam is metabolized by the cytochrome oxidase system. Oral midazolam is subject to hepatic first-pass metabolism. An alteration in this system results in a higher and more sustained midazolam plasma level. Erythromycin, protease inhibitors, and grapefruit juice alter this cytochrome oxidase system.[84,85]

Higher dosages of oral midazolam (0.75 to 1.0 mg/kg) are associated with a greater incidence of side effects. These include loss of head control, blurred vision, and dysphoria. A paradoxical reaction may also occur, in which the patient becomes more excited as opposed to sedated. This is more common in children and adolescents than in adults.[86]

Inhalational Agents

The ideal properties of an inhalational agent include sufficient potency, pleasant or no odor, limited cardiorespiratory effects, low blood and tissue solubility, and lack of organ toxicity. The primary benefit of an inhalational agent in the pediatric patient is the ability to use mask induction. The suitability of the agent for inhalational mask induction is dependent on a lack of pungent odor and sufficient potency. Of the available agents, nitrous oxide, halothane, and sevoflurane have a pleasant odor. An awake child usually will tolerate breathing these agents with minimal respiratory complications (e.g., coughing, breath-holding, laryngospasm).[87-89]

Nitrous oxide has anxiolytic, analgesic, amnestic, and sedative effects.[90,91] Nitrous oxide, while not a potent anesthetic agent, possesses a wide margin of safety and has few (if any) residual side effects. An advantage of nitrous oxide is its low solubility, which allows rapid equilibration between the pulmonary alveoli and the blood and the blood and the brain. This results in both rapid onset and anesthetic emergence.

Nitrous oxide may also be combined with other anesthetic agents. A deep sedative or general anesthetic state may be established by administration of nitrous oxide and an oral or parenteral agent. While nitrous oxide may potentiate the effect of another simultaneously administered agent, its low solubility provides rapid reversal and promotes a rapid emergence.[92-94]

While nitrous oxide lacks sufficient potency to induce general anesthesia, both halothane (minimum alveolar concentration [MAC], 0.77) and sevoflurane (MAC, 2.05) have sufficient potency to be used for mask induction of general anesthesia. All potent inhalational agents depress ventilation in a dose-dependent manner. This is seen clinically as a decrease in minute ventilation with a resultant increase in $Paco_2$. The change in minute ventilation is a consequence of a decrease in tidal volume. A slight increase in respiratory rate may occur. Halothane produces less respiratory depression than sevoflurane.[95] Acceptable respiratory parameters during spontaneous ventilation, however, can be maintained with all inhalational agents. All inhalational agents produce bronchial dilation and are advantageous in the management of the patient with bronchospastic disease.

The inhalational agents have cardiovascular depressant effects. Halothane produces the most myocardial depression, causing hypotension and bradycardia. The most problematic cardiovascular effect of halothane is that it sensitizes the heart to catecholamines, with resultant dysrhythmias. One study reported that 48% of the pediatric patients anesthetized with halothane had arrhythmias compared with 16% of the pediatric patients given 8% sevoflurane. Patients who had an incremental induction of sevoflurane had even fewer arrhythmias. Ventricular arrhythmias accounted for 40% of the arrhythmias in the children who received halothane and 1% of the arrhythmias in the children who received sevoflurane.[96] The common ventricular arrhythmias occurring with halothane included ventricular tachycardia, bigeminy, and couplets. Arrhythmias with sevoflurane usually included single ventricular ectopic beats.

Epinephrine contained in the local anesthetic solution has the potential to induce arrhythmias in patients receiving potent inhalational anesthetic agents. However, halothane is the only inhalational agent that is associated with arrhythmias when using clinical dosages of local anesthesia with epinephrine. A limit of 1.0 µg/kg of epinephrine in patients receiving halothane is recommended.[97-99]

Speed of induction and emergence from anesthesia are important criteria for ambulatory surgery. For an inhalational anesthetic agent, these properties are related to its blood and tissue solubility. Agents that have a low solubility in blood should have a more rapid induction and shorter emergence time. The blood gas solubility coefficients of desflurane, nitrous oxide, sevoflurane, isoflurane, and halothane are 0.42, 0.47, 0.6, 1.4, and 2.3, respectively.

Recovery from anesthesia is also dependent on the duration of the anesthetic. Sevoflurane has been shown, although not consistently, to be associated with a more rapid anesthetic emergence after intermediate-duration and long-duration anesthetics when compared with halothane. However, a typical office anesthetic for a pediatric dental procedure is brief, lasting less than 10 minutes. Clinical studies comparing sevoflurane and halothane for pediatric dental extractions lasting from 4 to 6 minutes have not demonstrated a more rapid recovery with sevoflurane. In one study in which children were subjected to a 4-minute anesthetic duration, time to eye opening was 102 seconds with halothane and 167 seconds with sevoflurane.[100,101]

The last factor that should be considered in selecting an anesthetic agent for the office is the toxicity of each drug. Halothane is metabolized in the liver to a trifluoroacetylated product, which binds liver proteins, promoting an immunologic response resulting in hepatic injury.[102,103] The incidence, which may be as high as 1 in 6,000 anesthetized adults, is significantly lower in the pediatric population. Sevoflurane, however, has been associated with potential renal toxicity.[104,105] First the drug undergoes hepatic metabolism, producing inorganic fluoride. The production of the fluoride within the liver (in contrast to methoxyflurane, which is metabolized in the kidneys), as well as the rapid elimination of sevoflurane, minimizes the renal fluoride exposure. This probably accounts for the lack of clinical renal dysfunction, despite some studies reporting patients with serum fluoride levels greater than 50 µmol/L. Renal injury also has been associated with the formation of compound A, which is a product of the reaction between sevoflurane and carbon dioxide absorbents. Most of the data, however, suggest that compound A does not induce renal toxicity in humans.

Halothane has for years provided the anesthetist with an agent that facilitated mask induction in the pediatric patient. However, the drug is associated with arrhythmias, and the incidence of halothane hepatitis is not fully known in the pediatric population. Sevoflurane, introduced in 1995 in North America, is an agent that is comparable in its ability to facilitate mask induction. Importantly, the agent is without known toxicity and is not associated with potentially lethal arrhythmias. It has, therefore, become the drug of choice for office pediatric anesthesia.

CONCLUSION

In this chapter we have suggested guidelines for pediatric office deep sedation and anesthesia. It should be emphasized that any surgeon undertaking such management in children must be familiar with and comfortable managing pediatric emergencies and pediatric resuscitation. Proper pediatric monitoring devices should be used and the surgeon should always keep in mind the much smaller margin for error in children.

REFERENCES

1. Alen NA, Rowbotham DJ, Nimmo WS: Hypoxemia during outpatient anaesthesia, *Anaesthesia* 61:498P, 1988.
2. Bone ME, Galler D, Flynn PJ: Arterial oxygen saturation during general anaesthesia for paediatric dental extractions, *Anaesthesia* 42:879, 1987.
3. Takahashi E, Atsumi H: Age differences in thoracic form as indicated by thoracic index, *Hum Biol* 27:65, 1955.
4. Davies G, Reid L: Growth of the alveoli and pulmonary arteries in childhood, *Thorax* 25:669, 1970.
5. Dunnil MS: Postnatal growth of the lung, *Thorax* 17:329, 1962.

6. Thurlbeck WM: Postnatal human lung growth, *Thorax* 37:564, 1982.

7. Gerhardt T, Reifenberg L, Hehre D, et al: Functional residual capacity in normal neonates and children up to 5 years of age determined by a N2 washout method, *Pediatr Res* 20:668, 1986.

8. Benumof JL, Dagg R, Benumof R: Critical hemoglobin desaturation will occur before return to an unparalyzed state following 1 mg/kg intravenous succinylcholine, *Anesthesiology* 87:979, 1997.

9. Kinouchi K, Fukumitsu K, Tashiro C, et al: Duration of apnoea in anaesthetized children required for desaturation of haemoglobin to 95%: comparison of three different breathing gases, *Pediatr Anaesth* 5:115, 1995.

10. Xue FS, Luo LK, Tong SY, et al: Study of the safe threshold of apneic period in children during anesthesia induction, *J Clin Anesth* 8:568, 1996.

11. Farmery AD, Roe PG: A model to describe the rate of oxy-haemoglobin desaturation during apnoea, *Br J Anaesth* 76:284, 1996.

12. Keenan RL, Shapiro JH, Kane FR, et al: Bradycardia during anesthesia in infants: an epidemiologic study, *Anesthesiology* 80:976, 1994.

13. Pang LM, Liu LMP, Cote CJ: Premedication and induction of anesthesia. In Cote CJ, Todres ID, Goudsouzian NG, Ryan JF, editors: *A practice of anesthesia for infants and children*, ed 3. Philadelphia, 2001, WB Saunders.

14. Kain ZN, Mayes LC, O'Connor TZ, et al: Preoperative anxiety in children: predictors and outcomes, *Arch Pediatr Adolesc Med* 150:1238, 1996.

15. Borland LM, Sereika SM, Woelfel SK, et al: Pulmonary aspiration in pediatric patients during general anesthesia: incidence and outcome, *J Clin Anesth* 10:95, 1998.

16. Olsson GL, Hallen B, Hambraeus-Jonzon K: Aspiration during anesthesia: a computer aided study of 185,358 anesthetics, *Acta Anaesthesiol Scand* 30:84, 1986.

17. Tiret L, Nivoche Y, Hatton F, et al: Complications related to anaesthesia in infants and children: a prospective survey of 40,240 anaesthetics, *Br J Anaesth* 61:263, 1988.

18. Maekawa N, Mikawa K, Yaku H, et al: Effects of two-, four-, and twelve-hour fasting intervals on preoperative gastric fluid pH and volume, and plasma glucose and lipid homeostasis in children, *Acta Anaesthesiol Scand* 37:783, 1993.

19. Splinter WM, Stewart JA, Muir JG: The effect of preoperative apple juice on gastric contents, thirst, and hunger in children, *Can J Anaesth* 36:55, 1989.

20. Splinter WM, Stewart JA, Muir JG: Large volumes of apple juice preoperatively do not affect gastric pH and volume in children, *Can J Anaesth* 37:36, 1990.

21. Splinter WM, Schaefer JD, Zunder IH: Clear fluids three hours before surgery do not affect the gastric fluid contents of children, *Can J Anaesth* 37:498, 1990.

22. Splinter WM, Schaefer JD: Ingestion of clear fluids is safe for adolescents up to three hours before anesthesia, *Br J Anaesth* 66:48, 1991.

23. Roberts R, Shirley M: Reducing the risk of acid aspiration during cesarean section, *Anesth Analg* 53:859, 1974.

24. Raidoo DM, Marszalek A, Brock-Utne JG: Acid aspiration in primates (a surprising experimental result), *Anaesth Intensive Care* 16:375, 1988.

25. Cate TR, Roberts TS, Russ MA, et al: Effect of common cold on pulmonary function, *Am Rev Respir Dis* 108:858, 1973.

26. Fridy WW Jr, Ingram RH Jr, Hierholzer JC, et al: Airway function during mild viral respiratory illnesses, *Ann Intern Med* 80:150, 1974.

27. Horner GJ, Gray FD Jr: Effect of uncomplicated, presumptive influenza on the diffusion capacity of the lung, *Am Rev Respir Dis* 108:866, 1973.

28. Mier-Jedrzejowicz A, Brophy C, Green M: Respiratory muscle weakness during upper respiratory tract infections, *Am Rev Respir Dis* 138:5, 1988.

29. Dueck R, Prutow R, Richman D: Effect of parainfluenza infection on gas exchange and FRC response to anesthesia in sheep, *Anesthesiology* 74:1044, 1991.

30. Parnis SJ, Barker DS, Van Der Walt JH: Clinical predictors of anaesthetic complications in children with respiratory tract infections, *Paediatr Anesth* 11:29, 2001.

31. Cohen MM, Cameron CB: Should you cancel the operation when a child has an upper respiratory tract infection? *Anesth Analg* 72:282, 1991.

32. DeSoto H, Patel RI, Soliman IE, et al: Changes in oxygen saturation following general anesthesia in children with upper respiratory infection signs and symptoms undergoing otolaryngological procedures, *Anesthesiology* 68:276, 1988.

33. Levy L, Pandit UA, Randel GI, et al: Upper respiratory tract infections and general anaesthesia in children: perioperative complications and oxygen saturation, *Anaesthesia* 47:678, 1992.

34. Olsson GL, Hallen B: Laryngospasm during anesthesia: a computer-aided incidence study in 136,929 patients, *Acta Anaesthesiol Scand* 28:567, 1984.

35. Olsson GL: Bronchospasm during anesthesia: a computer aided incidence study of 136,929 patients, *Acta Anaesthesiol Scand* 31:244, 1987.

36. Tait AR, Reynolds PI, Gutstein HB: Factors that influence an anesthesiologist's decision to cancel elective surgery for the child with an upper respiratory tract infection, *J Clin Anesth* 7:491, 1995.

37. Tait AR, Malviya S, Voepel-Lewis T, et al: Risk factors for perioperative adverse respiratory events in children with upper respiratory tract infections, *Anesthesiology* 95:299, 2001.

38. Tait AR, Knight PR: The effects of general anesthesia on upper respiratory tract infections in children, *Anesthesiology* 67:930, 1987.

39. Martin LD: Anesthetic implications of an upper respiratory infection in children, *Pediatr Clin North Am* 41:121, 1994.

40. Pang LM, Liu LMP, Cote CJ: Premedication and induction of anesthesia. In Cote CJ, Todres ID, Goudsouzian NG, Ryan JF, editors: *A practice of anesthesia for infants and children*, ed 3. Philadelphia, 2001, WB Saunders.

41. Badalaty MM, Houpt MI, Koenigsberg SR, et al: A comparison of chloral hydrate and diazepam sedation in young children, *Pediatr Dent* 12:33, 1990.

42. Brzustowicz RM, Nelson DA, Betts EK, et al: Efficacy of oral premedication for pediatric outpatient surgery, *Anesthesiology* 60:475, 1984.

43. Cote CJ, Notterman DA, Karl HW, et al: Adverse sedation events in pediatrics: a critical incidence analysis of contributing factors, *Pediatrics* 107(6):1494, 2001.

44. Hilger PA: *Fundamentals of otolaryngology, a textbook of ear, nose, and throat disease*, ed 6. Philadelphia, 1989, WB Saunders.

45. Malinovsky JM, Populaire C, Cozian A, et al: Premedication with midazolam in children: effect of intranasal, rectal, and oral routes on plasma midazolam concentrations, *Anesthesia* 50:351, 1995.

46. Walbergh EJ, Wills RJ, Eckhert J: Plasma concentrations of midazolam in children following intranasal administration, *Anesthesiology* 74:233, 1991.

47. Harris D, Robinson JR: Drug delivery via the mucosa membranes of the oral cavity, *J Pharm Sci* 81:1, 1991.

48. Kitahata LM, Taub A, Kosaka Y: Lamina specific suppression of dorsal-horn unit activity by ketamine hydrochloride, *Anesthesiology* 38:4, 1973.

49. White PF, Way WL, Trevor AJ: Ketamine—its pharmacology and therapeutic uses, *Anesthesiology* 56:116, 1982.

50. Smith DJ, Bouchal RL, deSanctic CA, et al: Properties of the interaction between ketamine and opiate binding sites in vivo and in vitro, *Neuropharmacology* 26:1253, 1987.

51. White PF, Ham J, Way WL: Pharmacology of ketamine isomers in surgical patients, *Anesthesiology* 52:231, 1980.

52. Hollister GR, Burn JMB: Side effects of ketamine in pediatric-anesthesia, *Anesth Analg* 53:264, 1974.

53. Meyers EF, Charles P: Prolonged adverse reactions to ketamine in children, *Anesthesiology* 49:39, 1978.

54. Drummond GB: Comparison of sedation with midazolam and ketamine: effects on airway muscle activity, *Br J Anaesth* 76:663, 1996.

55. Shulman D, Beardsmore CS, Aronson HB, et al: The effect of ketamine on the functional residual capacity in young children, *Anesthesiology* 62:551, 1985.

56. Smith JA, Santer LJ: Respiratory arrest following intramuscular ketamine injection in a 4-year-old child, *Ann Emerg Med* 22:613, 1993.

57. Carson IW, Moore J, Balmer JP, et al: Laryngeal competence with ketamine and other drugs, *Anesthesiology* 38:128, 1973.

58. Penrose BH: Aspiration pneumonitis following ketamine induction for general anesthesia, *Anesth Analg* 51:41, 1972.

59. Green SM, Johnson NE: Ketamine sedation for pediatric procedures: part 2, review and implications, *Ann Emerg Med* 19:1033, 1990.

60. Olsson GL, Hallen B: Laryngospasm during anaesthesia: a computer-aided incidence study in 136,929 patients, *Acta Anaesthesiol Scand* 28:567, 1984.

61. Corssen G, Gutierrez J, Reves JG, et al: Ketamine in the anesthetic management of asthmatic patients, *Anesth Analg* 51:588, 1972.

62. Strube PJ, Hallam PL: Ketamine by continuous infusion in status asthmaticus, *Anaesthesia* 41:1017, 1986.

63. Green SM, Nakamura R, Johnson NE: Ketamine sedation for pediatric procedures: part 1, a prospective study, *Ann Emerg Med* 19:1024, 1990.

64. Jackson APF, Dhadphale PR, Callaghan ML: Haemodynamic studies during induction of anaesthesia for open-heart surgery using diazepam and ketamine, *Br J Anaesth* 50:375, 1978.

65. White PF: Pharmacological interactions of midazolam and ketamine in surgical patients, *Clin Pharmacol Ther* 31:280, 1982.

66. Cartwright PD, Pingel SM: Midazolam and diazepam in ketamine anaesthesia, *Anaesthesia* 39:439, 1984.

67. Reich DL, Silvay G: Ketamine: an update on the first twenty-five years of clinical experience, *Can J Anaesthsiol* 35:186, 1989.

68. Pruitt JW, Goldwasser MS, Sabol SR, et al: Intramuscular ketamine, midazolam, and glycopyrrolate for pediatric sedation in the emergency department, *J Oral Maxillofac Surg* 53:13, 1995.

69. Epstein FB: Ketamine dissociative sedation in pediatric emergency medical practice, *Am J Emerg Med* 11:180, 1993.

70. Ryhanen P, Kangas T, Rantakla S: Premedication for outpatient adenoidectomy: comparison between ketamine and pethidine, *Laryngoscope* 90:494, 1980.

71. Morgensen F, Muller D, Valentin N: Glycopyrrolate during ketamine/diazepam anaesthesia: a double-blind comparison with atropine, *Acta Anaesthesiol Scand* 30:332, 1986.

72. Toft P, Romer UD: Glycopyrrolate compared with atropine in association with ketamine anaesthesia, *Acta Anaesthesiol Scand* 31:438, 1987.

73. Qureshi FA, Mellis PT, McFadden MA: Efficacy of oral ketamine for providing sedation and analgesia to children requiring laceration repair, *Pediatr Emerg Care* 11:93, 1995.

74. Grant IS, Nimmo WS, McNichol LR, et al: Ketamine disposition in children and adults, *Br J Anaesth* 55:1107, 1983.

75. Grant IS, Nimmo WS, Clements JA: Pharmacokinetics and analgesic effect of IM and oral ketamine, *Br J Anaesth* 53:805, 1981.

76. Alfonzo-Echeverri EC, Berg JH, Wild TW, et al: Oral ketamine for pediatric dental surgery sedation, *Pediatr Dent* 15:182, 1993.

77. Warner DL, Cabaret J, Velling D: Ketamine plus midazolam, a most effective paediatric oral premedicant, *Paediatr Anaesth* 2:293, 1995.

78. Rosenberg M: Oral ketamine for deep sedation of difficult-to-manage children who are mentally handicapped: case report, *Pediatr Dent* 13:221, 1991.

79. Rainey L, van der Walt JH: The anaesthetic management of autistic children, *Anaesth Intensive Care* 26:686, 1998.

80. Litman RS, Kottra JA, Berkowitz RJ, et al: Breathing patterns and levels of consciousness in children during administration of nitrous oxide after oral midazolam premedication, *J Oral Maxillofac Surg* 55:1372, 1997.

81. Litman RS: Airway obstruction after oral midazolam, *Anesthesiology* 85:1217, 1996.

82. Litman RS, Kottra JA, Berkowitz RJ, et al: Upper airway obstruction during midazolam/nitrous oxide sedation in children with enlarged tonsils, *Pediatr Dent* 20:318, 1998.

83. McMillan CO, Spahr SI, Sikich N, et al: Premedication of children with oral midazolam, 39:545, 1992.

84. Hiller A, Olkkola KT, Isohanni P, et al: Unconsciousness associated with midazolam and erythromycin, *Br J Anaesth* 65:826, 1994.

85. Bailey DG, Malcolm J, Arnold O, et al: Grapefruit juice–drug interactions, *Br J Clin Pharmacol* 46:101, 1998.

86. van der Bijl P, Roelofse JA: Disinhibitory reactions to benzodiazepines: a review, *J Oral Maxillofac Surg* 49(5):519-523, 1991.

87. Epstein RH, Stein AL, Marr AT, et al: High concentration versus incremental induction of anesthesia with sevoflurane in children: a comparison of induction times, vital signs, and complications, *J Clin Anesth* 10:41, 1998.

88. Kern C, Erb T, Frei FJ: Haemodynamic responses to sevoflurane compared with halothane during inhalational induction in children, *Paediatr Anaesth* 7:439, 1997.

89. Sigston PE, Jenkins AM, Jackson EC, et al: Rapid inhalation induction in children: 8% sevoflurane compared to 5% halothane, *Br J Anaesth* 78:362, 1997.

90. Jastak JT, Donaldson D: Nitrous oxide, *Anesth Prog* 38:142, 1991.

91. Kaufman E, Chastain DC, Gaughan AM, et al: Staircase assessment of the magnitude and time course of 50% nitrous oxide analgesia, *J Dent Res* 71:1598, 1992.

92. Litman RS, Berkowitz RJ, Ward DS: Levels of consciousness and ventilatory parameters in young children during sedation with oral midazolam and nitrous oxide, *Arch Pediatr Adolesc Med* 150:671, 1996.

93. Litman RS, Kottra JA, Berkowitz RJ, et al: Breathing patterns and levels of consciousness in children during administration of nitrous oxide after oral midazolam premedication, *J Oral Maxillofac Surg* 55:1372, 1997.

94. Litman RS, Kottra JA, Verga KA, et al: Chloral hydrate sedation: the additive sedative and respiratory depressant effects of nitrous oxide, *Anesth Analg* 86:724, 1998.

95. Doi M, Ikeda K: Respiratory effects of sevoflurane, *Anesth Analg* 66:241, 1987.

96. Blayney MR, Malins AF, Cooper GM: Cardiac arrhythmias in children during outpatient general anaesthesia: a prospective randomized trial, *Lancet* 354(9193):1864-1866, 1999.

97. Johnson RR, Eger EI II, Wilson C: A comparative interaction of epinephrine with enflurane, isoflurane, and halothane in man, *Anesth Analg* 55:709, 1976.

98. Moore MA, Weiskopf RB, Eger EI II, et al: Arrhythmogenic doses of epinephrine are similar during desflurane or isoflurane anesthesia in humans, *Anesthesiology* 79:943, 1993.

99. Navarro R, Weiskopf RB, Morre MA, et al: Humans anesthetized with sevoflurane or isoflurane have similar arrhythmogenic response to epinephrine, *Anesthesiology* 80:545, 1994.

100. Ariffin SA, Whyte JA, Malins AF, et al: Comparison of induction and recovery between sevoflurane and halothane supplementation of anaesthesia in children undergoing outpatient dental extractions, *Br J Anaesth* 78:157, 1997.

101. Paris ST, Cafferkey M, Tarling M, et al: Comparison of sevoflurane and halothane for outpatient dental anaesthesia in children, *Br J Anaesth* 79:280, 1997.

102. Kenna JG, Jones RM: The organ toxicity of inhaled anesthetics, *Anesth Analg* 81:S51, 1995.

103. Njoku D, Laster MJ, Gong DH, et al: Biotransformation of halothane, enflurane, isoflurane, and desflurane to trifluoroacetylated liver proteins: association between protein acylation and hepatic injury, *Anesth Analg* 84:173, 1997.

104. Malan TP Jr: Sevoflurane and renal function, *Anesth Analg* 81:S39, 1995.

105. Ebert EI II, Messana LD, Uhrich TD, et al: Absence of renal and hepatic toxicity after 1.25 minimum alveolar anesthetic concentration sevoflurane anesthesia in volunteers, *Anesth Analg* 86:662, 1998.

Perioperative Anesthetic and Metabolic Care of Children and Adolescents

Erik S. Shank

The pediatric oral and maxillofacial surgery (OMFS) patient presents important anesthetic management challenges for the anesthesiologist and surgeon. Safe administration of anesthesia for these patients requires rational decisions about airway management, nutrition, and fluid and electrolyte replacement. In addition, the anesthesiologist often is asked to provide deliberate hypotension to improve the operative field and to decrease blood loss. This chapter discusses our approach to these issues.

AIRWAY MANAGEMENT
Face Mask Ventilation

The pediatric airway differs significantly from that of the adult. These differences include size of the anatomic structures, compressibility of the underlying soft tissues, prominence of the occiput which causes neck flexion in the supine position, and relatively large size of the tongue and tonsils. All these factors contribute to the difficulty of establishing a mask airway in a healthy child. A child with a maxillofacial skeletal (e.g., micrognathia, midface deficiency) or soft tissue deformity or with bony or soft tissue pathology may be even more challenging (Figure 8-1).

The first order of importance is to select the appropriately fitting mask. Pediatric face masks come in various sizes to accommodate the tremendous physical variation in size, from 500 g premature neonates to fully developed adolescents larger than 100 kg (Figure 8-2). The mask should fit over the patient's mouth and nose, without compressing the orbits. In cases of severe facial deformity, insertion of gauze sponges (as a seal) may be required to obtain a good mask fit. In other cases, oral or nasal mask ventilation alone may be possible while occluding the orifice not being ventilated.

The patient should be positioned supine on the operating room table with the head in a neutral (no neck flexion or extension) position. In infants, this usually requires one or more blankets under the shoulder blades to negate the relatively prominent occiput. The flexed neck compromises the airway and may make ventilation difficult.

The mask should be held snugly on the patient's face with the index finger and thumb, while the middle and ring fingers perform a jaw lift on the angle of the mandible (Figure 8-3). It is essential in infants and young children that the soft tissues adjacent to the mandible are not compressed,[1] because this force may be transmitted to the oropharynx, obstructing ventilation (Figure 8-4).

Infants are obligate nasal breathers, so an oral airway (Figure 8-5) is often a useful adjunct to optimize face mask ventilation. Placement of an appropriate-size oral airway lifts the tongue off the back of the oropharynx,

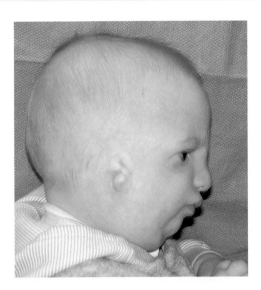

Figure 8-1

Lateral photograph of 5-month-old boy with Treacher Collins syndrome. Note the severely retrognathic mandible abutting the neck and the tracheostomy. (Courtesy Dr. L.B. Kaban and Dr. M.J. Troulis.)

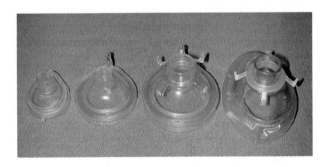

Figure 8-2

Pediatric face masks varying in size to accommodate a 500 g premature neonate to a fully developed adolescent.

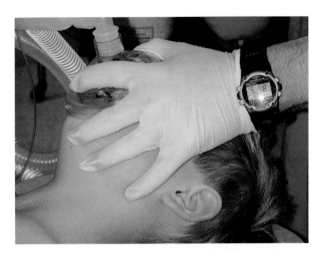

Figure 8-3

The face mask should be held to fit snugly over the patient's mouth and nose, with the index finger and thumb. Note that the middle and ring fingers are positioned on the angle and mandible and used to perform a jaw lift.

must be exercised to avoid aggressive positive pressures. It is generally accepted that a pressure greater than 20 cm of water will exceed the pressure of the lower esophageal sphincter and result in insufflation of gas into the stomach. As gastric pressure increases, risk of gastric reflux and aspiration increase. Pulmonary compliance decreases because of reduced diaphragmatic excursion.

Patients with maxillofacial pathology are frequently difficult to ventilate by mask.[2,3] It is important to recognize this and to ensure that people skilled in airway

thus opening up the hypopharyngeal passage. If the inserted airway is too large, it may aggravate obstruction by compressing the palate and closing off the nasopharyngeal passage. A poor-fitting oral airway may also cause damage to pharyngeal structures. An oral airway must never be placed in a conscious patient because it may trigger gag reflexes, vomiting, or laryngospasm secondary to pharyngeal stimulation.

When ventilating an infant with a face mask, it is important to recognize that the airway is not protected from stomach contents or other substances (e.g., blood or saliva). The only devices that can reliably protect the airway from aspiration are endotracheal or tracheostomy tubes. When ventilating a child with either a bag-mask-valve device (e.g., "ambu") or anesthesia circuit, care

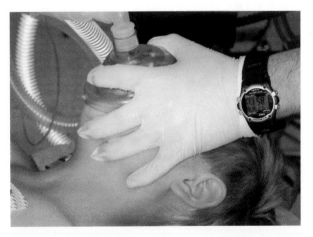

Figure 8-4

When using the face mask, it is important that the fingers do not compress the soft tissues adjacent to the mandible, as is seen in this photograph.

management are available. A dedicated "difficult airway cart" should be ready in areas where these patients are anesthetized, sedated, and recovering. This cart should contain an assortment of laryngoscopy tools, as well as a fiberoptic laryngoscope and equipment for emergent jet ventilation (14 gauge angiocatheter, pediatric endotracheal tube adapter, 3 ml syringe).

Laryngeal Mask Airway

The laryngeal mask airway (LMA) is a relatively new device, having been introduced in 1988. It has quickly become an indispensable tool in pediatric airway management (Figure 8-6). The LMA is a latex-free, silicone-based device that is inserted orally and conforms to the shape of the hypopharynx, with a ventilation outlet (when properly placed) directly over the larynx. It has proved very useful as an adjunct and alternative to face mask ventilation.[4] Use of the LMA is easily learned, the device is easy to place, and it may establish an airway rapidly in a patient who is difficult to ventilate by mask due to external (e.g., facial dysmorphism such as micrognathia)[5,6] or internal factors (e.g., large tongue). These attributes have earned the LMA a place in the American Society of Anesthesiologists' *Difficult Airway Algorithm* (Figure 8-7).[7]

In pediatric LMA studies, successful placement was achieved in approximately 90% of first and close to 100% of second attempts. The well-placed LMA is a useful guide for fiberoptic visualization of the larynx.[8] An endotracheal tube (placed on the fiberscope) can be advanced through the LMA (Table 8-1). This technique has been employed in patients with significant micrognathia as in Pierre Robin sequence[9,10] and Treacher Collins syndrome.[11] Alternatively, a technique has been described in which a wire stent is placed into the trachea, via the LMA-directed fiberscope. The LMA and fiberscope are then withdrawn, and an endotracheal tube is placed into the trachea using the stent for

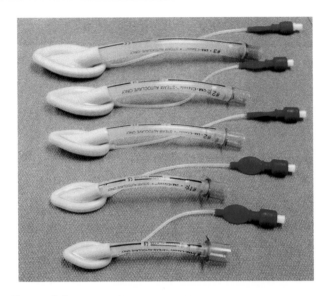

Figure 8-6

Laryngeal mask airways are available in a variety of sizes and are useful in the management of the pediatric airway.

guidance. This technique requires considerable practice for the clinician to use it successfully and dependably.

It is important to note that the LMA is not without potential problems. It is not a device that protects the lungs from gastric contents or blood. It is more invasive than the face mask and may result in trauma to the hypopharynx. It is relatively nonstimulating but may elicit a gag reflex or laryngeal reflex in patients who are not fully anesthetized. Lastly, for many oral and maxillofacial procedures it is not suitable because of its bulk and because it can be dislodged during complex or lengthy procedures.

Endotracheal Tubes

The endotracheal tube is the most reliable method for protecting the lungs from gastric aspiration or saliva

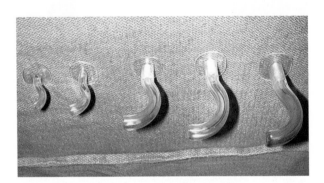

Figure 8-5

Oral airways are available in a variety of sizes to accommodate children, from infants to adolescents.

TABLE 8-1 Standards of Endotracheal Tubes Advanced Through the LMA

LMA Size	Pediatric Size	ETT	Fiberscope
1	Neonate up to 5 kg	3.5 ID mm	2.7 mm
1.5	Infants 5-10 kg	4.0	3.0
2	10-20 kg	4.5	3.5
2.5	20-30 kg	5.0	4.0
3	30-50 kg	6.0 cuffed	5.0

LMA, Laryngeal mask airway; *ETT,* endotracheal tube; *ID,* internal diameter.

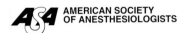

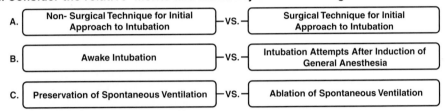

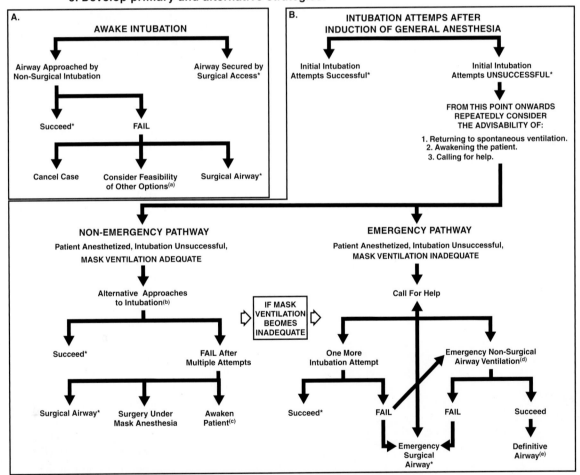

Figure 8-7

The American Society of Anesthesiologists' *Difficult Airway Algorithm.*

and blood during an oral or maxillofacial surgical procedure. The common endotracheal tubes include straight, oral, and nasal RAE tubes (Ring, Adire, Elwyn manufactured by Mallinckrodt, St. Louis) (Figure 8-8). All of these must be placed through the vocal cords (VC) into the laryngeal inlet. Techniques for placement of the tube include direct visualization of the VC via a laryngoscope (Figure 8-9) or a fiberoptic scope, LMA-assisted placement,[12] and nonvisualized (sometimes called *blind*) placement. Any time that instruments are introduced into the larynx there is a potential for dangerous laryngeal reflexes (i.e., laryngospasm), as well as trauma to the laryngeal structures. Therefore, it is important that only people skilled in these techniques attempt to intubate a pediatric patient.

The standard endotracheal tube usually is placed orally, exiting to the right or left of the mouth. The tube must be secured either by tape to the skin, with surgical steel wire (26 gauge) around a tooth, or with a circummandibular wire. Tube selection needs to be appropriate for the size and age of the child. Any endotracheal tube in a pediatric patient that does not leak with 30 cm, or greater, water pressure should be replaced with a smaller tube.

The oral RAE tube is useful for surgical procedures on the maxilla because it exits the mouth and travels caudally over the mandible. The oral RAE tube can be wired to teeth or taped to the jaw or chin. The appropriate diameter of this tube must be evaluated as above (i.e., measure leak pressures). However, it is also imperative to assess the length of the tube from the tip to the curve. This distance must be adequate to ensure that there is sufficient tube in the trachea past the VC but not past the carina (resulting in a left or right "main stem" intubation) when the tube is secured in its desired position.

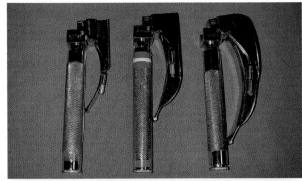
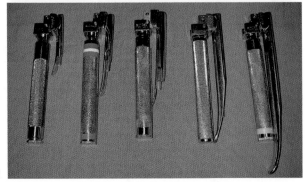

Figure 8-9
Laryngoscopes come in a variety of sizes and with either curved (**A**) or straight (**B**) blades.

Nasal intubation is beneficial when the surgeon requires unobstructed access to the oral cavity to perform the operation. The nasal RAE tube is also useful when the anesthesia circuit must come over the forehead with a low profile (Figure 8-10). For placement of a nasoendotracheal tube, the same sizing considerations as for an oral tube apply. In addition, the size of the patient's nares and nasal passages must be evaluated. The nasal septum and turbinates should be assessed because they affect the patency of the nasal airway. The clinician should occlude one nostril and ask the patient to breathe, then repeat for the other nostril. The more patent nasal passage is chosen for the endotracheal tube. The site and the side of the surgical procedure also determine which nostril is preferable.

Premedication with a topical nasal spray (e.g., phenylephrine) or a local anesthetic (e.g., cocaine) improves ease of passage of the endotracheal tube by producing vasoconstriction of the nasal mucosa. Even with premedication, there is a significant risk of bleeding if the nasal mucosa is traumatized. This risk must be appreciated, and suction should be immediately available for both intubation and extubation. Nasoendotracheal tubes may be secured with tape to the nose or, preferably, sutured through the cartilaginous nasal septum, taking care not to secure the suture to the columella.

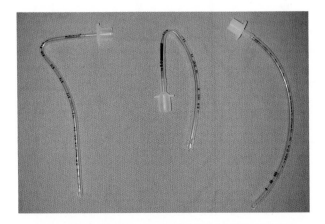

Figure 8-8
Commonly used pediatric endotracheal tubes. Note the lack of a balloon. From left to right: nasal RAE, oral RAE, and straight tubes. (Mallinckrodt, St Louis.)

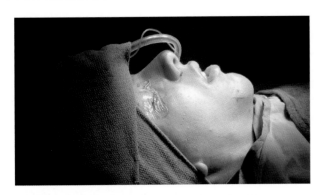

Figure 8-10

Lateral photograph of anesthetized patient, nasally intubated and draped. The nasal RAE tube is secured to the cartilaginous nasal septum with a 2-0 resorbable suture.

MANAGEMENT OF THE DIFFICULT AIRWAY

Patients with syndromic and nonsyndromic congenital deformities and those with severe acquired maxillofacial deformities are often difficult to ventilate by mask and to intubate. This should be anticipated, and the anesthesiologist and surgeon should plan in advance for these challenging cases.[13] This includes optimizing any coexisting diseases of the patient, having the proper airway management equipment immediately available, and having skilled personnel available to secure a surgical airway (tracheostomy), if necessary. Specific techniques for management of the child with an anticipated difficult airway vary widely, depending on the training and skill of the anesthesia and surgical teams. They include awake intubation, awake sedated intubation, and awake intubation with topical local anesthesia or laryngeal nerve block or both. Alternatively, the patient may be intubated while asleep with spontaneous breathing or asleep with assisted ventilation. Tools that may be employed include LMAs,[14,15] fiberoptic[16] and fiberoptic-enabled laryngoscopes,[17] and jet ventilation. Cricothyroidotomy and tracheotomy should be considered in the patient with a high-risk, difficult airway.

HYPOTENSIVE ANESTHESIA

In attempt to decrease the morbidity associated with maxillofacial reconstruction, clinicians and investigators have turned to controlled hypotension.[18-26] The potential benefits of controlled hypotension include decreased blood loss; clearer surgical field leading to more accurate surgery; decreased anesthesia and surgical time, decreased postoperative edema, and postoperative infection rates; and increased patient comfort. The effects of hypotensive anesthesia on both blood loss and operative time during orthognathic surgery have been reported.

The data indicate that the hypotensive technique results in decreased blood loss, a perception by the surgeon of improved surgical field, but no shortening of operative time.[19,20,27,28]

In general, deliberate hypotension is described as a 30% decrease in mean arterial pressure compared with baseline levels or systolic pressures in the 80 to 90 mm Hg range. This controlled hypotension can be achieved by a number of different pharmacologic techniques. They include inhalational anesthetics,[20,29] β-blockers,[19] calcium-channel blockers, and direct-acting vasodilators like nitroglycerin and sodium nitroprusside.[30] For most OMFS cases, deliberate hypotension is achieved easily and safely with high levels of inhalational anesthetics. Potential disadvantages of this technique include delayed emergence from anesthesia and decreased ability to monitor evoked potentials (usually not an issue with OMFS procedures). Inhalational anesthetics are contraindicated in children with a history of malignant hyperthermia.

The use of deliberate hypotension in healthy patients does not require any alterations in the anesthetic monitoring techniques. An invasive arterial line is usually not necessary to safely administer this technique, although many studies do advocate the use of one.[19,27,29,31] However, a Foley catheter should be used to monitor urine output. Relative contraindications to the practice of controlled hypotension include patients who demand a high systemic vascular resistance, such as those with intracardiac pressure-directed shunts or with compromised perfusion to vital organs.[32]

Steroids

Another adjuvant (to hypotensive anesthesia) used to decrease the morbidity associated with maxillofacial reconstruction is the use of perioperative steroids. Multiple protocols exist, but at Massachusetts General Hospital we use 12 mg dexamethasone IV before induction of anesthesia and then 12 mg Decadron every 12 hours for two doses and 8 mg on postoperative day 2. The benefits of perioperative steroids include decreased postoperative edema,[33-35] less postoperative trismus, and increased patient comfort. Additionally, perioperative steroids have a useful antiemetic function. It has also been reported that global changes in anesthetic and surgical technique (including perioperative steroids and controlled hypotension) significantly decreased the length of hospital stay.[36]

PHARMACOLOGIC ISSUES IN THE PEDIATRIC PATIENT

The pharmacokinetics and pharmacodynamics of drugs differ in pediatric patients versus adults. This is due to differences in *active* (e.g., rates of metabolism or excretion) and *passive* properties (e.g., water content and blood protein concentrations) by age.

The metabolism and elimination of most drugs is accomplished by the action of the liver or kidneys or both. Neonates and premature infants may have difficulty with conjugation reactions, which are a major pathway for the conversion of lipophilic drugs to hydrophilic drugs. This conversion makes drugs more water soluble and more easily excreted by the kidneys. An example of this phenomenon is the "jaundice of the newborn." Most hepatic functions improve with age, up to a peak during childhood, before beginning a progressive decline.

Renal function displays a similar pattern. Premature infants and neonates have decreased glomerular filtration rate (GFR) and tubular function. This makes them very susceptible to hypovolemia when fluids are restricted preoperatively, because they have an inability to concentrate the urine. The GFR and tubular processes rapidly improve, becoming fully developed at around 2 years of age.

The neonate and infant have a higher percentage of total body water compared with the older child and adolescent or adult. This implies that a larger dosage of water-soluble drugs, such as succinylcholine and many antibiotics, will be required. Additionally, these same patients may have decreased fat and muscle mass, so drugs with a clinical response that is usually terminated by redistribution (e.g., sodium thiopental) may have longer durations of action.

A premature infant or neonate with diminished hepatic function may also have diminished plasma protein levels. Many medications commonly employed in the operating room setting (barbiturates, local anesthetics, antibiotics, and anxiolytics) may have a more potent effect in these individuals because levels of unbound (usually more pharmacologically active) drug will be higher. Neonates may also be more susceptible to hypnotics, sedatives, and analgesics secondary to a relatively permeable blood-brain barrier.[37]

Both the *active* and *passive* differences between the neonate and the older child and adolescent or adult demand that heightened vigilance be employed when using these medications. An important concept when these drugs are required in children is to *titrate to effect.*

ANESTHETIC AGENTS

Intravenous agents should be titrated according to the hepatic and renal function of the patient,[38] as well as body composition (e.g., fat content, volume of distribution issues), as discussed above. As in adults, all anesthetics, including local anesthetics, also have potential to elicit allergic responses.[39]

Inhalational agents are, for the most part, not metabolized or excreted by the infant but rather eliminated by ventilation. Neonates have a decreased *minimum alveolar concentration (MAC)* when compared with children, whereas children have a higher MAC than adults. A healthy child may have an MAC that is 30% greater than that of an adult. It is important to recognize this physiologic difference between children and adults to avoid under-dosing these anesthetics.[40]

NONANESTHETIC MEDICATIONS

Most oral surgical procedures require perioperative antibiotics. Routine protocols include penicillin (100,000 U/kg/day), oxacillin (50 to 100 mg/kg/day), clindamycin (20 to 40 mg/kg/day), or cefazolin (20 to 50 mg/kg/day). All dosages are given as total per day and are administered in divided doses intravenously. Choice of antibiotic depends on the site and the procedure being performed. For all dental and oral procedures, children with heart murmurs require prophylaxis for bacterial endocarditis (see Chapter 1, Table 1-2).[41] The standard regimen is amoxicillin 50 mg/kg by mouth, 1 hour before the procedure. For children unable to take oral medications, ampicillin 50 mg/kg is administered either intramuscularly or intravenously 30 minutes before the operation. For children allergic to penicillin, clindamycin (20 mg/kg) is administered either orally 1 hour before or intravenously 30 minutes before the procedure.

METABOLIC MANAGEMENT

It is important to appreciate the child's overall state of hydration before any operation. Factors that influence fluid volume status include the amount of time the patient has been on restricted oral intake (i.e., "npo status"), age, and coexisting disease states (e.g., sepsis, diabetes insipidus, diarrhea, and nausea or vomiting) that may result in disruption of fluid balance. In addition to a thorough history, physical examination may yield important clues for fluid management. These include vital signs such as tachycardia, hypotension, widened pulse pressures, and orthostatic changes. Other physical signs include sunken fontanels in the neonate, decreased capillary refill time, or loss of skin membrane moisture or skin turgor. It must be noted that a child may be severely hypovolemic before many of these signs are appreciated. Laboratory studies may help confirm hypovolemia, but they usually are not ordered routinely during the immediate preoperative period.

The pediatric patient arriving for an OMFS procedure usually will have some degree of hypovolemia due to oral intake restriction during the preoperative period. Recent trends have been to relax these fluid restrictions compared with the antiquated "nothing by mouth after midnight" requirement. At the Massachusetts General Hospital for Children, pediatric patients may have clear fluids ad lib up to 2 hours before an operation. This policy has decreased the incidence of hypotension on induction of general anesthesia, without an apparent increase in aspiration of gastric contents.

The kidneys of premature infants and neonates are not fully matured; thus, special care must be paid to their preoperative volume status. The immature kidney cannot effectively concentrate urine or conserve sodium. Additionally, this age population has the poorest compensatory mechanisms for hypovolemia. A neonate or premature infant should have an intravenous line begun preoperatively, to avoid hypovolemia. By 1 year of age, the kidneys have achieved most of the homeostatic mechanisms seen in older children and adults.

A patient awaiting surgery still has insensible fluid losses. There are mandatory fluid losses from the kidneys, gastrointestinal tract, lungs, and skin. These ongoing losses during the fasting preoperative period commonly are referred to as the patient's *fluid deficit*. To estimate a patient's deficit, the number of hours fasting is multiplied by the patient's hourly fluid maintenance requirement. Calculations of maintenance fluid requirements for a pediatric patient are based on the studies of Holiday and Segar: 100 ml of fluid is required for each 100 calories metabolized. Translating this to weight generates the standard "4.2.1" rule of pediatric maintenance fluids: that is, 4 ml/kg for the first 10 kilograms, 2 ml/kg for the next 10 kilograms, and 1 ml/kg for the remaining kilograms. The patient's deficit commonly is replaced intraoperatively by administering one half the calculated deficit the first hour and the remaining deficit spread out over the next 2 hours. Generally, a patient does not require the full deficit replaced because there are compensatory mechanisms (e.g., concentration of urine, decreased extremity perfusion) that conserve fluids when a patient is fasting. It is, however, important to evaluate each patient individually for dehydration (Table 8-2).

Intraoperatively, maintenance fluids are supplied in addition to the calculated deficits. Finally, blood and third-space losses must be considered. Blood usually is replaced with isotonic crystalloid solutions in a 3:1 ratio (3 ml of crystalloid for each ml of blood) or 1:1 if blood or other colloidal solution is used for replacement.

Third-space losses are fluids that exit the circulating blood via capillary leak and surgical trauma and reside in extravascular compartments. These losses must also be replaced with crystalloids or colloids. Third-space losses for oral and maxillofacial procedures are usually in the range of 2 to 5 ml/kg/hr.

Blood loss over a certain threshold should be replaced by blood (usually as packed red blood cells). Thresholds for transfusion vary. Additional factors that influence this decision include co-morbidity of the patient (e.g., the child with congenital heart disease may require greater oxygen carrying capacity than a healthy child) and likelihood of further blood loss, either intraoperatively or postoperatively. However, whatever the threshold for transfusion, the *maximal allowable blood loss* (MABL) can be calculated as follows:

MABL = (estimated blood volume × [initial hematocrit – threshold hematocrit]) / initial hematocrit. MABL is dependent on age and weight.

A rough estimate is 100 ml/kg for the premature infant, 90 ml/kg for the term infant, 80 ml/kg for a toddler, and 70 ml/kg for the older child. This formula obviously has significant variability, and the MABL should always be verified by an actual hematocrit, especially if the threshold for transfusion hematocrit is a relatively low number.

TABLE 8-2   Estimating Dehydration

Signs and Symptoms	Mild Dehydration	Moderate Dehydration	Severe Dehydration
Percentage of blood loss	<20	20-40	>40
Percentage of weight loss	5	10	15
Turgor of skin	Normal	Normal/decreased	Decreased
Appearance of mucous membranes	Normal	Dry	Parched
Tears	Present	+/–	Absent
Anterior fontanelles	Flat	+/–	Sunken
Orthostatic blood pressure changes	None	Postural drops	Postural drops
Behavior	Normal	Restlessness	Irritable, agitated, or lethargic
Thirst	Slight	Moderate	Intense
Urinary output	Normal	Decreased	Markedly decreased

Modified from Herrin J: Fluid and electrolytes. In Graef J, editor: *Manual of pediatric therapeutics*, ed 6, Philadelphia, 1997, Lippincott-Raven.

Techniques for minimizing the need for transfusion include preoperative crystalloid infusion (so the "blood" being lost has a relatively lower hematocrit) and deliberate hypotension (discussed earlier).

The specific choice of crystalloid solution for parenteral fluid replacement remains somewhat controversial. However, most clinicians believe that isotonic salt solutions should be used. The reasons for this include that ongoing volume losses (blood and third-space losses) are isotonic and large volumes of hypotonic solutions (e.g., free water, 5% dextrose in water) cause intracellular entry of fluid, causing edema and potential electrolyte changes. Additionally, endogenous release of antidiuretic hormone results in selectively increased retention of water versus sodium if inadequate amounts of sodium are supplied.

Dextrose-containing solutions usually are discouraged because the brain is less tolerant of hypoxic insult in a hyperglycemic state. However, pediatric patients, especially neonates and premature infants, may be prone to hypoglycemia, which is also dangerous and detrimental. A reasonable compromise for long cases in young infants is a "maintenance" drip of dextrose-containing solution at 3 ml/kg/min, and the remaining replacement fluid as lactated Ringer's or normal saline solution.

When planning postoperative fluid management, it is imperative to consider intraoperative blood loss, intraoperative volume replacement, third-space fluid loss, renal function, and urine output. Ongoing issues such as continued bleeding, fluid losses through drains or gastric tubes, and decreased oral intake must be incorporated into the assessment of the patient's volume requirements. Although generally uncommon in the pediatric surgery population, pathologic volume responses (e.g., syndrome of inappropriate antidiuretic hormone release, renal failure, and cirrhosis) may grossly alter the child's ability to regulate fluid balance.

Preoperative and intraoperative fluid alterations must guide postoperative fluid management. Additional information obtained by the postoperative physical examination(s), intake-output fluid balance sheets, and laboratory studies of serum and urine electrolyte values must be taken into account.

Fluid overload may manifest itself during the postoperative period as generalized edema or, in rare occurrences, pulmonary edema. This diagnosis may be evident during the immediate postoperative period or may appear slowly over the first 24 to 36 hours, as third-space losses gradually mobilize into the systemic circulation. Management of fluid overload includes sodium and water restriction, as well as diuretic agents. In extreme cases, with renal or heart failure, dialysis may be necessary to remove the excess fluid.

CONCLUSION

Successful pediatric OMFS requires an understanding and appreciation of pediatric airway management, as well as the metabolic demands and alterations of the infant and child throughout the perioperative period.

REFERENCES

1. Reber A, Wetzel SG, Schnabel K, et al: Effect of combined mouth closure and chin lift on upper airway dimensions during routine magnetic resonance imaging in pediatric patients sedated with propofol, *Anesthesiology* 90(6):1617-1623, 1999.
2. Vaughan C: Anesthetic management of children with craniofacial anomalies, *CRNA* 8(4):123-134, 1997.
3. Ferguson DJ, Barker J, Jackson IT: Anesthesia for craniofacial osteotomies, *Ann Plast Surg* 10(4):333-338, 1983.
4. Todd DW: A comparison of endotracheal intubation and use of the laryngeal mask airway for ambulatory oral surgery patients, *J Oral Surg* 60:2-4, 2002.
5. Barnes SD: Emergent intubation of the difficult pediatric airway using the laryngeal mask airway, *Am J Crit Care* 5(5):376-378, 1996.
6. Markakis DA, Sayson SC, Schreiner MS: Insertion of the laryngeal mask airway in awake infants with the Robin sequence, *Anesth Analg* 75(5):822-824, 1992.
7. Benumof JL: Laryngeal mask airway and the ASA difficult airway algorithm, *Anesthesiology* 84(3):686-699, 1996.
8. Levy RJ, Helfaer MA: Pediatric airway issues, *Crit Care Clin* 16(3):489-504, 2000.
9. Myer CM, Reed JM, Cotton RT, et al: Airway management in Pierre Robin sequence, *Otolaryngol Head Neck Surg* 118(5):630-635, 1998.
10. Hansen TG, Joensen H, Henneberg SW, Hole P: Laryngeal mask airway guided tracheal intubation in a neonate with the Pierre Robin syndrome, *Acta Anaesthesiol Scand* 39(1):129-131, 1995.
11. Inada T, Fujise K, Tachibana K, Shingu K: Orotracheal intubation through the laryngeal mask airway in paediatric patients with Treacher-Collins syndrome, *Paediatr Anaesth* 5(2):129-132, 1995.
12. Heard CM, Caldicott LD, Fletcher JE, Selsby DS: Fiberoptic-guided endotracheal intubation via the laryngeal mask airway in pediatric patients: a report of a series of cases, *Anesth Analg* 82(6):1287-1289, 1996.
13. Sofferman RA, Johnson DL, Spencer RF: Lost airway during anesthesia induction: alternatives for management, *Laryngoscope* 107(11 Pt 1):1476-1482, 1997.
14. Stocks RM, Egerman R, Thompson JW, Peery M: Airway management of the severely retrognathic child: use of the laryngeal mask airway, *Ear Nose Throat J* 81(4):223-226, 2002.
15. Selim M, Mowafi H, Al-Ghamdi A, Adu-Gyamfi Y: Intubation via LMA in pediatric patients with difficult airways, *Can J Anaesth* 46(9):891-893, 1999.
16. Blanco G, Melman E, Cuairan V, et al: Fiberoptic nasal intubation in children with anticipated and unanticipated difficult intubation, *Paediatr Anaesth* 11(1):49-53, 2001.
17. Brown RE Jr, Vollers JM, Rader GR, Schmitz ML: Nasotracheal intubation in a child with Treacher Collins syndrome using the Bullard intubating laryngoscope, *J Clin Anesth* 5(6):492-493, 1993.
18. Tobias JD: Controlled hypotension in children: a critical review of available agents, *Paediatr Drugs* 4(7):439-453, 2002.
19. Dolman RM, Bentley KC, Head TW, English M: The effect of hypotensive anesthesia on blood loss and operative time during Le Fort I osteotomies, *J Oral Surg* 58(8):834-840, 2000.
20. Lessard MR, Trepanier CA, Baribault JP, et al: Isoflurane-induced hypotension in orthognathic surgery, *Can J Anaesth* 37(4 Pt 2): S42, 1990.

21. Yaster M, Simmons RS, Tolo VT, et al: A comparison of nitroglycerin and nitroprusside for inducing hypotension in children: a double-blind study, *Anesthesiology* 65(2):175-179, 1986.

22. Sanders GM, Sim KM: Is it feasible to use magnesium sulphate as a hypotensive agent in oral and maxillofacial surgery? *Ann Acad Med Singap* 27(6):780-785, 1998.

23. Praveen K, Narayanan V, Muthusekhar MR, Baig MF: Hypotensive anaesthesia and blood loss in orthognathic surgery: a clinical study, *Br J Oral Maxillofac Surg* 39(2):138-140, 2001.

24. Gardner WJ: The control of bleeding during operation by induced hypotension, *JAMA* 132:172, 1946.

25. Gallagher DM: Induced hypotension for orthognathic surgery, *J Oral Surg* 37:47-51, 1979.

26. Fromme GA, MacKenzi RA, Gould AB Jr, et al: Controlled hypotension for orthognathic surgery, *Anesth Analg* 65:683-686, 1986.

27. Precious DS, Splinter W, Bosco D: Induced hypotensive anesthesia for adolescent orthognathic surgery patient, *J Oral Surg* 54:680-684, 1996.

28. Samman N, Cheung LK, Tong AC, Tideman H: Blood loss and transfusion requirements in orthognathic surgery, *J Oral Surg* 54:21-24, 1996.

29. Enlund MG, Ahlstedt BL, Andersson LG, Krekmanov LI: Induced hypotension may influence blood loss in orthognathic surgery, but it is not crucial, *Scand J Plast Reconstr Surg Hand Surg* 31(4):311-317, 1997.

30. Hack H, Mitchell V: Hypotensive anaesthesia, *Br J Hosp Med* 55(8):482-485, 1996.

31. Gourdeau M, Martin R, Lamarche Y, Tetreault L: Oscillometry and direct blood pressure: a comparative clinical study during deliberate hypotension, *Can Anaesth Soc J* 33(3 Pt 1):300-307, 1986.

32. Kick O, Van Aken H, Wouters PF, et al: Vital organ blood flow during deliberate hypotension in dogs, *Anesth Analg* 77(4):737-742, 1993.

33. Schaberg SJ, Kelly JF, Terry BC, et al: Blood loss and hypotensive anesthesia in oral-facial corrective surgery, *J Oral Surg* 34:147-156, 1976.

34. Gersema L, Baker K: Use of corticosteroids in oral surgery, *J Oral Maxillofac Surg* 50(3):270-277, 1992.

35. Hooley JR, Hohl TH: Use of steroids in the prevention of some complications after traumatic oral surgery, *J Oral Surg* 32(11):864-866, 1974.

36. Juvet LM, Dodson TD, Kaban LB, et al: Variables affecting hospital length of stay in orthognathic surgery patients, *J Dent Res* 81(A):A-397, 2002.

37. Miller RI: Anesthesia, ed 5, St Louis, 2000, Churchill Livingstone.

38. Cillo JE Jr: Propofol anesthesia for outpatient oral and maxillofacial surgery, *Oral Surg Oral Med Oral Pathol Oral Radiol Endod* 87(5):530-538, 1999.

39. Wilson AW, Deacock S, Downie IP, Zaki G: Allergy to local anaesthetic: the importance of thorough investigation, *Br Dent J* 188(3):120-122, 2000.

40. Cote CJ, Ryan JF, Todres ID, Goudsouzian NG: *A practice of anesthesia for infants and children*, ed 2, Philadelphia, 1993, WB Saunders.

41. Dajani AS, Taubert KA, Wilson W, et al: Prevention of bacterial endocarditis. Recommendations by the American Heart Association, *JAMA* 277(22):1794-1801, 1997.

Ancillary Surgical Procedures

Leonard B. Kaban, Michael T. Longaker, and Maria J. Troulis

The ancillary operations most frequently employed in pediatric oral and maxillofacial surgery consist of intravenous access procedures, bone graft harvesting, and tracheotomy. Intravenous access may be a problem, particularly in infants and toddlers, requiring altered percutaneous or surgical vascular access. Bone grafts are used commonly to repair alveolar clefts, to fill osteotomy gaps, and to reconstruct other osseous defects (e.g., full-thickness defects after tumor resection). Finally, when a tracheotomy is required in children, the surgeon must be aware of anatomic characteristics that are somewhat different from those in adults.

INTRAVENOUS ACCESS
General Considerations

Intravenous access generally is required for fluid and electrolyte replacement, drug therapy, and short and long-term nutritional support. The oral and maxillofacial surgeon is concerned most commonly with short-term fluid replacement and intravenous drug administration. The technique and anatomic location chosen for intravenous cannulation depend on the age of the patient, indications for intravenous therapy, and expertise of the surgeon.[1]

Neonates and infants have considerable subcutaneous fat and very small veins. Venous access sites on the dorsum of the hand or in the antecubital fossa, commonly available in adults, are usually not possible in this age group. Hair on the scalp is sparse and veins are visible; therefore, scalp veins are used frequently. The dorsum of the foot and ankle are other common access sites for infants and small children (less than 3 years). In toddlers and older children, the hand and antecubital fossa often are available for venous cannulation.

When large fluid volumes are required, or if percutaneous access in the scalp or upper extremity has been unsuccessful, the saphenous vein may be cannulated, either percutaneously or by cutdown. If necessary, a long cannula can be placed as a central venous line from the saphenous vein. Finally, the external jugular vein may be used either percutaneously or by cutdown.

Technique

Scalp Vein Access. The scalp hair is clipped but not shaved, and the skin is prepared with povidone-iodine 10% or other antiseptic. The patient is placed in the Trendelenburg position, and the needle is inserted.

Temporal or forehead veins are the most commonly used vessels. The entry site is protected with antibiotic ointment and an occlusive tape dressing. A paper or plastic cup may be taped over the intravenous site for additional safety (Figure 9-1).

Percutaneous Foot or Ankle Access. A tourniquet is placed above the ankle, and the skin is prepared with povidone-iodine 10% solution. A scalp vein butterfly or 1.5-inch venous catheter (Angiocath) is inserted into the dilated vein (Figure 9-2). The wound is covered with an occlusive dressing, and the foot is immobilized (Figure 9-3).

Saphenous Vein Cutdown. It is helpful to use loupe magnification for this procedure. General anesthesia usually is required, because it is difficult for children to cooperate under local anesthesia for this operation. A tourniquet is applied proximally, and the foot and ankle are prepared with povidone iodine 10% and draped for sterility. A horizontal incision is made approximately one finger breadth (1.0 to 1.5 cm) above and medial to the medial malleolus.

With a hemostat, spreading parallel to the tibia, the dissection is carried bluntly down to the superficial fascia of the malleolus. The hemostat is then elevated with the full thickness of subcutaneous tissue; the vein is in this pad of tissue. The vein is identified and dissected free, and proximal and distal ligatures are placed. The distal ligature is tied; a venotomy incision is made, and the catheter is threaded proximally, using the proximal tie to place traction on the vein. The proximal ligature is then tied securely around the vein, sealing the catheter (see Figure 9-2).

The wound is closed with 5-0 nylon sutures and the catheter is secured to the skin with a 4-0 nylon stitch. Antibiotic ointment and an occlusive dressing are placed over the intravenous site (see Figure 9-3).

External Jugular Venous Access. The external jugular vein is cannulated percutaneously or by cutdown when intravenous access is necessary for more than a few days or when it is undesirable, or not possible, to have a catheter in an extremity. This access is particularly appropriate for the patient who needs long-term parenteral antibiotics or intravenous nutrition. A pediatric surgeon usually is consulted to perform an elective external jugular cutdown; general anesthesia is required.

The patient is placed in the Trendelenburg position. The neck is prepared with povidone-iodine 10% solution and draped for sterility. The vein is identified, and percutaneous cannulation is performed (Figure 9-4, *A*). For cutdown, a horizontal incision is made in the overlying skin. The dissection is carried bluntly to the vein, and the vessel is dissected free circumferentially. Proximal and distal ligatures are placed and the distal one tied. A venotomy is made and the catheter is threaded centrally into the superior vena cava. The proximal ligature is tied securely.

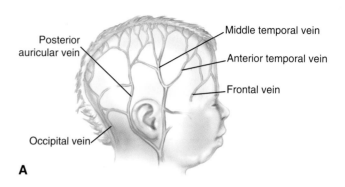

A

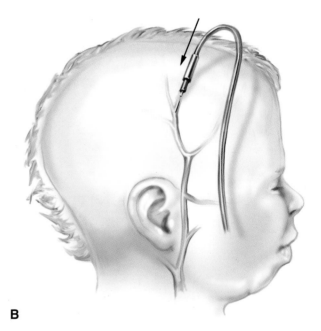

B

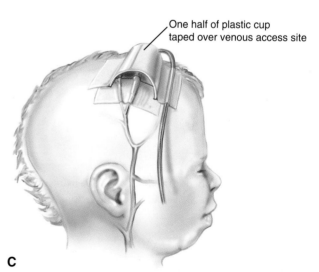

C

Figure 9-1 ▬▬▬▬

Scalp vein access. **A,** Venous architecture of the scalp. **B,** Schematic of infant with a right temporal scalp vein intravenous catheter. **C,** Note the occlusive dressing over the access site and the plastic cup, which prevents the cannula from being inadvertently dislodged.

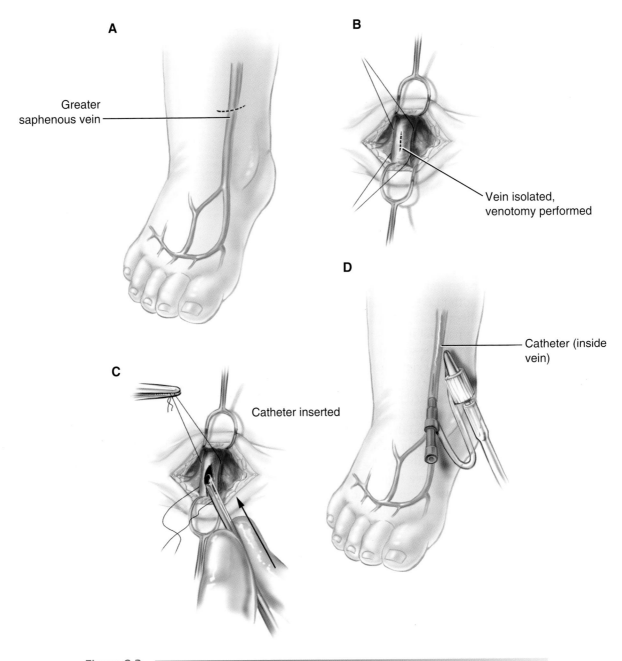

Figure 9-2
Saphenous vein access. **A,** Drawing of a child's right foot shows the position of the saphenous vein. **B,** Isolation of saphenous vein. **C,** Insertion of catheter. **D,** Catheter with two-port access.

When a percutaneous or cutdown catheter is to remain for a long period, it is tunneled under the skin to exit far from the venotomy, minimizing infection or dislodgment (Figure 9-4, *B*). The skin is closed with 5-0 nylon sutures, and the catheter is secured with 4-0 nylon. The intravenous site is covered with antibiotic ointment and an occlusive tape dressing.

TRACHEOTOMY
General Considerations

In the 1950s and 1960s the incidence of tracheotomy in children increased significantly because of improvements in surgical technique and the development of soft, pliable plastic tubes.[2] The number of tracheotomies decreased after the mid-1960s because of widespread

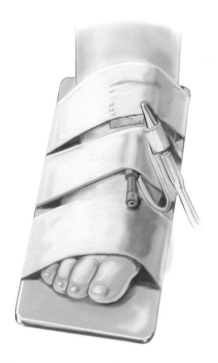

Saphenous vein access. Whether percutaneous or cutdown access is obtained, an occlusive dressing is used for the access site, and the foot is immobilized by taping it to an IV board.

use of endotracheal intubation.[3-5] Indeed, from 1970 to 1985, short-term endotracheal intubation for airway obstruction from acute infections and long-term intubation for patients on ventilators replaced early tracheotomies for these conditions. In one study, the number of tracheotomies decreased from 73 to 55 to 25 during the three 5-year periods from 1970 to 1985.[4] Carter and Benjamin[5] found that 60% of tracheotomies

were for acute inflammatory airway obstruction between 1972 and 1975, compared with 15% for this indication between 1979 and 1981. These trends remain reflective of surgical practice today.

An artificial airway (nasoendotracheal, oroendotracheal, or tracheostomy tube) may be required for one or more of three basic reasons: (1) to bypass an obstruction of the airway, (2) to aid in pulmonary toilet, and (3) to facilitate assisted ventilation.[6] In pediatric oral and maxillofacial surgery, the most common indication for elective tracheotomy is to provide a temporary airway for intraoperative ventilation or to prevent postoperative airway obstruction in major craniofacial and orthognathic operations. Children with micrognathia and first and second branchial arch deformities (Treacher Collins syndrome, hemifacial microsomia, bilateral craniofacial microsomia), Pierre Robin sequence, or syndromic craniosynostosis (e.g., Crouzon or Apert syndromes) may have a permanent tracheostomy because of airway obstruction during infancy. Emergency tracheotomy is performed occasionally for airway obstruction after maxillofacial trauma, although fiberoptic endotracheal intubation has replaced tracheotomy almost totally for this indication.

The trachea should be entered with a midline vertical incision through three adjacent tracheal rings. A short tracheal incision is dangerous, because pressure from a tight fit causes deformation of adjacent tracheal rings when decannulation is carried out.[3] Cartilage should not be excised in children; a flap tracheostomy opening, sometimes used in adults, is contraindicated because it results in instability of the airway upon decannulation or obstruction by displacement of the flap.[5,6] The tube should fit comfortably without being tight. In most instances, inflation of the cuff need be only intermittent.

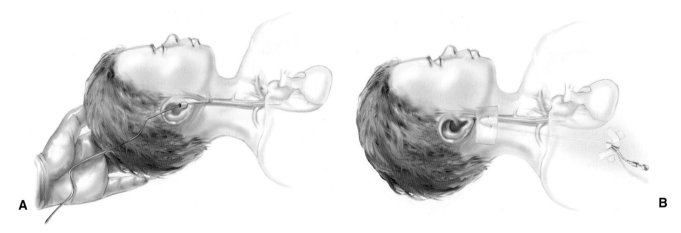

A   **B**

External jugular vein access. **A,** Percutaneous external jugular cannulation. **B,** Introducer and sheath are removed in preparation for tunneling of catheter to exit far from venotomy site.

If possible, tracheotomy should be avoided in infants and children because of potential problems with tracheal stenosis and chronic airway obstruction. Aberdeen and Downes,[3] however, have demonstrated that with a sufficiently long vertical incision (three rings), without removing cartilage when opening the trachea and with the use of a soft tube, the stricture problem can be virtually eliminated. Carter and Benjamin[5] also found no cases of tracheal stenosis in a review of 164 pediatric tracheotomies. A tracheostomy, however, presents a major psychosocial challenge to the patient and family. Finally, tracheostomy in young children may result in poor or abnormal speech and communication development.[7]

Technique

The patient is placed on the operating table in the supine position. General anesthesia is administered via an endotracheal tube. A roll is placed under the shoulders, and the head is positioned in a "donut" or ring. The proper size tracheostomy tube is selected, and the cuff is tested, by inflating it under water, *before* beginning the operation.

A horizontal incision is made one to two fingerbreadths above the sternal notch. The dissection is continued transversely through the subcutaneous tissue and the platysma muscle (Figure 9-5, *A*). The strap muscles are separated in the midline, by blunt dissection through the pretracheal fascia, to expose the trachea. Few vessels are encountered in this dissection. The thyroid isthmus, which rarely has to be divided, is elevated and retracted superiorly.

The tracheal rings are then counted, and the trachea is retracted with a hook placed below the second ring. Silk sutures (4-0) are placed through the fourth tracheal ring on either side of the planned tracheotomy incision; they are knotted with long loops and used for traction intraoperatively (Figure 9-5, *B*). Should the tube become dislodged postoperatively, these sutures are used to open the airway for recannulation.

A vertical incision is made in the trachea, usually through the third, fourth, and fifth tracheal rings (Figure 9-5, *B* and *C*). The endotracheal tube is identified, slowly withdrawn, and replaced by the tracheostomy tube (Figure 9-5, *D*). The tube is secured to the skin with sutures (4-0 nylon) and tracheal tape while the head is in a flexed position. The incision is closed partially and the wound dressed with an antibiotic ointment and a gauze sponge.

Postoperative Care

Postoperatively, the child should breathe warm, humidified air and oxygen and should be observed in an intensive care unit for 72 hours. Tracheal suctioning, preced-

ed by hand ventilation with 100% oxygen, is done with a sterile catheter whenever there are excessive secretions or signs of airway obstruction. The cuff is deflated as often as possible but at least every hour for 5 minutes. A spare tracheostomy tube should always accompany a child being transferred.

RIB HARVESTING
General Considerations

The chest is an excellent donor site, with a plentiful supply of bone and cartilage. Rib resection is technically easy, and perioperative and long-term morbidity are low.[8-10] The bone can be split longitudinally, cut into corticocancellous chips, or used full thickness with or without the costochondral junction.

In the past, ribs were used commonly for contour augmentation of the forehead, zygoma, and anterior maxilla. However, in more recent years, calvarial bone grafts have become more favored for contour augmentation because there is reportedly less postoperative resorption and loss of contour. A full-thickness rib with costochondral junction is the method of choice to replace or construct the mandibular condyle and proximal ramus.

Long-term and short-term complications resulting from the rib donor site are uncommon.[8-10] Laurie et al.[8] reviewed donor site morbidity and found a 9% incidence of pleural tears requiring chest tube drainage. This complication usually occurred when two or three ribs were harvested and rarely occurred in those patients from whom one rib was taken. Patients had a moderate degree of postoperative donor site pain, lasting a mean of 2 weeks (1 to 8 weeks).

Long-term follow-up revealed that most patients had a visible mild chest wall contour defect; none had a palpable bony defect in the regenerated rib. However, when harvested a second time, the regenerated rib was usually thin and not suitable for use as a graft. More than 2 years postoperatively, 3 of 44 patients had persistent pleuritic pain with exercise.

Sawin et al.[10] reported an overall complication rate of 3.7% including pneumonia, atelectasis, and superficial wound dehiscence. Pneumothorax, intercostal neuralgia, and chronic chest wall pain were not encountered in 300 patients. This low complication rate probably reflects the fact that rib only, without costal cartilage, was harvested. The rib donor site morbidity in this study was significantly less than that of iliac crest.

Technique

The patient is placed in the supine position, with a blanket roll elevating the ipsilateral chest. The incision is made 2.5 cm from the margin of the nipple-areolar

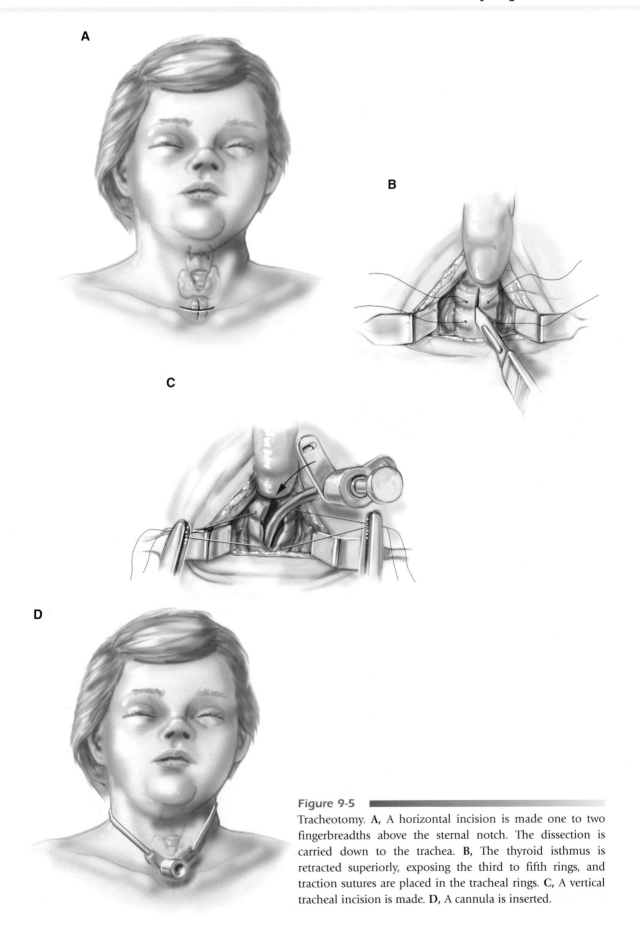

Figure 9-5

Tracheotomy. **A,** A horizontal incision is made one to two fingerbreadths above the sternal notch. The dissection is carried down to the trachea. **B,** The thyroid isthmus is retracted superiorly, exposing the third to fifth rings, and traction sutures are placed in the tracheal rings. **C,** A vertical tracheal incision is made. **D,** A cannula is inserted.

complex. This is important to avoid nipple retraction and to ensure that the incision lies in the inframammary fold at the completion of growth (Figure 9-6, *A*).

The dissection is continued with electrocautery. The chest wall muscles are divided, the rib exposed, and the periosteum incised. An Alexander elevator is used to reflect the periosteum (Figure 9-6, *B*). When the superior and inferior surfaces of the rib are reached, an Overholt elevator is used to dissect over the edges to the pleural side of the rib (Figure 9-6, *C*). Next, a Doyen elevator is used to strip the remaining deep periosteum (Figure 9-6, *D*). When a costochondral junction is needed, the perichondrium and periosteum on the superficial side of the graft, across the junction, are left in place. In this way, it is less likely that the cartilage will separate from the bone. Two millimeters of cartilage is harvested with the bone.[11,12] The cartilage is incised with a no. 15 blade, protecting the posterior tissues with the Doyen retractor.

When cartilage is not required, the rib is divided near the costochondral junction with a guillotine rib cutter. It is then retracted, and a right-angled cutter is used to make the second (posterior) osteotomy (Figure 9-6, *E*). The rib is removed and the wound is irrigated. To detect any air leak (pleural tear), positive pressure (25 mm Hg) breaths are administered by the anesthesiologist. The wound is closed in layers: 2-0 chromic for the muscle periosteal layer, 4-0 Vicryl (Ethicon, Cincinnati, Ohio) for the dermis, and 5-0 nylon or a buried 5-0 Monocryl (Ethicon, Cincinnati, Ohio) for the skin. No attempt is made to close the periosteum as a separate layer (Figure 9-6, *F*).

If a pleural tear is detected at the time of the operation, a small red rubber catheter is placed in the pleural cavity through the opening. A purse-string suture is placed around the tube and, with the anesthesiologist administering positive pressure breaths, the tube is placed on suction and withdrawn while tying the suture. If this is not successful in reinflating the lung, a chest tube is placed.

A chest radiograph is obtained postoperatively. If a pneumothorax of greater than 10% is detected, a chest tube is inserted and suction applied. When the lung is reinflated, the chest tube attached to a water seal. When no leak is demonstrated for 24 to 48 hours, the tube is removed.

ILIAC CREST BONE HARVESTING
General Considerations

Iliac crest is perhaps the most versatile and commonly used bone graft donor site. It is a source of corticocancellous blocks and large quantities of particulate marrow. Iliac bone is easy to manipulate, and it can be used to provide contour augmentation and stability across osteotomy gaps, to fill alveolar clefts, and to replace missing bone (e.g., full-thickness mandibular defects). Disadvantages of the iliac donor site include (1) blood loss, (2) postoperative pain, and (3) postoperative gait problems.[13] When a full-thickness graft is harvested, 250 to 500 ml of blood may be lost intraoperatively. An additional 250 ml (ranging from 42 to 493 ml) may be lost during the first 24 hours postoperatively.[13] Most patients have moderate to severe pain lasting from 2 to 8 weeks. Patients who have had both rib and iliac donor sites harvested complain significantly more about the hip than the chest.[8,10,14] Paresthesia of the lateral femoral cutaneous nerve, temporary or permanent, is also a well-known complication occurring in approximately 5% of patients. Meralgia paresthetica is an unusual but very troublesome complication.[13-17] Finally, a contour defect may develop in the crest, particularly troublesome in thin patients.[18-23] Harvesting small grafts for orthognathic surgery or pure marrow grafts for alveolar clefts is accompanied by a very low morbidity rate.[13]

Technique

Particulate Marrow. This technique is used to obtain bone marrow for grafting alveolar clefts or to augment the alveolar ridge for implants.[8,23] The patient is in the supine position, with a roll under the gluteus muscle to elevate the hip. An incision is made lateral to the iliac crest (Figure 9-7, *A*). The dissection is carried through the skin and subcutaneous tissue to the iliac crest. The crest, with its cartilaginous cap, the attachments of the gluteus maximus and tensor fascia lata laterally, and the iliacus muscle medially are identified (Figure 9-7, *B*).

With an osteotome, a 2.5-cm sagittal cut is made through the crest into the marrow space. The crest is then wedged apart with the osteotome and the marrow cavity is exposed (Figure 9-8). Occasionally, in older children, a cut must be made perpendicular to the sagittal osteotomy anteriorly to allow for opening of the crest. This should be done at least 1 cm posterior to the anterior superior iliac spine to avoid the lateral femoral cutaneous nerve. Marrow is harvested with bone curettes and stored in blood mixed with a small volume of Ringer's lactate. The marrow should *not* be soaked in an antibiotic solution.

The crest is reapproximated with 3-0 Prolene (Ethicon, Cincinnati, Ohio) interrupted stitches, and the wound is closed in layers with 3-0 chromic, 4-0 Vicryl for the dermis, and 5-0 nylon suture for the skin. No drain is placed.

Full-Thickness Graft. A lateral incision is used, and the dissection is carried down to the iliac crest as described above. An incision is made at the attachment of the gluteus muscle. The muscle is dissected off the bone, exposing the lateral surface of the ilium. The iliacus

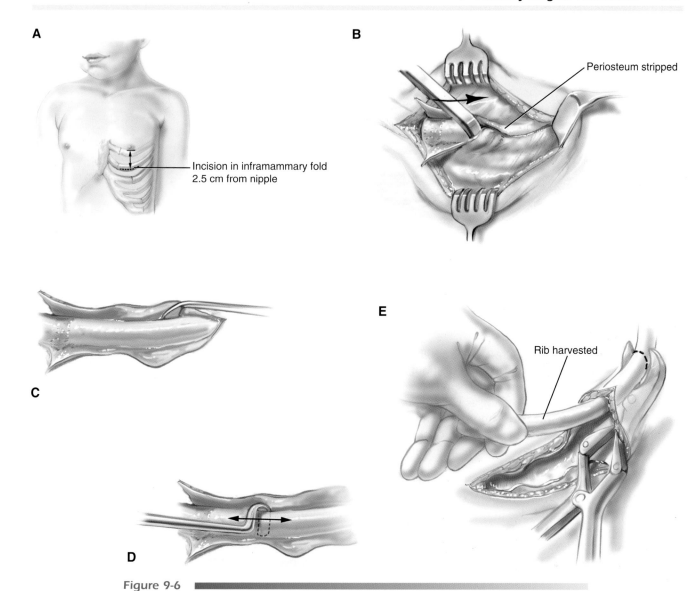

A, Incision in inframammary fold 2.5 cm from nipple

B, Periosteum stripped

E, Rib harvested

Figure 9-6

Rib graft harvesting procedure. **A,** Diagram of an incision 2.5 cm from the margin of the nipple-areolar complex. **B,** An Alexander elevator is used to complete a subperiosteal dissection, exposing the costochondral junction and rib. Note the direction of the elevator, stripping periosteum up, on the down side of the periosteal reflection, and down, on the up side of the periosteal reflection. **C,** An Overholt elevator is used to dissect over the edges to the pleural side of the rib. **D,** A Doyen elevator is used to complete the deep periosteal dissection, thereby freeing up the rib. **E,** An angled rib cutter is used to make the posterior cut while the rib is stabilized with the other hand or a bone holder. The wound is closed in layers.

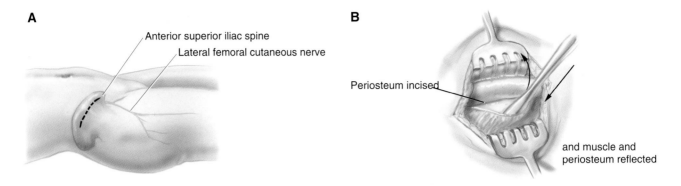

Figure 9-7
Iliac crest harvesting procedures. **A,** Incision markings are drawn on the right iliac region. Note the relationship of the anterior superior iliac spine and lateral femoral cutaneous nerve. Usually, the lateral incision is used, lateral to the crest and perpendicular to the skin striae. **B,** The periosteum is incised and is reflected along with the muscle.

muscle is left attached to the crest (Figure 9-9, *A*). An osteotomy is made across the iliac crest about 1 cm posterior to the anterior superior iliac spine. A second vertical cut is made as far posterior as possible on the crest. The two osteotomies are connected with a full-thickness subcrestal osteotomy. The iliac crest is then elevated, pedicled to the iliacus muscle as a composite muscle-bone flap.

The segment of bone to be removed is excised using a power saw or osteotomes. The bone cuts are made so as to leave a 5- to 10-mm ledge in the ilium. The crestal bone flap is returned to its original position and wired with 26-gauge stainless steel sutures (Figure 9-9, *B*). A suction drain is placed. The wound is closed in layers:

3-0 chromic, 4-0 Vicryl for the dermis, and 5-0 nylon for the skin.

An alternative method is to leave the crest intact and harvest the segment of bone from the lateral aspect.

The technique for iliac bone graft harvesting described here incorporates modifications to minimize donor site morbidity.[13] The incision is made lateral to the crest to minimize the potential for dehiscence. To avoid excessive muscle dissection, the lateral skin wound is shifted to lie directly over the crest. When using a medial incision, it should be placed at least 2 cm medial to the crest. When the patient stands, the skin moves inferiorly and laterally; thus, the medial incision may come to lie directly over the crest. Contour defects of the bony crest

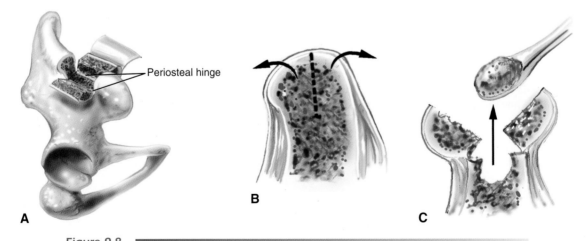

Figure 9-8
Harvest of particulate marrow from iliac crest. **A,** Diagram of the sagittal osteotomy, which allows opening of the crest, which remains attached to the medial and lateral muscles. **B,** The crested is wedged open like a book. **C,** Particulate marrow is scooped out with a bone curette.

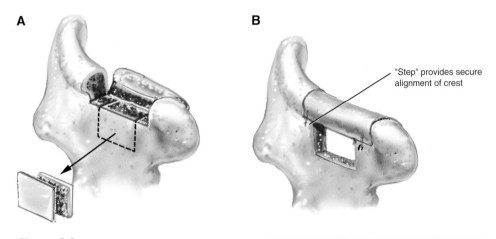

Figure 9-9

Iliac crest full-thickness graft. **A,** Diagram of the technique recommended for harvesting full-thickness iliac crest using a subcrestal osteotomy to provide a crestal flap of bone, periosteum, and muscle. **B,** After a full-thickness graft is removed, the crest is returned and wired in place.

can be avoided by elevating the crest as a flap attached to the iliacus muscle or by leaving the crest completely intact and harvesting bone from below. Acetabular fracture is unlikely if bone cuts are performed only after adequate exposure is developed and if the surgeon does not use excessive force or leverage to free and deliver the graft.

CALVARIAL BONE HARVESTING
General Considerations

The skull is an excellent source of bone. There is a plentiful quantity of graft material available, the scalp incision is not visible, and there is minimal donor site pain. In craniofacial operations, a separate donor site incision is not required.

In pediatric patients with a normal skull, the quantity of bone compares favorably with other donor sites. Cranial bone provides excellent stability across osteotomy gaps or discontinuity defects, because it is predominantly cortical in nature. It has been claimed that when calvarial bone is used for augmentation, as in zygomatic reconstruction, there is less resorption and better long-term maintenance of graft volume.[24-28] The skull may be used as a full-thickness or partial-thickness (inner or outer table) graft or may be morselized into corticocancellous chips.[25-33] Finally, calvaria may be harvested attached to temporalis muscle and transferred as a muscle-bone composite flap in cases of soft tissue and bony deficiency.[34,35]

When the patient has an abnormal skull, such as in craniosynostosis, hypertelorbitism, trauma, or secondary to increased intracranial pressure, harvesting is more

difficult and the quantity of bone may be inadequate. In general, however, complications are rare. Jackson and colleagues[24] reported 17 complications in 307 cranial bone grafts during a 6-year period: hematoma (6), seroma (4), scalp wound dehiscence (2), dural tear (2), arachnoid bleed (1), and scalp wound infection (2).

Technique

When bone is being harvested as part of a craniofacial operation or repair of midface, orbital, or nasoethmoidal fractures, the coronal incision and dissection provide access and no additional incisions are required. When small amounts of bone are needed, the incision and dissection may be limited to one side and the entire temporalis need not be detached.

A neurosurgeon should attend the harvest of full-thickness calvarial grafts. The skull is exposed, burr holes are made, and the dura is dissected off the undersurface of the skull with Penfield and Freer elevators. A power drill with a guarded bit is used to connect the burr holes. When the osteotomy is completed, the portion of skull is removed, carefully dissecting the remaining dura off the graft. The bone is split and the inner table returned to the donor site; the outer cortex is used to construct or augment the forehead, zygoma, anterior maxilla, or mandible. A straight graft can be harvested from the parietal bone, a curved graft for the zygoma from the temporoparietal region.

Partial thickness calvarial grafts are harvested more commonly in pediatric maxillofacial reconstruction. The shape of the graft is outlined with a sterile marking pencil, and then a drill is used to create a trough into the diploë. Bleeding occurs when the correct depth is reached. An osteotome can then be inserted into the marrow cavity and gently tapped to separate the outer table (Figure 9-10). Hemostasis is achieved with bone wax or microfibrillar collagen (Avitene, Bard, Murray Hill, NJ), and the edges of the donor site are smoothed with a burr. Split-thickness calvarial grafts commonly are used for osteotomy gaps (e.g., Le Fort I osteotomy), posttraumatic orbital and zygomatic defects, and for reconstruction of a variety of craniofacial congenital

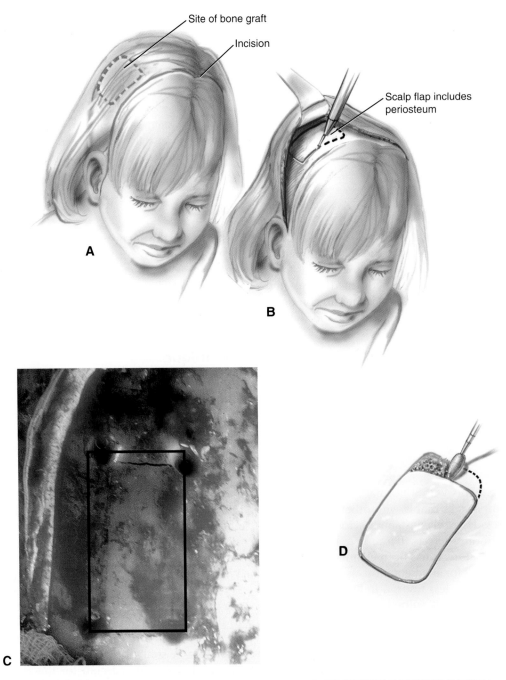

Figure 9-10

Calvarial bone graft harvesting. **A,** Diagram of coronal incision and bone graft donor site. Diagram **(B)** and intraoperative photograph **(C)** of completed dissection and outline of bone to be harvested. Note the partial-thickness burr holes, in photograph, which will be connected to make a partial-thickness trough **(D).**

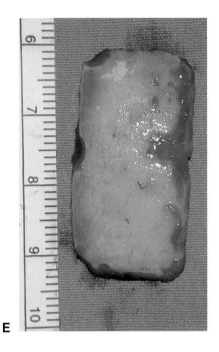

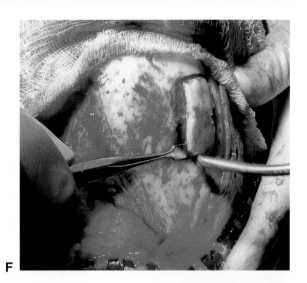

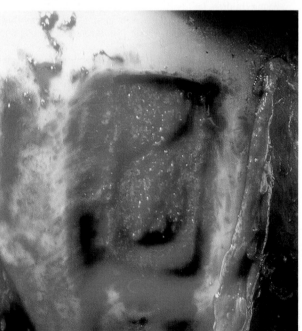

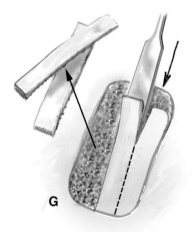

Figure 9-10—*continued*

E, Intraoperative photograph of split-thickness graft. Intraoperative photograph **(F)** and diagram **(G)** of split-thickness bone strips being harvested. **H,** Intraoperative view of intact inner table after the strips are harvested. (**C** and **E** courtesy Dr. T. Dodson.)

and acquired contour deficiencies. They are also useful as a source of corticocancellous chips for alveolar clefts, although iliac marrow remains the graft of choice for this indication.

Vascularized Calvarial Grafts. These are full-thickness or partial-thickness portions of the skull attached to the temporalis muscle and fascia. The dissection is the same, except that the temporalis muscle is left attached to the skull and provides blood supply for the graft flap.[24,34,35]

CONCLUSION

In this chapter, we reviewed the common ancillary surgical procedures used in pediatric oral and maxillofacial surgery practice. The most common procedures involve intravenous access and bone graft harvesting. Particular attention was paid to anatomic considerations, techniques unique to children, and donor site morbidity.

REFERENCES

1. Filler RM, Eraklis A, Das B: Fluids, electrolytes and intravenous nutrition. In Gans SL, editor: *Surgical pediatrics,* New York, 1973, Grune and Stratton.
2. Beatrous WP: Tracheostomy (tracheotomy): its expanded indications and its present status. Based on an analysis of 1000 consecutive operations and a review of the recent literature, *Laryngoscope* 78:3-55, 1968.
3. Aberdeen E, Downes II: Artificial airways in children, *Surg Clin North Am* 54:1155-1170, 1974.
4. Line WS, Hawkins DB, Kahlstrom EI, et al: Tracheotomy in infants and young children: the changing perspective 1970-1985, *Laryngoscope* 96:515, 1986.
5. Carter P, Benjamin B: Ten-year review of pediatric tracheotomy, *Ann Otol Rhinol Laryngol* 92:398-400, 1983.
6. Aberdeen E, Johnson DG: Tracheostomy. In Welch KI, Randolph IG, Ravitch MM, et al., editors: *Pediatric surgery,* Chicago, 1986, Year Book Medical Publishers.
7. Kaslon KW, Stein RE: Chronic pediatric tracheotomy: assessment and implications for habilitation of voice, speech and language in young children, *Int J Pediatr Otorhinolaryngol* 9:165-171, 1985.
8. Laurie SWS, Kaban LB, Mulliken JB, et al: Donor site morbidity after harvesting rib and iliac bone, *Plast Reconstr Surg* 73:933-938, 1984.
9. Gurley JM, Pilgram T, Perlyn CA, Marsh JL: Long-term outcome of autogenous rib graft and reconstruction, *Plast Reconstr Surg* 108:1895-1905, 2001.
10. Sawin PD, Traynelis VC, Menezes AH: A comparative analysis of fusion rates and donor-site morbidity for autogeneic rib and iliac crest bone grafts in posterior cervical fusions, *J Neurosurg* 88:255-265, 1998.
11. Kaban LB, Perrott DH: Commentary: unpredictable growth pattern of costochondral grafts, *Plast Reconstr Surg* 90:887-889, 1992.
12. Perrott DH, Umeda H, Kaban LB: Costochondral construction/reconstruction of the ramus condyle/unit: long-term follow-up, *Int J Oral Maxillofac Surg* 23:321-328, 1994.
13. Keller EE, Triplett WW: Iliac bone grafting: review of 160 consecutive cases, *J Oral Maxillofac Surg* 45:11-14, 1987.
14. Hoard MA, Bill TJ, Campbell RJ: Reduction in morbidity after iliac crest bone harvesting: the concept of preemptive analgesia, *J Craniofac Surg* 9:448-451, 1998.
15. Cockin J: Autologous bone grafting—complications at the donor site, *J Bone Joint Surg (Br)* 53:153, 1971.
16. Edelson JG, Nathan H: Meralgia paresthetica: an anatomical interpretation, *Clin Orthop* 122:255, 1977.
17. Weikel AM, Habal MB: Meralgia paresthetica: a complication of iliac procurement, *Plast Reconstr Surg* 60:572, 1977.
18. Hill NM, Horne JG, Devane PA: Donor site morbidity in the iliac crest, *Aust N Z J Surg* 69:726-728, 1999.
19. Hardy SP, Wilke RC, Doyle JF: Advantages of percutaneous hollow needle technique for iliac bone harvest in alveolar cleft grafting, *Cleft Palate Craniofac J* 36:252-255, 1999.
20. Boustred AM, Feranandes D, van Zyl AE: Minimally invasive iliac cancellous bone graft harvesting, *Plast Reconstr Surg* 99:1760-1764, 1997.
21. Dawson KH, Egbert MA, Myall RW: Pain following iliac crest bone grafting of alveolar clefts, *J Craniomaxillofac Surg* 24:151-154, 1996.
22. Canady JW, Zeitler DP, Thompson SA, Nicholas CD: Suitability of the iliac crest as a site for harvest of autogenous bone grafts, *Cleft Palate Craniofac J* 30:579-581, 1993.
23. Beirne JC, Barry HJ, Brady FA, Morris VB: Donor site morbidity of the anterior iliac crest following cancellous bone harvest, *Int J Oral Maxillofac Surg* 25:268-271, 1996.
24. Jackson IT, Helden G, Marx R: Skull bone grafts in maxillofacial and craniofacial surgery, *J Oral Maxillofac Surg* 44:949-955, 1986.
25. Tessier P: Autogenous bone grafts taken from the calvarium for facial and cranial applications, *Clin Plast Surg* 9:531, 1982.
26. Zins IE, Whitaker LA: Membranous versus endochondral bone: implications for craniofacial reconstruction, *Plast Reconstr Surg* 72:778, 1983.
27. Smith ID, Abramson M: Membranous vs. endochondral bone autografts, *Arch Otolaryngol* 99:203, 1974.
28. Denny AD, Talisman R, Bonawitz SC: Secondary alveolar bone grafting using milled cranial bone graft: a retrospective study of a consecutive series of 100 patients, *Cleft Palate Craniofac J* 36:144-153, 1999.
29. Kortebein MJ, Nelson CL, Sadove AM: Retrospective analysis of 135 secondary alveolar cleft grafts using iliac or calvarial bone, *J Oral Maxillofac Surg* 49:493-498, 1991.
30. Barone CM, Jimenez DF: Split-thickness calvarial grafts in young children, *J Craniofac Surg* 8:43-47, 1997.
31. Frodel JL: Calvarial bone graft harvest in children, *Otolaryngol Head Neck Surg* 121:78-81, 1999.
32. Cheney ML, Gliklich RE: The use of calvarial bone in nasal reconstruction, *Arch Otolaryngol Head Neck Surg* 121: 643-648, 1995.
33. Koenig WJ, Donovan JM, Pensler JM: Cranial bone grafting in children, *Plast Reconstr Surg* 95:1-4, 1995.
34. McCarthy JG, Zide BM: The spectrum of calvarial bone grafting: introduction of the vascularized calvarial bone flap, *Plast Reconstr Surg* 74:10, 1984.
35. McCarthy JG, Cutting CB, Shaw WW: Vascularized calvarial flaps, *Clin Plast Surg* 14:37-48, 1987.

PART II

ORAL SURGICAL PROCEDURES

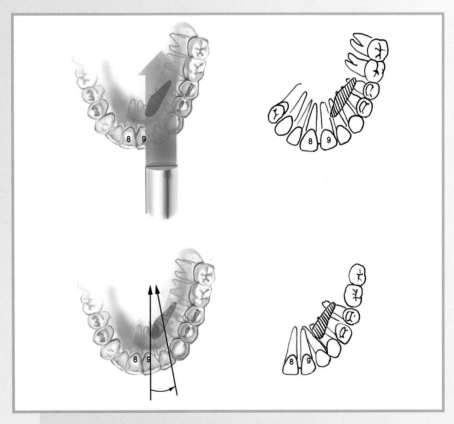

Diagram of the tube-shift technique

CHAPTER 10

Dentoalveolar Surgery

Leonard B. Kaban and Maria J. Troulis

CHAPTER OUTLINE

The pediatric patient presents with a variety of minor oral surgical problems that differ from those seen in adults. For example, the most commonly impacted teeth for which oral surgeons are consulted in children are maxillary canines, followed by maxillary central incisors and mandibular second premolars; in teenagers and adults, the most commonly impacted teeth are third molars. In preteenage children, a mesiodens is the supernumerary tooth most frequently requiring extraction, whereas in teenagers fourth molars and extra mandibular premolars predominate. Delayed or failed eruption of normal teeth (e.g., 6-year and 12-year molars) is another problem more common in children. It is important to understand the timing and techniques for management of late eruption.

Odontogenic and nonodontogenic dentoalveolar lesions that occur in childhood differ from those seen in adults. In children, complex and compound odontomas, cementomas, and small fibroosseous lesions are common, as are traumatic or hemorrhagic bone cysts. In adults, dentigerous cysts and ameloblastomas predominate.

Behavioral aspects of pediatric care in the hospital and office setting were discussed previously (see Chapters 3, 6, and 7). Management of common dentoalveolar problems in childhood is the subject of this chapter. The techniques described here are not necessarily new or unique, but they are ones with which we have had extensive clinical experience.

IMPACTED TEETH

Teeth may fail to erupt because they are mechanically obstructed by a supernumerary tooth, cyst, or odontogenic tumor or because there is insufficient space in the dental arch, either of skeletal (micrognathia) or dental (premature loss of deciduous teeth or tooth–arch size discrepancy) origin.[1] Failure of eruption also may be associated with syndromes of the head and neck (e.g., cleidocranial dysostosis, craniosynostosis)[2] or genetic[3,4] and endocrine abnormalities. Hypothyroidism and hypopituitarism are the two most commonly encountered examples of the latter.[5,6] In most cases, however, the etiology of eruption failure is unknown. Trankmann[7] found a 0.07% incidence of unerupted permanent teeth exclusive of third molars in a prospective study of 14,021 randomly selected males and females. These teeth, in order of frequency, were maxillary canine, mandibular second premolars, and maxillary incisors. Failure of eruption of permanent molars was noted to be very rare.

IMPACTED MAXILLARY CANINES
General Considerations

Inadequate space with dental crowding frequently contributes to failure of eruption of the maxillary canine. When an impacted canine is encountered, the choices of management are: (1) surgical exposure of the tooth, followed by orthodontic movement to its proper place in the dental arch, (2) extraction, or (3) autotransplantation (i.e., extraction and replantation into the normal position). The ideal treatment is prevention by close observation of the child's eruption pattern and jaw and dental development. When necessary, space is created by serial extraction of deciduous teeth and permanent premolars or by orthodontic therapy, or by both.

An impacted canine must be treated in the context of the patient's overall dental development and orthodontic status. Before any procedure is carried out, the orthodontic plan should be established; in most cases, orthodontic appliances should be in place. For example, in the patient who requires premolar extractions for space and alignment of teeth, a deeply impacted canine might be sacrificed because the prognosis for orthodontic movement is poor or because it is desirable (for medical or behavioral reasons) to shorten treatment time. The first premolar is then used in the canine position. Alternatively, if extraction is not appropriate, it might be necessary to surgically move an impacted canine to its proper position (Figure 10-1).

Root development of the canine is also important. If the root is fully developed and the apex is closed, there is little chance for spontaneous movement into the arch after exposure (Figure 10-2). If, however, root development is incomplete and the canine is vertical in orientation, significant spontaneous movement often occurs. The ideal time for exposure of an impacted canine (if one is sure the tooth will not erupt naturally) is when the root is developed but before the apex is closed. In very high impactions, exposure can be carried out when there is approximately two-thirds root development.

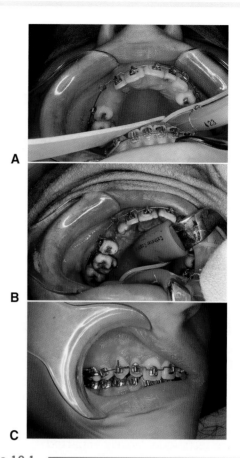

Figure 10-1

A, Teenage patient who had four premolars extracted and exposure of an impacted canine. The tooth was ankylosed and would not respond to orthodontic forces. Extraction was contraindicated at this time. **B,** The tooth was surgically moved into the dental arch. **C,** Eighteen months later, the tooth was stable, and there was no sign of root resorption.

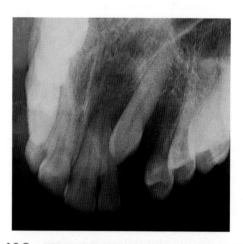

Figure 10-2

This patient had an overretained deciduous canine extracted 6 months before this radiograph at age 26. There was no spontaneous movement of the canine, although it was vertically oriented and there was adequate space, because the root apex was completely closed.

Treatment

The first critical step in management is radiographic evaluation of the anatomy of the impacted canine and its location in the maxilla. Occlusal radiographs are used because they allow full visualization of the root structure and the relationship of the canine to the maxillary alveolus and nasal cavity. The first radiograph is taken directly in the midline, and a second is taken with the beam shifted toward the side of the impacted tooth. Using Clark's rule, otherwise known as the *tube-shift* or *buccal-shift technique*, an impacted canine located on the palate will appear to move in the same direction as the x-ray beam, while one on the labial aspect of the ridge will move in the opposite direction (SLOB, *s*ame *l*ingual, *o*pposite *b*uccal) (Figures 10-3 and 10-4). An impacted canine located in the middle of the alveolus will *not* appear to change its location in the two radiographs. This is because the alveolar ridge is the center about which the beam is rotating.

The axial orientation of the tooth and its location (i.e., labial or palatal) may be demonstrated nicely on a lateral radiograph (an occlusal film placed over the anterior region of the maxilla parallel to the midsagittal plane or a lateral cephalogram) (Figure 10-5). This technique is particularly useful to localize teeth near the midline of the maxilla. Occasionally, a computed tomographic scan is helpful if the canine is very high and plain films cannot localize it definitively.

It is imperative to determine the location of an impacted canine before operating. The procedure may be unnecessarily long and of great magnitude if the position of the tooth is in doubt or assessed inaccurately.

Exposure Technique: Palatally Impacted Canines

The standard exposure technique for palatally impacted canines is to excise the overlying soft tissue with elec-

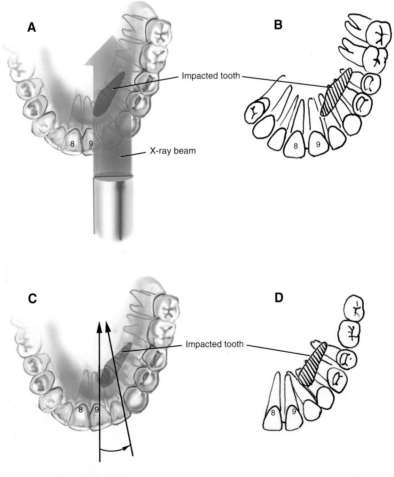

Figure 10-3

Diagram of the tube-shift technique. **A,** X-ray beam in midline. **B,** Appearance of palatally impacted canine. **C,** X-ray beam shifted around arch, toward patient's left side. **D,** Impacted canine appears to move off the left central incisor and onto the left lateral incisor in the same direction as the beam.

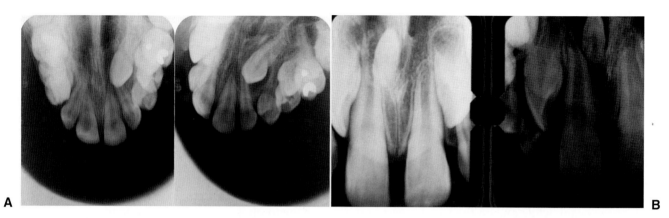

Figure 10-4

A, Occlusal radiographs of an impacted canine on the palate. When the tube is moved from its central position *(left)* toward the side of the impacted tooth *(right)*, the tooth appears to move in the same direction as the tube. **B,** Periapical radiographs of labial-impacted mesiodens. *Left,* The x-ray beam is directed in the midline. *Right,* As the tube moves to the patient's right, the mesiodens appears to move to the patient's left.

trocautery. To locate the crown, bone is removed with a hand chisel or rongeur. The remaining bone covering the tooth is then removed to the cervical margin. With electrocautery, remnants of the dental follicle are excised. A bracket-hook with a gold chain is then etched to the crown and the chain is connected to the orthodontic arch wire. The wound can be left open or dressed with periodontal packing. The latter is left in place for 4 to 5 days. The canine is allowed to move spontaneously for 6 to 8 weeks before active orthodontic forces are applied (Figures 10-5 and 10-6).

The advent of bonded brackets has allowed considerable flexibility in the exposure technique.[8] The need for a crown former to cover the exposed tooth has been eliminated. In addition, a single surface of the crown may be exposed if the impacted canine is adjacent to the palatal aspect of the central and lateral incisors. In these cases, exposure of the entire crown is not feasible. A bracket can simply be bonded to the exposed surface and orthodontic treatment begun.

Exposure Technique: Labially Impacted Canines

Canines impacted on the labial aspect of the ridge are exposed by using an apically repositioned flap.[9] Use of electrocautery to uncover labially impacted canines should be avoided because this procedure often results in a lack of attached gingiva, requiring a secondary grafting procedure (Figure 10-7). The flap is outlined in the

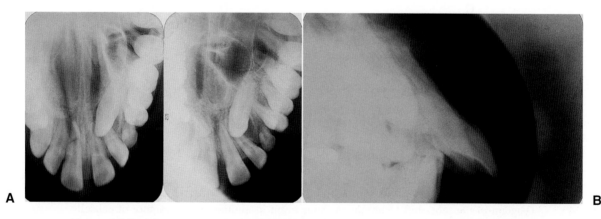

Figure 10-5

A, Occlusal radiographs exhibit tube-shift technique. **B,** Lateral radiograph. Both types of radiographs demonstrate impacted canine on the palate.

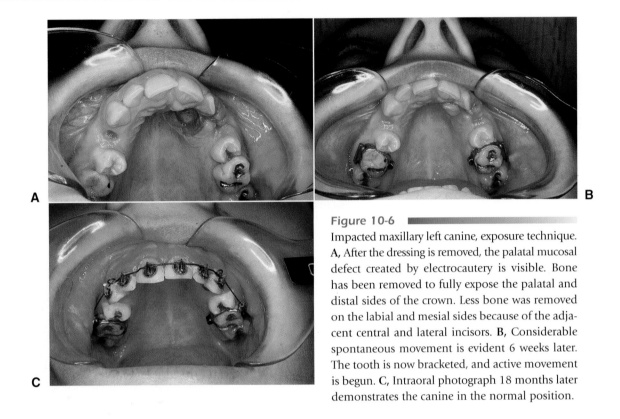

Figure 10-6

Impacted maxillary left canine, exposure technique. **A,** After the dressing is removed, the palatal mucosal defect created by electrocautery is visible. Bone has been removed to fully expose the palatal and distal sides of the crown. Less bone was removed on the labial and mesial sides because of the adjacent central and lateral incisors. **B,** Considerable spontaneous movement is evident 6 weeks later. The tooth is now bracketed, and active movement is begun. **C,** Intraoral photograph 18 months later demonstrates the canine in the normal position.

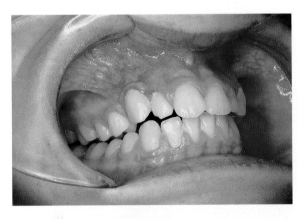

Figure 10-7

Intraoral photograph shows narrow band of attached gingiva that resulted from electrocautery exposure of labially impacted canine.

soft tissue overlying the tooth and then elevated to the depth of the labial sulcus (Figure 10-8). Bone is removed to the cervical margin, and then the remnants of the follicle are excised with electrocautery. The flap is repositioned apically and sutured in place with 5-0 chromic catgut. The distal edge of the flap is positioned at the cervical margin of the canine. A bracket-hook with gold chain is bonded to the exposed tooth and connected to the orthodontic arch wire. The wound usually is left open but may be covered with a periodontal pack dressing for 5 days. Again, no active orthodontic movement is started for 6 to 8 weeks.

Surgical Movement of Impacted Canines

When the maxillary canine is deeply impacted and the prognosis for orthodontic movement is poor, the tooth may be sacrificed and the first premolar used in its place. If extractions are not indicated, the impacted canine can be moved surgically into place or extracted and replanted (see Figure 10-1). The long-term prognosis for such surgically replanted canines is good.[10,11] Both Moss[10] and Pogrel[11] reported approximately 70% survival rates of autotransplanted canines. Pogrel found 102 of 162 autotransplanted canines to be present in the arch without external root resorption after at least 2 years of follow-up. Teeth that were lost were most often extracted within the first 2 years after transplantation. When the donor tooth was removed atraumatically, with preservation of the periodontal membrane, the success rate was 94%. There is some evidence that endodontic treatment with calcium hydroxide may arrest or slow external root resorption, and this is recommended when root resorption begins to develop.[12]

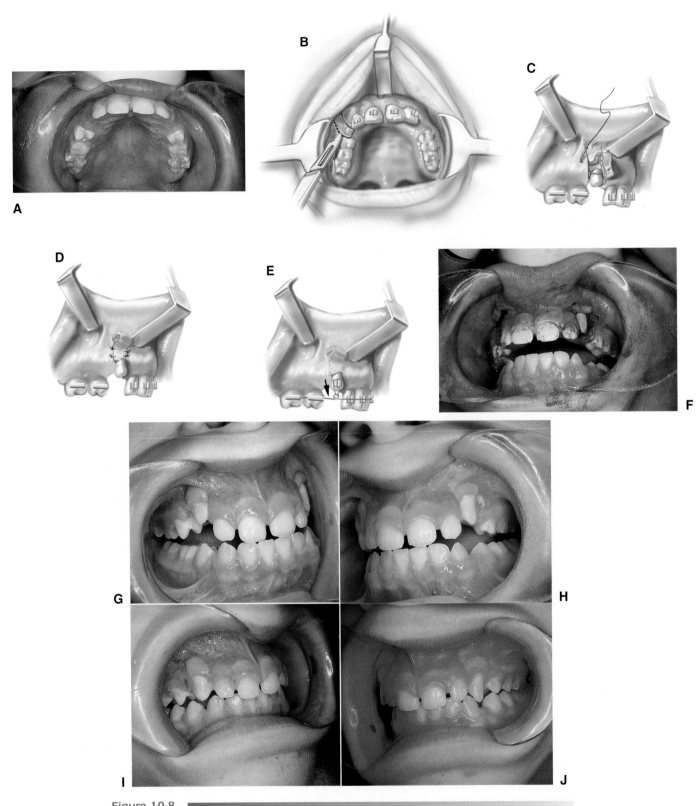

Figure 10-8

A, Bilateral labially impacted maxillary canines. **B,** Flap design. **C,** Flap elevated and first suture being placed to position the flap edge at cervical margin. **D,** Flap sutured in place. **E,** Diagrammatic representation of flap in place and gold chain attached to the arch wire *(arrow).* **F,** Intraoperative photograph of apically repositioned flap. **G** and **H,** Right and left sides 1 month postoperatively. **I** and **J,** Postoperative views of flaps at 1.5 years. Note the wide band of attached gingiva.

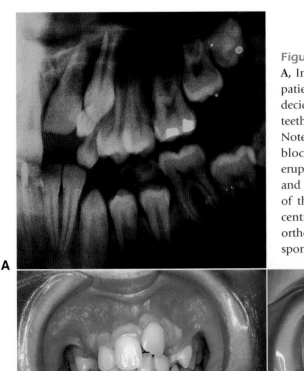

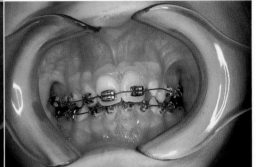

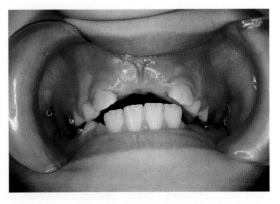

Figure 10-9

A, Impacted maxillary left central incisor in a patient with a history of traumatic intrusion of deciduous central and lateral incisors. These teeth were eventually lost because of infection. Note the abnormal impacted lateral incisor blocking the normal central incisor from erupting. **B,** The abnormal tooth was extracted, and there was some spontaneous movement of the central incisor. **C,** One year later, the central incisor was brought into the arch orthodontically, and the canine is visible with spontaneous eruption.

IMPACTED MAXILLARY INCISORS
General Considerations

In our experience, after maxillary canines, maxillary incisors are the most frequently impacted teeth seen in pediatric patients. This differs from Trankmann's[7] report in which he found premolars most frequent after canines. It is possible that the children the authors see, in an inner-city tertiary care hospital, have a higher caries and trauma rate in the maxillary anterior region. This results in early loss of deciduous incisors and a higher rate of permanent incisor impaction. A single impacted maxillary central incisor usually occurs with a history of trauma or infection in the deciduous dentition. The deciduous incisor might have been intruded, loosened, partially or totally avulsed, or lost secondary to infection; presumably, some damage occurred to the alveolus and follicle of the developing permanent incisor (Figure 10-9). When multiple deciduous maxillary incisors have been lost before age 5, soft tissue over the alveolus becomes hypertrophic and fibrotic, preventing eruption of the permanent central incisors (Figure 10-10). Impacted supernumerary teeth, as well as odontogenic cysts or tumors, may also prevent eruption of the maxillary incisors.

The patients often seek treatment around the age of 9 or 10, well after the permanent incisors normally erupt. At this time, the roots are fully developed, and the teeth have little spontaneous eruption potential (Figures 10-11 and 10-12). Ideally, the primary care dentist should determine that there is a problem earlier, by

Figure 10-10

Failure of eruption of permanent incisors as a result of early loss of deciduous incisors with resultant fibrosis of the alveolar ridge.

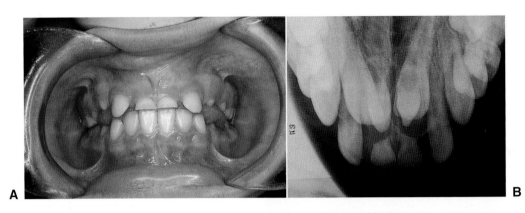

Figure 10-11

A, Overretained deciduous maxillary incisors. **B,** Radiograph demonstrates impacted supernumerary incisors blocking eruption of the normal teeth. The central incisor roots were fully developed; prognosis for spontaneous movement therefore was poor.

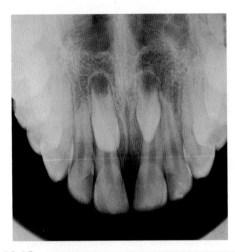

Figure 10-12

Radiograph demonstrates that supernumerary incisors do not always block eruption of the permanent teeth. Therefore one should wait until the permanent incisor roots are at least two thirds developed before removing the supernumeraries.

monitoring the child's dental development pattern. If possible, the impacted incisor is exposed when the root is two-thirds developed or, at the latest, before closure of the apex. In this way, there is potential for some spontaneous eruption postoperatively (Figure 10-13). Once the central incisor roots are fully developed, it may be difficult to get these teeth into the arch, even with significant orthodontic forces.

Technique

Before the procedure, an impacted incisor is located radiographically as described above for impacted canines. A lateral radiograph (occlusal size film) of the anterior maxilla is the radiograph of choice. Most impacted incisors are on the palatal aspect of the ridge or in the middle of the alveolus.

A full-thickness mucoperiosteal flap is elevated, and bone is removed to uncover the tooth to the cervical

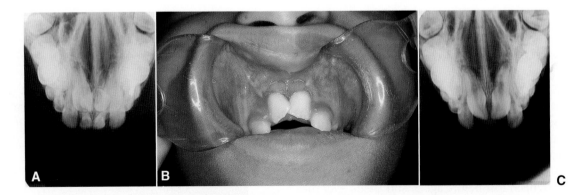

Figure 10-13

A, Overretained deciduous incisors, impacted supernumeraries, and central incisors with two-thirds root development. **B,** Partial spontaneous eruption after extraction of the extra incisors. **C,** Radiograph corresponding to clinical photograph. Orthodontic appliances will be used to complete the movement of the teeth.

margin. Dental follicle remnants are excised with electrocautery. Hypertrophic gingiva on the crest of the ridge is removed, leaving a path of eruption for the impacted tooth. Brackets can be bonded to the incisors and connected to the orthodontic arch wire at this time. If the incisor roots are not fully developed, the teeth can be allowed to erupt spontaneously. However, most impacted incisors, even with incomplete root development, require orthodontic therapy to be brought into the dental arch.

IMPACTED MAXILLARY AND MANDIBULAR PREMOLARS
General Considerations

Impacted premolars occur more frequently in the mandible than the maxilla. On the maxilla, they almost always are located on the palate, whereas on the mandible they are most frequently in the middle of the ridge or lingual. The teeth can be localized radiographically by Clark's rule or the tube-shift technique. If there is adequate space and no extractions are planned, surgical exposure of the premolar is the treatment of choice. This should be done before completion of root development.

Technique

A flap is reflected, bone and follicular tissue are removed to uncover the tooth to the cervical margin, and a bracket or hook is bonded to the tooth (Figures 10-14 and 10-15). The flap is then sutured in place, with tissue excised on the occlusal surface to provide a path of eruption. When a premolar is located on the palate, it is exposed exactly as described for a palatally impacted canine.

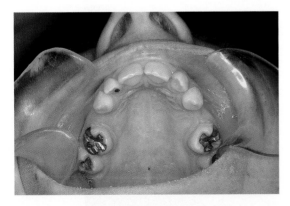

Figure 10-14

A mentally retarded 13-year-old girl with missing premolars. Orthodontic treatment was not possible. Previous extraction of first premolars did not result in second premolar eruption.

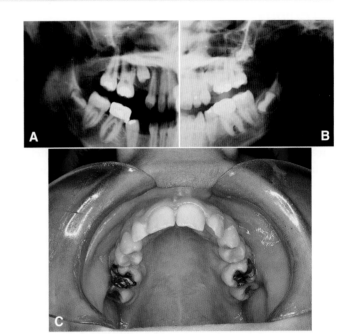

Figure 10-15

A and **B,** Panoramic radiographs show impacted premolars. **A,** On the patient's right side, the root apex was open. **B,** On the left side, the root was two thirds developed. **C,** Intraoral photograph 18 months after exposure illustrates the potential for spontaneous eruption if root development is not complete.

Root development and clinical eruption are followed carefully. If the tooth does not begin to erupt spontaneously in 2 months, orthodontic forces are used to move the tooth into the arch.

IMPACTED MOLARS
General Considerations

Pediatric and adolescent patients occasionally have unerupted 6-year or 12-year molars. Failure of eruption of adult molar teeth results in significant occlusal and periodontal sequelae. Management of these teeth after root development is complete and adaptive movements of adjacent teeth have occurred is difficult and the prognosis is poor. Therefore, early diagnosis and treatment are imperative.[1] If a single permanent molar fails to erupt when the other three have done so on schedule, the patient should be evaluated by radiographs. Once the roots have developed more than 50%, the impacted tooth should be exposed and gently luxated to allow spontaneous eruption. Kaban et al.[1] noted that patients with impacted molar teeth, treated by surgical exposure and luxation, had successful clinical results when the procedure was carried out before closure of root apices. Conversely, exposure and luxation carried out after complete root development was less successful.

Technique

A flap is reflected and bone and follicular tissue are removed to the cervical margin. The tooth is luxated gently into an upright position below the occlusal plane and allowed to erupt actively into occlusion (Figure 10-16). If treatment is delayed, the follicle of an impacted molar root may begin to curve along the inferior border of the mandible and develop parallel to it, the path of least resistance. This curvature of the follicle results in hooked or dilacerated roots. Early treatment prevents this deformation of the follicle and roots, which necessitates extraction of the tooth (Figure 10-17).

Treatment of pain, infection, and other pathology associated with third molars, as well as surgical removal of these teeth, constitutes a significant part of oral and maxillofacial surgery practice. The literature on this subject is voluminous, and the problems most commonly occur during the late teens—an age beyond the focus of this book. Therefore, wisdom teeth are not discussed except as they become significant in tooth transplantation.

IMPACTED SUPERNUMERARY TEETH

The most commonly impacted supernumerary tooth is the mesiodens (see Figure 10-4, *B*), followed by supernumerary maxillary incisors (Figure 10-18), fourth molars (Figure 10-19), and supernumerary mandibular premolars (Figure 10-20). Mesiodens and impacted supernumerary incisors may prevent eruption of the permanent maxillary incisors. These supernumerary teeth are best removed when the permanent incisors exhibit 50% of their root development. This ensures safety of the normal permanent teeth and prevents interference with their eruption. The mesiodens and supernumerary incisors are localized by radiographs preoperatively. A lateral radiograph of the anterior maxilla with an occlusal film or a lateral cephalogram are useful in this regard.

Fourth molars usually are removed at the same time as third molar extraction. If maxillary fourth molars are especially high on the posterior wall of the maxilla, they are left in place to erupt spontaneously after the third molars are removed. They can then be extracted in a second stage.

Supernumerary mandibular premolars should be removed when they can be distinguished from the adjacent normal premolars. Root development in the normal tooth is usually significantly ahead of that in the abnormal tooth. When a supernumerary premolar is extracted before its root is fully developed, the procedure is technically much easier and requires less bone removal than if done after the root is completely formed.

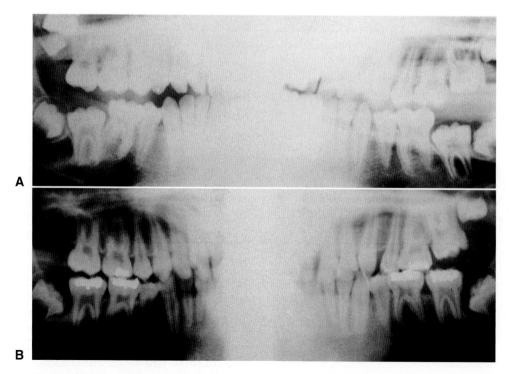

Figure 10-16 Patient with bilateral unerupted lower 12-year molars. **A**, Preoperative radiograph. **B**, Radiograph 1 year later. The teeth were exposed and luxated.

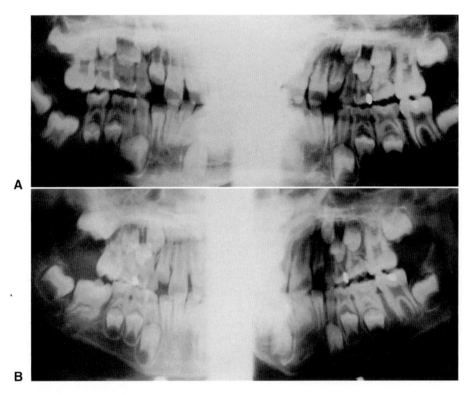

Figure 10-17

Preoperative **(A)** and postoperative **(B)** radiographs of a patient with an unerupted lower right, 6-year molar. The roots were beginning to deform at the inferior border at the time of surgery. Had treatment been delayed, the roots would have become dilacerated, and extraction would have been necessary.

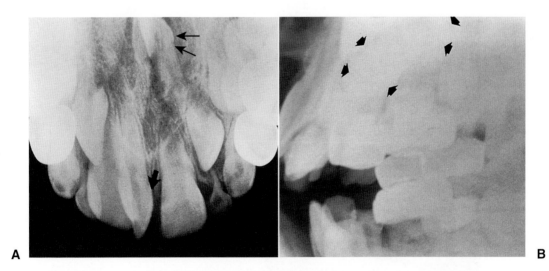

Figure 10-18

A, Occlusal radiograph demonstrating mesiodens *(arrow)* and inverted supernumerary incisor *(arrows).* **B,** Lateral radiograph shows the palatal position of the inverted tooth *(arrows).*

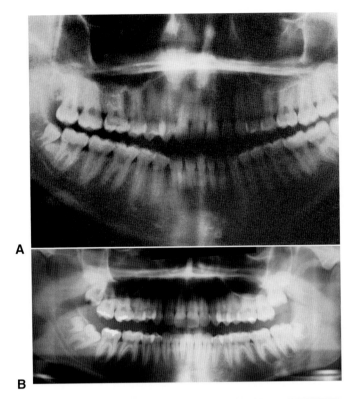

Figure 10-19

A, Mandibular fourth molars. B, Maxillary and mandibular fourth molars.

TRANSPLANTATION OF TEETH
General Considerations

The field of organ transplantation has blossomed since the early 1950s, when the first successful kidney transplant was performed. Use of organ transplants has been stimulated greatly by the development of immunosuppressive drugs to combat rejection. In general, allogeneic tooth transplantation has not become a widely applicable procedure. The antigenic stimulus of the periodontal membrane ultimately leads to rejection, and the complications of immunosuppression make it impractical for dental transplantation.

Autologous tooth transplantation, however, is feasible and quite useful, particularly in adolescents. The two most common autografts are impacted canines, when orthodontic movement is not feasible, and impacted third molars transplanted to first or second molar sites.[11,13]

Transplantation of impacted canines has been reviewed earlier in this chapter. Transplantation of a third molar to the first molar position is the next most common procedure (Figure 10-21). It can be carried out in any quadrant or from the maxillary third molar to the opposite mandibular molar site. The most common indication is loss of a 6-year molar due to caries. The patient may not have the financial means to obtain endodontic treatment, or the carious tooth may be

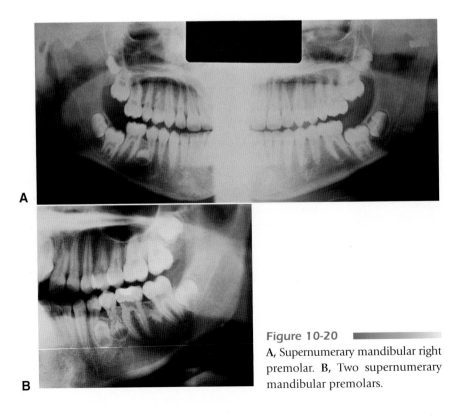

Figure 10-20

A, Supernumerary mandibular right premolar. B, Two supernumerary mandibular premolars.

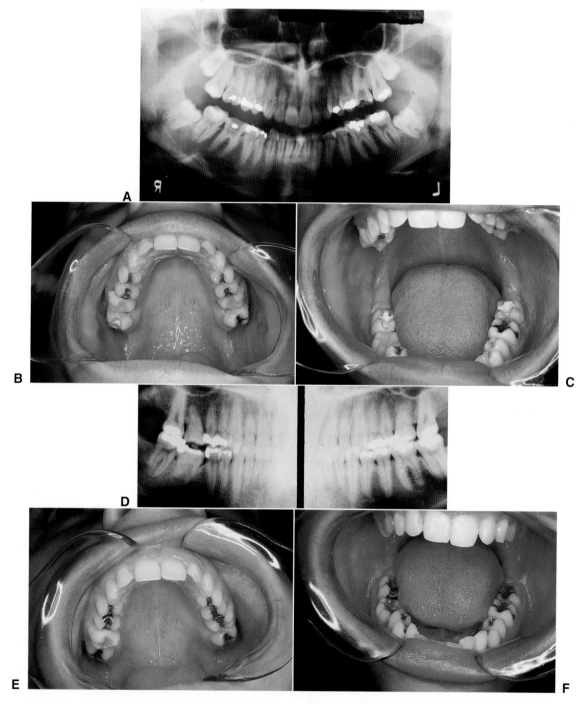

Figure 10-21

A, Panoramic radiograph shows large carious lesions in the upper right and left and lower right first molars. **B** and **C,** Intraoral photographs 1 month after the third to first molar transplants of the upper right and left and lower right third molars to the corresponding first molar sockets. **D,** Panoramic radiograph 5 years postoperatively demonstrates good root development, no external resorption, and amalgam restorations in two of the three transplants. **E** and **F,** Intraoral photographs 5 years postoperatively.

prosthetically unrestorable. The donor third molar roots should be no less than one-half and preferably about two-thirds developed.

Autologous tooth transplants carried out at the proper time in root development, in the absence of acute infection and with meticulous technique, have a high success rate. Defining success as the tooth being clinically firm and with normal color, with no clinical or radiographic evidence of resorption, ankylosis, or periapical pathology, Pogrel[11] reported an overall success rate of 72%. This included all transplants in a series of 400 cases followed for at least 2 years. Natiella et al.,[13] reviewing over 2000 tooth transplants and replants in the literature from 1950 to 1970, reported a similar success rate. The largest single factor in failure was damage to the periodontal membrane of the donor tooth during the procedure. When the transplant was removed atraumatically, with an intact periodontal membrane, and was transferred within 3 minutes to a well-fitting socket, the success rate was 94%.[11] Failure occurred either very early if the transplant became infected, or late if it became ankylosed and exhibited external root resorption. However, in Pogrel's series, all failures were evident within the first 2 years. Teeth that showed no evidence of ankylosis, resorption, or periapical pathology after 2 years did not develop these problems at longer follow-up intervals of up to 10 years. There is some evidence that external root resorption may be stopped or at least slowed down by prophylactic endodontic treatment.[13] Even in the case of failure over a period of 5 to 7 years, the patient has had a physiologic replacement and space maintainer and still has the option of obtaining a bridge or an implant.

Technique

Acute infection is controlled with antibiotics and drainage when indicated. If there is a significant periapical radiolucency, the infected molar is removed and the transplant carried out 2 to 4 weeks later. Care is taken not to damage the recipient site or to remove significant amounts of bone from the socket during the extraction. The donor-impacted third molar is extracted with careful bone removal by hand instruments. Extraction is done with forceps, or with a wire ligature around the tooth, and traction. Great care is taken not to damage the periodontal membrane of the transplant by using dental elevators.

The recipient socket is irrigated, and the third molar is inserted and firmly depressed to a level below the occlusal plane. The only modification of the recipient socket usually required is excision of the interfering septal bone. The wound is sutured with 3-0 silk in the interdental papillae and tied over the transplant in a figure-of-eight fashion. The wound is covered with periodontal packing, and the patient is placed on penicillin 250 mg by mouth four times per day (erythromycin in penicillin-allergic patients) for 7 days. The dressing is removed after 1 week, and the patient remains on a soft diet for 2 additional weeks. The tooth slowly erupts into the occlusal plane once the dressing is removed (see Figure 10-21).

OSSEOINTEGRATED IMPLANTS

Since the publication of Kaban's *Pediatric Oral and Maxillofacial Surgery* in 1990, the use of osseointegrated implants to replace teeth in adults has become commonplace, and the success rates are extraordinarily high. Dental implants also have been used in children with success. However, the field has been somewhat hampered by misconceptions regarding the indications and timing.

In children requiring the replacement of missing teeth, the ideal restoration is a fixed prosthesis achieved with osseointegrated implants. Loaded implants help to ensure maintenance of ridge height, prevent supraeruption of opposing teeth, and maintain a stable occlusion. Furthermore, children often do not use removable appliances, and hence supraeruption and loss of the free-way space occurs. However, the use of implants in children has been controversial.[14]

The arguments against the placement of implants in children relate to growth and bone remodeling. Osseointegrated implants have been reported to migrate.[14-17] The implants may become submerged as the alveolar bone grows vertically. Furthermore, osseointegration of mandibular implants is lost as the implant becomes lingually displaced by appositional growth of the mandible.[17-20]

Despite these concerns, there is a growing body of research that demonstrates the successful use of osseointegrated implants in the growing child.[14-16,21] Submersion of dental implants can be prevented by delaying implant placement until the adjacent permanent dentition has erupted. In general, by age 12 (eruption of 12-year molars) vertical alveolar growth of the jaws is nearly complete. Implants placed after the permanent dentition has erupted, therefore, do not become submerged. Furthermore, in long, bone-grafted segments, which have little potential for vertical growth, the implants maintain bone height and there is little chance for submersion to occur. If necessary, the prosthesis can be modified over time. Furthermore, on the mandible, implants are placed as buccally as possible to prevent lingual displacement. Finally, a prosthesis should never cross the midline sutures. In a recent case series published by our group, 23 implants were placed in seven growing children ages 3.5 to 16 years (mean age, 8 years), successfully restored and without any complications (Figure 10-22). If these considerations are respected, the restoration of a child's dentition with a fixed prosthesis is achievable.

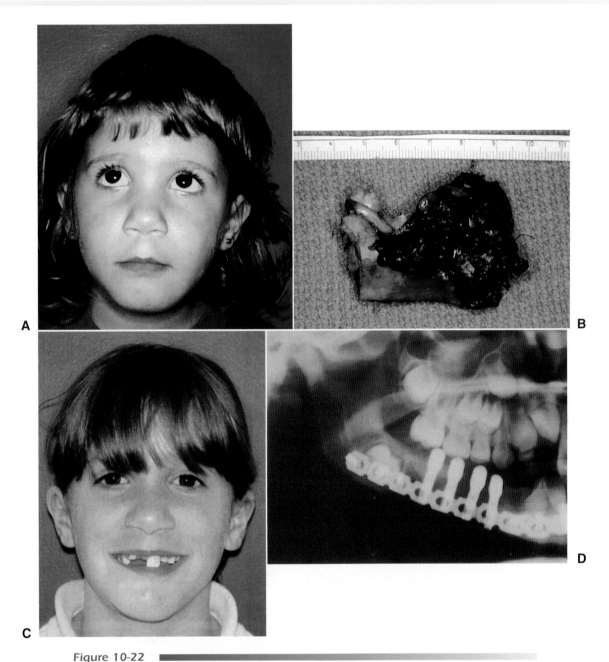

Figure 10-22
A, Frontal photograph of 3-year-old girl with a desmoplastic fibroma of the right mandible (see Chapter 15). The child underwent a right partial mandibulectomy. **B,** Photograph of specimen. Approximately 6 months later the patient had an iliac bone graft to the mandible and subsequently had implant placement for restoration of her occlusion. Frontal photograph **(C)** and panoramic radiograph **(D)** after the second stage of implant surgery.

LESIONS OF THE ALVEOLAR RIDGE

Benign odontogenic tumors of mesenchymal origin (complex and compound odontomas, cementomas) and odontogenic and nonodontogenic cysts are common in pediatric patients. They are often small and slow growing and are discovered on a routine follow-up radiograph or during the diagnostic workup of an unerupted tooth. Primary jaw tumors are discussed in Chapter 15.

ODONTOGENIC TUMORS

Odontoma

The most common odontogenic tumors seen in the pediatric population are varieties of odontomas. These tumors are usually asymptomatic, small, and slow growing and have a very low recurrence rate after curettage. They are excised frequently in the office and usually are not reported in large series of odontogenic tumors.[22,23]

The tumor is discovered on routine follow-up examination or during the diagnostic workup of an unerupted tooth. It may appear as a radiolucent, radiopaque, or mixed lesion on the radiograph. There is usually no destruction of surrounding bone or resorption of adjacent tooth roots. Displacement of the roots of adjacent teeth is the most commonly associated radiographic finding. The tumor may be present in the normal location of a missing deciduous or permanent tooth (Figure 10-23) or may appear to be a failed attempt at formation of a supernumerary tooth. There is no associated pain or paresthesia and no tenderness to palpation.

Odontomas are well encapsulated and can be enucleated easily from the surrounding bone.[22,23] Adjacent teeth that have been displaced are usually vital and are separated from the odontoma by a septum of bone. They are, therefore, not harmed by the excision, and endodontic therapy usually is not required (Figures 10-23 and 10-24).

Cementoma

Cementomas usually occur at the apices of teeth, most commonly in the mandible. These are very slow-growing asymptomatic lesions discovered on routine radiographic survey. The affected tooth is usually vital. A cementoma may appear as a periapical radiolucency, in which case it has to be differentiated from an abscess, granuloma, or fibro-osseous lesion. Treatment is not necessary unless the lesion begins to grow.[22,24] Cementomas, especially those that exhibit a large increase in size, may be related to fibro-osseous lesions and are discussed in Chapter 15.

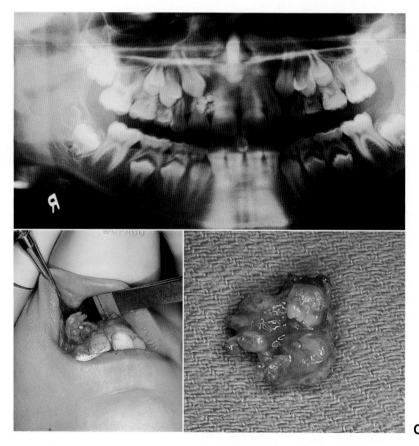

B **C**

Figure 10-23

A, Radiograph of odontoma between the maxillary right lateral incisor and canine—perhaps an aborted supernumerary tooth. **B,** Tumor in situ covered by a thin shell of bone. **C,** Specimen reveals small toothlike structures.

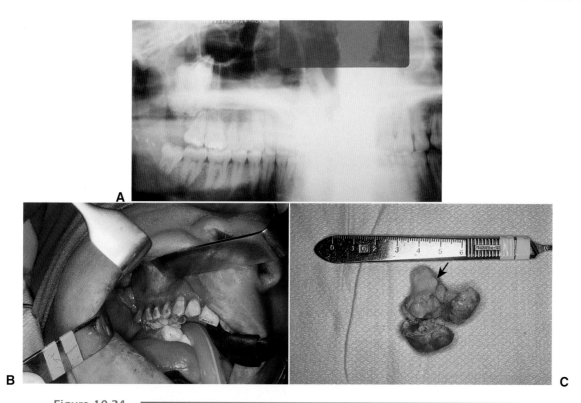

Figure 10-24

A, Odontoma associated with an impacted maxillary right third molar. **B,** At operation, the alveolus was considerably expanded. **C,** Specimen consisting of an impacted third molar *(arrow)* and attached odontoma.

Ameloblastic Fibroma

Ameloblastic fibroma is a benign neoplasm of odontogenic origin composed of epithelium and mesenchyme. It appears as an asymptomatic radiolucency and can be associated with an unerupted tooth, usually in the mandible. The lesion can be unilocular or mutilocular, usually with a sclerotic rim.[25] It is more common in children than adults. Ameloblastic fibromas are not associated with bone destruction or resorption of adjacent tooth roots. The histology demonstrates mostly myxoid connective tissue with strands of epithelium.[25] Calcified dental elements may also be present, referred to as an *ameloblastic fibroodontoma,* making the distinction between this lesion and an odontoma difficult on gross examination. The treatment of choice for ameloblastic fibroma is enucleation and curettage; recurrence is rare (Figure 10-25).

DEVELOPMENTAL ODONTOGENIC CYSTS

Odontogenic cysts in children, as in adults, are frequently associated with impacted teeth. In pediatric patients, however, maxillary canine dentigerous cysts are involved more frequently than third molar cysts. In the late mixed and early permanent dentition, cysts may be associated with impacted premolars and 12-year molars. In teenagers, impacted wisdom teeth account for most dentigerous cysts. Follicular cysts are found most commonly in the mandibular premolar region in children, whereas they are found most often in the third molar region in teenagers and adults. Lateral periodontal and residual cysts are rare in childhood.

Odontogenic cysts usually are discovered when a permanent tooth has not erupted on schedule. Radiographs reveal a radiolucent lesion associated with an impacted normal or supernumerary tooth. Whenever a tooth is missing, the diagnostic radiograph should encompass the entire alveolus. A panoramic radiograph is most useful to avoid missing a cyst with a deeply impacted tooth (Figure 10-26).

The most common odontogenic cyst is the dentigerous cyst. Treatment consists of enucleation of the cyst and removal of the impacted tooth. If an impacted canine associated with a dentigerous cyst is positioned favorably for orthodontic movement, it may be saved.

The odontogenic keratocyst represents approximately 10% of odontogenic cysts. Reported recurrence rates with this cyst type are zero to 62.5%.[26-28] Although

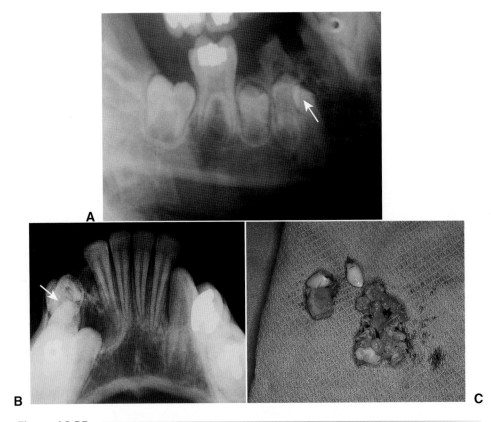

Figure 10-25

Lateral (**A**) and occlusal (**B**) views of an expansile lesion of the mandible. Radiographically, this appears to be a mixed radiolucent and radiopaque lesion with small toothlike structures within *(arrows)*. **C**, The surgical specimen was predominantly fibrous tissue, but toothlike elements were also present. The pathologic diagnosis was ameloblastic fibroma.

more rare than in adults, odontogenic keratocysts do occur in children. Especially common in children are multiple keratocysts as a component of nevoid basal cell carcinoma syndrome.[29] Keratocysts that occur as part of the nevoid basal cell carcinoma syndrome have a higher recurrence rate (35%), as compared with isolated keratocysts (10%).[29] In children with more than one keratocyst, this syndrome must be considered.

It is helpful to differentiate between dentigerous cyst or keratocyst preoperatively. August et al.[30] demonstrated that modified fine-needle aspiration with cytokeratin-10 staining provides a quick (usually within 24 hours) definitive diagnosis. Children older than 7 to 8 years usually tolerate this procedure easily with some local anesthesia.

Definitive management for keratocysts includes enucleation, enucleation with adjuvant therapy (cryotherapy, Carnoy's solution, peripheral ostectomy),[31-34] and en bloc or marginal resection.[35] More recently, the minimally invasive technique of decompression, placement of a stent, and irrigation has been shown to have a good cure and low recurrence rate.[30,36,37] Furthermore, this technique causes less surgical morbidity, and anatomic

structures such as the inferior alveolar nerve and developing teeth are less vulnerable to damage.[30] Decompression and irrigation is a useful strategy in children with multiple cysts (nevoid basal cell carcinoma syndrome) because bone and dental structures are preserved, and the multiple necessary interventions over time are less marked (Figure 10-27).

NONODONTOGENIC CYSTS
Hemorrhagic Bone Cyst

The most common nonodontogenic cyst in childhood is the traumatic or hemorrhagic bone cyst. The patient has an asymptomatic radiolucent lesion of the mandible in the symphysis or premolar-molar region. Hemorrhagic cysts are more common in males than females and the presumed etiology is trauma, although there may be no history of a significant blow to the mandible.

A traumatic bone cavity is not a true epithelial-lined cyst but, rather, an arrest of the normal healing process of bone. Intraosseous hemorrhage, as a result of trauma to the jaw, is resorbed without being infiltrated by inflammatory cells, followed by fibroblasts and,

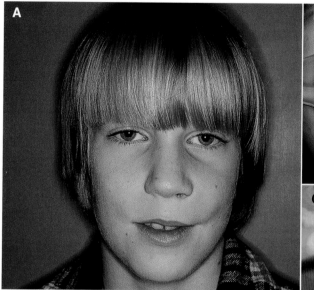

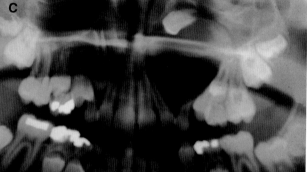

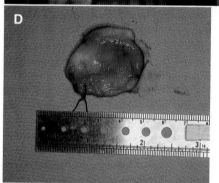

Figure 10-26

A, A teenage boy was referred for evaluation of left facial and intraoral swelling thought to be secondary to an infected deciduous canine tooth. Facial photograph shows swelling of the left maxillary and alar base regions but no erythema. **B,** Intraoral view shows fullness in the left maxillary labial sulcus. **C,** Panoramic radiograph shows a large dentigerous cyst related to the maxillary left canine. Note the spreading of the roots of the lateral incisor and deciduous canine. With a small periapical film, this was mistaken for an abscessed deciduous canine. **D,** Specimen with canine tooth *(arrows)* at the top of the cyst.

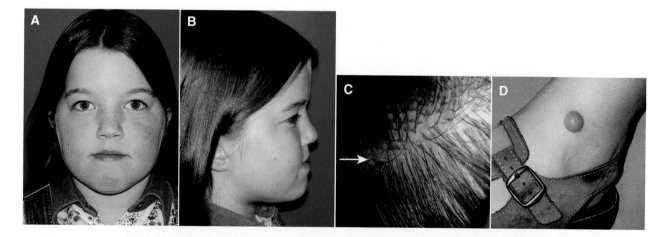

Figure 10-27

Frontal **(A)** and lateral **(B)** photographs of 10-year-old child with multiple maxillary and mandibular keratocysts. These were successfully treated with decompression and irrigation. At the time of presentation the examination also revealed a scalp lesion **(C)** (histologic examination revealed basal cell carcinoma) and a cystic lesion on the left ankle **(D)** (histologic examination revealed sebaceous cyst). The child was diagnosed with nevoid basal cell carcinoma syndrome.

eventually, bone-forming cells. The result is an empty bone cavity.

Management consists of exploration and curettage. This is a diagnostic maneuver to rule out an epithelial-lined cyst or jaw tumor. It also serves as definitive therapy by producing bleeding in the cavity. The fresh blood is then replaced by normal bone as it is resorbed. In cysts larger than 5 cm, or when the inferior border or condylar head becomes very thin, a bone graft is indicated (Figures 10-28 to 10-30).

Aneurysmal Bone Cyst

Aneurysmal bone cysts may be confused with traumatic cysts, odontogenic and nonodontogenic tumors, and vascular lesions.[22] They occur in children more commonly than in adults, in females more frequently than males, and most commonly in the mandibular molar region. The patient exhibits an enlarging jaw swelling without pain or paresthesia. There is often a history of trauma. Radiographs show cortical thinning and displacement of adjacent tooth roots, as well as a multilocular lucency with a soap-bubble appearance.[22]

During exploration there may be brisk bleeding, but this is controllable with pressure and usually slows down considerably after the cyst is removed by curettage. A fibrous lining, with many septa across the cavity, is usually encountered. Histologically, there are no epithelial cells lining the cyst. These lesions fill in spontaneously with bone after curettage and the recurrence rate is 10% to 15%. Aneurysmal bone cysts are part of a spectrum of vascular lesions and are associated with jaw tumors (ABC+) (see Chapters 15 and 17).

CONCLUSION

In this chapter we examined the common minor oral surgical problems that occur in the dentoalveolar segments. The most common dentoalveolar procedures in the pediatric age group relate to impacted permanent and supernumerary teeth. An understanding of the principles of timing of treatment and the potential to prevent problems by early diagnosis and treatment are fundamental differences between the care of children and adults with these problems.

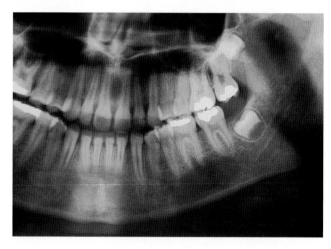

Figure 10-29
Traumatic bone cyst in the mandibular molar region.

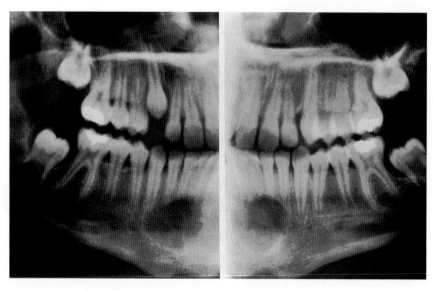

Figure 10-28
Traumatic bone cyst in the mandibular symphysis region.

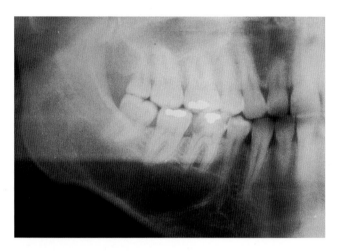

Figure 10-30

Traumatic bone cyst. Note the large carious lesion in the adjacent first molar. Again, with a small periapical film, this could be mistaken for a periapical abscess.

REFERENCES

1. Kaban LB, Needleman HL, Hertzberg J: Idiopathic failure of eruption of permanent molar teeth, *Oral Surg Oral Med Oral Pathol* 42:155-163, 1976.
2. Gorlin RJ, Pindborg JJ: *Syndromes of the head and neck,* New York, 1964, McGraw-Hill.
3. Reid DJ: Incomplete eruption of the first permanent molar in two generations of the same family, *Br Dent J* 96:272-273, 1954.
4. Heizer E, Harvey MC: Impacted molars: a new lethal in cattle, *J Hered* 28:123-128, 1937.
5. Downs WG: An experimental study of the growth effects of the anterior lobe of the hypophysis on the teeth and other tissues and organs, *J Dent Res* 10:601-654, 1930.
6. Baume LJ, Becks H, Evans HM: Hormonal control of tooth eruption, *J Dent Res* 33:80-114, 1954.
7. Trankmann J: The frequency of retention of permanent teeth, *Dtsch Zahnarztl Z* 28:415-420, 1973.
8. Boyd RL: Clinical assessment of injuries in orthodontic movement of impacted teeth I. Methods of attachment, *Am J Orthod* 82:478-486, 1982.
9. Boyd RL: Clinical assessment of injuries in orthodontic movement of impacted teeth II. Surgical recommendations, *Am J Orthod* 86:407-418, 1984.
10. Moss JP: Autogenous transplantation of maxillary canines, *Br J Oral Surg* 26:775, 1968.
11. Pogrel MA: Evaluation of over 400 autogenous tooth transplants, *J Oral Maxillofac Surg* 45:205-211, 1987.
12. Tronstad L, Andreason JO, Hasselgren G, et al: Ph changes in dental tissues after root canal filling with calcium hydroxide, *J Endodont* 7:17, 1987.
13. Natiella JR, Armitage JE, Greene GW: The replantation and transplantation of teeth. A review, *Oral Surg Oral Med Oral Pathol* 29:397-413, 1970.
14. Kearns G, Sharma A, Perrott D, et al: Placement of endosseous implants in children and adolescents with hereditary ectodermal dysplasia, *Oral Surg Oral Med Oral Pathol Oral Radiol Endod* 88(1):5-10, 1999.
15. Bergendal B, Bergendal T, Hallonsten AL, et al: A multidisciplinary approach to oral rehabilitation with osseointegrated implants in children and adolescents with multiple aplasia, *Eur J Orthod* 18(2):119-129, 1996.
16. Perrott D, Sharma AB, Vargervik K: Endosseous implants for pediatric patients, *Oral Maxillofac Surg Clin N Am* 6(1):79-88, 1994.
17. Thilander B, Odman J, Grondahl K, Lekholm U: Aspects on osseointegrated implants inserted in growing jaws. A biometric and radiographic study in the young pig, *Eur J Orthod* 14(2):99-109, 1992.
18. Cronin RJ, Oesterle LJ, Ranly DM: Mandibular implants and the growing patient, *Int J Oral Maxillofac Implants* 9(1):55-62, 1994.
19. Odman J, Grondahl K, Lekholm U, Thilander B: The effect of osseointegrated implants on the dento-alveolar development. A clinical and radiographic study in growing pigs, *Eur J Orthod* 13(4):279-286, 1991.
20. Thilander B, Odman J, Grondahl K, Friberg B: Osseointegrated implants in adolescents. An alternative in replacing missing teeth? *Eur J Orthod* 16(2):84-95, 1994.
21. Troulis MJ, Kaban LB: Staged protocol for resection, skeletal reconstruction and oral rehabilitation of children with jaw tumors, *J Oral Maxillofac Surg* 2003 (in press).
22. Kaban LB, Chuong R: Nonmucosal neoplasms of the maxillofacial region. In Peterson DE, Elias EH, Sonis ST, editors: *Head and neck management of the cancer patient,* New York, 1986, Martinus Nijhoff.
23. Chuong R, Kaban LB: Diagnosis and treatment of jaw tumors in children, *J Oral Maxillofac Surg* 43:323-332, 1985.
24. Hamner JE, Scofield HH, Cornyn J: Benign fibroosseous jaw lesions of periodontal membrane origin: an analysis of 249 cases, *Cancer* 22:861-878, 1968.
25. Regezi JA, Sciubba J: Odontogenic tumors. In Regezi JA, Sciubba J, editors: *Oral pathology clinical-pathologic correlations,* Philadelphia, 1993, WB Saunders.
26. Bataineh AB, Al Qudah M: Treatment of mandibular odontogenic keratocysts, *Oral Surg Oral Med Oral Pathol Oral Radiol Endod* 86:42, 1998.
27. Dammer R, Niederdellmann H, Dammer P, et al: Conservative or radical treatment of keratocysts: a retrospective review, *Br J Oral Maxillofac Surg* 35:46, 1997.
28. Voorsmit RA, Stoelinga PJ, van Haelst UJ: The management of keratocysts, *J Oral Maxillofac Surg* 9:228, 1981.
29. Regezi JA, Sciubba J: Cysts of the oral region. In Regezi JA, Sciubba J, editors: *Oral pathology clinical-pathologic correlations,* Philadelphia, 1993, WB Saunders.
30. August MA, Faquin WC, Troulis M, Kaban LB: Differentiation of odontogenic keratocysts from nonkeratinizing cysts by use of fine-needle aspiration biopsy and cytokeratin-10 staining, *J Oral Maxillofacial Surg* 58:935-940, 2000.
31. Stoelinga PJW: Long-term follow-up on keratocysts treated according to defined protocol, *Int J Oral Maxillofac Surg* 30:14, 2001.
32. Schmidt BL, Pogrel MA: The use of enucleation and liquid nitrogen cryotherapy in the management of odontogenic keratocysts, *J Oral Maxillofac Surg* 59:720, 2001.
33. Hsun-Tau C: Odontogenic keratocyst. A clinical experience in Singapore, *Oral Surg Oral Med Oral Pathol Oral Radiol Endod* 86:573, 1998.
34. Irvine GH, Bowerman JE: Mandibular keratocysts: surgical management, *Br J Oral Maxillofac Surg* 23:204, 1985.
35. Brondum N, Jensen VJ: Recurrence of keratocysts and decompression treatment. A long-term follow-up of forty-four cases, *Oral Surg Oral Med Oral Pathol Oral Radiol Endod* 72:265, 1991.
36. Marker P, Brondum N: Treatment of large odontogenic keratocysts by decompression and later cystectomy. A long-term follow-up and a histologic study of 23 cases, *Oral Surg Oral Med Oral Pathol Oral Radiol Endod* 82:122, 1996.
37. August M, Faquin WC, Troulis MJ, Kaban LB: Dedifferentiation of odontogenic keratocyst epithelium after cyst decompression, *J Oral Maxillofac Surg* 61:678, 2003.

CHAPTER 11

Intraoral Soft Tissue Abnormalities

Leonard B. Kaban and Maria J. Troulis

CHAPTER OUTLINE

Oral and maxillofacial surgeons, pediatric dentists, pediatricians, and family dentists frequently encounter intraoral soft tissue abnormalities. In the adult population, most nonhealing oral lesions are neoplasms; in children, they are often infectious or developmental abnormalities. The purpose of this chapter is to familiarize the reader with common intraoral soft tissue problems seen in a pediatric oral and maxillofacial surgery referral center. These problems include (1) the prominent frenum: maxillary labial frenum, mandibular labial frenum, lingual frenum ("tongue-tie"), (2) soft tissue lesions: salivary gland (mucocele, ranula), pyogenic granuloma, irritation fibroma, papilloma, vascular lesions, eruption cysts, drug-induced gingival hyperplasia, and (3) macroglossia. Other intraoral soft tissue pathology is presented in the chapters dealing with maxillofacial infection (Chapter 12), inflammatory salivary gland disease (Chapter 13), salivary gland tumors (Chapter 14), malignant head and neck tumors (Chapter 16), and vascular anomalies (Chapter 17).

PROMINENT FRENUM
Maxillary Labial Frenum

General Considerations. The labial frenum is a band of fibroelastic tissue that originates in the lip and inserts in the attached gingiva at the midline of the maxilla.[1] A prominent maxillary labial frenum, inserting on the crest of the alveolar ridge and incisive papilla, may be a normal finding in infants (Figure 11-1). The attachment on the ridge relocates apically with normal vertical growth of the alveolus.[2]

A prominent frenum in young children is of concern for parents, pediatricians, and pediatric dentists because of its appearance and because it may be associated with

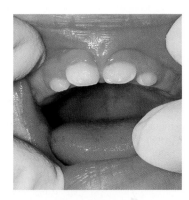

Figure 11-1

Intraoral photograph of a patient with a prominent maxillary labial frenum associated with a diastema. This is normal in an infant.

a diastema between the deciduous or permanent maxillary central incisors. It is important to reassure parents that a midline diastema may be normal in the deciduous dentition or in the permanent dentition before eruption of the maxillary canine teeth.[2-6] When a labial frenum is indeed contributing to the persistence of a diastema, the band usually crosses the alveolus and inserts into the incisive papilla. When the lip is stretched, the papilla blanches (Figure 11-2). Histologically, a frenum is composed of mucosa and connective tissue with a significant quantity of elastic fibers. It is thought that the prominent elastic component of a frenum, not excessive muscle pull, contributes most to persistence of a diastema.[1]

Other possible etiologic factors for a diastema should be ruled out before surgical correction of a prominent maxillary labial frenum. These include thumb sucking, tongue thrusting, supernumerary teeth, cystic lesions, notching of alveolar bone between the incisors, a true midline bony cleft, or primary bone pathology such as fibrous dysplasia.[2]

Frenectomy should not be performed before the permanent maxillary central and lateral incisors have erupted and the maxillary canines are erupting actively. Occlusal and anterior movement of the erupting canines often leads to partial or complete closure of the diastema. If orthodontic treatment is anticipated, frenectomy may be carried out before canine eruption, if necessary to facilitate orthodontic tooth movement. However, most orthodontists and pedodontists recommend frenectomy, if the diastema has failed to close, after the six maxillary anterior teeth have erupted.[2,5]

When a diastema occurs in the presence of a midline bony cleft, frenectomy and orthodontic treatment may not provide a stable result. Permanent orthodontic retention, or excision of the fibrous tissue in the bony cleft

with segmental osteotomy or bone graft, may be required to eliminate the diastema[7] (Figure 11-3).

Techniques

Standard Frenectomy. To eliminate a prominent frenum successfully and to allow closure of a diastema, the fibro-elastic band must be excised. Simply cutting or incising the mucosal band results in a high rate of recurrence for both the frenum and the diastema.

An incision is made across the base of the frenum, at its attachment to the incisive papilla. The dissection is carried down to the periosteum (Figures 11-2, 11-4, and 11-5), and the incision is then extended along both sides of the frenum to its attachment on the labial mucosa. The specimen is placed on traction and excised from the lip. This results in a bell-shaped defect. The edges of the wound are undermined for several millimeters and relaxing incisions are made at the mucogingival line. The labial flaps are then advanced and the wound closed with 5-0 chromic catgut sutures. The diamond-shaped defect in the attached gingiva is allowed to heal by secondary intention. No dressing is used and antibiotics are unnecessary. The patient is placed on a soft diet for several days. Normal tooth brushing with a soft brush is resumed immediately after the procedure.

Laser Frenectomy. The labial frenum is excised easily using a carbon dioxide laser. The procedure takes less time than the standard technique, produces less swelling and less discomfort, and the wound does not require suturing. However, when the procedure is done in the office setting, nitrous oxide and oxygen cannot be used because of the fire hazard. Furthermore, the patient must be cooperative enough to ensure laser safety.

Standard laser safety precautions must be followed: (1) room doors closed with a large sign warning that a laser is in use, (2) no oxygen or other flammable gases, (3) protective eyewear for the patient and all personnel, (4) isolated field with protection of adjacent structures, and (5) all personnel must be trained and certified in laser treatment.

The lip is stretched to delineate the frenum as in the standard technique (Figure 11-6). Using a carbon dioxide laser (NovaPulse, Luxar Company, Bothell, Washington) set at 7 watts in the pulsating mode, the frenum is outlined. Then the laser is set to the continuous mode and the band is excised to the periosteum. Relaxing incisions are made at the mucogingival line. Hemostasis is achieved by defocusing the beam and then applying laser to the wound in the pulsating mode. This leaves a dry, brown-black char. No sutures are placed and the wound is allowed to heal by epithelialization and contraction. The postoperative instructions are the same as for the standard technique.

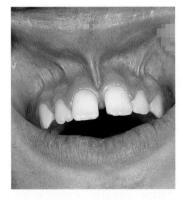

Figure 11-2 ▬▬▬▬▬
Intraoral photograph of a patient with a prominent maxillary labial frenum associated with a diastema. Note the attachment of the frenum into the incisive papilla on the palate.

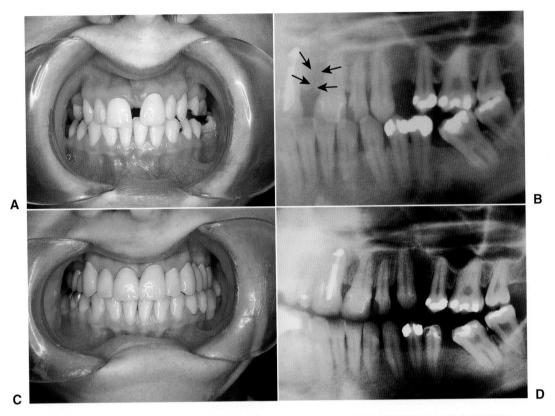

Figure 11-3   **A,** Large diastema with thick labial frenum in an adult. Several attempts at orthodontic closure with frenectomy failed because of the bony cleft. **B,** Panoramic radiograph demonstrating diastema and bony cleft *(arrows)* extending to the floor of the nose. **C,** One year after excision of fibrous tissue in the cleft and an anterior maxillary osteotomy with a midline split. Closure of the diastema is stable. **D,** Postoperative radiograph.

Mandibular Labial Frenum

General Considerations. The midline mandibular labial frenum is a normal anatomic landmark. However, when it attaches high on the interdental papilla, between the lower incisors, it creates an adverse periodontal environment (Figure 11-7). Movement of the lip during function results in traction on the interdental papilla, pulling it away from the teeth. This results in trapping of food and accumulation of plaque. The patient develops chronic inflammation, a periodontal pocket, and recession of the attached gingiva. Failure to eliminate this abnormal frenum pull may lead to bone loss and mobility of the central incisors. It should be kept in mind, however, that control of gingival inflammation by proper oral hygiene techniques, as well as scaling, curettage, and root planing, is of great importance. The patient should demonstrate an ability to cooperate with an oral hygiene program preoperatively. Powell and McEniery[8] followed for 2 years 42 children (ages 6 to 8 years) with isolated gingival recession of the mandibular central incisor region. They found that control of gingival inflammation was the most important prognostic factor in these patients. In fact, when inflammation was controlled, the abnormal frenum pull became less prominent.

Techniques

Excision. The frenum is excised as described for the maxillary labial frenum (Figure 11-8). The wound edges are undermined, relaxing incisions are made, and wound closure is carried out also as described for the maxillary frenum.

Excision and Z-Plasty Closure. The mandibular labial frenum also may be treated successfully by excision of the band and wound closure using Z-plasty rotation flaps (Figure 11-9). Postoperative care is the same as for a maxillary frenectomy.

Laser Excision. Finally, excision of the frenum using the carbon dioxide laser is possible, also. The considerations, safety procedures, and technique are exactly as described for the maxillary labial frenum above.

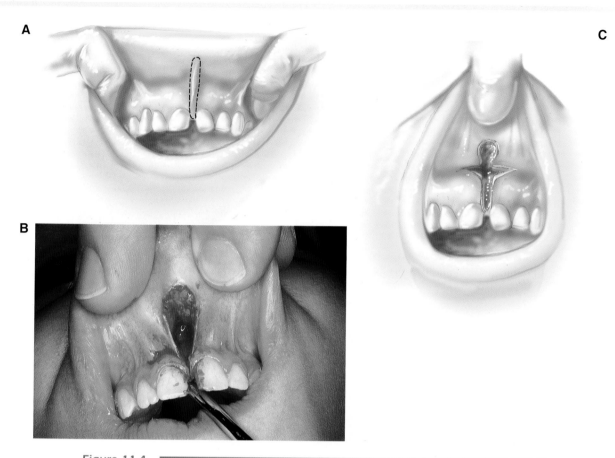

Figure 11-4

A, Diagram of frenum excision that results in a bell-shaped defect. **B,** Intraoperative view showing defect after excision. **C,** Diagram illustrating relaxing incisions at the mucogingival line and the resultant shape of the wound. *The ungloved fingers in the picture are those of the patient's father.*

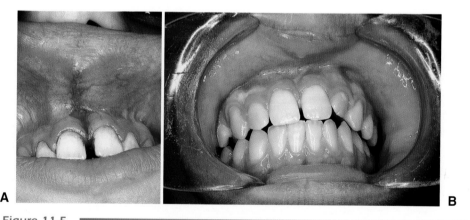

Figure 11-5

A, Immediate postoperative result. **B,** A similar patient who had significant spontaneous closure of a diastema 1 year after frenectomy.

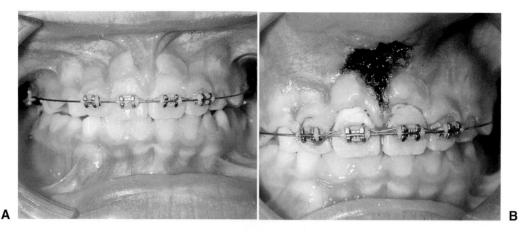

Figure 11-6

A, Prominent labial maxillary frenum in a 14-year-old. **B,** Intraoperative view after laser excision.

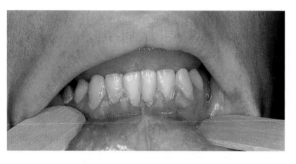

Figure 11-7

A mandibular labial frenum with high attachment producing gingival inflammation and recession. Note the loss of attached gingiva at both central incisors.

Rapid, dramatic improvement in the periodontal condition usually is achieved after the frenectomy, regardless of the technique. This is especially true in the patient who cooperates by using proper hygiene techniques. In the pediatric patient, a free gingival graft is almost never required. Wound healing by secondary intention on the alveolar ridge provides an adequate band of attached gingiva.

Lingual Frenum or Tongue-Tie

General Considerations. A prominent lingual frenum, attached high on the lingual alveolar ridge, is seen commonly in infants. This causes great concern on the part of parents and pediatricians because of decreased

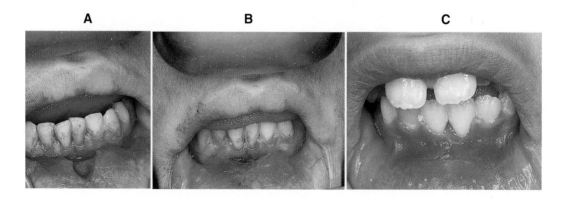

Figure 11-8

A, A similar patient as the one shown in Figure 11-7 with frenum excised, relaxing incisions made, and flaps undermined. **B,** Immediate postoperative view showing wound closure with resultant defect on the alveolar ridge, which will heal by secondary intention. **C,** Another patient 6 weeks postoperatively. This photograph shows the excision of the frenum; attached gingiva has reformed in the diamond-shaped raw surface. The interdental papilla is no longer loose.

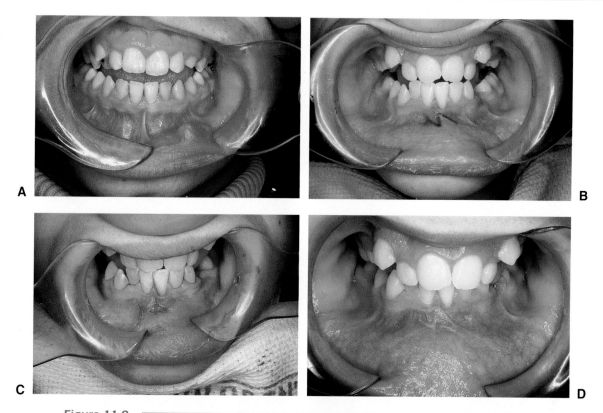

Figure 11-9

A, Mandibular labial frenum exerting abnormal pull on the interdental papilla. **B,** The proposed Z-plasty incisions have been outlined in Malachite green. **C,** Incisions are made. **D,** Well-healed wound and resolved periodontal problem 6 months later.

tongue mobility and the fear of future speech impairment. The lingual frenum usually becomes less prominent during the first 2 to 5 years of life, as the alveolar ridge grows in height and teeth begin to erupt. Speech problems on the basis of tongue-tie are uncommon in infants and toddlers, and early frenectomy in this age group rarely is indicated.[9,10]

Children in the mixed dentition may complain of difficulty moving the tongue; they are particularly bothered by an inability to protrude it from the mouth. They complain of the bifid appearance of the tongue, which may lead them to be teased by other children. A lingual frenum with a high attachment on the alveolus may contribute to gingival inflammation and recession in relation to the central incisors. Finally, there may be a continuous fibroelastic band, from the tongue across the alveolus and into the lip, which produces a tongue-tie, a mandibular diastema, and gingival inflammation. Lingual frenectomy is performed more commonly for one of the preceding indications rather than for articulatory speech problems related to tongue-tie.

A simple incision or "snipping" of a tongue-tie results in a high rate of relapse in all but the most minor varia-

tions. Subsequent procedures are more difficult because of postoperative scarring in an area where the submandibular ducts open. Therefore excision, with V-Y lengthening of the ventral surface of the tongue, or Z-plasty release, are the procedures of choice for correction of tongue-tie (Figure 11-10). It is also possible to use the laser for tongue-tie release in the milder forms of the condition.

Techniques

Excision and V-Y Closure. The operation requires a general anesthetic except in cooperative children with milder forms of tongue-tie. The frenum is cut from the attachment on the alveolar ridge. Then traction is applied with forceps. Parallel incisions, extending along the floor of the mouth and ventral surface of the tongue, are made and the band of tissue is removed. Relaxing incisions are then made at the junction of the floor of the mouth and the ventral surface of the tongue, converting the straight-line defect to a "V." The defect is then closed as a "Y" with 4-0 and 5-0 chromic catgut sutures. This procedure accomplishes excision of the frenum and simultaneous lengthening of the lingual sulcus (Figure 11-10).

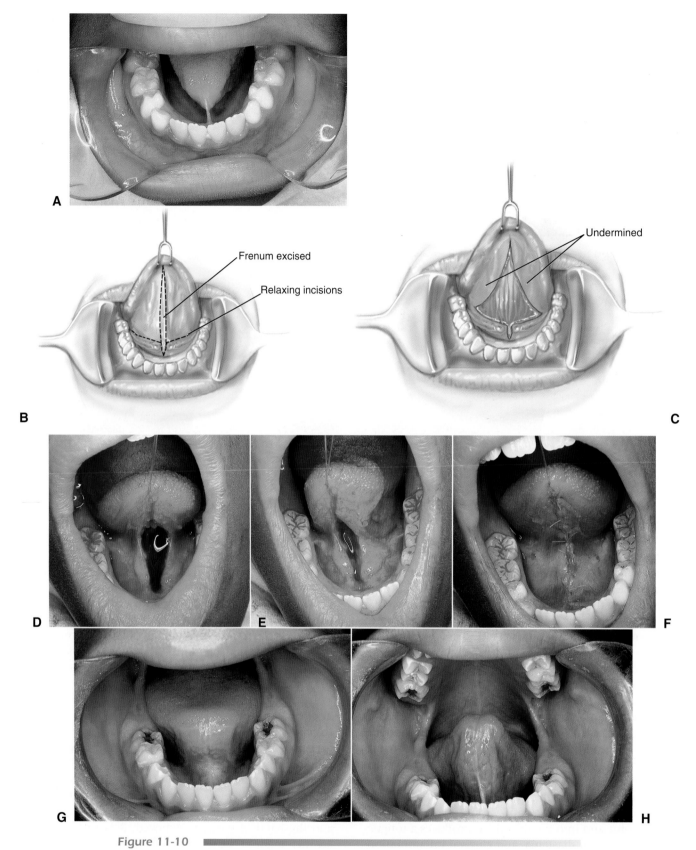

Figure 11-10

A, Intraoral view of a child with tongue-tie—a short lingual frenum from the tip of the tongue to the alveolar ridge. **B,** Diagram showing incisions for frenectomy and the development of flaps in the floor of the mouth. Note that the frenum is completely excised, including its insertion into the tip of the tongue. Diagram **(C)** and intraoperative photograph **(D)** of wound resulting from frenectomy and relaxing incisions at the junction of the floor of the mouth and ventral surface of the tongue. **E,** Resultant mobility of the tongue. **F,** Wound closure and immediate postoperative result. One year postoperatively the patient is able to retract **(G)** and elevate **(H)** her tongue.

Excision and Z-Plasty Closure. An excellent alternative operation is a frenectomy (excision of the band) with single or multiple Z-plasties to lengthen the ventral surface of the tongue (Figures 11-11 to 11-13). The frenum is excised as described above. Two large triangular flaps are created on the ventral surface of the tongue, away from the junction of the tongue and floor of the mouth. The flaps are transposed as a Z-plasty. This improves tongue mobility without endangering the submandibular ducts. The area on the alveolar ridge is allowed to heal by secondary intention. Occasionally, multiple small Z-plasties are used. When there is a single, continuous lingual-labial band, it is excised and the reconstruction is carried out as described previously for the lingual and labial sides of the alveolar ridge.

Laser Excision. Tongue-tie may also be corrected using the carbon dioxide laser. The standard laser safety rules as outlined above must be observed. Traction is applied to the tongue to identify the frenum. With the laser set at 7 watts in the pulsating mode, the frenum is outlined. Then, using the continuous mode, the frenum is excised. Relaxing incisions are made at the junction of the floor of the mouth and ventral surface of the tongue. Hemostasis is achieved by defocusing the beam and lasering the bed. No sutures are required. Although it is said that applying laser to the submandibular duct orifices does not lead to scarring or obstruction, it is best to avoid these structures (Figure 11-14).

INTRAORAL SOFT TISSUE LESIONS
Salivary Gland Lesions
Mucocele
General Considerations. The most common benign salivary gland problem in childhood is the mucous retention cyst, or mucocele. The lesion is a pseudocyst and does not have an epithelial lining; the etiology is usually trauma.[11] The most frequent location is the lower lip, the result of an accidental self-inflicted bite (Figures 11-15 to 11-17). Mucoceles frequently occur in the buccal mucosa, near the occlusal plane, and less commonly on the upper lip of children. The ranula is also a salivary pseudocyst. The lip lesions are often a result of local trauma to the face, from a fall or being struck by a blunt object. In adults, fluid-filled lesions on the upper lip are rarely mucoceles; they are more commonly benign mixed tumors.[12]

The pathogenesis is extravasation of saliva from a minor salivary gland into the surrounding soft tissues. The fluid eventually becomes walled off with a fibrous lining, forming a pseudocyst.[12,13]

The patient characteristically has a history of weeks to months of intermittent swelling and drainage on the lower lip or cheek mucosa. When the lesion drains, the fluid is either dark red and bloodlike or a thick, viscous, mucoid-type secretion. Typically, the parents and child remember no local trauma to the lip. The lesion is usually not painful. It may be clear or bluish in color or pale and fibrotic, if it has been present for months. In the latter cases, it is hard to distinguish a mucocele from a fibroma.

The treatment of choice is surgical excision. Drainage alone is accompanied by a high recurrence rate.[13]

Techniques
Standard. A circular incision is made around the lesion. The dissection is continued in the plane adjacent to the capsule, down to the muscle layer of the lip, and the cyst is removed. All remaining minor salivary glands in the field, down to the muscle, should be excised to prevent or minimize the chance of recurrence. Careful hemostasis is achieved with electrocautery. When the lip is allowed to relax, the circular wound becomes elliptical and it is oriented perpendicular to the pull of the orbicularis oris muscle fibers. The wound edges are undermined gently and the wound closed with 4-0 chromic catgut sutures.

Laser. To minimize bleeding and to facilitate removal of adjacent minor glands, the carbon dioxide laser is an excellent alternative method of excision. Lesions on the lower lip can be vaporized with the laser, but those on the upper lip should be excised to obtain a specimen for pathologic analysis. The excision is carried out in a circular pattern as described for the standard technique. Remaining minor glands in the field should be vaporized or excised. Hemostasis is achieved by defocusing the beam, and a char is formed in the base of the wound. The carbon dioxide laser is set at 7 watts in the pulsating mode to start and then changed to the continuous mode. Mucocele excision using the laser is especially advantageous in children, because sutures are not necessary and there is less postoperative pain and swelling when compared with excision using a scalpel or electrocautery (see Figures 11-16 and 11-17).

Ranula
General Considerations. The ranula is another common salivary retention cyst seen in children. Ranulas appearing in infants and toddlers are congenital, a result of dilation of sublingual or submaxillary gland ducts in the floor of the mouth. Those appearing in older children or teenagers are usually posttraumatic. The name *ranula* is derived from the Latin, *Ranula pipiens* (i.e., frog). Elevation of the tongue by the fluid-filled pseudocyst is reminiscent of the appearance of a frog's tongue and floor of mouth. Ranulas must be differentiated from lymphatic malformations because the treatment and prognosis are quite different.

A lymphatic malformation (see Chapter 17) is usually present at birth and grows proportionately with the

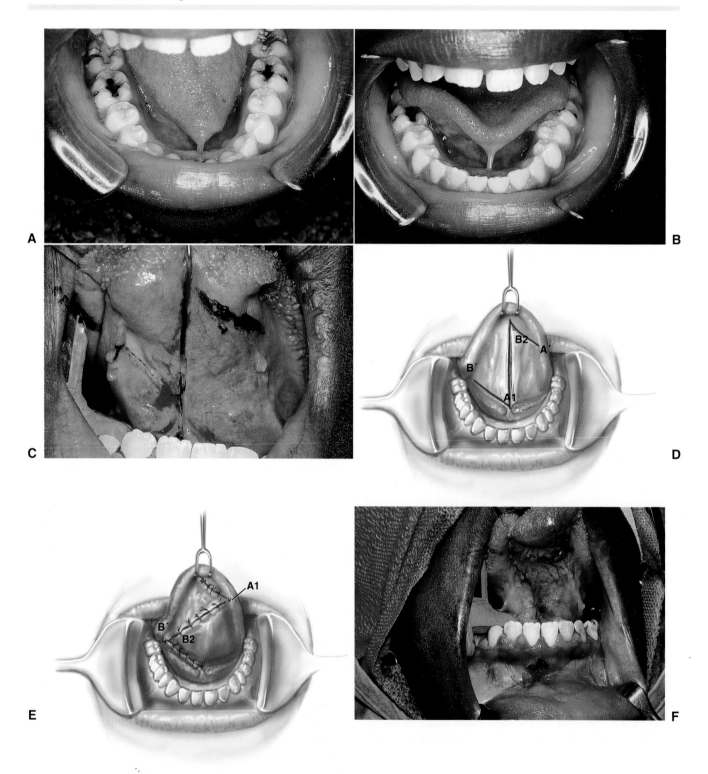

Figure 11-11

A, Patient with severe tongue-tie. **B,** Intraoral view, attempting to elevate the tongue. Note the high attachment on the lingual alveolus. **C,** Intraoperative view of incisions drawn on the elevated tongue after frenectomy. **D,** Diagram of Z-plasty triangular rotation flaps. Diagram **(E)** and photograph **(F)** of transposition of flaps and wound closure. Note the resultant reorientation of B2-A1. The distance from the tongue-tip to the alveolus is now 60% larger.

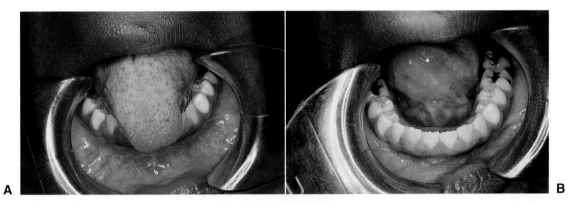

Figure 11-12

Tongue protrusion (**A**) and elevation (**B**) 1 year postoperatively of patient shown in Figure 11-11.

patient. It rarely drains spontaneously and does not disappear completely. It may increase in size during an upper respiratory infection or with crying or other Valsalva maneuvers. Lymphatic malformations occasionally become infected secondarily. In contrast, ranulas are rarely present at birth. They often increase in size, drain spontaneously, disappear, and then reappear weeks to months later. Ranulas rarely become infected and do not change in size with upper respiratory infection or a Valsalva maneuver.

Ranulas characteristically are located in the sublingual space between the mylohyoid muscle and the lingual mucosa (Figures 11-18 and 11-19). Occasionally the swelling extends into the submental or submandibular space by perforating through the mylohyoid muscle, a "plunging ranula" (Figures 11-20 and 11-21).

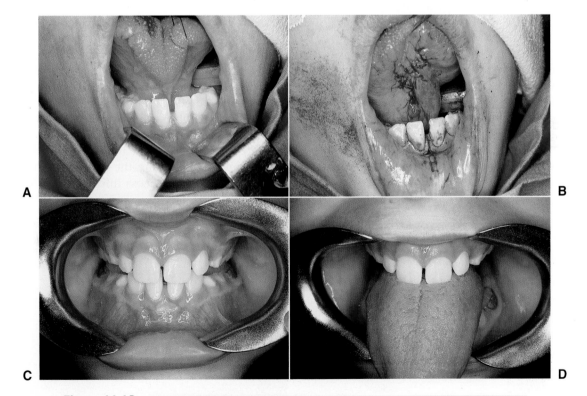

Figure 11-13

A, Lingual frenum and mandibular diastema. **B,** Immediate postoperative view of Z-plasty frenectomy and mandibular labial frenectomy. **C,** View of labial frenum region 1 year postoperatively. **D,** Tongue protrusion 1 year postoperatively.

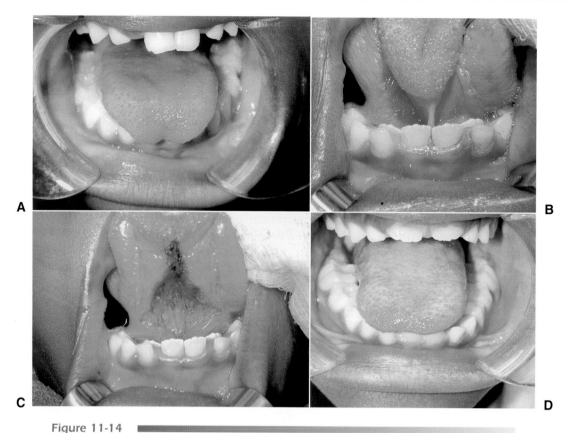

Figure 11-14

A and B, Intraoral photographs show severe tongue-tie in a young child. C, Intraoperative view after laser release of the tongue-tie. Note the resultant diamond-shaped wound. D, Same child protruding tongue 6 months later.

Small ranulas can be excised; however, large ones should be observed for several months until the lining is mature. Then the lesion is marsupialized to allow free drainage and to avoid damage to the submandibular ducts, sublingual glands, blood vessels, and nerves in the floor of the mouth. Plunging and recurrent ranulas often require excision of the sublingual gland to prevent recurrence.

Techniques

Marsupialization. Before marsupialization, a ranula should be allowed to mature for at least several months while a distinct fibrous lining develops. The roof of the pseudocyst is then excised, the cavity drained, and the mature lining is identified and sutured to the raw edge of the mucosa. With time, the circular wound edge contracts, but a mature mucosa-lined pathway for drainage

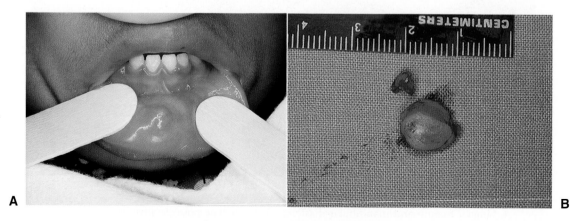

Figure 11-15

A, Mucocele of the lower lip. B, Specimen after excision.

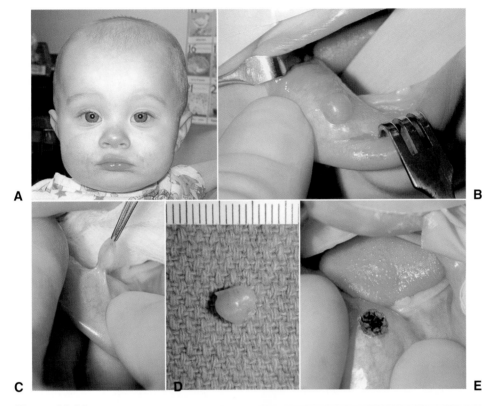

Figure 11-16

A, Frontal view of an infant with a sessile-appearing lesion **(B)** on the lower right lip (as seen in this intraoperative view). **C,** The lesion was pedunculated. **D,** Photograph of a specimen after the lesion was excised at the stalk. **E,** The bed after laser treatment. Pathology was consistent with a mucocele.

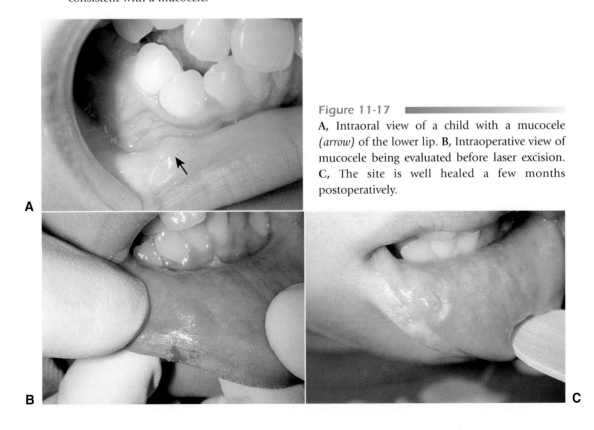

Figure 11-17

A, Intraoral view of a child with a mucocele *(arrow)* of the lower lip. **B,** Intraoperative view of mucocele being evaluated before laser excision. **C,** The site is well healed a few months postoperatively.

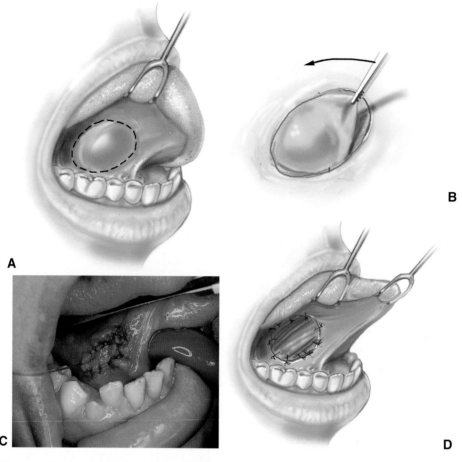

Figure 11-18

A, Drawing of an intraoperative view of a ranula in the right posterior floor of the mouth. The tongue has been placed on traction and a marsupialization incision marked. **B,** Diagram of the planned excision. Postoperative intraoral view **(C)** and diagram **(D)** of the postoperative result. The fibrous lining is sutured to the mucosa to complete marsupialization.

forms (see Figures 11-18 and 11-19). It is important, when marsupializing a ranula, to have the submandibular duct identified and cannulated (see Figure 11-19, *C*). This prevents traumatic injury and subsequent obstruction of the submandibular duct leading to submandibular sialadenitis and recurrence of the ranula.

Sublingual Gland Excision. Sublingual gland excision is accomplished via an intraoral approach (Figure 11-22). The submandibular duct is cannulated with a silicone rubber catheter that is sutured in place for identification during the dissection. An incision is made in the floor of the mouth lateral to the submandibular duct. With blunt dissection, the sublingual gland is identified. The posterior aspect of the gland is placed under traction and elevated. This allows for identification of the lingual nerve. The gland is then dissected free of surrounding tissue, keeping the lingual nerve and submandibular duct in view. The wound is closed loosely with 4-0

chromic catgut sutures. The catheter is left in the submandibular duct for 10 days (Figure 11-23).

Irritation Fibroma

After salivary pseudocysts, fibromas of the lower lip, buccal mucosa, and tongue are the most common intraoral soft tissue lesions seen in children. These tumors are benign and grow very slowly. However, recurrent trauma (e.g., during chewing or talking) may result in ulceration, bleeding, and pain (Figure 11-24).

The lesions usually are excised under local anesthesia. General anesthesia may be required in young children. A circular incision is made around the lesion, and the mass is dissected free and removed. Hemostasis is achieved with needlepoint electrocautery. The tissue is relaxed and the wound becomes elliptical and oriented perpendicular to the direction of contraction of the

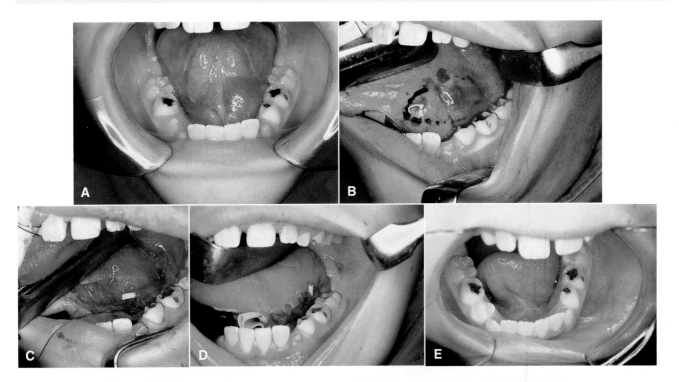

Figure 11-19
A, Intraoral view of a ranula in the left floor of the mouth. B, With the tongue on traction, the incision is marked. C, The submandibular duct has been identified and cannulated. D, Closure was obtained over a Penrose drain. E, Four months postoperatively.

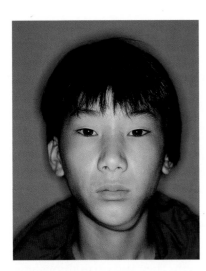

Figure 11-20
Facial photograph of submental swelling caused by a "plunging" ranula.

underlying muscle. The wound is closed with 4-0 or 5-0 chromic catgut sutures. The laser is quite useful as an alternative approach to these lesions for the same reasons described above for mucoceles.

Papillomas or Warts

Papillomas commonly occur on the labial or buccal mucosa, tongue, gingiva, and palate. They are pale to whitish in color and have an exophytic surface texture with numerous fingerlike projections.[13] The child characteristically has warts on the fingers, which must also be removed if the oral papillomas are to be cured; the lesions are spread by contact. The common skin wart, verruca vulgaris, is similar to the oral papilloma. A high percentage of the skin lesions are of viral etiology; oral papillomas may have a similar viral etiology.[13,14]

Oral papillomas are best removed with electrocautery. After the lesion is excised, the bed is cauterized, thus killing any remaining viruses. The lesions on the fingers should also be treated. The dermatologist may remove them chemically or with cryotherapy.

Pyogenic Granuloma

Pyogenic granuloma is a well-known lesion that occurs in the gingival papilla or marginal gingiva of children.[15] Foreign material may be found in the gingival crevice or interproximal region.[16] As the name suggests, pyogenic granuloma, sometimes called *peripheral giant cell reparative granuloma,* is an exuberant tissue response to local

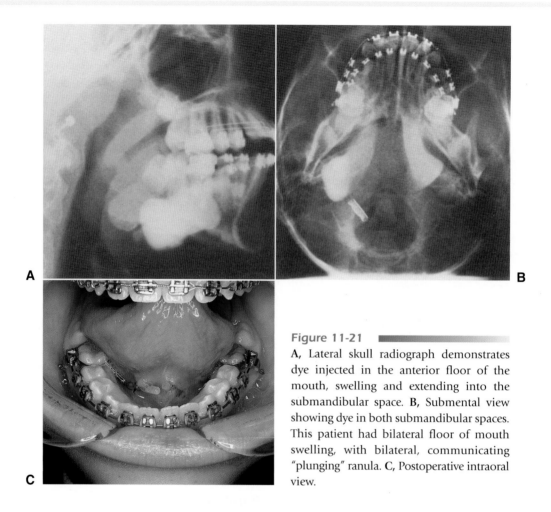

Figure 11-21

A, Lateral skull radiograph demonstrates dye injected in the anterior floor of the mouth, swelling and extending into the submandibular space. **B,** Submental view showing dye in both submandibular spaces. This patient had bilateral floor of mouth swelling, with bilateral, communicating "plunging" ranula. **C,** Postoperative intraoral view.

irritation. It should not be confused with central giant cell reparative granuloma or giant cell tumor of childhood. These lesions are true neoplasms and are discussed in Chapter 15.

Pyogenic granulomas are bluish to purple in color and resemble hemangiomas. They bleed easily and may be tender. There is usually no significant bone loss in the early stages of the lesion but, with time, a radiolucent defect may develop in the bone. This exuberant tissue response to local irritation has a tendency to recur after excision. For this reason, it is important to determine the exact etiology.

The teeth should be scaled and roots planed. The lesion is excised with electrocautery or with the laser to minimize bleeding and improve hemostasis.

Vascular Lesions

Chapter 17 is devoted entirely to vascular lesions. In the context of this discussion, however, small intraoral hemangiomas of the buccal mucosa and alveolar ridge that may appear in infants should be considered. They are usually not present at birth but appear within the first few months of life. They grow for several months, remain stable in size for weeks to months, and then begin to regress.[17] Hemangiomas may be mistaken for mucoceles or eruption cysts of natal teeth. Small lesions may be followed clinically until they regress, or they may be excised easily if they cause problems with feeding or bleeding.[17]

Eruption Cysts and Natal Teeth

Eruption cysts occur in newborn infants in association with natal teeth. They also occur throughout childhood in association with the eruption of deciduous and permanent teeth.[18] The reported incidence of natal teeth varies from 1 in 3392 live births in retrospective studies[17] to 1 in 716 live births in a series of 7155 infants personally examined by the investigators.[19] Kates et al.[19] found that 95% of the natal and neonatal teeth were normal primary central incisors and 5% were supernumerary incisors. For this reason, it was recommended to observe these teeth and extract them only if they are extremely

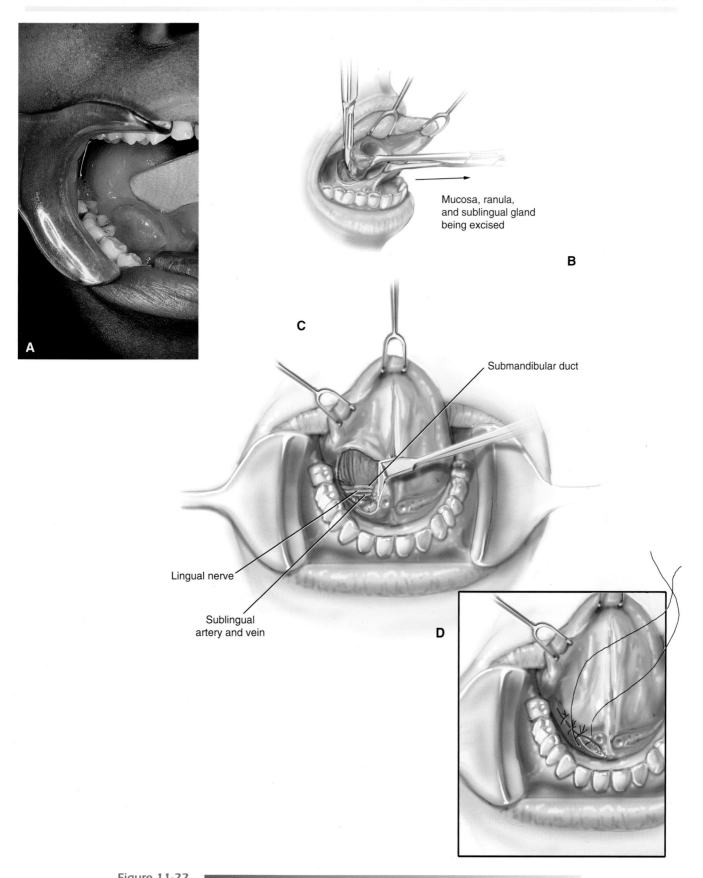

Figure 11-22
Diagram of sublingual gland excision through an intraoral approach (see text for details of procedure). **A,** Ranula visualized with tongue placed on traction. **B,** Mucosa and ranula excised, exposing sublingual gland. **C,** Wound after removal of the gland. **D,** Closure.

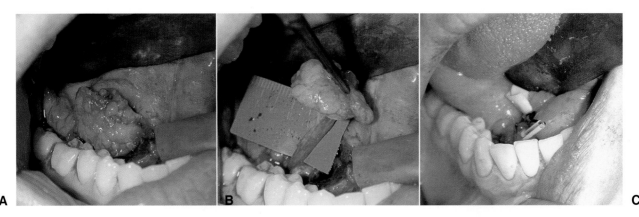

Figure 11-23

A, Intraoperative view of sublingual gland excision. **B,** The gland is elevated, and the submandibular duct clearly identified. **C,** The submandibular duct has been cannulated, a Penrose drain placed in the floor of the mouth, and closure obtained.

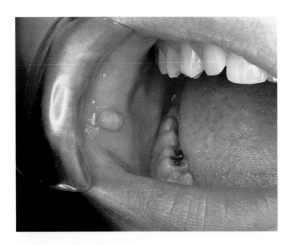

Figure 11-24

Intraoral view of a fibroma.

mobile. In many cases, the teeth stabilize in a short period of time as root development proceeds.[20]

Eruption cysts appear on the crest of the alveolar ridge as clear or blood-tinged, fluid-filled masses. They are not painful, but they may be a nuisance in feeding or bleed intermittently when traumatized. Often, they can be observed to disappear when the underlying tooth erupts. If the lesion becomes painful or infected or if the lesion bleeds, it can be unroofed and drained. Natal teeth are removed, at the time the cyst is unroofed, if they are mobile and if development of a periodontal attachment is unlikely.

Drug-Induced Gingival Hyperplasia

General Considerations. Gingival hyperplasia is associated with a number of drugs, the most common of which are diphenylhydantoin (Dilantin) and phenobarbital. It has also been reported recently in association with nifedipine.[21] The primary abnormality in these patients is not epithelial hyperplasia but, rather, fibrous tissue overgrowth not unlike keloids that form in skin.[13,22] Diphenylhydantoin hyperplasia does not occur in all patients taking the drug. There may be a biochemical interaction between the drug and an abnormal receptor in gingival mesenchymal cells, or diphenylhydantoin may interfere with enzymatic reactions within the cell.[22,23] Superimposed on the primary reaction is an inflammatory component that is more or less severe depending on the state of oral hygiene. This component may be particularly significant because many of the patients are cognitively challenged or have other handicaps that make oral hygiene procedures difficult. Dilantin also affects the periodontal membrane and the underlying bone.[24] The teeth are often mobile and may become malpositioned under the stress of normal occlusal forces.

Proper instructions for oral hygiene are obviously important. Scaling, curettage, and root planing may improve the inflammatory component, especially if the patient is able to cooperate and maintain meticulous oral hygiene. If possible, the neurologist should consider changing the medication at least temporarily while an attempt is made to control gingival hyperplasia.

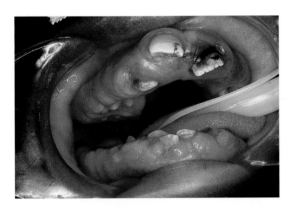

Figure 11-25

Severe phenytoin (Dilantin) hyperplasia in a mentally retarded patient.

Technique. Excision of diphenylhydantoin hyperplasia using standard gingivectomy techniques may result in a large volume of blood loss and a high recurrence rate. The best success has been achieved using either electrocautery or the laser. Electrocautery excision can be achieved with minimal blood loss. The gingiva is easily contoured and recurrence of hyperplasia is delayed in comparison with results after standard scalpel gingivectomy (Figures 11-25 to 11-27). The disadvantage of electrocautery is the post-operative pain that occurs while the wound is healing secondarily. Laser excision, by contrast, can also be achieved with minimal blood loss, and the resultant wound is less painful during the healing phase. When excising severe gingival hyperplasia with the carbon dioxide laser, the surgeon must take care not to damage the teeth.

Macroglossia

True macroglossia is an uncommon condition. In the child who is thought to have macroglossia causing a speech problem or drooling, it must be differentiated from: (1) forward posturing of the tongue as in reverse swallowing or tongue thrusting, (2) relative macroglossia in the presence of micrognathia, (3) midface hypoplasia with airway obstruction, and (4) neurologically flaccid tongue. Pressure from the family for an operation to reduce the size of the tongue must be resisted until the correct diagnosis is established.[25]

General Considerations. Very rarely a newborn or infant exhibits macroglossia and partial or intermittent airway obstruction.[26-28] This is usually in association with a small mandible (e.g., Pierre Robin sequence) and insufficient space for the tongue in the oral cavity. The base of the tongue then impinges on the nasopharyngeal and oropharyngeal airway. An older child may complain of difficulty in chewing or swallowing. Poor control of saliva, which leads to drooling, becomes a source of teasing by other children and criticism by adults. Speech impairment is rare, but occasionally a patient will have a lisp with sibilant sounds.[29]

Vogel et al.[25] proposed a classification system in an attempt to improve understanding of the problem and to aid in diagnosis and treatment planning. They divided macroglossia into congenital and acquired forms. Congenital macroglossia is the most common form. Muscular hypertrophy and enlargement of the tongue due to vascular malformation are the most frequent causes. Congenital macroglossia is subdivided into generalized or localized enlargement.

Generalized tongue enlargement in the newborn may be associated with the condition of hemihypertrophy, in which all structures on one side of the body are enlarged. In patients with hemihypertrophy, the tongue enlargement may be unilateral or bilateral. Hemihypertrophy may be associated with Wilms' tumor, adrenocortical carcinoma, and primary hepatocellular carcinoma in infants. Tongue enlargement may also be associated with endocrine or metabolic disease.[30] Macroglossia occurs in association with hypothyroidism, Beckwith-Wiedemann syndrome, and inherited mucopolysaccharidoses (Hurler's, Hunter's and Scheie's syndromes)[22,27] (Figure 11-28).

Macroglossia frequently is associated with Down's syndrome,[31,32] but it is not clear whether the apparent large tongue in these patients is anatomically enlarged or functionally enlarged as a result of an abnormal forward posture. The narrow maxilla that results in lack of space for the tongue in the roof of the mouth may also contribute to forward posture of the tongue. Oster[33] found that 57% of patients with Down's syndrome had enlarged tongues, while Singh[34] reported 67% to 92% of these patients had protruding tongues. One study reported reversal of tongue protrusion in Down's syndrome with 5-hydroxytryptophan, which suggests that the problem was secondary to oral hypotonia and not an anatomically large tongue.[35] In a radiographic study of acromegalics, Ardran et al.[36] demonstrated macroglossia, but they were unable to document tongue enlargement in a series of children they examined with Down's syndrome.

Localized macroglossia is a morphologic abnormality in the tongue without systemic disease. The most common etiology is a vascular lesion—frequently, a lymphatic malformation or a combined venous-lymphatic malformation.[17] The anterior two thirds of the tongue is affected most commonly, but the base of the tongue may also be abnormal. Lymphatic malformation of the tongue usually is noted at birth and grows proportional to the child. It may become enlarged intermittently in the presence of upper respiratory or oral

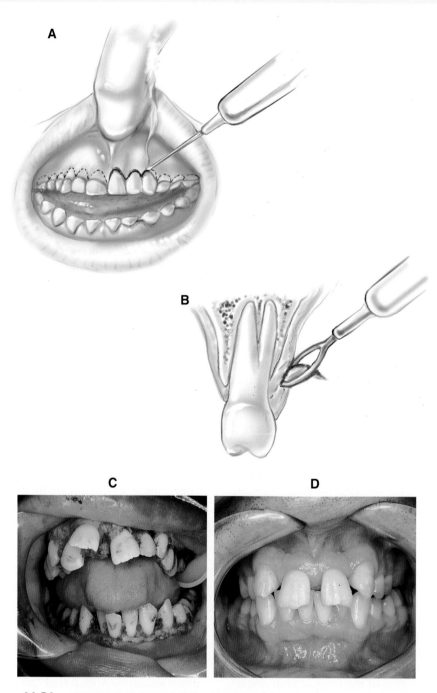

Figure 11-26

Diagram illustrating the technique of gingivectomy. (This technique was used in the patient shown in Figure 11-25). **A,** Level of cervical margin is marked with a needle point electrocautery. **B,** Tissue is then shaved down with a loop blade (5 to 10 mm diameter). Sculpting is completed with the needle point. **C,** Immediate postoperative result. **D,** Postoperative view 1 year later.

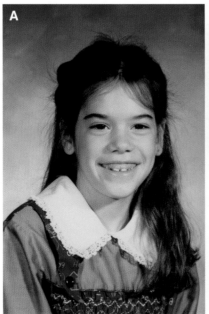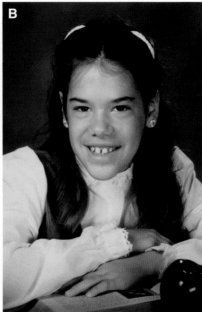

Figure 11-27

A, Preoperative photograph of a young patient with seizure disorder who was taking phenytoin (Dilantin). **B,** One year after excision of phenytoin hyperplasia by electrocautery technique.

infection. Physical examination reveals an enlarged tongue with an irregular, pebbly surface containing clear, bluish vesicles. The blue vesicles contain blood from ruptured capillaries. Lymphatic malformations of the tongue may coexist with similar lesions in the floor of the mouth or neck (previously called *cystic hygroma*) (see Chapter 17). Macroglossia may also be secondary to neurofibromatosis.

Acquired macroglossia may be acute or chronic.[25] The acute forms usually result from (1) allergic reactions, (2) hemorrhage (systemic coagulopathy or trauma), or (3) infection. The tongue may be enlarged primarily by intramuscular infiltration of edema fluid, blood, or purulent material or may be enlarged secondarily by infiltration of the floor of the mouth and elevation of the tongue, or a combination of both.

Chronic tongue enlargement usually is associated with a systemic disease. Primary or secondary amyloidosis, acromegaly, gigantism (excessive somatotrophic hormone), and hypothyroidism[30] are all associated with macroglossia.

Relative macroglossia may result from orthognathic surgery, as in correction of open bite or mandibular prognathism (Figure 11-29). Bell[37] has estimated that problems with tongue adaptation may occur in 10% of patients who have orthognathic surgical correction, and this may result in instability of the occlusal result or problems with the oropharyngeal airway. It is rarely

necessary, however, to surgically reduce the tongue in orthognathic surgery patients.

The indications for surgical correction of macroglossia are (1) obstruction of the oropharyngeal airway, (2) speech difficulty (i.e., lingual lisp), (3) dentoalveolar protrusion with or without open bite, with crenations on the peripheral border of the tongue, (4) esthetics (i.e., inability to hold the tongue in the mouth because of size), (5) drooling secondary to macroglossia, and (6) recurrence of open bite or bimaxillary protrusion and interdental spaces when the tongue is large.

The operation is designed to correct the anatomic deformity. If the tongue is long and not particularly wide, then an anterior wedge resection is done. If the tongue is both long and wide, a wedge resection is done in combination with an elliptical excision on the dorsum of the tongue (see Figures 11-28 and 11-29).

Technique. The operation is done under general anesthesia. The tongue is mobilized with three stay sutures of 3-0 silk: one in the tip and one on each side of the tongue proximal to the borders of the wedge excision (see Figures 11-28 and 11-29). The wedge is marked with malachite green, making sure both limbs of the wedge are equal in length. The dorsal ellipse is marked similarly to provide adequate narrowing of the tongue, if necessary. The tongue is then infiltrated with

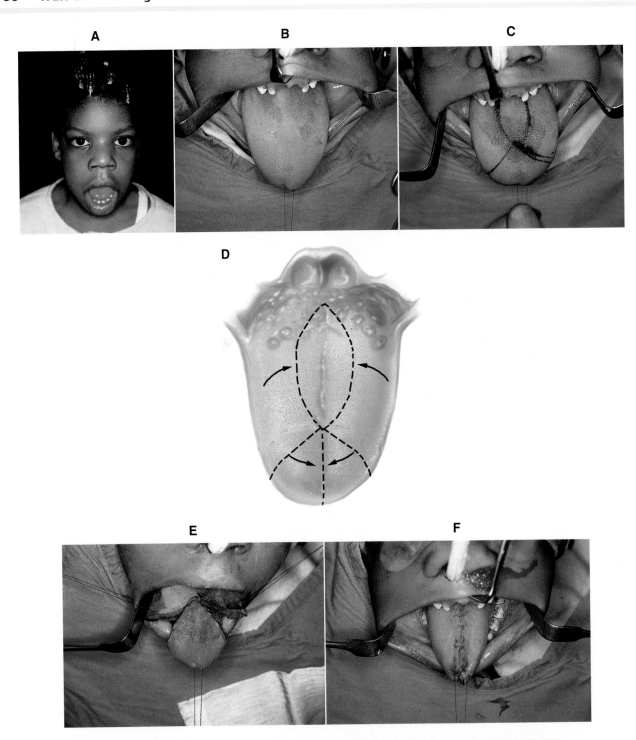

Figure 11-28

A, Frontal view of a patient with Beckwith-Weidemann syndrome and macroglossia. The patient keeps her mouth open and protrudes the tongue for lack of space. This produces a problem with control of secretions and drooling. **B,** Intraoral photograph shows long and excessively wide tongue. **C** and **D,** Proposed excision is drawn on tongue and illustrated diagrammatically. **E,** Specimen is removed. **F,** Tongue is closed in three layers with chromic catgut suture: muscle layer first, ventral surface of tongue second, dorsal surface last.

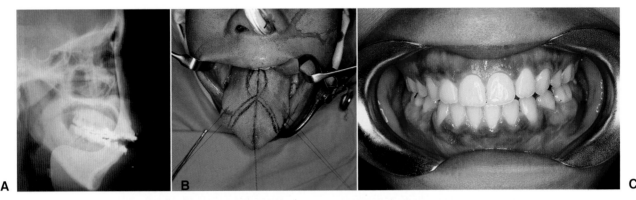

Figure 11-29
Lateral cephalogram showing open bite. The patient had vertical maxillary excess but also had significant macroglossia. She was treated with a Le Fort I osteotomy and advancement "jumping" genioplasty (to advance and shorten the chin). After the intermaxillary fixation was removed, the open bite began to recur, and spaces opened between the maxillary and mandibular teeth. **B,** Tongue reduction outlined. **C,** Two years after orthognathic surgery and orthodontic treatment were completed; 1 year after the reduction glossectomy. The result remained stable.

lidocaine 0.5% with epinephrine 1:200,000. The excision is carried out with electrocautery to minimize blood loss. The muscle layer is closed with 3-0 chromic catgut sutures. Once this is completed, the junction of the ventral and dorsal surfaces of the tongue is approximated at the tip with a 4-0 Vicryl vertical mattress suture, which is cut long to be used for traction. The ventral and dorsal surfaces are also closed with interrupted 4-0 Vicryl vertical mattress sutures. The vertical mattress sutures, double layer closure, and electrocautery excision help keep bleeding and swelling to a minimum (see Figure 11-28).

The same operation may be accomplished using the carbon dioxide laser with less bleeding and less swelling. If reduction glossectomy is being done for a vascular lesion, horizontal mattress, through-and-through stay sutures are placed in the tongue proximal to the borders of the wedge excision. This helps to control intraoperative bleeding. The rest of the operation is identical to that described above.

CONCLUSION

In this chapter, we discussed minor intraoral soft tissue problems that are seen commonly in children. Some of this material is related to that presented in other chapters (e.g., vascular lesions and salivary gland disease in Chapters 17 and 13, respectively). However, most conditions discussed here, the frenum, mucocele, ranula, and small pathologic lesions, are seen and treated in the office or ambulatory setting and are therefore grouped together for convenience.

REFERENCES

1. Henry SW, Levin MP, Tsaknis PJ: Histologic features of the prominent superior labial frenum, *J Periodontol* 47:25-28, 1976.
2. Edwards JG: The diastema, the frenum, the frenectomy: a clinical study, *Am J Orthod* 71:489-508, 1977.
3. Taylor JE: Clinical observation relating to the normal and abnormal frenum labii superioris, *Am J Orthod Oral Surg* 25:646-650, 1939.
4. Dewel BF: The normal and abnormal labial frenum: clinical differentiation, *J Am Dent Assoc* 33:318-329, 1946.
5. Finn SB: *Clinical pedodontics*, Philadelphia, 1973, WB Saunders.
6. Baum AT: The midline diastema, *J Oral Med* 21:30, 1966.
7. Bell WH: Surgical-orthodontic treatment of interincisal diastemas, *Am J Orthod* 57:158-163, 1970.
8. Powell RN, McEniery TM: A longitudinal study of isolated gingival recession in the mandibular central incisor region of children aged 6-8 years, *J Clin Periodontol* 9:357-364, 1982.
9. Horton CE, Crawford HH, Adamson JE, Ashbell TS: Tongue-tie. Presented at the 67th Annual Meeting of American Cleft Palate Association, 1969.
10. Mason RM: Principles and procedures of orofacial examination, *Int J Oral Myol* 6(2):3-19, 1980.
11. Bhaskar SN, Bolden TE, Weinman JP: Pathogenesis of mucoceles, *J Dent Res* 35:863, 1956.
12. Batsakis JG: *Tumors of the head and neck*, Baltimore, 1979, Williams & Wilkins.
13. Shafer WG, Hine MK, Levy BA: *A textbook of oral pathology*, Philadelphia, 1974, WB Saunders.
14. Lutzner M, Kuffer R, Blanchet-Bardon C, et al: Different papilloma viruses as the cause of oral warts, *Arch Dermatol* 118:393-399, 1982.
15. Kfir Y, Buchner A, Hansen LS: Reactive lesions of the gingiva: a clinicopathologic study of 741 cases, *J Periodontol* 51:655-661, 1980.
16. Moriconi ES, Popowich LD: Alveolar pyogenic granuloma: review and report of a case, *Laryngoscope* 94:807-809, 1984.
17. Kaban LB, Mulliken JB: Vascular anomalies of the maxillofacial region, *J Oral Maxillofac Surg* 44:203-213, 1986.
18. Leung AK: Natal teeth, *Am J Dis Child* 140:249-251, 1986.
19. Kates GA, Needleman HL, Holmes LB: Natal and neonatal teeth: a clinical study, *J Am Dent Assoc* 109:441-443, 1984.

20. Cohen RL: Clinical perspectives on premature tooth eruption and cyst formation in neonates, *Pediatr Dermatol* 1:301-306, 1984.

21. Lederman D, Lumerman H, Reuben S, Freedman PD: Gingival hyperplasia associated with nifedipine therapy: report of a case, *Oral Surg* 57:620-622, 1984.

22. Barbanell RL, Lian IB, Keith DA: Structural proteins of the connective tissues. In Shaw IH, Sweeney EA, Cappucino CC, Meller SM: *Textbook of oral biology*, Philadelphia, 1978, WB Saunders.

23. Vittek I, Hernandez MR, Wenk EI, et al: Specific estrogen receptors in human gingiva, *J Clin Endocrinol Metab* 54:608-612, 1982.

24. Hahn TI: Bone complications of anticonvulsants, *Drugs* 12:201-211, 1976.

25. Vogel IE, Mulliken IB, Kaban LB: Macroglossia: a review and nosologic approach, *Plast Reconstr Surg* 78:715-723, 1986.

26. Bronstein RP, Abelson SM, Iaffe RH, vonBonin IG: Macroglossia in children, *Am J Dis Child* 54:1328, 1937.

27. Bell GW, Millar RG: Congenital macroglossia, *Surgery* 24:125, 1948.

28. Bell WH, Proffit WR, White RP: *Surgical correction of dentofacial deformities*. II. Philadelphia, 1980, WB Saunders.

29. Colby RA, Kerr DA, Robinson HBG: *Color atlas of oral pathology*, Philadelphia, 1961, Lippincott.

30. Coleman M: Serotonin levels in infant hypothyroidism, *Lancet* 2:365, 1970.

31. Hendrick IW: Macroglossia or giant tongue, *Surgery* 39:674, 1956.

32. Cohen MM, Winer RA, Schwartz S, Shklar G: Oral aspects of mongolism, *Oral Surg* 44:92, 1961.

33. Oster I: *Mongolism: a clinicogenealogical investigation comprising 526 Mongols living on Sealand and neighboring islands in Denmark*, Copenhagen, 1953, Danish Scientific Press.

34. Singh DN: Down's syndrome: a study of clinical features, *J Natl Med Assoc* 68:521, 1976.

35. Tukiainen E, Tuomisto I, Westermarck T, Kupiainen H: Nature of lowered 5-hydroxytryptamine uptake by blood platelets of patients with Down syndrome, *Acta Pharmacol Toxicol* 49:365, 1980.

36. Ardran GM, Harker P, Kemp FH: Tongue size in Down's syndrome, *J Ment Defic Res* 16:160, 1972.

37. Bell WH: Adjunctive surgical procedures: reduction of the tongue. In Bell WH, Proffit WR, White RP, editors: *Surgical correction of dentofacial deformities*, Philadelphia, 1980, WB Saunders.

PART III

PEDIATRIC MAXILLOFACIAL SURGERY

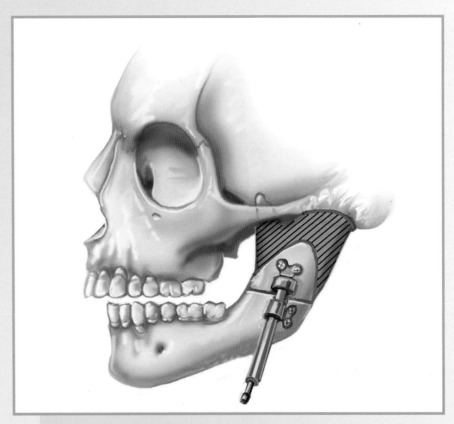

Placement of distractor in the mandible

CHAPTER 12

Infections of the Maxillofacial Region

Thomas B. Dodson and Leonard B. Kaban

Diagnosis and treatment of maxillofacial infections account for a significant part of oral and maxillofacial surgery (OMFS) training and practice. To manage pediatric infections successfully, the surgeon must obtain an accurate history and physical examination and appropriate imaging studies. Empiric antibiotic therapy, covering the appropriate organisms, is started, and timely operative intervention is performed, when indicated.

This subject is usually discussed according to the type of infection: odontogenic, sinus, salivary gland, or skin. This is an unrealistic approach, particularly in the pediatric age group. Children may not give an accurate history, they do not come to the surgeon with a specific known diagnosis, and the clinical findings are similar regardless of the type of infection. Therefore, in this chapter, the subject of maxillofacial infections is presented as an exercise in differential diagnosis based primarily on the child's age, location of swelling, presence of fever, trismus, or, occasionally, a chronic, nonhealing wound.

Concepts of differential diagnosis are important, because multiple contiguous structures in the head and neck may be the source of acute or chronic infection. Determination of the primary anatomic source and bacterial etiology provide a guide for initial empiric therapy. This is especially critical in children because they have a greater tendency to become rapidly dehydrated and systemically ill than do adults. In addition, a variety of infections may exhibit similar initial signs and symptoms. For example, in the pediatric age group, in which upper respiratory infection is common, it may be difficult to differentiate between primary maxillary sinusitis and an acute odontogenic infection. Likewise, tumors of childhood may occur with rapid onset of swelling and pain in a manner very similar to that of acute infection.

Pediatric facial infections are uncommon, and they represent a field of overlap among several dental and medical specialties. As such, it is unusual for any one practitioner to have extensive clinical experience in the evaluation and management of these infections. Furthermore, there is little data addressing this subject in the literature. The conceptual approach in this chapter is based on the authors' experience with pediatric maxillofacial infections in tertiary care hospitals during the past 25 years.

Since the first edition of this book, four important updates have been incorporated into this chapter. First, the evaluation and management protocol outlined in the first edition, based on location of infection, i.e., upper versus lower face, has been evaluated at different institutions and continues to be a useful diagnostic model.[1-6] Second, the introduction of *Haemophilus influenzae* type b (Hib) vaccine has changed dramatically the nature of pediatric maxillofacial infections. In the first edition of this book, one of the more common and serious diagnoses was facial cellulitis of unknown origin due to *H. influenzae* infection and its associated risks for bacteremia and meningitis. In 2004, facial cellulitis due to *H. influenzae* is virtually nonexistent. In its place is the growing prevalence of facial cellulitis due to *Streptococcus pneumoniae*, with its increasing prevalence of penicillin resistance. Third, improvements in microbiologic techniques have resulted in the identification of new organisms and reclassification of known organisms. It has also been recognized that most facial infections are polymicrobial and composed frequently of penicillin-resistant organisms. As such, in many situations the choice of antibiotic therapy is the same regardless of the etiology. Finally, several new chemotherapeutic agents have been introduced since the first edition.

INFECTIONS OF THE UPPER FACE
Evaluation and Differential Diagnosis

Upper face infections are defined as infections characterized by upper face swelling or originating from anatomic structures of the upper face, such as the skin or skin appendages of the upper face, including the parotid duct and structures up to the level of the periorbital region, maxillary sinus, orbits, maxillary teeth, and parotid gland.[1]

The introduction of Hib vaccine in 1987 has changed dramatically the epidemiologic and microbiologic spectrum of upper face infections.[7,8] Previously, the most prevalent diagnosis associated with children hospitalized for management of upper face infections was periorbital or facial cellulitis of unknown origin due to *H. influenzae*. This was a very serious diagnosis, because *H. influenzae* bacteremias produced a low, but finite, rate of central nervous system infection (meningitis). After the introduction of Hib vaccine to the United States, the most prevalent causes of pediatric upper face infections that required hospitalization were those with known sources of organisms, in contiguous structures such as skin, sinuses, ocular structures, and teeth. The emphasis in management is to identify the most likely source of infection and to direct empiric antibiotic therapy toward the organisms associated with the source.

Since the advent of Hib vaccine, *S. pneumoniae* has become the most common cause of facial cellulitis. *S. pneumoniae* is associated with an increased risk for bacteremia but has a lower risk for meningitis when compared with *H. influenzae*.[8] Therefore, blood cultures should be obtained for children with upper face infection of unknown etiology. Lumbar puncture and cerebral spinal fluid cultures, however, are of limited value.[7,8] As with *H. influenzae*, risk factors for *S. pneumoniae* include a recent history of upper respiratory infection or otitis media. Historically, *S. pneumoniae* has been universally penicillin sensitive, but there is an increasing

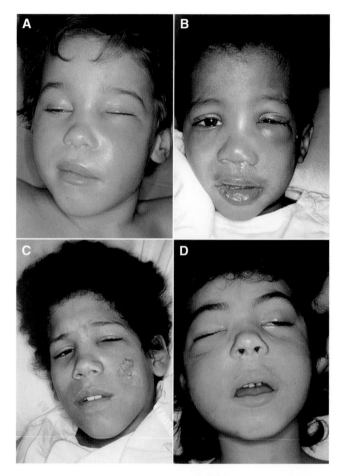

Figure 12-1

Upper face swelling, differential diagnosis. **A,** Frontal photograph of a 9-year-old child with left upper lip, alar base, cheek, and periorbital erythema and edema due to an odontogenic source. **B,** Frontal view of a 6-year-old patient with erythema and swelling over the left cheek and periorbital region. The patient was recovering from an upper respiratory infection; there was no dental, sinus, or other identifiable source of infection. The diagnosis was erysipelas due to β-streptococcal infection and responded well to penicillin therapy. **C,** A 12-year-old patient with left cheek and periorbital swelling. The skin ulceration was an infected burn, the source of the facial cellulitis. **D,** A young child with right cheek and periorbital swelling. The right anterior maxillary region was tender to palpation. No dental pathology was evident. The diagnosis was acute sinusitis.

prevalence of penicillin resistance (10% to 15%).[8] A previous course of antibiotics effective against a β-lactamase producing (BLP) organism is associated with an increased risk for penicillin resistance.

It is well recognized that most facial infections are caused by mixed microbiologic flora. Additionally, these mixed infections are composed of an increasing proportion of anaerobic and BLP organisms. Therefore most empiric antibiotic management recommendations for nonodontogenic infection include the use of broad-spectrum antibiotics with coverage for BLP organisms, especially when antibiotic therapy has already been attempted.

Clinical Picture. Children with upper face infections commonly suffer from similar signs and symptoms regardless of the etiology (Figure 12-1). Patients frequently complain of facial pain, swelling, fever, malaise, and an inability to eat or drink. If the source of infection is a maxillary tooth, there is usually a history of antecedent toothache. If there is a primary maxillary sinusitis, it is often preceded by an upper respiratory infection or a history of chronic sinus drainage. The patient may complain of headache.[9] In many children, there is no history of a prior dental or maxillary sinus problem, but there may be a history of otitis media, upper respiratory infection, local trauma (e.g., insect bite or a minor burn on the skin), or a recent episode of varicella.[9,10]

The patient's age is helpful as a guide to determining the source of infection and bacterial etiology.[1,3,5,11,12] Upper face infections, especially preseptal (periorbital)

cellulitis, are most common in children under age 5, whereas lower face infections are more common in those between ages 6 and 12. In the younger age group (deciduous dentition or earlier), the exact source of infection is less likely to be found, and these patients have a higher incidence of *S. pneumoniae* or *Staphylococcus aureus* growing from blood or wound cultures. In the older age group (mixed dentition or later), the infections are more likely to be odontogenic in origin and caused by penicillin-sensitive organisms. The common bacteria contributing to pediatric maxillofacial infections are listed in Box 12-1.

Physical examination findings may be remarkably similar, regardless of the etiology of infection (see Figure 12-1). Swelling and erythema of the upper lip, cheek, nasolabial fold, and periorbital region are accompanied by tenderness to palpation. The eyelids may be partially closed by edema and cellulitis. Evidence of proptosis, chemosis, changes in visual acuity, or complaints of photophobia suggest an orbital cellulitis or abscess. Intraorally, there may be swelling of the buccal sulcus. In the case of odontogenic infection, one or more offending teeth are usually obvious because of

---

BOX 12-1	Microbiology of Pediatric Facial Infections

Gram-Positive Aerobic/Facultative Species
Staphylococcus aureus
S. epidermidis
Streptococcus pneumoniae
Streptococcus pyogenes (ß-Hemolytic streptococcus)
Groups A, B, and F *Streptococcus* sp.
α-Hemolytic streptococcus *(Streptococcus viridans)*
Streptococcus milleri
Arachnia sp.
Corynebacterium diphtheria

Gram-Negative Aerobic/Facultative Species
Pseudomonas aeruginosa
Enterobacter sp.
Escherichia coli
Klebsiella pneumonia
Moraxella catarrhalis

Gram-Positive Anaerobic Species
Peptostreptococcus sp.
Peptococcus sp.
Bifidobacteria sp.
Actinomyces sp.
Propionibacterium sp.
Clostridia sp.
Eubacterium sp.

Gram-Negative Aerobic/Facultative Species
Haemophilus influenzae
H. parainfluenzae
Eikenella corrodens

Gram-Negative Anaerobic/Facultative Species
Bacteroides sp.
Prevotella melaninogenica (formerly *Bacteroides melaninogenicus*)
Porphyromonas sp.
Pasteurella multocida
Veillonella sp.
Fusobacterium sp.

caries, periodontal disease, or injury and tenderness to percussion. In patients with primary maxillary sinusitis, there is usually no acute dental pathology, but there may be sensitivity to percussion and drainage in the gingival sulcus of multiple maxillary teeth in the corresponding quadrant (Figure 12-2). In addition, the anterior maxilla, palpated extraorally, is frequently tender.[13] Transillumination of the sinus is helpful in older children (over 10 years) when most of the permanent teeth have erupted.[10] An antrum filled with fluid does not transilluminate. Risk factors for sinusitis include systemic disorders, such as recent upper respiratory infection, allergies, cystic fibrosis, effects of second-hand smoke, and local problems including mechanical obstruction due to deviated septum, mucosal swelling, polyps, and foreign bodies.[14] Imaging studies include dental and panoramic radiographs when appropriate and computed tomo-

graphic (CT) scans. The role of magnetic resonance imaging is limited to those cases in which intracranial spread (e.g., cavernous sinus thrombosis) is suspected.

In children 6 years of age or under, imaging studies to confirm a diagnosis of sinusitis are not necessary.[10] For children over 6 years of age or patients with severe symptoms, the role of imaging is controversial. An upright Waters' view radiograph demonstrates the maxillary, frontal, and ethmoid sinuses. This helps to differentiate pansinusitis from localized sinus disease, which is more likely to be secondary to odontogenic infection. A panoramic radiograph is used to demonstrate dental pathology and fluid in the maxillary sinus. If the panoramic radiograph is inadequate to demonstrate suspected dental pathology, an intraoral radiograph is taken. However, the child may be too uncomfortable to cooperate for this study. Plain or

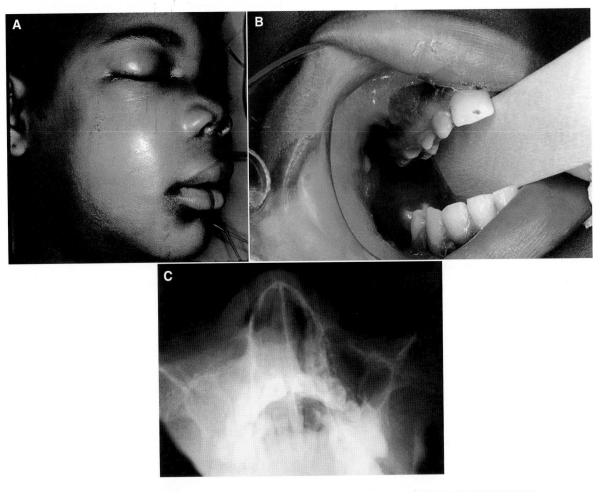

Figure 12-2 ▮
A, Patient with pain and swelling involving the right upper lip, alar base, cheek, and periorbital region. All the teeth in the right upper quadrant ached and were sensitive to percussion. **B,** Intraoral view shows buccal sulcus swelling and drainage around multiple teeth in the upper right quadrant. **C,** Waters' view confirms the diagnosis of acute right maxillary sinusitis.

panoramic radiographs can be less effective in children. CT imaging can aid in delineating the extent of sinus involvement and is recommended if operative intervention is being considered.[10] Normal findings on sinus radiographs are powerful evidence that bacterial sinusitis is not the cause of clinical symptoms. Endoscopic examination of the sinus and endoscopic sampling for culture is of unproved efficacy.

Anatomic Pathways

Because of the intimate anatomic relationship of multiple contiguous structures in the face, it is important to understand the anatomic pathways by which acute and chronic infections spread through the tissue planes[15,16]

(Figures 12-3 and 12-4). This allows the clinician to make a more accurate assessment of the source of infection during the diagnostic workup. Although the oral and maxillofacial surgeon most commonly sees children with primary odontogenic infection, the path of spread through the anatomic planes of the upper face is similar, regardless of the etiology.

Maxillary molar infections may dissect laterally from the roots, inferior to the buccinator attachment, and perforate the buccal plate into the mucobuccal fold; they may spread above the buccinator attachment into the soft tissues of the cheek. The former path of spread results in intraoral swelling, whereas the latter results in swelling of the cheek and periorbital tissues (see Figure 12-3).

A

B

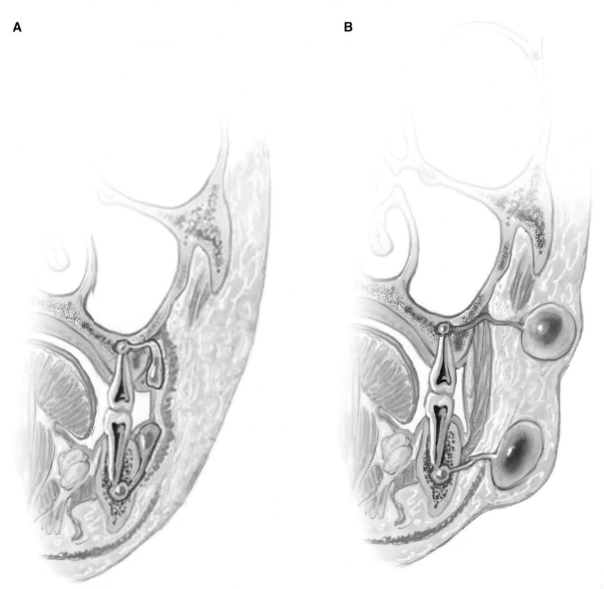

Figure 12-3
The path of spread of infection from the upper and lower premolar teeth medially (**A**) and laterally (**B**) in relation to the buccinator muscle attachments.

The roots of the maxillary premolars and molars are closely related to the maxillary sinuses. Infection in these teeth may produce secondary maxillary sinusitis with swelling of the cheek and buccal sulcus, as well as drainage through the nose. Finally, maxillary molar infections may spread posteriorly, in the buccal space, to the pterygopalatine fissure and infratemporal fossa. Infection may then reach the orbit via the inferior orbital fissure. In such cases, the patient exhibits periorbital swelling in addition to swelling of the cheek and buccal sulcus. The orbit or periorbital tissues or both may become secondarily infected from the maxillary anterior teeth by direct spread through local tissue planes or by retrograde spread through the valveless anterior facial, angular, and ophthalmic veins[15-19] (see Figures 12-4 and 12-5).

When a patient with periorbital swelling is evaluated, one must also consider the paranasal sinuses as a source. Drainage of veins or lymphatic vessels from the sinuses becomes obstructed, and infectious phlebitis and edema ensue. Inflammatory cells and bacteria infiltrate the orbit retrograde and cellulitis develops.[19-24]

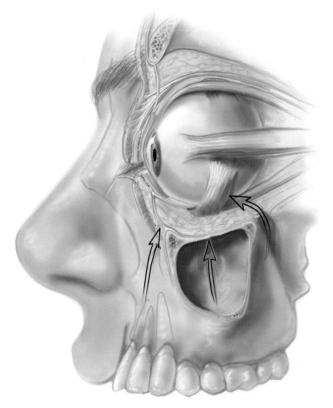

Figure 12-4

The path of spread of infection from the skin, teeth, and maxillary sinus to the orbit. Note that the orbit may become involved through the infratemporal fossa via the inferior orbital fissure.

Treatment

To develop a differential diagnosis for upper face infections, consider first the anatomic source, including teeth, paranasal sinuses (especially the antrum), overlying skin and its appendages and, occasionally, the parotid gland. It is important to note that carious deciduous teeth may produce serious odontogenic infections, with secondary cellulitis and systemic toxicity, in a manner similar to those caused by carious permanent teeth. Second, consider other risk factors such as a history of trauma, including recent insect or animal bites, burns, upper respiratory infection, or otitis media.

Once the location and source of the primary infection are determined, empiric therapy can be started (Table 12-1). When a fluctuant swelling is present, it should be drained or aspirated for Gram stain and culture before starting antibiotics. Unfortunately, in an uncomfortable, crying, febrile, dehydrated child, this is not always possible.[1] The child should be kept well hydrated, using the guidelines for fluid and electrolyte replacement described in Chapter 8. Indications for admitting pediatric patients to the hospital include (1) signs of sepsis, such as fever, lymphadenopathy, elevated white blood cell count, (2) poor oral intake, (3) doubt about the care they will receive at home, (4) the need for an operation, and (5) failure of outpatient management to resolve the infection.

In the case of odontogenic infection, the patient is started on oral or intravenous penicillin (25 to 50 mg/kg/day po q6-8h or 100,000 to 250,000 units/kg/day IV q4h). If the child is already receiving antibiotics and not responding, or if the child has been previously treated, coverage for BLP-producing organisms must be considered. A penicillinase-resistant antibiotic such as clindamycin (20 to 30 mg/kg/day po q6h or 25 to 40 mg/kg/day IV q6-8h), amoxicillin-clavulanate (40 mg/kg/day of amoxicillin component po q8-12h), or ampicillin-sulbactam (50 mg/kg/day of ampicillin component IV q8h), should be substituted. Operative intervention, such as tooth extraction with or without incision and drainage, commonly is indicated to resolve odontogenic infections. In general, this is not true for upper face infections from most other sources. In some cases, however, the patient may respond adequately to medical therapy and the tooth saved with endodontic treatment.

If maxillary sinusitis is thought to be secondary to odontogenic infection, penicillin remains the drug of choice for initial therapy. In patients with acute maxillary sinusitis who have had an antecedent upper respiratory infection, the most likely responsible organisms are *S. pneumonia* (35% to 42%), nontypeable *H. influenzae* (21% to 28%), *Moraxella catarrhalis* (21% to 28%) and, occasionally, *S. aureus* or anaerobic organisms.[25] Over the last 5 years, *S. pneumonia* has become a BLP organism with increasing frequency. Almost 100% of *M. catarrhalis*

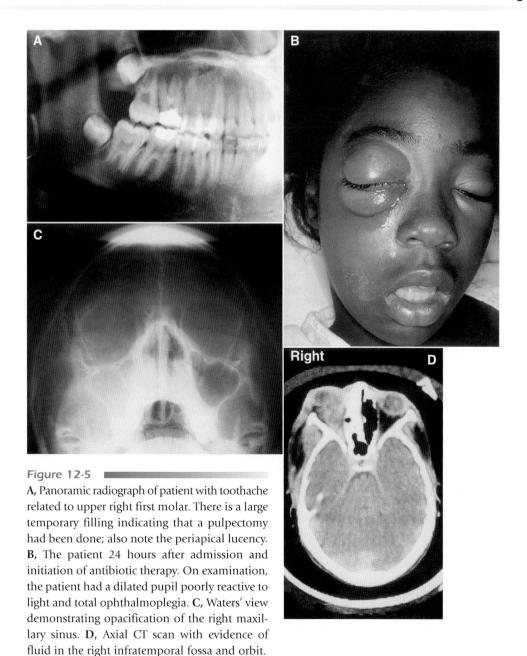

Figure 12-5 ▬▬▬▬▬

A, Panoramic radiograph of patient with toothache related to upper right first molar. There is a large temporary filling indicating that a pulpectomy had been done; also note the periapical lucency. **B,** The patient 24 hours after admission and initiation of antibiotic therapy. On examination, the patient had a dilated pupil poorly reactive to light and total ophthalmoplegia. **C,** Waters' view demonstrating opacification of the right maxillary sinus. **D,** Axial CT scan with evidence of fluid in the right infratemporal fossa and orbit.

are BLP organisms. Initial management includes nasal vasoconstrictors (e.g., phenylephrine nasal drops or spray) and humidification. The appropriate antibiotic therapy is initiated and continued until the patient is free of symptoms plus an additional 7 days.[10] Hospitalization should be considered for patients with severe symptoms, such as temperature of 102° F (39° C) or above and concurrent purulent nasal discharge for at least 3 to 4 days in a child who appears ill.[10] In the absence of risk factors, most children (80%) will respond to amoxicillin (25 to 50 mg/kg/day po q8-12h). In penicillin-allergic patients consider clarithromycin (15 mg/kg/day po q12h), azithromycin (12 mg/kg/day po q24h), or clindamycin as alternatives.[10] In the presence of other risk factors, including recent treatment (within 30 days) or failure to improve, other antibiotics to consider are amoxicillin-clavulanate, cefdinir (7 mg/kg/day po q12h), cefuroxime, or cefpodoxime (10 mg/kg/day po q12h). There is a limited role for operative intervention in the acute setting.[14]

Chronic maxillary sinusitis is defined as episodes of inflammation of the paranasal sinuses lasting more than 90 days. Risk factors for chronic sinusitis include allergies, cystic fibrosis, and local intranasal problems

TABLE 12-1   Alphabetical Listing of Antibiotics Used in Pediatric Maxillofacial Infections

Generic	Route	Dosage	Interval
Ampicillin	IV, IM	100-400 mg/kg/day	4-6 hr
Ampicillin/sulbactam	IV	50 mg/kg/day of ampicillin component	8 hr
Amoxicillin	po	25-50 mg/kg/day	8-12 hr
Amoxicillin/potassium clavulanate	po	40 mg/kg/day of amoxicillin component	8 hr
Azithromycin	po	12 mg/kg/day	24 hr
Cefaclor	po	40 mg/kg/day	8-12 hr
Cefadroxil monohydrate	po	30 mg/kg/day	12 hr
Cefamandole nafate	IV, IM	100-150 mg/kg/day	4-6 hr
Cefazolin sodium	IV, IM	50-100 mg/kg/day	8 hr
Cefdinir	po	7 mg/kg/day	12 hr
Cefixime	po	8 mg/kg/day	12-24 hr
Cefotaxime sodium	IV, IM	100-200 mg/kg/day	6-8 hr
Cefoxitin sodium	IV, IM	80-160 mg/kg/day	4-6 hr
Cefpodoxime	po	10 mg/kg/day	12 hr
Cefprozil	po	15-30 mg/kg/day	24 hr
Ceftazidime	IV, IM	100-150 mg/kg/day	8 hr
Cefuroxime	IV, IM	50-100 mg/kg/day	6-8 hr
Clarithromycin	po	15 mg/kg/day	12 hr
Clindamycin (HCl hydrate or palmitate HCl)	po	20-30 mg/kg/day	6 hr
Clindamycin phosphate	IV, IM	25-40 mg/kg/day	6-8 hr
Cloxacillin	po	50-100 mg/kg/day	6 hr
Dicloxacillin monohydrate sodium	po	12-25 mg/kg/day	6 hr
Erythromycin	po	40 mg/kg/day	6 hr
Imipenem/cilastatin	IV	60-100 mg/kg/day (imipenem component)	6 hr
Methicillin, sodium	IV, IM	150-200 mg/kg/day	6 hr
Metronidazole	po	15-35 mg/kg/day	6 hr
Nafcillin monohydrate, sodium	IV, IM	150 mg/kg/day	6 hr
Oxacillin sodium	po	50-100 mg/kg/day	6 hr
Penicillin G (potassium)	po	25-50 mg/kg/day	6-8 hr
Penicillin G (procaine)	IM	25,000-50,000 units/kg/day	12-24 hr
Penicillin G (sodium)	IV, IM	100,000-250,000 units/kg/day	4 hr
Penicillin V	po	25-50 mg/kg/day	6-8 hr
Ticarcillin/clavulanate	IV	200-300 mg/kg/day	4-6 hr
Trimethoprim/sulfamethoxazole	po	6-10 mg/kg/day (trimethoprim component)	12 hr
Vancomycin HCL	IV	40 mg/kg/day	6 hr

blocking sinus or nasal drainage. The infection is commonly polymicrobial in nature with a significant anaerobic component, including *Veillonella* species, *Peptococcus* species, *Propionibacterium acnes,* and anaerobic non–spore-forming gram-positive bacteria. Many of the latter are BLP bacteria.[10,26] A second-generation cephalosporin or clindamycin is an excellent choice for initial therapy.[26] Operative intervention is a more frequent consideration for chronic maxillary sinusitis.[26]

Skin infections are commonly polymicrobial and composed of aerobic (*S. aureus, S. pyogenes,* or other streptococcal species) and anaerobic flora.[27,28] The antibiotics of choice include penicillinase-resistant drugs such as amoxicillin-clavulanate, clindamycin, nafcillin (150 mg/kg/day IV q6h), oxacillin (50 to 100 mg/kg/day po q6h), cefoxitin (80 to 160 mg/kg/day IV q4-6h), or metronidazole (15 to 35 mg/kg/day po q6h) in combination with a BLP-resistant pencillin.[27] In the case of dog, cat, or human bite wounds that become infected, appropriate wound management (assessment of rabies and tetanus status and cleansing, debridement, and drainage) is indicated. Amoxicillin-clavulanate is the drug of choice for both prophylaxis and outpatient management of a minor bite wound infection. It is active against most animal and human bite pathogens, including capnocytophaga (dog), *Pasteurella multocida* (dog and cat), *S. aureus*, *S. viridans*, and *Eikenella corrodens* (human). The choice of agents for human bite wounds in penicillin-allergic patients is problematic because *E. corrodens* is resistant to erythromycin and variably resistant to the cephalosporins, penicillinase-resistant penicillins, and clindamycin. Trimethoprim-sulfamethoxazole (6 to 10 mg/kg/day trimethoprim component po q12h) and clindamycin in combination is an appropriate empiric regimen for both animal or human bite wounds in the penicillin-allergic patient. Prophylaxis should be given for a total of 5 days, as long as the wound does not become infected.

For hospitalized patients with major or significantly infected bite wounds, initiate antimicrobial therapy using ampicillin-sulbactam or ticarcillin-clavulanate (200 to 300 mg/kg/day ticarcillin component IV q4-6h). If the patient is penicillin allergic, trimethoprim-sulfamethoxazole or clindamycin in combination is an appropriate choice. Infected bite wounds should be cultured from the deep portion of the wound at the time of initial evaluation. Empiric antibiotic therapy can then be adjusted once the results of sensitivity testing are known. Antibiotic treatment for localized cellulitis or abscess should be administered for 10 to 14 days after initial drainage and debridement. If parenteral therapy is initiated, a switch to oral antibiotics is reasonable after 5 to 10 days or after significant improvement is noted.[29]

Any fluctuant swelling is drained as soon as possible. If local anesthesia cannot be administered because of swelling or lack of patient cooperation, then the child is made npo in preparation for a general anesthetic to be delivered (see Chapter 8 for details of preparing a child for anesthesia).

Complications

The common systemic complications of maxillofacial infections in childhood are sepsis and dehydration. Children may deteriorate rapidly after developing a toothache and local swelling. Cellulitis, fever, chills, and dehydration often develop after only a few hours. For this reason, it is critical to follow pediatric patients very closely, especially if they are being treated at home. The child may be uncooperative in taking oral antibiotics and fluid, and the parents may not appreciate the potential complications. When in doubt, a child should be admitted to the hospital for observation, hydration, and parenteral antibiotics.

Regardless of etiology, serious complications of upper face infections (e.g., cavernous sinus thrombosis, other central nervous system complications such as meningitis or brain abscess, and blindness) have become very rare during the antibiotic era. These complications occur when the infection spreads to the central nervous system or orbit through local tissue planes or retrograde through the valveless facial and angular veins.[15,16,21-24,30,31] Brook and others[30] reported on eight patients (6 to 15 years of age) who had periorbital cellulitis and other complications of sinusitis. Subdural empyema occurred in four patients, in one case accompanied by brain abscess and in another by meningitis. It is of note that alveolar abscesses in the upper incisors of two children resulted in maxillary and ethmoid sinusitis and then spread to the orbit.

Periorbital infections are classified by their relationship to the orbital septum, which is a periosteal reflection from the infraorbital rim to the tarsal plate (Figure 12-6). The septum separates the lids from the orbital contents and acts as a barrier to the spread of infection from the skin into the orbit. Preseptal cellulitis involves the tissues superficial to the orbital septum, whereas orbital cellulitis involves tissues deep to the septum. Both conditions are manifest by erythema, edema, and warmth of the eyelids, whereas orbital cellulitis is more likely to show proptosis, chemosis, limitation and pain with eye movement, and loss of visual acuity.[22-24] Frank orbital abscess causes symptoms similar to those of orbital cellulitis.

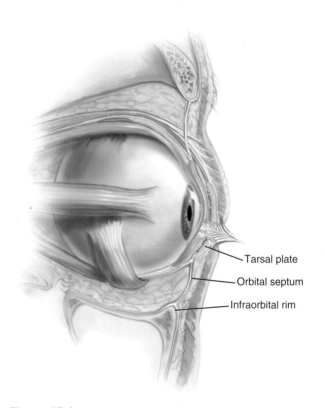

Tarsal plate
Orbital septum
Infraorbital rim

Figure 12-6

Lateral view of the orbit demonstrating the relationship of the orbital septum to the orbital cavity and showing overlying lid and skin.

It is sometimes difficult to make the clinical distinction between these three entities (periorbital cellulitis, orbital cellulitis, orbital abscess), but it is important to do so because prompt surgical drainage of orbital cellulitis or abscess may be necessary to prevent central nervous system complications and to preserve vision. The CT scan is useful in this differential diagnosis (see Figure 12-5). It illustrates the soft tissue contents of the orbits and distinguishes them from the surrounding bones and paranasal sinuses.[16,20,32]

Orbital cellulitis or abscess is a rare condition. In a recent review of periorbital and orbital cellulitis in childhood, Smith and others[33] found that only 2 of 39 patients had true orbital cellulitis. Orbital cellulitis developed after trauma in one case and after spread from a local infection in another case. Kaban and McGill[16] reported a case of orbital cellulitis resulting from a maxillary molar infection. One to three percent of patients with acute sinusitis will develop orbital cellulitis. Conversely, 70% of cases of orbital cellulitis are associated with a coexisting sinusitis.[34] In patients with preseptal cellulitis, the cause is usually spread from infection of a contiguous structure or from a preexisting upper respiratory infection.

During the preantibiotic era, orbital and periorbital cellulitis and cavernous sinus thrombosis were well-known sequelae of dental infection and were reported frequently in the literature.[17,35,36] The advent of antibiotics has reduced greatly the incidence of this problem. No mention was made of dental infection in the etiology of periorbital or orbital cellulitis in several large series.[21-23,31,37,38] However, isolated cases continue to be reported in the literature.[16,39,40] In the series from San Francisco General Hospital, 5 out of 35 patients with periorbital cellulitis had an identifiable dental source.[1] This underscores the importance of constant and close follow-up of pediatric patients with orofacial infections.

In the patient reported by Kaban and McGill[16] (see Figure 12-5), infection rapidly progressed from the maxillary first molar to the maxillary and ethmoid sinuses, infratemporal fossa, and the posterior portion of the bony orbit. The orbital cavity became involved through the inferior orbital fissure. The persistent proptosis, decreased visual acuity, chemosis, limitation of extraocular muscle movement, and the dilated pupil seen in this patient made it imperative to determine the extent of infection in the orbit and adjacent structures. A CT scan was used to demonstrate the muscle cone, optic nerve, and globe in relation to the less dense surrounding fat. The scan may be used to distinguish a variety of orbital conditions such as tumors, neuritis, Grave's disease, and acute inflammation.[41] Inflammatory exudate may be localized to the anterior or posterior aspect of the orbit, and the relationship of the fluid to the optic nerve can

be demonstrated. In the patient under discussion, the CT scan clearly showed fluid in the infratemporal fossa, ethmoid sinus, and posterior aspect of the orbit surrounding the optic nerve (see Figure 12-5). This localization of the inflammatory process led the authors to drain the orbit by decompressing the infratemporal fossa.[16] If the purulent exudate had been more anteriorly located in the orbit, drainage would have been carried out through an incision in the orbital septum.

The signs and symptoms of cavernous sinus thrombosis are similar to those of orbital cellulitis: periorbital edema, chemosis, proptosis, and limitation of extraocular movements. In addition, there is no consensual pupillary response to light in the opposite eye and there is decreased sensation in the distribution of the first division of the trigeminal (fifth) nerve. Potential sequelae of cavernous sinus thrombosis are meningitis and brain abscess. Management consists of high-dose intravenous antibiotics and definitive treatment of the underlying cause.

LOWER FACE INFECTIONS
Evaluation and Differential Diagnosis

Infections of the lower face are defined as those localized to the buccal space or arising from structures of the lower face, including skin or skin appendages inferior to the parotid duct, mandibular teeth, submandibular or sublingual salivary glands, lymph nodes, and structures of the floor of the mouth.[1,3] Patients with lower face infections suffer from pain, swelling, and trismus. When infection involves the buccal or masseteric spaces, the predominant swelling is visible extraorally, and it rarely spreads superiorly to involve the eyelids. Involvement of the pterygoid space and infratemporal fossa, medial to the mandibular ramus, produces swelling in the region of the pterygomandibular raphe, soft palate, and lateral pharyngeal wall; there is little extraoral swelling (Figure 12-7). The predominant findings are pain and trismus (Figures 12-8 and 12-9). Infection in the sublingual space results in pain and elevation of the tongue, whereas in the submandibular space the patient develops extraoral swelling. When the sublingual and submandibular spaces on both sides of the midline are involved, the infection is known as *Ludwig's angina* (Figure 12-10).

As in the upper face, determination of the location of the primary site of infection and associated etiology is the first step in evaluation. The common sources of infection in the lower face are teeth, skin and its appendages, local lymph nodes, and salivary glands. Dodson and colleagues[1,3] found that dental infection was the most common primary diagnosis in patients with lower facial swelling. These infections usually were produced by penicillin-sensitive organisms. The remaining etiologies, in order of frequency, were trauma, skin

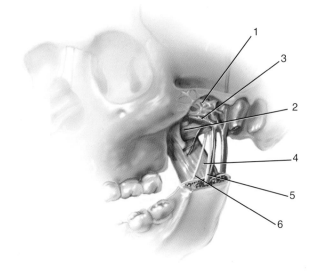

Figure 12-7

Infratemporal fossa. The presence of the inferior alveolar *(5)* and lingual *(6)* nerves and medial *(4)* and lateral *(2)* pterygoid and temporalis muscles explains the severe pain and trismus, with little visible swelling in patients with an infection in the infratemporal space. Internal maxillary artery *(3)* and pterygoid venous plexus *(1)* are also illustrated.

appendages (cysts), burns, and insect bites. In those patients who did not respond to penicillin, the most common organism cultured was a resistant *S. aureus.*

Neck infections related to local lymph nodes are common in pediatric patients. There is a history of recent or multiple upper respiratory infections with generalized lymphadenopathy. After the patient recovers, a submandibular or masseteric swelling remains, the result of a secondarily infected lymph node.

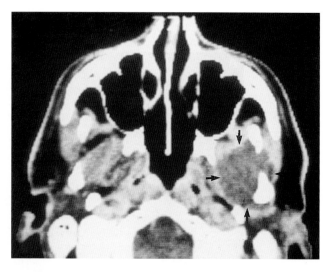

Figure 12-9

Axial CT scan of patient with minimal facial swelling but severe pain and trismus. The scan demonstrates a large fluid-filled mass (abscess) in the infratemporal fossa *(arrows)*.

Anatomic Pathways

Infection spreads from the mandibular molars into the infratemporal fossa (posteriorly and medially) or into the buccal space (posteriorly and laterally) (see Figures 12-3 and 12-7). Medial spread of infection results in swelling of the floor of the mouth and elevation of the tongue. Ludwig's angina results from confluent infection in the sublingual and submandibular spaces (see Figure 12-10). Mandibular premolar infection may spread medially to the sublingual space and medially and inferiorly into the submylohyoid (submandibular) space. When the submylohyoid space is involved, the

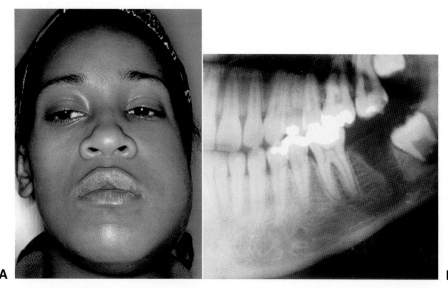

Figure 12-8

A, Teenager with pain, trismus, and swelling in left buccal space. **B,** Panoramic radiograph demonstrating recent lower left second molar extraction socket—the source of this infection.

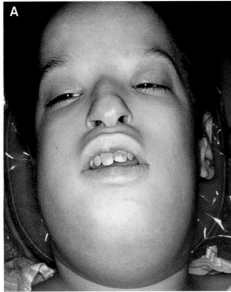

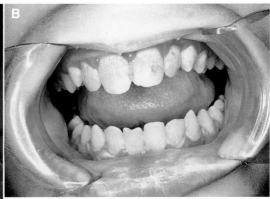

Figure 12-10
A, Nine-year-old boy with Ludwig's angina of odontogenic origin, infected mandibular right 6-year molar. **B,** Intraoral view demonstrating elevated tongue.

patient experiences an extraoral swelling. The mandibular incisors and canine teeth may produce infection in the sublingual or submylohyoid spaces. In addition, if the infection spreads to perforate the labial cortex, the chin becomes swollen. Infections of the submandibular and submental lymph nodes may spread to produce cellulitis of the corresponding spaces. Likewise, infection in the lymph nodes overlying the masseter muscle may spread to the buccal space.

Treatment and Complications

The principles of treatment are similar to those described for infections of the upper face. However, there is the additional consideration of potential airway obstruction resulting from trismus, swelling, and elevation of the tongue. When in doubt, the patient should be admitted to the hospital for intravenous antibiotic therapy (see Table 12-1) and careful observation of the airway and breathing. Close monitoring of the situation may allow elective endotracheal intubation, if necessary, rather than emergency tracheotomy.

The patient is treated with antibiotics as described for odontogenic infections of the maxilla. Fluids and electrolytes are replaced as needed, using the guidelines in Chapter 8.

A fluctuant swelling requires drainage, and infected teeth require extraction or pulp extirpation. Anesthetic considerations are the same as those for upper face infections. However, the presence of trismus and swelling of the floor of the mouth may make airway management more difficult. Resolution of lower face infections may take longer than those of the upper face because of the lack of natural gravity drainage, less diffuse blood supply, and more bulky overlying soft tissue.

CHRONIC INFECTIONS
Nonhealing Wound

Patients with chronic infection often complain of a draining or nonhealing intraoral or extraoral wound, with little or no pain, swelling, trismus, or fever. One must consider local and systemic etiologies in the differential diagnosis.

The most common local etiology for a nonhealing wound is persistent mechanical, thermal, or chemical trauma. For example, children who place foreign bodies (sharp or pointed toys or sticks) in their mouths may produce a nonhealing, ulcerating wound. Persistent trauma to the adjacent cheek from orthodontic brackets or wires may also result in a traumatic ulcer. The pyogenic granuloma is another typical nonhealing, reactive lesion that occurs in children. Finally, one must consider local benign or malignant tumors in the differential diagnosis of a nonhealing wound (Figures 12-11 and 12-12).

A variety of systemic diseases may result in intraoral nonhealing wounds. Histiocytosis and acute leukemia, for example, are the two most common causes of nonhealing, intraoral wounds in children (Figure 12-13). Often, this is the first sign of systemic disease. Patients taking systemic drugs such as phenytoin or cyclosporine may also have chronic nonhealing inflammatory disease of the gingiva. When an intraoral wound or infection does not respond in the expected way to treatment, an underlying systemic illness should be considered in the differential diagnosis.

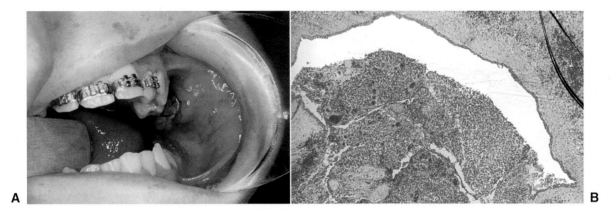

Figure 12-11
A, Intraoral view of a nonhealing ulceration of the left cheek presumed to be related to the orthodontic band on the molar tooth. After removing the band, the ulceration enlarged. A biopsy was performed. **B,** This is a photomicrograph of a hematoxylin and eosin stained biopsy specimen. The diagnosis was undifferentiated sarcoma of the parotid duct.

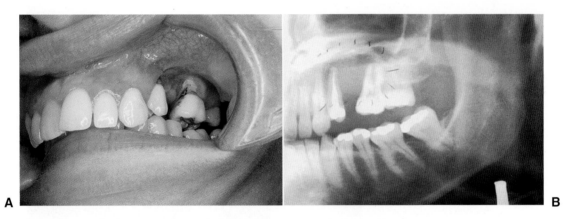

Figure 12-12
Intraoral view (**A**) and radiograph (**B**) of upper left quadrant in a patient with a 1-year history of a persistent "infection" in this area. The problem did not resolve despite multiple efforts of scaling and curettage, endodontic treatment and, ultimately, extraction. Biopsy revealed an ameloblastoma.

Chronic Draining Skin Lesions of Dental Origin

Patients with draining lesions on the face often are referred to dermatologists and general or plastic surgeons. The differential diagnosis includes local skin infections, such as carbuncles and infected sebaceous cysts, traumatic lesions, and basal or squamous cell carcinomas.[15] The possibility of skin drainage from a chronically infected tooth often is overlooked in the evaluation, resulting in recurrence of the lesion after treatment.

The case report illustrates the chronic, insidious nature of odontogenic infections that can spread to the face, producing orocutaneous fistulas. Frequently, the patient is asymptomatic relative to the teeth, and the skin drainage is distant from the source.[42-44] The patients are often unaware of any intraoral problems, and they do not appreciate the relationship of the teeth to the skin lesion. The surgeon must, therefore, be aware of this relationship and pursue it in differential diagnosis.[15] When the diagnosis of odontogenic infection is made, a dye may be injected, or a needle or gutta percha point inserted into the tract to demonstrate its relationship to the tooth apex. The tooth is treated as indicated, using endodontic therapy or extraction. Postoperatively, drainage ceases and the tract closes spontaneously. The scar is revised later, if necessary.

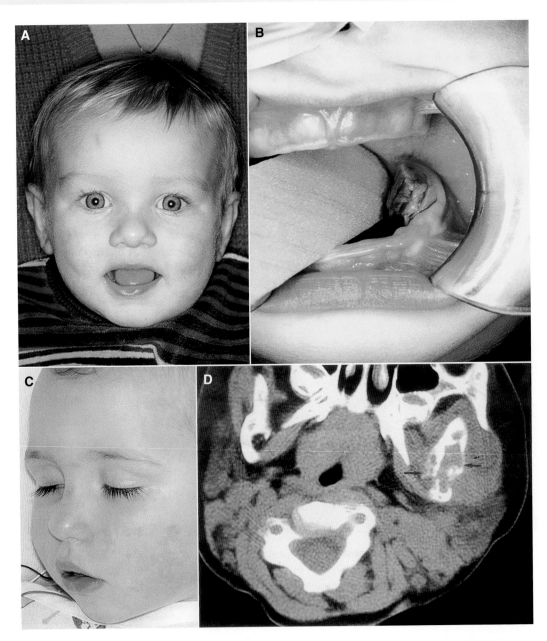

Figure 12-13

Three-year-old boy with left mandibular swelling (**A**), intraoral ulceration (**B**), and fever. The differential diagnosis was tumor versus infection. Biopsy revealed histiocytosis. Lateral photograph (**C**) and axial CT scan (**D**) of a 19-month-old girl with swelling and erythema over the left cheek. The CT scan demonstrates the expansile radiolucent lesion. Pathologic evaluation of the tissue specimen revealed Langerhans cell histiocytosis.

CONCLUSION

In this chapter, we have discussed management of pediatric maxillofacial infections. The approach of differential diagnosis of swelling, pain, trismus, and a nonhealing wound was used because it more closely reflects the clinical situation in pediatric patients.

Early diagnosis and treatment of head and neck infections in pediatric patients are important because of the tendency for children to deteriorate rapidly and become systemically ill. Upper face infections occur in younger children (usually less than age 5). Often, a specific source or etiology cannot be identified in younger children,

CASE REPORT 12-1

A 10-year-old patient was followed over a period of 12 months in the pediatric surgery clinic for a chronic draining lesion on the chin (Figure 12-14). She was treated with antibiotics, and the drainage ceased, only to recur several weeks later. The lesion was then excised and the pathology report indicated "chronic and acute inflammation." An anteroposterior radiograph of the mandible was read as negative for abnormalities.

When the drainage recurred after excision, she was referred to the oral and maxillofacial surgery clinic. The patient had been hit in the mouth while playing with her brother several years previously. She denied any history of a toothache or intraoral swelling.

Examination showed a discolored lower left central incisor fractured into the dentin, and the "negative" anteroposterior mandibular radiograph revealed a radiolucency at the apex of this tooth. The nonvital tooth was treated endodontically and the sinus tract excised.

The postoperative course was uneventful, and the patient has had no recurrence during 5 years of follow-up.

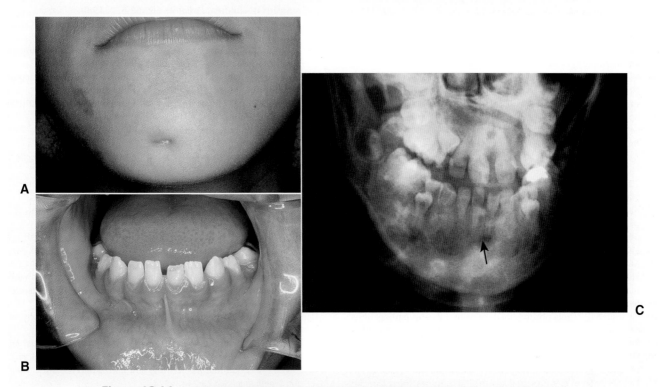

Figure 12-14

A, Draining orocutaneous fistula on chin. **B,** Intraoral view demonstrates fractured mandibular left central incisor. **C,** Anteroposterior radiograph reveals a radiolucent lesion *(arrow)* at the apex of the mandibular left central incisor. (From Kaban LB: *Plast Reconstr Surg* 66: 711-717, 1980.)

and they are more likely to exhibit a penicillin-resistant organism, especially if they have received antibiotic therapy previously. Lower face infections occur more frequently in the mixed dentition. They are more likely to be of odontogenic origin and are usually caused by a penicillin-sensitive organism.

REFERENCES

1. Dodson T, Perrott OH, Kaban LB: Pediatric maxillofacial infections: a retrospective study of 113 cases, *J Oral Maxillofac Surg* 47:327-330,1989.
2. Dodson TB, Barton JA, Kaban LB: Predictors of outcome in children hospitalized with maxillofacial infections: a linear logistic model, *J Oral Maxillofac Surg* 49:838-842, 1991.

3. Biederman GA, Dodson TB: Epidemiologic review of facial infections in hospitalized pediatric patients, *J Oral Maxillofac Surg* 52:1042-1045, 1994.

4. Dodson TB, Kaban LB: Diagnosis and management of pediatric facial infections, *Oral Maxillofac Surg Clin North Am* 6:13-20, 1994.

5. Scutari P Jr, Dodson TB: Epidemiologic review of pediatric and adult maxillofacial infections in hospitalized patients, *Oral Surg Oral Med Oral Pathol* 81:270-274, 1996.

6. Unkel JH, McKibben DH, Fenton SJ, et al: Comparison of odontogenetic and nonodontogenic facial cellulitis in a pediatric hospital population, *Am Acad Pediatr Dent* 19:476-479, 1997.

7. Donahue SP, Schwartz G: Preseptal and orbital cellulitis in childhood. a changing microbiologic spectrum, *Ophthalmology* 105:1902-1906, 1998.

8. Givner LB, Mason EO Jr, Barson WJ, et al: Pneumococcal facial cellulitis in children, *Pediatrics* 106:E61, 2000, http://www.pediatrics.org/cgi/content/full/106/5/e61, accessed June 13, 2003.

9. Wald ER, Milmoe GJ, Bowen A, et al: Acute maxillary sinusitis in children, *N Engl J Med* 304:749-754, 1981.

10. Wald ER and the Subcommittee on Management of Sinusitis and Committee on Quality Improvement: Clinical practice guidelines: management of sinusitis, *Pediatrics* 108:798-808, 2001.

11. Spires JR, Smith RJH: Bacterial infections of the orbital and periorbital soft tissues in children, *Laryngoscope* 96:763-767, 1986.

12. Brook I: Microbiology of abscesses of the head and neck in children, *Ann Otol Rhinol Laryngol* 96:429-433, 1987.

13. Herz G, Gfeller J: Sinusitis in paediatrics, *Chemotherapy* 23:5-57, 1977.

14. Nash D, Wald E: Sinusitis, *Pediatr Rev* 22:111-117, 2001.

15. Kaban LB: Draining skin lesions of odontogenic origin: the path of spread of chronic odontogenic infection, *Plast Reconstr Surg* 66:711-717, 1980.

16. Kaban LB, McGill T: Orbital cellulitis of dental origin, *J Oral Maxillofac Surg* 38:682-685, 1980.

17. Haymaker W: Fatal infections of the central nervous system and meninges after tooth extraction, *Am J Orthod* 31:117, 1945.

18. Sicher H: *Oral anatomy*, ed 4, St Louis, 1965, CV Mosby.

19. Chandler JR, Langenbrunner DJ, Stevens ER: The pathogenesis of orbital complications in acute sinusitis, *Laryngoscope* 80:1414-1428, 1970.

20. Goldberg F: Differentiation of orbital cellulitis from preseptal cellulitis by computed tomography, *Pediatrics* 62:1000-1005, 1978.

21. Lessner A, Stern GA: Preseptal and orbital cellulites, *Infect Dis Clin North Am* 6:933-953, 1992.

22. Donahue SP, Khoury JM, Kowalski RP: Common ocular infections: a prescriber's guide, *Drugs* 52:526-540, 1996.

23. Uzcategui N, Warman R, Smith A, Howard CW: Clinical practice guidelines for the management of orbital cellulites, *J Pediatr Ophthalmol Strabismus* 35:73-79, 1998.

24. Jain A, Rubin PAD: Orbital cellulitis in children, *Int Ophthalmol Clin* 41:71-86, 2001.

25. Poole MD, Jacobs MR, Anon JB, et al: Antimicrobial guidelines for the treatment of acute bacterial rhinosinusitis in immunocompetent children, *Int J Pediatr Otorhinolaryngol* 63:1-13, 2002.

26. Brook I, Yocum P: Antimicrobial management of chronic sinusitis in children, *J Laryngol Otol* 109:1159-1162, 1995.

27. Brook I: Microbiology of infected epidermal cysts, *Arch Dermatol* 125:1658-1661, 1989.

28. Brook I: Antimicrobial therapy of skin and soft tissue infection in children, *J Am Podiatr Med Assoc* 83:398-405, 1993.

29. Endom EE: Animal and human bites in children, *UpToDate Online*, version 10.3, 2002.

30. Brook I, Friedman EM, Rodriguez WJ, et al: Complications of sinusitis in children, *Pediatrics* 66:568-572, 1980.

31. Watters EC, Waller PH, Hiles DA, et al: Acute orbital cellulites, *Arch Ophthalmol* 94:785-788, 1976.

32. Haynes RE, Cramblett HG: Acute ethmoiditis: its relationship to orbital cellulites, *Am J Dis Child* 114:261-267, 1967.

33. Smith TF, O'Day D, Wright PF: Clinical implications of preseptal cellulitis in childhood, *Pediatrics* 62:1006-1009, 1978.

34. Hunger DG, Trucksis M: Orbital complication of cellulites, *UpToDate Online*, version 10.3, 2002.

35. Gamble RC: Acute inflammation of the orbits in children, *Arch Ophthalmol* 10:483-497, 1933.

36. Green J: Management of orbital infections, *Am J Ophthalmol* 14:196-201, 1931.

37. Gellady AM, Shulman ST, Ayoub EM: Periorbital and orbital cellulitis in children, *Pediatrics* 61:272-277,1978.

38. Healy GB, Strong MS: Acute periorbital swelling, *Laryngoscope* 82:1491-1498, 1972.

39. Gold RS, Sager E: Pansinusitis, orbital cellulitis, and blindness as sequelae of delayed treatment of dental abscess, *J Oral Surg* 32:40-43, 1974.

40. Limongelli WA, Clark MS, Williams AC: Panfacial cellulitis with contralateral orbital cellulitis and blindness after tooth extraction, *J Oral Surg* 35:38-43,1977.

41. Gyldensted C, Lester J, Fledelius H: Computed tomography of orbital lesions, *Neuroradiology* 13:141-150, 1970.

42. Endelman J: *Special dental pathology. a treatise for students and for practitioners of dentistry and medicine*, ed 2, St Louis, 1927, Mosby.

43. Green J Jr: Inflammatory swellings simulating dacryocystitis, *Trans Am Ophthalmol Soc* 22:244, 1924.

44. Blair VP: *Surgery and diseases of the mouth and jaws: a practical treatise on the surgery and diseases of the mouth and allied structures*, ed 3, St Louis, 1920, Mosby.

CHAPTER 13

Salivary Gland Inflammatory Disorders in Children

Oded Nahlieli

Inflammatory salivary gland disease represents more than one third of salivary gland pathology in childhood.[1,2] Because salivary gland disorders are encountered infrequently in children, there are relatively few papers in the literature dealing with these problems. In this chapter, we discuss salivary gland inflammatory conditions of childhood, diagnostic methods, and treatment.

DIAGNOSTIC METHODS
Clinical Evaluation

Accurate history and physical examination are crucial components of the evaluation. Children usually complain of pain and swelling occurring minutes to several hours after a meal. The swelling often will recede slowly with time, and often the parents and child relate that massage of the gland relieves the symptoms. The child may have a history of multiple episodes, treated with and responding to antibiotic therapy.

Visual scanning of submandibular, preauricular, and postauricular regions is the first step in assessing swelling and erythema (Figure 13-1, A). This is followed by intraoral examination. Surgical magnification loops (2.5 to 3.5) are very useful to improve visualization of the orifice of Wharton's and Stensen's ducts. The orifice may be red and edematous and appear as a papilla. Plaques or whitish secretions from the duct may represent frank infection. Sometimes a small stone can be found in the orifice; occasionally, the white-yellow color of a stone can be seen through the translucent mucosa (Figure 13-1, B and C). Bimanual palpation is particularly important when examining the submandibular gland and duct. It helps to differentiate the gland from adjacent lymph nodes, inferior to the gland, and to ascertain the presence of any firm mass in the take-off of Wharton's duct from the hilum of the gland.

For the parotid gland, manual palpation allows the surgeon to determine the consistency of the gland. One should also massage the gland to milk and inspect the saliva.

Salivary Imaging

There are a variety of newly available imaging methods to detect tumors and inflammatory diseases of the salivary glands. In this section we focus on those techniques most suitable for children.

Submandibular Gland Imaging. The most effective imaging methods for inflammatory conditions of the submandibular and parotid glands are plain radiographs (occlusal, occlusal oblique, panoramic), sialography (if possible), ultrasonography, and computed tomography. Sialoendoscopy is a newly developed

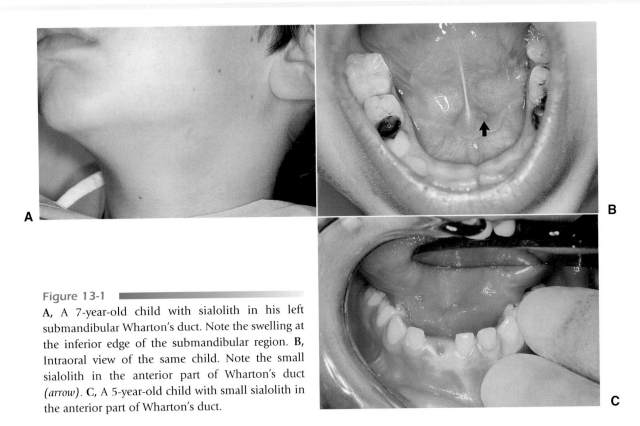

Figure 13-1

A, A 7-year-old child with sialolith in his left submandibular Wharton's duct. Note the swelling at the inferior edge of the submandibular region. **B,** Intraoral view of the same child. Note the small sialolith in the anterior part of Wharton's duct (*arrow*). **C,** A 5-year-old child with small sialolith in the anterior part of Wharton's duct.

technique that is useful for imaging and treatment. It is discussed separately.

Plain Radiography. Most of the obstructive pathologies of the salivary glands are radiopaque and will, therefore, be visible on plain radiographs.[3] Occlusal, occlusal oblique, and panoramic radiographs are excellent for ruling out any calcification in the submandibular region (Figure 13-2, *A* and *B*). In young children there is not enough space to insert the conventional occlusal film. A simple solution is to use ordinary periapical film for this purpose. The cooperation needed from the child for the success of these plain radiographs is minimal. In the case of infants, parents are often able to assist the child to allow completion of the image.

Sialography. Sialography in children is often impossible and is reserved, if necessary, for selected cooperative patients. In the past, when there were no alternatives, this technique was accomplished under general anesthesia. Reducing the discomfort during sialography may be achieved by applying topical anesthesia to Wharton's duct papilla or by lavaging the gland through the orifice with lidocaine 2% before the injection of the water-soluble dye. Sialography provides images of the morphology of the ductal system and allows the diagnosis of strictures, dilations, and filling defects. This technique also provides information on glandular function.

Ultrasonography. High-resolution ultrasonography (above 10 MHz) is a good imaging method to assess the salivary glands in children. It is noninvasive and there is no associated discomfort. It is useful to distinguish the submandibular gland from surrounding lymph nodes and to locate calculi. The portion of Wharton's duct that leads from the hilum of the gland toward the floor of the mouth, precisely after the penetration of the mylohyoid muscle, is difficult to identify.[4]

Computed Tomography. The CT scan is especially useful for evaluating inflammatory conditions of the submandibular gland. Sialoliths are readily identified on CT imaging (Figure 13-2, *C*). The standard images should be 1-mm cuts with 3-dimensional reconstruction. In this way the glands and ducts can be visualized in all planes and stones are less likely to be missed.

Parotid Gland Imaging. Most inflammatory conditions of the parotid glands are not a consequence of sialolithiasis. Therefore, the imaging techniques are directed toward documenting changes in Stensen's duct morphology and size and changes in the substance of the gland. The most effective imaging methods for inflammatory parotid conditions in childhood are sialography, ultrasonography, and sialoendoscopy.

Sialography. This is an excellent imaging technique to demonstrate changes in the parenchyma (sialectasis),

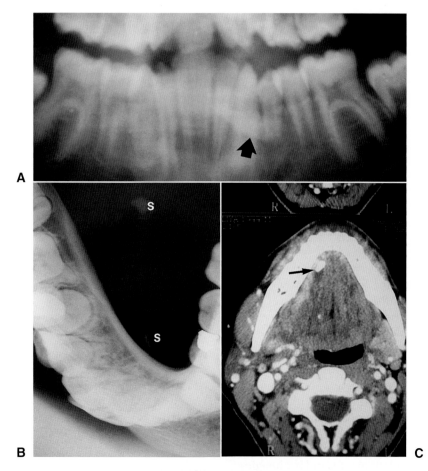

Figure 13-2

A, Panorex radiograph reveals *(black arrow)* large calculus in a 10-year-old child. **B,** Occlusal radiograph of 10-year-old boy demonstrating two sialoliths *(S)* in the anterior and middle third of Wharton's duct. **C,** CT scan demonstrating calculus *(arrow)* in the anterior part of the right Wharton's duct.

and small strictures and dilations in the main and secondary ducts. As noted for the submandibular gland, discomfort during the dye injection is a limiting factor. Topical anesthesia and lidocaine 2% lavage may be used, but in young children the procedure requires general anesthesia (Figure 13-3).

Ultrasonography. Ultrasonography is useful to demonstrate parenchymal changes such as sialectasis and morphologic alterations of the parotid duct. The same advantages for ultrasonography noted in the submandibular gland apply for the parotid (Figure 13-4).

Laboratory Data

Laboratory studies are helpful in the diagnosis of viral and bacterial infections, as well as noninfectious inflammatory disorders. Complete blood count with differen-

tial white blood cell count is helpful to distinguish viral from bacterial infection. In the former there will often be lymphocytosis, whereas in the latter leukocytosis is seen. Serum amylase and serum antibody titers are helpful in the acute phase of mumps. Secretions or drainage from the salivary ducts should be sampled for Gram stain and sent for anaerobic and aerobic culture and sensitivity testing. This is especially helpful during the acute stages of sialadenitis. As in adults, *Staphylococcus aureus* is the most common pathogen isolated from the parotid gland, and *Streptococcus viridans* from the submandibular gland.

SIALOENDOSCOPY

Sialoendoscopy is a novel technique that has added a significant new dimension to the surgeon's armamen-

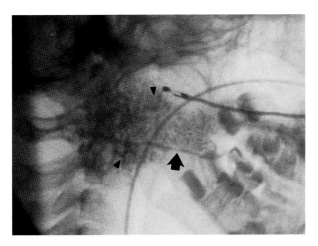

Figure 13-3

Sialography using a constant fluoroscopy technique under general anesthesia demonstrating the ductal system of the right parotid gland of a 7-year-old child with recurrent acute parotitis. Note presence of a stricture in the middle of Stensen's duct *(arrow)* and multiple sialectasis *(arrowheads)*.

tarium for diagnosis and management of inflammatory salivary disease. Obstructive sialadenitis, with or without sialolithiasis, represents the most common inflammatory disorder of the major salivary glands. The diagnosis and treatment of this problem traditionally has been hampered by the limitations of standard imaging techniques. Satisfactory management depends on the surgeon's ability to reach a precise anatomic diagnosis and, in the case of sialoliths, to locate accurately the obstruction.

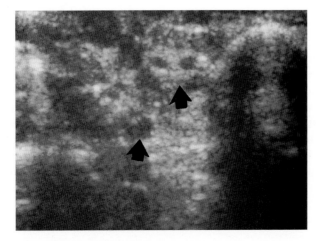

Figure 13-4

Ultrasonograph of parotid gland affected with recurrent acute parotitis. Note the demonstration of multiple areas of sialectasis *(arrows)*.

In the past, there were two options for treatment: (1) intraoral removal of stones from Wharton's or Stensen's ducts when accessible from the mouth or (2) excision of the gland when the stone was not accessible or when there was obstruction without identification of a stone. Sialoendoscopy has not only improved the diagnosis of intraductal obstructions, but has also provided a minimally invasive surgical treatment to successfully manage stones or anatomic abnormalities (e.g., strictures) not accessible by standard intraoral techniques.[5-9]

History

Konigsberger,[10] in 1990, was the first to introduce a mini flexible endoscope combined with an intracorporeal lithotripter for fragmentation of calculi. Katz,[11] in 1991, published his technique. He introduced a mini-flexible endoscope into the ductal system of the major salivary glands. He used a 0.8-mm flexible endoscope for diagnosis and extraction of calculi with a Dormia basket using a blind technique.

In 1994, Nahlieli[5] described the use of a mini rigid endoscope for diagnosis and treatment of salivary gland obstruction. Intermediate-term and long-term experiences with this technique were reported subsequently.[7-9] Marchal et al.[12] reported a similar experience with sialoendoscopic techniques in 2000.

Instrumentation

The recommended endoscope is 1 mm in diameter (100 mm in length) with two channels: an exploration unit with an outer sleeve of 1.3 mm and a surgical unit with a sleeve of 2.3 mm by 1.3 mm (Karl Storz, GmbH, Germany). This unit has three channels for introducing the scope, instruments, and irrigation (Figure 13-5). The surgical instruments must have a diameter of 3 Fr (1 mm) or less.

Useful tools include grasping forceps, basket, grasper, and balloonlike Fogarty or Sialoballoon catheter (Sialotechnology, Israel), biopsy forceps, intracorporeal electrohydraulic lithotripter probes, and erbium-YAG and holmium-YAG laser probes. It is best to work under direct vision, but occasionally in children it is necessary to work in a semi-blind manner because of size constraints of the duct. In this case, the obstruction is identified with the endoscope, and then the telescope is removed to make room for the working instrument. In the near future there will be a 1 mm surgical unit that will include both the endoscope of 0.5 mm and a surgical port.

Indications

1. To remove stones in the posterior portion of Wharton's duct, where proximity to the lingual

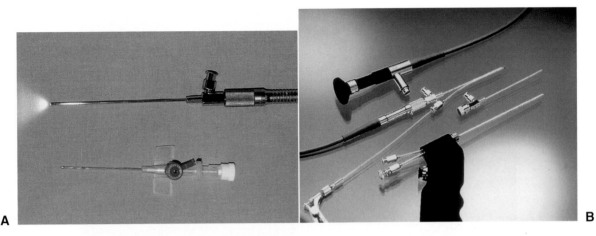

Figure 13-5
A, Sialoendoscopic exploration unit (1.3 mm with irrigation port). **B,** Nahlieli Sialoendoscope system. (Karl Storz, Germany.)

nerve makes the conventional intraoral approach hazardous
2. To remove stones in Stensen's duct posterior to its sigmoid bend around the masseter muscle
3. To screen the ductal system to rule out any residual calculi after sialolithotomy in either the submandibular or parotid ducts
4. To explore and dilate the duct when there is evidence of ductal dilation or stenosis on sialography or ultrasonography
5. To explore the ductal system when there are recurrent episodes of major salivary gland swelling without obvious cause

Technique

In children, the procedure is done under general anesthesia. There are four possible techniques for introducing the endoscope into the ductal lumen:
1. The endoscope can be introduced into the natural orifice after dilation with a lacrimal duct probe.
2. The papillotomy procedure is performed with a carbon dioxide laser immediately posterior to the orifice of the duct, thus enlarging the opening.
3. A ductal cutdown involves surgical dissection and exposure of the anterior portion of the duct using loop magnification. The duct is then incised longitudinally to allow the intraluminal insertion of the endoscope. If there are any difficulties in introducing the endoscope in the anterior part (e.g., stricture, too narrow ductal lumen), it may be necessary to expose the duct

more posteriorly to arrive at a location where the diameter will accommodate the endoscope.
4. Via a sialolithotomy opening, the endoscope can be inserted through the same opening in the duct from which the stone was extracted.

Irrigation

Irrigation is crucial in every endoscopy procedure. The cavity must be filled with fluid to allow free movement of the instrument, and the area needs to be lavaged to permit good visualization. Isotonic saline is the fluid of choice. An intravenous bag containing isotonic saline is connected to the irrigation port and the endoscope is moved forward, accompanied by a gentle flow of saline. Four milliliters of 2% lidocaine is injected through this port, resulting in the anesthesia of the entire ductal system.

Sialolithotomy

When a sialolith is encountered, its diameter is estimated using the caliber of the endoscope as a reference. The sialolith is removed by one or a combination of the following techniques:
1. Removal in one piece with a mini grasper forceps, basket, grasper, balloon (Figure 13-6)
2. Crushing the calculus with forceps and then removing the pieces using irrigation
3. Fragmentation with Er-YAG or holmium-YAG laser lithotriptor or intracorporeal lithotripter (Calcutript, Karl Storz, GmbH, Germany) (Figure 13-7)

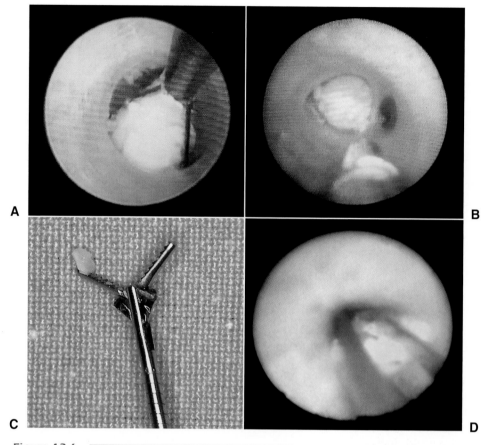

Figure 13-6
A, Grasper removal of stone from the submandibular hilum. **B,** Miniforceps grasper removal of stone from submandibular hilum. **C,** The sialolith on the prong of the miniforceps grasper after its removal. **D,** Basket retrieval of sialolith from Stensen's duct.

4. Combined lithotripsy plus basket plus grasper forceps

The first choice is to remove the calculus in one piece. If this fails, the second choice is crushing, and the last choice would be intracorporeal lithotripsy. Occasionally, particularly in cases in which lithotripsy has been used or multiple sialoliths were encountered, it has been necessary to perform a second sialoendoscopy to clear the involved gland of all obstructions. In cases of chronic sialadenitis without sialolithiasis, copious lavage with isotonic saline is used as a therapeutic measure.

Choosing the Appropriate Instrument. A calculus that can be bypassed usually is best handled with the basket. When the calculus cannot be bypassed due to the size of the duct, it can be handled with a grasper forceps or grasper. The grasper forceps is well controlled and the stone can be held and maneuvered easily by this instrument. Lithotripter probes are used to fragment the calculus when removal by the other instruments has failed. Balloons are good tools, espe-cially for strictures, but also for soft small calculi. Biopsy forceps are used for polyps.

Postoperative Management

Following endoscopy, a temporary polymeric stent (Sialotechnology, Israel) in the diameter of the inner part of the duct is introduced into the duct and kept in place (Figure 13-8).

Ideally, a 2-week period of retention of the stent is desirable. Its purpose is to prevent obstruction of the ductal lumen from postoperative edema and to allow any particles of calculus to be washed out by the saliva. The stent may also reduce the possibility of stenosis. Ductal marsupialization, consisting of suturing the incised ductal margins to the overlying incised mucosal margins, can act as a supplement to provide added assurance of retaining the ductal opening. All patients are treated postoperatively with age-appropriate doses of amoxicillin (see Table 12-1).

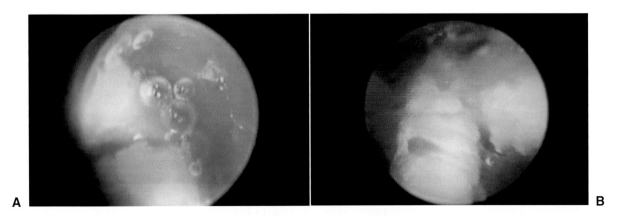

Figure 13-7

A, Intracorporeal lithotripsy procedure. Note the crack in the stone. **B,** Multiple fragments of same stone on completion of procedure.

In conclusion, sialoendoscopy is a promising new minimally invasive method for use in diagnosis and management of sialolithiasis and sialadenitis. The only absolute contraindication to this technique is the presence of acute sialadenitis.

PATHOLOGY AND TREATMENT
Viral Infections

Mumps (Viral Parotitis). Before the widespread use of vaccination, mumps (paramyxovirus) was the most common salivary gland disease in children. Mumps-measles-rubella vaccination programs have reduced the frequency of mumps by 90% in the United States. The incubation period is between 14 and 21 days, and the clinical symptoms are enlargement of the major salivary glands, especially the parotid glands, with pain and tenderness, fever, malaise, chills, and sore throat. The parotid swelling can be unilateral or bilateral. Up to 40% of the cases are asymptomatic.[13] Mumps can be distinguished from other forms of parotid inflammation by the clinical picture and by laboratory tests. There is absence of neutrophil leukocytosis and presence of lymphocytosis, and elevation of serum amylase levels. The enzyme-linked immunosorbent assay (ELISA) is the usual test for viral antigen.

Complement fixation is used for quantification of the antibody responses to the S and V antigenic components. Antibodies to the S antigen usually reach a peak within a week from the onset of symptoms; complement fixation antibodies to the V component reach a peak after 2 to 3 weeks and slowly decline but stay at low levels for years.

The virus is transmitted by infected salivary secretions and urine. Complications include pancreatitis, orchitis,

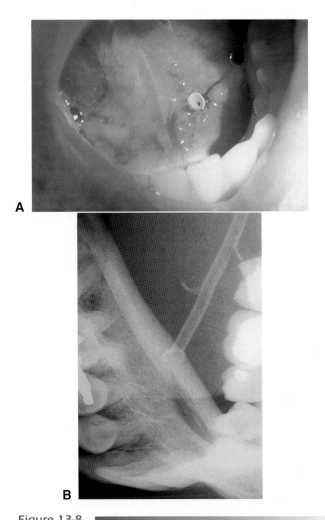

Figure 13-8

A, The polymeric stent is inside the duct. **B,** Occlusal radiograph of the same stent. Note flaps holding stent in place.

mumps, and meningitis (meningoencephalitis). Orchitis occurs with mumps in approximately 20% of adults.

Mumps resolves spontaneously after 5 to 10 days. There is no specific treatment, but prevention of dehydration and symptomatic relief of pain and fever is necessary.

Other Causes of Viral Infections. Parotitis caused by other viruses rarely occurs in children.[13] Coxsackie, enteric cytopathic human orphan (ECHO) virus, cytomegalovirus, Epstein-Barr virus, influenza A, parainfluenza 1 and 3, and human immunodeficiency virus (HIV) have been reported.[14] In the case of HIV-positive children, xerostomia, lymphadenopathy, and lymphoepithelial cysts also occur.

Recurrent Acute Parotitis (Juvenile Recurrent Parotitis). Recurrent acute parotitis (RAP) is the second most common salivary gland disease in children after mumps. In young children it is difficult to differentiate between the two. RAP is defined as *recurrent, nonobstructive, nonsuppurative parotid inflammation*. The condition is characterized by swelling of the parotid gland, usually accompanied by pain and systemic symptoms such as fever and malaise.

It is commonly unilateral, but bilateral exacerbation can occur. When the symptoms are bilateral, they are usually more prominent on one side. Swelling appears suddenly over a period of a few hours and may be accompanied by xerostomia. The disease can start at any age between 3 months and 16 years, with a peak after 5 to 7 years. Exacerbation lasts for several days, and the episodes may recur over many years with variable frequency. RAP is self-limiting, and after puberty the symptoms usually subside and the disease may resolve completely. However, the morbidity during the years of active disease can be significant, with multiple recurrences, days lost from school, and the requirement for antibiotics and supportive therapy.

Histopathologic evaluation of the diseased gland reveals a lymphocytic infiltrate that tends to form lymphoid follicles and small ductal dilations. These intraductal cystlike dilations are demonstrated clearly by sialography and are called sialectasis or sialectasia. Sialectasis is usually present in the asymptomatic contralateral gland, as well.[15] These sialographic changes remain unaltered in adult life. Ultrasonographic examinations demonstrate multiple small hypoechogenic areas and punctate calcifications, corresponding to the sialectasis demonstrated by sialography. Results of routine laboratory tests are normal.[15] Autoimmune antibody titers are negative.[15]

A variety of etiologic factors have been considered for RAP: congenital ductal malformations, hereditary and genetic factors,[16] viral or bacterial infection, allergy, and local manifestation of an autoimmune disease. The self-limiting nature of the disease, the reports of a male predilection, and the absence of immunoglobulin abnormalities indicate that RAP is probably not an autoimmune disease. Nevertheless, primary Sjögren's syndrome must be considered when recurrent parotitis is assessed, despite the rarity of this condition.[17]

Ericson et al.[15] found no evidence to support the suggestion that RAP is an allergic condition. Reid et al.[16] found a pattern consistent with autosomal dominant inheritance with incomplete penetrance suggesting that, at least in some cases, genetic factors are involved. One particularly attractive explanation for the pathogenesis of RAP is retrograde infection. This might occur as a result of upper respiratory infection when a child typically becomes dehydrated. This would produce a decrease in salivary secretion and decreased salivary flow in the parotid gland. Increased viscosity of the mucoid saliva in combination with decreased flow might result in bacterial infection.[19]

Cohen et al.[18] demonstrated a deficiency in salivary (secretory) immunoglobulin A (IgA) in patients who suffer from recurrent parotitis. This deficiency did not relate necessarily to low serum IgA concentrations. They reported that sialectasis appears to be secondary to recurrent infections but may also occur rarely in early, well-treated, recurrent parotitis. Kaban et al.[2] reported that sialectasis occurred in both affected and contralateral totally asymptomatic parotid glands.

The results reported by Ericson strongly indicate that sialectasis in patients with RAP precedes the infection, and that these areas constitute a site of decreased resistance.[15] Congenital ectasia and retrograde infection from the mouth are reasonable explanations of the pathogenesis of RAP. Treatment of the acute phase of RAP is observation, supportive care, and antibiotic therapy. Cohen et al.[18] recommend low-dose penicillin treatment or prophylactic administration early in an attack, when a deficiency in salivary IgA is observed. Antibiotic treatment prevents further damage to the glandular parenchyma. Kaban et al. reported that patients with RAP respond to penicillin therapy and hydration.

Between episodes a regimen of massage, encouragement of fluid intake, application of heat, use of chewing gum or sour candy, and sialogogues have been advocated. Intermittent duct probing and dilation, as well as over-filling of the gland during sialography, have also been recommended.[22] Other treatment methods mentioned in the literature include duct ligation to produce glandular atrophy, parotidectomy, and tympanic neurectomy.[20]

Nahlieli et al.[21] reported on 26 children with symptomatic recurrent acute parotitis, which they called juvenile recurrent parotitis (JRP), treated by endoscopic surgery. There were 14 males and 12 females with a mean age of 7 years (range, 2.5 to 13 years). The mean age at the time of initial symptoms was 3.8 years. The patients all had at least two episodes of infection during a 12-month period. A predominant gland was usually affected, although the contralateral gland was affected in 19 of 26 patients. One of the patients who was referred from another center after left superficial parotidectomy, due to JRP, developed contralateral gland swelling a short time after surgery (Figure 13-9).

All of the procedures were performed bilaterally and under general anesthesia.[21] The endoscope was used to examine the main duct and secondary ducts, as possible. Through the endoscope, the gland was lavaged thoroughly with 60 milliliters of normal saline. The duct system was dilated with saline under pressure and, when necessary, with a balloon. Follow-ing the lavage and the dilation, hydrocortisone 100 mg was injected into the duct system. All the patients were treated with amoxicillin-clavulanic acid or clindamycin for 1 week, along with frequent massage of the glands.

The following clinical, imaging, and endoscopic findings were encountered in this research (Figures 13-10 to 13-12):

1. Wide orifice of Stensen's duct
2. Sialectasis, strictures, and kinks in the main and secondary ducts
3. White appearance of the main duct, without the natural proliferation of blood vessels as seen in a healthy gland.

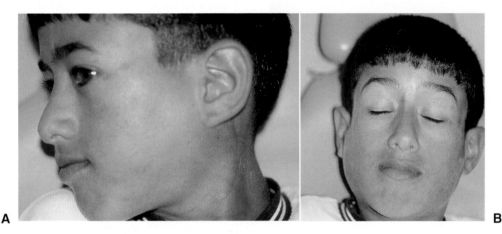

Figure 13-9

A, A 12-year-old child with recurrent acute parotitis 6 months after left superficial parotidectomy. **B,** Note swelling of contralateral right parotid gland.

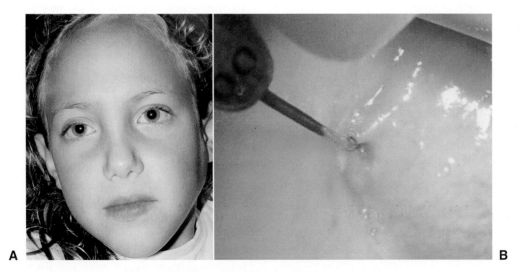

Figure 13-10

A, A 7-year-old girl suffering from recurrent acute parotitis. Note swelling of her left preauricular region. **B,** Close-up of Stensen's duct of a 7-year-old child; lacrimal probe is inside the duct. Note the wide opening of the orifice.

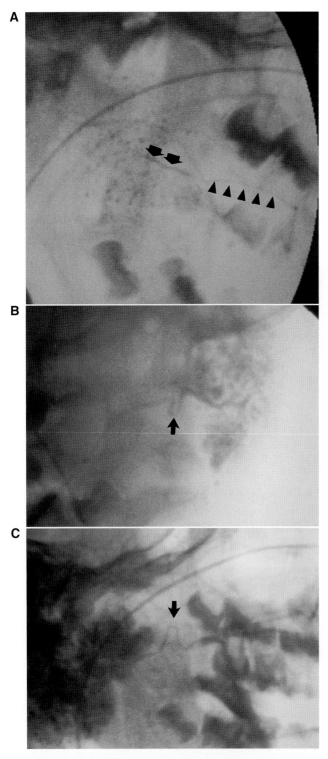

Figure 13-11

A, Sialogram of 6-year-old boy suffering from recurrent acute parotitis. Note multiple sialectasis, dilation of the duct *(two black arrows)*, and the stricture *(small arrowheads)*. **B** and **C,** Demonstration of kinks in patient with recurrent acute parotitis *(arrow)*.

These findings support the theory that ductal malformation is responsible for the formation of JRP.

After the endoscopic procedure, 24 of the 26 patients remained symptom free during the follow-up period of 36 months. During the first few hours following the procedure, bilateral swelling of the parotid glands was noticed due to the irrigation (Figure 13-13). The swelling resolved spontaneously within 12 hours after the procedure.

In conclusion, a variety of factors have been cited as contributing to RAP (JRP); most of these factors have been excluded in recent studies. The possibility of ductal malformation as the main cause for RAP (JRP) has been cited in a recent paper. The possibility of investigating and treating the affected gland endoscopically would allow a conservative and safe way to treat this entity.

Obstructive Sialadenitis. Sialolithiasis is a well-known entity, with about 1% of the population having suffered from this disease at one time or another.[23] In children, salivary gland calculi are uncommon. A review of the English literature revealed sporadic cases of sialolithiasis of the submandibular gland in children ages 3 weeks to 15 years.[24-33] According to the literature, it is assumed that 3% of all sialolithiasis cases are in children.[34]

Nahlieli et al.,[3] in 2000, reported on 15 children with symptomatic salivary gland obstructive disease. Of the children included in the study, 13 patients were male (87%) and 2 (13%) were female. The ages of the patients ranged between 5 and 14 years (mean, 8 years). Follow-up was performed up to 36 months postoperatively. Detection of the sialoliths was aided by routine radiography—panoramic, occlusal, occlusal oblique, and ultrasonographic. For three cases with parotid gland pathology, posteroanterior radiographs were added. Sialography was reserved only for cooperative patients. In this series, sialoendoscopy was performed on all patients, nine under general anesthesia and six under local anesthesia. Three cases occurred in the parotid and 12 in the submandibular duct.[3]

Three cases of parotid sialolithiasis were detected in Stensen's duct. Submandibular sialolithiasis occurred in the remaining 12 cases. Two were associated with foreign bodies, one with a hair follicle (Figure 13-14), one with a particle of plant *(Phytobezoar)*, and one with intraductal evagination (Figure 13-15). Thirteen calculi (from 12 patients) were found in Wharton's duct, eight of them located in the anterior third of the duct, three in the middle third, and two in the hilar region. In 10 of the 15 cases, the calculi were visible as radiopaque objects on radiographic film. In the other five cases we could not perform precise intraoral radiographs due to the young age of the patients, but the calculus could be diagnosed clinically in the anterior part of the duct (Figure 13-16). During the follow-up period, between 6 to 36 months, there were no complications and there was no recurrence of the disease.

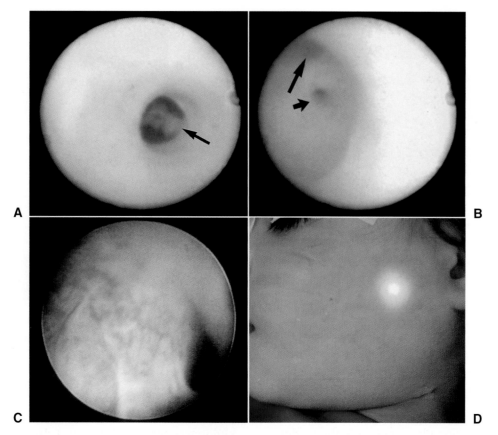

Figure 13-12

A, Endoscopic appearance of the duct of a 5-year-old child diagnosed with recurrent acute parotitis. Note the white avascular appearance of the duct and a cloudy plaque *(arrow)*. **B,** Endoscopic appearance of the same child near the hilum of the gland *(arrows)*. **C,** Endoscopic view of normal appearance of Stensen's duct mucosa. **D,** Intraoperative figure demonstrating endoscope inside the gland. Note transillumination effect. It helps to locate the site of the endoscope tip.

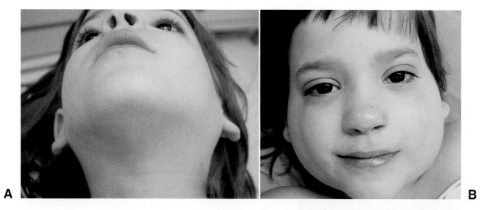

Figure 13-13

A, A 6-year-old girl with recurrent acute parotitis. Note bilateral swelling. This girl suffered 30 attacks of swelling episodes during 1 year. **B,** Immediately after endoscopic exploration and lavage with bilateral swelling.

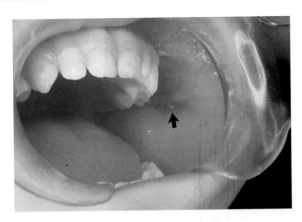

Figure 13-14
A 5-year-old child with a hair follicle in the left Stensen's duct (*arrow*).

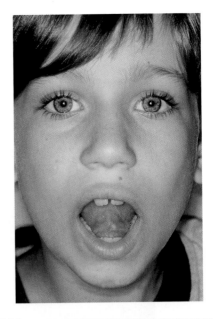

Figure 13-16
Calculus in orifice of Wharton's duct in a 7-year-old child.

Sialolithiasis is a relatively common condition in adults but rarely is found in children. Nevertheless, it must be included in the differential diagnosis of facial swelling and intermittent pain in youngsters. The main complaint is unilateral swelling. Historically, authors suspected that congenital anomalies and foreign bodies were the etiologic factors for most cases of sialolithiasis.[3,35] Endoscopic findings support this hypothesis. Finally, another striking phenomenon is the predominance of males in the reported series of sialolithiasis.[24-26] There is no current explanation for this.

In conclusion, pediatric sialolithiasis is a well-known but uncommon problem. Sialoendoscopy is a promising new technique for its management. The procedure is minimally invasive, and preliminary results suggest that excision of the gland can be avoided in most cases.

Acute Suppurative Parotitis. Acute suppurative parotitis is a rare entity. It usually occurs in very young children or infants who are systemically ill or immunosuppressed. As with acute suppurative parotitis of adults, dehydration in a patient with debilitating illness is the primary etiology. Kaban et al.[2] have identified specific predisposing factors: sepsis, surgery, glomerulonephritis, chemotherapy, and immunosuppression. HIV-infected patients are another group particularly at risk.[36]

A closely related entity is neonatal suppurative parotitis. This is a very rare condition, with only 111 cases reported in the literature. Known risk factors are premature birth, malnutrition, and dehydration.[37] Physical examination reveals tender swelling involving both the preauricular and postauricular regions and extending to the mandibular angle. The skin is erythematous and tender. Stensen's papilla is usually enlarged, and purulent material often can be expressed from the duct spontaneously or after massaging the gland. *Staphylococcus aureus* is the most common organism cultured from the gland, but in rare cases *Escherichia coli* and *Pseudomonas* spp. have been isolated. The treatment is aggressive management of the associated illness, rehydration, and antibiotic therapy.

Submandibular Sialadenitis. Submandibular sialadenitis without obstruction of the gland is a very rare condition in childhood. Most of the submandibular infections in children are caused and associated with obstruction of Wharton's duct.[35] Nonobstructive inflammatory disease is a diagnosis of exclusion using all the diagnostic modalities discussed previously.

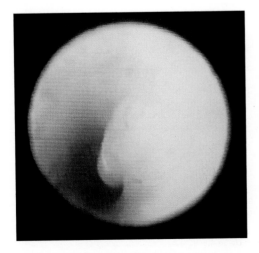

Figure 13-15
Endoscopic view after retrieval of sialolith. Note the formation of intraductal evagination.

Management in the acute phase is hydration and antibiotics (penicillin). The most common causative organism is *Streptococcus viridans*. Care must be taken not to confuse submandibular gland infections with submandibular space infection or lymphadenitis of dental origin.

Rare Conditions That Produce Salivary Gland Swelling. Although rare, the following specific conditions may cause salivary gland infection and swelling or mimic infection in children: pneumoparotid, juvenile Sjögren's syndrome, atypical mycobacteria, tuberculosis, actinomycosis, acquired immunodeficiency syndrome, hemangioma, lymphangioma, and vascular malformation.

Pneumoparotid. This is a rare condition of the parotid gland in which it is inflated with air as a result of positive air pressure inside the mouth (up to 150 mm Hg). Physical examination reveals parotid enlargement, usually unilateral but also bilateral. Palpation of the affected gland produces crepitus.[38,39] The best imaging technique is CT scan, which will show air in the parotid gland, Stensen's duct and, occasionally, in the surrounding tissue (Figure 13-17). Pneumoparotid can be classified as occupational (glassblowers and players of wind instruments like trumpets) or nonoccupational. Nonoccupational pneumoparotid is self-induced. In childhood most of the cases are self-induced but a few are accidental, such as from blowing up a balloon, aggressive blowing of the nose, inflating a bicycle tire inner tube without a pump, or inveterate gum chewing.

The management of pneumoparotid depends on its etiology. Management of accidental cases requires prophylactic antibiotics to prevent secondary infection. Clindamycin is the drug of choice. Recurrent self-induced pneumoparotid cases require psychological evaluation and management. Other therapeutic options include the Wilkie antidrooling approach to divert the ductal orifice.

Juvenile Sjögren's Syndrome. Sjögren's syndrome in childhood is very rare and only a few cases have been described in the literature.[17,40,41] The syndrome should be considered in the differential diagnosis of children with recurrent parotitis, keratoconjunctivitis sicca, or early dental caries associated with xerostomia.

Atypical Mycobacteria. Atypical mycobacterial infections have been identified as an important cause of infection in the head and neck in children.[42] The parotid and submandibular gland can be affected, as can the neighboring lymph nodes. The clinical appearance is swelling of the affected gland and sometimes spontaneous drainage. Diagnosis relies upon culture, histology, chest radiography, and purified protein derivative. Long-term antibiotic therapy with azithromycin and ciprofloxacin is needed.

Tuberculosis. Tuberculosis of the salivary gland in children can develop primarily or secondary to pul-

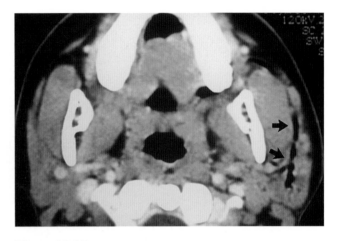

Figure 13-17
CT scan of 12-year-old girl with self-induced bilateral pneumoparotid. Arrows on left side indicate air inside Stensen's duct and parenchyma.

monary tuberculosis.[41,43] The parotid gland is affected more often than the submandibular gland and the clinical picture is a firm swelling, sometimes with a draining fistula. Diagnostic tests of suspected cases include chest radiograph, purified protein derivative skin test, and acid-fast staining from drainage material and from tissue. It should be remembered that calcification of infected lymph nodes and salivary tissue can be identified in patients with tuberculosis. The calcified tissue can mimic sialoliths (Figure 13-18).

Actinomycosis. Actinomycotic infections can affect the salivary glands; 10% of orofacial infections are in the salivary glands.[41] Actinomycosis can be acute or chronic and the definitive diagnosis is made by cultures.

Acquired Immunodeficiency Syndrome. Children infected with HIV develop salivary gland enlargement in 18% of cases.[44] The prognosis of children with salivary gland enlargement is poor. The life expectancy of this group is 5.4 years.[44]

Hemangioma, Lymphangioma, Vascular Malformation. These are discussed in Chapters 14 and 17.

CONCLUSION

Inflammatory disorders in childhood are far more common than neoplastic salivary gland pathology. The most common inflammatory condition is mumps, followed by recurrent acute parotitis and then obstructive sialadenitis. Acute suppurative parotitis and submandibular sialadenitis (without obstruction) are very rare conditions in children.

Infections of the salivary glands in children, without stone obstruction, occur most frequently in the parotid glands. Calculi are far more common in the submandibular glands. Another striking feature is the predominance

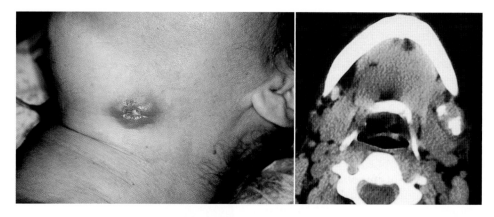

Figure 13-18

Tuberculosis of the left submandibular gland appearing as sialolithiasis. **A,** Draining fistula from the left submandibular gland. **B,** CT scan demonstrating calcification of the gland.

of sialolithiasis and RAP in boys. Sialoendoscopy is a promising new technique for minimally invasive access, diagnosis, and management of this group of salivary gland diseases.

REFERENCES

1. Welch KJ, Trump DS: The salivary glands. In Mustard WT, Ravitch MM, Snyder WH Jr, et al, editors: *Pediatric surgery,* Chicago, 1969, Year Book.
2. Kaban LB, Mulliken JB, Murray JE: Sialadenitis in childhood, *Am J Surg* 135:570-576, 1978.
3. Nahlieli O, Eliav E, Hasson O, et al: Pediatric sialolithiasis, *Oral Surg Oral Med Oral Pathol* 90:709-712, 2000.
4. Koischwitz D, Gritzmann N: Ultrasound of the neck, *Radiol Clin North Am* 38:1029-1045, 2000.
5. Nahlieli O, Neder A, Baruchin AM: Salivary gland endoscopy: a new technique for diagnosis and treatment of sialolithiasis, *J Oral Maxillofac Surg* 52:1240-1242, 1994.
6. Nahlieli O, Baruchin AM: Sialoendoscopy—three years experience as a diagnostic and treatment modality, *J Oral Maxillofac Surg* 55:912-918, 1997.
7. Nahlieli O, Baruchin AM: Endoscopic technique for the diagnosis and treatment of obstructive salivary gland diseases, *J Oral Maxillofac Surg* 57:1394-1401, 1999.
8. Nahlieli O, Baruchin AM: Long-term experience with endoscopic diagnosis and treatment of salivary gland inflammatory diseases, *Laryngoscope* 110:988-994, 2000.
9. Nahlieli O: Development and application of microsalivary gland endoscopy. In MacGurk M, Renehan A, editors: *Controversies in the management of salivary gland disease,* Oxford, 2001, Oxford University Press.
10. Konigsberger R, Feyh J, Goetz A, et al: Endoscopic controlled laser lithotripsy in the treatment of sialolithiasis, *Laryngorhinootologie* 69:322-323, 1990.
11. Katz PH: Endoscopie des glands salivires [Endoscopy of the salivary glands], *Ann Radiol (Paris)* 34:110-113, 1991.
12. Marchal F, Becker M, Dulguerov P, Lehmann W: Interventional sialendoscopy, *Laryngoscope* 110:318-320, 2000.
13. McQuone SJ: Acute viral and bacterial infection of the salivary glands, *Otolaryngol Clin North Am* 32:793-811, 1999.
14. Goldberg MH: Infections of the salivary glands. In Topazian RG, Goldberg MH, editors: *Oral and maxillofacial infections,* ed 3, Philadelphia, 1994, WB Saunders.
15. Ericson S, Zetterlund B, Ohman J: Recurrent parotitis and sialectasis in childhood. Clinical, radiologic, immunologic, bacteriologic and histologic study, *Ann Otol Rhinol Laryngol* 100:527-535, 1991.
16. Reid E, Douglas F, Crow Y, et al: Autosomal dominant juvenile recurrent parotitis, *J Med Genet* 35:417-419, 1998.
17. Hearth-Holmes M, Baethge BA, Abreo F, Wolf RE: Autoimmune exocrinopathy presenting as recurrent parotitis of childhood, *Arch Otolaryngol Head Neck Surg* 119:347-349, 1993.
18. Cohen HA, Gross S, Nussinovitch M, et al: Recurrent parotitis, *Arch Dis Child* 67:1036-1037, 1992.
19. Chitre VV, Premchandra DJ: Recurrent parotitis, *Arch Dis Child* 77:359-363, 1997.
20. Mulcahy D, Isaacs D: Recurrent parotitis, *Arch Dis Child* 68(1):151, 1993.
21. Nahlieli O, Shacham R, Shlesinger M, Eliav E: Juvenile recurrent parotitis: a new method of diagnosis and treatment, *Pediatrics,* 2003.
22. Galili D, Marmary Y: Juvenile recurrent parotitis: clinicoradiological follow-up study and the beneficial effect of sialography, *Oral Surg Oral Med Oral Pathol* 61(6):550-556, 1986.
23. Rauch S, Gorlin RJ: Diseases of the salivary glands. In Gorlin RJ, Goldman HM, editors: *Thoma's oral pathology,* ed 6. St Louis, 1970, Mosby.
24. Myer C, Cotton RT: Salivary gland diseases in children. A review. Part 1. Acquired non-inflammatory disease, *Clin Pediatr* 25:314-322, 1986.
25. Woolley AL: Salivary gland diseases in children, *Curr Opin Otolaryngol Head Neck Surg* 335, 1964.
26. Bodner L, Fliss DM: Parotid and sub-mandibular calculi in children, *J Pediatr* 31:35-37, 1995.
27. Steiner M, Gould AL, Kushner GM, et al: Sialolithiasis of the submandibular gland in an 8-year-old child, *Oral Surg Oral Med Oral Pathol* 83:188, 1997.
28. Suuigura N, Kubo I, Negoro M, et al: A case of sialolithiasis in a two-year-old girl, *Shoni Shikagaku Zasshi* 28:741-746, 1990.
29. Zou ZJ, Wang SL, Zhu JR, et al: Chronic obstructive parotitis. Report of ninety-two cases, *Oral Surg Oral Med Oral Pathol* 73:434-440, 1992.
30. McCullom C, Lee CY, Blaustein DI: Sialolithiasis in an 8-year-old child: case report, *Pediatr Dent* 13:231-233, 1991.
31. Reuther J, Hausamen JE: Submaxillary salivary calculus in children, *Klin Padiatr* 188:285-288, 1976.
32. Di Felice R, Lombardi T: Submandibular sialolithiasis with concurrent sialoadenitis in a child, *J Clin Pediatr Dent* 20:57-59, 1995.

33. Shinohara Y, Hiromatsu T, Nagata Y, et al: Sialolithiasis in children: report of four cases, *Dentomaxillofac Radiol* 25:48-50, 1996.

34. Lustman J, Regev E, Melamed Y: Sialolithiasis: a survey on 245 patients and a review of the literature, *J Oral Maxillofac Surg* 19:135-138, 1990.

35. Kaban LB: Salivary gland disease. In Kaban LB, editor: *Pediatric oral and maxillofacial surgery,* Philadelphia, 1990, WB Saunders.

36. Chaloryoo S, Chotpitayasunondh T, Chiengmai PN: AIDS in ENT in children, *Int J Pediatr Otorhinolaryngol* 10:103-107, 1998.

37. Sabatino G, Verrotti A, de Martino M, et al: Neonatal suppurative parotitis: a study of five cases, *Eur J Pediatr* 158:312-314, 1999.

38. Martin-Granzio R, Herrera M, Gacia-Gonzalez D, Mas A: Pneumoparotid in childhood: report of two cases, *J Oral Maxillofac Surg* 57:1468-1471, 1999.

39. Curtin JJ, Ridley NTF, Cumberworth VL, et al: Pneumoparotitis, *J Otolaryngol* 106:178, 1992.

40. Stiller M, Golder W, Doring E, Biedermann T: Primary and secondary Sjögren syndrome in children—a comparative study, *Clin Oral Invest* 4:176-182, 2000.

41. Rice DH: Chronic inflammatory disorders of the salivary glands, *Otolaryngol Clin North Am* 32:813-818, 1999.

42. Jervs PN, Lee JA, Bull PD: Management of non-tuberculosis mycobacterial peri-sialadenitis in children: the Sheffield otolaryngology experience, *Clin Otolaryngol* 26:243-248, 2001.

43. Mert A, Ozaras R, Bilir M, et al: Primary tuberculosis of the parotid gland, *Int J Infect Dis* 4:229-230, 2000.

44. Magalhaes MG, Bueno DF, Serra E, Goncalves R: Oral manifestation of HIV positive children, *J Clin Pediatr Dent* 25:103-106, 2001.

Salivary Gland Tumors in Children

Robert A. Ord

Salivary gland tumors are uncommon in adults. They account for approximately 3% of all head and neck tumors. Only 5% of all salivary gland tumors occur in pediatric patients,[1-3] making these lesions exceedingly rare. It is very difficult to provide precise figures for percentages of individual neoplasms at particular sites because the literature lacks uniformity. In addition, in the larger reported series, authors have defined children differently, such as less than 15 to 20 years of age or, in some reports, just including infants. Other reviews have included nonneoplastic, as well as neoplastic, lesions or have included only epithelial neoplasms excluding mesenchymal tumors. Some authors reviewed only parotid tumors or major salivary gland tumors, while at least four separate reports have used entirely or partly the same Armed Forces Institute of Pathology (AFIP) material analyzed for different years or ages.[4-7]

In general, all papers document a preponderance of lesions in the parotid gland (as in adults). Furthermore, in children there is a greater percentage of malignant epithelial tumors than is seen in adults. In infants there is a higher incidence of mesenchymal tumors. Krolls et

al.[4] reviewed 9993 salivary gland lesions, of which 430 (4.3%) occurred in children. There were 262 nonneoplastic lesions and 168 neoplasms. The tumors included 114 benign lesions, of which 60 were epithelial and 46 mesenchymal (predominantly vascular). Of the 54 malignant lesions, 35 were epithelial in origin.

Jacques et al.[5] reported on 124 patients under 15 years of age with parotid tumors: 40 (32.3%) vascular, 50 (40.3%) benign epithelial, and 34 (27.5%) malignant epithelial neoplasms. Lack and Upton[8] report 80 cases of salivary tumors in children less than 18 years of age from the Boston Children's Hospital. Of these tumors, 25 were epithelial in origin, 10 (40%) were benign, and the others were malignant. There were 55 mesenchymal tumors, of which 47 (85.4%) were vascular lesions or lymphangiomas. The largest and most recent AFIP series (Ellis et al.)[7] included 494 salivary tumors in children under the age of 17 years: 210 (42.5%) benign epithelial tumors, 212 (42.9%) malignant epithelial tumors, and 72 (15.6%) mesenchymal tumors.

This chapter reviews the diagnosis and management of mesenchymal and epithelial tumors of the salivary glands in children.

MESENCHYMAL TUMORS

Vascular Tumors: Hemangioma and Hemangioendothelioma

Vascular salivary neoplasms accounted for 8.1%,[7] 23.2%,[4] 32.3%,[8] and 35%[5] of salivary tumors in four published series. These tumors include hemangiomas and hemangioendotheliomas, and virtually all of these tumors occurred in the parotid gland. The varying percentages may simply represent different age mixes because these tumors are most common in newborns, infants, and toddlers. Bhaskar and Lilly[6] reported 25 of

27 vascular tumors in children to be in those under 5 years of age (Figure 14-1). Another explanation is that the lower incidence in more recent series reflects a trend away from operative therapy during the last 20 years.

Vascular tumors of the parotid are reported most commonly in children under age 1 year. Many are noted at or soon after birth, and they are more frequent in females. Wawro et al.[9] reported 10 cases, of which seven were present at birth and three discovered during the first year of life. Eight of the 10 tumors occurred in females. Lack and Upton[8] reported a median age of 4 months in 27 cases, of which 19 patients were females. In general, reported cases are classified as hemangioendotheliomas occurring in patients younger than 6 months and exhibiting rapid growth and aggressive behavior, or slower growing capillary or cavernous hemangiomas in older children. These lesions are probably biologically similar and represent parotid variant of the soft tissue hemangioma of infancy and childhood.[10]

Scarcella et al.[11] reported regression and involution of rapidly growing infantile hemangioendotheliomas of the parotid in two cases. Other authors have also observed these lesions to undergo proliferative and involutional phases as seen in other hemangiomas. However, parotid lesions may be associated with slower involution or scarring.[12]

Clinical findings include a soft, compressible mass with a bluish tinge. Some lesions may extend to the skin, in which case the tumor may appear to be a superficial hemangioma. Following involution, phleboliths may occur and be seen radiographically in older children (Figure 14-2). High-frequency sonography has been recommended as the initial diagnostic imaging tech-

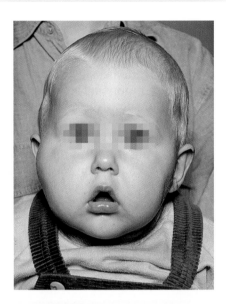

Figure 14-1

A 4-month-old infant with soft compressible swelling of the right parotid gland (hemangioendothelioma).

nique over magnetic resonance (MR) or red blood cell imaging.[13] Sonography has proven to be accurate and efficient and there is usually no need for sedation or anesthesia in uncooperative infants and young children.[13] Other authors, however, have recommended MR imaging for hemangioendothelioma of the parotid gland.[14]

Histologically, the infantile hemangioendothelioma is marked by a dominant solid endothelial component,

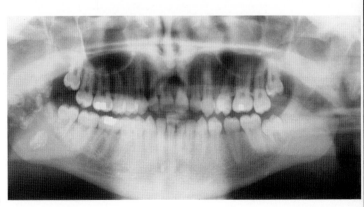

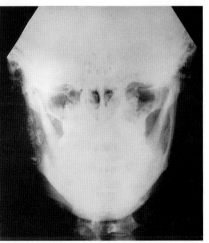

A

B

Figure 14-2

A, An 18-year-old with calcifications over the right ramus of the mandible on routine panoral radiograph to assess erupting wisdom teeth. **B,** Posteroanterior view of facial bones confirms calcified phleboliths to be in the right parotid gland.

while after 6 months of age well-formed vascular channels become increasingly prominent. These histologic findings correspond with those seen on imaging.

Management of parotid hemangioendothelioma has changed as the natural history and behavior have become better understood. Initially, radiation therapy was used successfully for rapidly growing tumors in infants.[15,16] However, risk of late secondary malignancies in irradiated children makes this treatment modality unacceptable at this time. Surgical excision was the mainstay of treatment for many years and is still sometimes necessary (Figure 14-3). However, resection of these lesions in infants and young children incurs high risk for complications. In Campbell's review of 60 cases,[17] 46 underwent resection: two infants died, nine had facial nerve

palsy, five had recurrence and were reoperated. Two of these children developed facial nerve palsy. Scarcella et al.[11] operated on three infants less than 3 months of age. One of these patients died. Two other infants who were treated by observation had complete regression of the tumors, one by 6 months and the other at 14 months of age. Most authors now recommend nonoperative treatment for infants based on the spontaneous regression of these tumors. However, large, rapidly growing tumors with potential complications such as Kasabach-Merritt syndrome[18,19] or cardiac failure[20] require treatment. In childhood hemangiomas, the efficacy of systemic steroid therapy is well documented.[12,21-23] Intralesional injections of triamcinolone have also been reported. In life-threatening lesions that do not respond

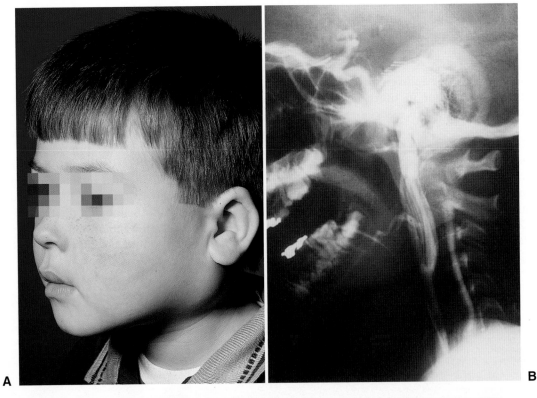

A   **B**

Figure 14-3

A, Lateral view of a 3-year-old boy with left parotid swelling, which is soft and compressible; the overlying skin has a bluish tinge. The parents are concerned about repeated swellings during upper respiratory tract infections. **B,** Doppler ultrasonography showed turbulent blood flow, and an angiogram confirmed a cavernous venous hemangioma (with probable lymphangiomatous component from the history). **C,** Diagram showing parotidectomy incision. Intraoperative photograph **(D)** and diagram **(E)** showing vascular tumor involving the posterior parotid inferior to the level of the nerve exposed by parotidectomy incision. Intraoperative diagram **(F)** and photograph **(G)** after the tumor was gently elevated and removed, preserving the nerve. **H,** Diagram after superficial parotidectomy; the facial nerve is preserved. Note in the diagram that the earlobe can be temporarily sutured to the helix. **I,** Specimen showing the size of the mixed vascular lesion and its relation to the parotid *(P)*. **J,** Closure is obtained in layers.

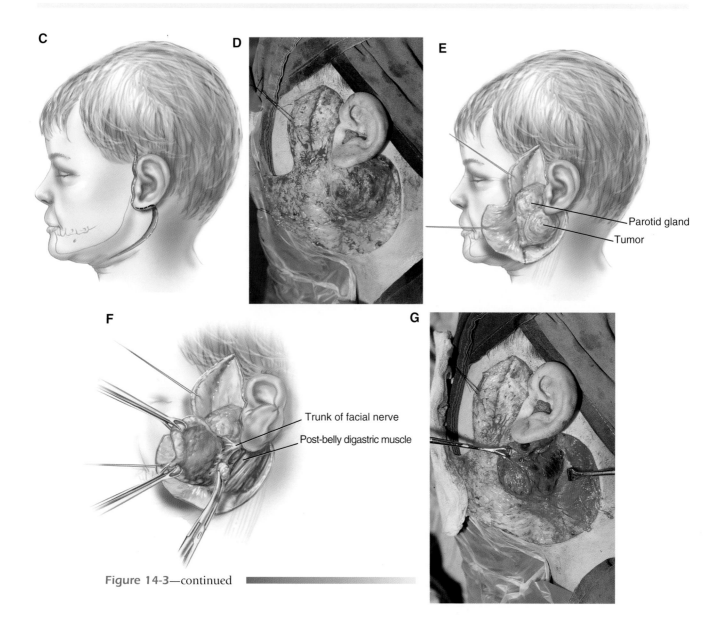

C

D

E
— Parotid gland
—Tumor

F
Trunk of facial nerve
Post-belly digastric muscle

G

Figure 14-3—continued

to steroids, interferon alfa-2a and alfa-2b have been used successfully.[24,25] However, medical therapy for parotid hemangiomas has not been as successful as for other hemangiomas.[26]

Hemangiomas and hemangioendotheliomas of the parotid in infants should be managed by observation, whenever possible, to await natural involution. When rapid growth or size dictate treatment, medical therapy as described is indicated. Surgical resection is reserved for recalcitrant lesions.

If parotidectomy is carried out in infants less than 4 months of age, it should be understood that the facial nerve is very superficial due to lack of development of the mastoid process (see Figure 14-3).

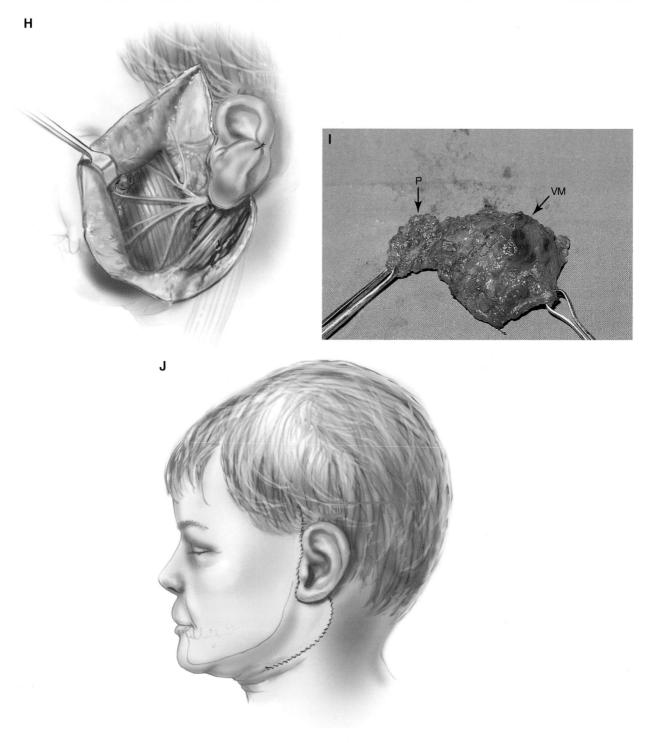

Figure 14-3—continued

Lymphatic Malformations

Lingeman[27] reported that 93% of lymphangiomas occur in the cervical region and that primary involvement of the parotid is rare. He described three varieties of lymphangioma: capillary, cavernous (both of which may be associated with neoplastic blood vessels), and cystic.

Because of the association with blood vessels, some authors have included lymphangiomas with vascular lesions. Krolls et al.[4] reported four of "39 vascular proliferations" of the parotid in children to be lymphangiomas. Ellis et al.[7] also found these neoplasms to be rare. Lymphangiomas accounted for five of 494

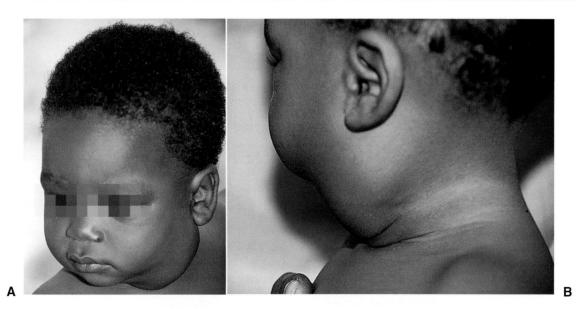

Figure 14-4
A, Lateral view of an 18-month-old infant with cystic lymphangioma of left parotid and upper neck present since birth. **B,** Posterior view.

pediatric tumors (1%). However, Lack and Upton[8] reported 19 of 80 pediatric parotid tumors to be lymphangiomas (24%). Lingeman[27] reported five cases from 8 months to 7 years and stated that these tumors are found most commonly in childhood and infancy (Figure 14-4). Lack and Upton[8] found that lymphangiomas appeared at a later age than hemangiomas, with the median age being 6 years (range, 2 months to 16 years). The authors found a 6:1 female-to-male ratio, which is similar to that found in hemangiomas. Occasionally, lymphatic malformations will increase in size rapidly during an upper respiratory tract infection.

Treatment advocated for lymphangioma (lymphatic malformation) has included observation, injection of sclerosing agents, and conservative surgery. Sclerosing agents are most successful in those lesions that have large cystic "lakes." However, injection of sclerosant agents may be hazardous close to the facial nerve. Therefore, in cases of infiltrative malformations resection is preferred.

Surgical excision with preservation of the facial nerve usually will not remove completely the abnormal lymphatic channels and microcysts. However, this "debulking" procedure appears clinically effective. The carbon dioxide laser can be a useful adjunct to surgery for lymphangiomas.

Neural Tumors

Neural tumors of the parotid may be divided into neurilemmomas, neurofibromas, and manifestations of neurofibromatosis (Figure 14-5). Ellis et al.[7] reported 10 benign neural tumors in a series of 494 pediatric parotid neoplasms (2%). There were three neurilemmomas and seven neurofibromas. They also reported two malignant neurilemmomas in this series. Lack and Upton[8] reported that six patients of 80 with parotid tumors (7.5%) had neural tumors, four of which involved the parotid, one the submandibular, and one the sublingual gland. The average age of these children was 7 years, with a range of 3 months to 15 years.

Of the children with neurofibromas, most had neurofibromatosis with a plexiform neurofibroma of the parotid. These tumors are difficult to remove completely because of their highly infiltrative nature manifested by multiple minute extensions. They can be debulked with parotidectomy, sparing the facial nerve.

EPITHELIAL SALIVARY TUMORS
General Considerations

Malignant epithelial salivary tumors are relatively more common in children (40% to 60% of total) than in adults (20% to 30%). In the series of salivary tumors at all sites reported by Ellis et al.,[7] 432 of 494 (85.4%) of tumors were of epithelial origin: 210 (42.5%) benign and 212 (42.9%) malignant. In these pediatric patients, 193 of the benign tumors were pleomorphic adenomas (39.1%), whereas in patients of all ages 52% were pleomorphic adenomas. In Lack and Upton's series,[8] pleomorphic adenoma represented 40% of all epithelial neoplasms, five of 10 in the parotid, four in the submandibular gland, and one in the minor glands.

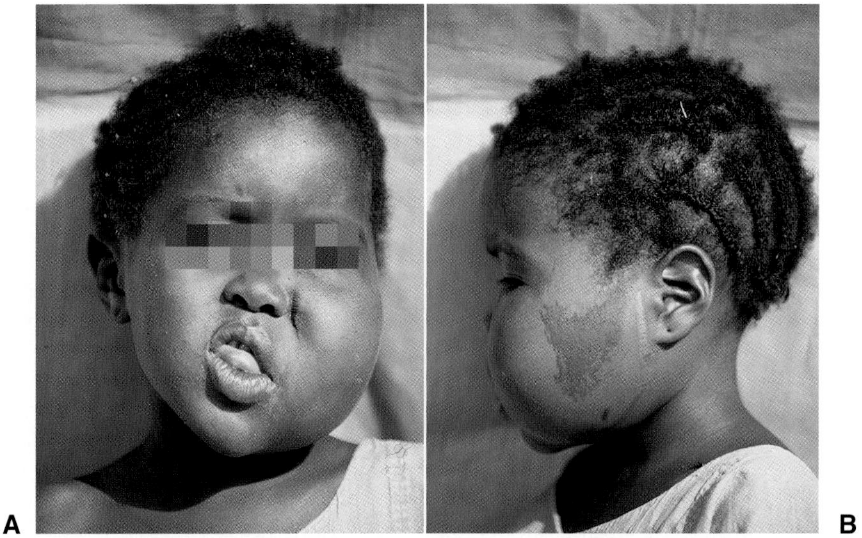

Figure 14-5

A, A 2-year-old boy with extensive plexiform neurofibroma of left parotid. Note scars from previous attempts at removal. **B,** Lateral view shows an obvious café au lait spot in this child with neurofibromatosis.

Callender et al.[28] reported six of 29 tumors (20.6%) were pleomorphic adenomas. Case series of pediatric salivary tumors reported from Europe[29] and Japan[30] show an incidence of malignant tumors to be 33.75% and 55%, respectively. A series of 38 cases of major salivary gland tumors in children from Memorial Sloan-Kettering reported 50% of tumors to be benign.[31] Mucoepidermoid carcinoma is the most commonly reported malignant salivary tumor in children. Hicks and Flaitz[32] report that these tumors represent 51% of pediatric malignant salivary tumors. However, in some series acinic cell or adenocystic carcinoma has a comparatively high incidence.

Parotid Tumors

Seifert et al.[29] reported 71% of pediatric salivary tumors occurred in the parotid. In combining three series in which location was documented[4,27,33] for 126 childhood salivary neoplasms, 87 (69%) occurred in the parotid, 22 (17.5%) in the submandibular gland, and 17 (13.5%) in minor glands. In contrast, in adults it is commonly held that approximately 80% of salivary tumors occur in the parotid; 80% of these are benign and 80% are pleomorphic adenoma.

Pleomorphic adenoma accounts for virtually all of benign pediatric neoplasms, Warthin's tumor and monomorphic adenoma being extremely rare.[4,30,34,35] In 166 children with epithelial parotid tumors, 93 (55%) tumors were benign and 73 (45%) were malignant.[5,27,30,31,36] In these five series, 47 of the 73

malignancies (64.4%) were mucoepidermoid carcinomas and 17 (23.3%) acinic cell carcinomas. Low-grade mucoepidermoid tumors were more common than high-grade. Only one group of authors examining salivary malignancies in children reported adenocystic carcinoma to be more common than mucoepidermoid carcinoma.[37] Thus, although the parotid gland is a slightly less common site for salivary tumors in children versus adults, there is a greater chance of malignancy.

The child with a firm parotid mass (Figure 14-6) is treated in the same manner as an adult. Fine-needle aspiration biopsy is useful for preoperative diagnosis, and MR or CT imaging may also be helpful. Superficial parotidectomy with preservation of the facial nerve is the basic operation for all tumors with no sign of malignancy and is curative for benign and low-grade malignant tumors. Measurement of proliferating cell nuclear antigen (PCNA) and Ki-67 levels may be helpful in predicting biologic behavior of mucoepidermoid carcinoma in children.[32]

Facial nerve sacrifice is performed only when necessary secondary to tumor invasion. Neck dissection is used for high-grade neoplasms or metastatic disease. Radiation may be indicated for positive margins and high-grade or recurrent cancers. However, the potential for interference with facial growth and later second primary cancers requires careful consideration prior to radiation in children. Five of eight children treated with adjunctive radiation for salivary gland cancer had complications: two with trismus, one extensive dental caries, one arrested dental development, and one with facial asymmetry.[27]

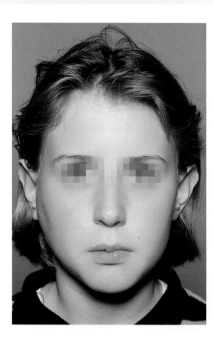

A rare malignant tumor of the parotid in infancy known as *congenital parotid salivary carcinoma*,[38] *embryoma*,[39] or *sialoblastoma*[40] is of interest because it may be impossible to differentiate clinically from the hemangioendothelioma. MR imaging can be useful in diagnosis of this extremely uncommon entity.[39]

Minor Salivary Gland Tumors

Minor salivary gland tumors account for approximately 10% of all salivary tumors,[41] and they appear to be rare in children. Waldron et al.[42] reported only 16 cases below 19 years of age in 424 tumors of the intraoral minor salivary glands. Of these 16 tumors, 13 were benign. As previously noted, 17 tumors[4,27,35] (13.5%) of 126 in three series occurred in minor salivary glands. Thirteen tumors were pleomorphic adenomas, two mucoepidermoid carcinomas, and two acinic cell carcinomas. The palate is the most frequent site. In a review of 80 intraoral minor salivary gland tumors[43] at the University of Maryland, there were six pediatric cases. All of these patients had malignant tumors (Table 14-1).

There is no literature specifically dealing with the management of pleomorphic adenoma of the palate in children. However, extracapsular wide removal, as advocated for adults,[44] is the best guarantee against recurrence. Mucoepidermoid carcinoma, although very rare, is the most common malignant tumor of the palate (Figures 14-7 and 14-8). Gustaffson et al.[45] in 1987 reviewed the literature and found only 17 cases of mucoepidermoid carcinoma of the palate in children.

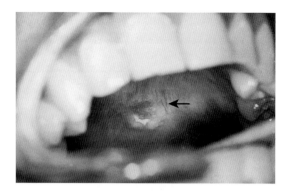

Figure 14-7
A 16-year-old boy with low-grade mucoepidermoid carcinoma at the junction of hard and soft palate *(arrow)*. (From Ord RA: Management of intra-oral salivary gland tumors. In Gold L, editor: *Oral and maxillofacial surgery,* vol 6, Philadelphia, 1994, WB Saunders.)

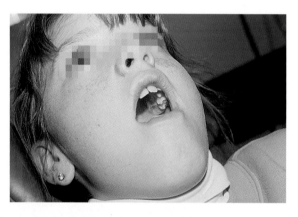

Figure 14-8
A 10-year-old girl with low-grade mucoepidermoid carcinoma of hard palate. (From Ord RA: Salivary diseases. In Fonsecca R, editor: *Oral and maxillofacial surgery,* vol 5, Philadelphia, 2000, WB Saunders.)

Fortunately, virtually all reported cases have been of low or intermediate grade. Caccamese and Ord[46] have advocated local excision, with a 1-cm margin. They recommend bone excision only if the periosteum is infiltrated and the bone shows invasion. Using this technique on four patients, there was 100% survival with 34 to 94 months of follow-up (average, 58 months). High-grade salivary malignancies do occur in children and need treatment as radical as for an adult patient (Figure 14-9).

CONCLUSION

Pediatric salivary tumors are rare. The parotid is the most common site but is less predominant than in adult patients. Mesenchymal tumors have a greater incidence, particularly in infants below 5 years of age.

TABLE 14-1	Review of Six Pediatric Cases of Salivary Gland Tumors at the University of Maryland			
Age	Race	Site	Diagnosis	Follow-up (yr)
14	W	Palate	Low-grade mucoepidermoid carcinoma	3 LFU
13	W	Palate	Low-grade mucoepidermoid carcinoma	7 AW
16	W	Soft palate/anterior pillar	Intermediate-grade mucoepidermoid carcinoma	5 AW
16	B	Hard/soft palate	Low-grade mucoepidermoid carcinoma	11 AW
17	H	Tuberosity/maxilla	Adenocystic carcinoma	5 AW
9	W	Left buccal mucosa	Low-grade mucus-producing adenocarcinoma	2 AW

W, white; *B*, black; *H*, Hispanic; *LFU*, lost to follow-up ; *AW*, alive and well.

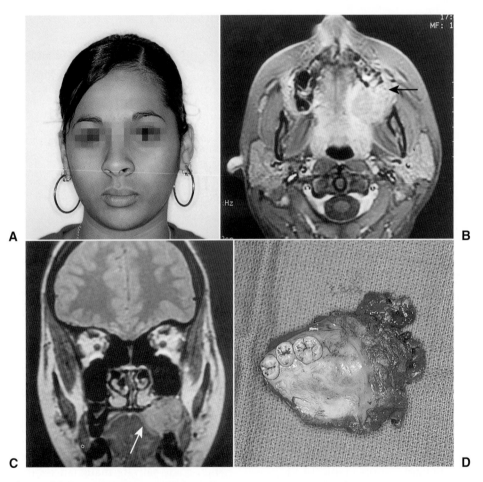

Figure 14-9

A, A 17-year-old Hispanic girl with mass, left tuberosity noted after extraction of upper wisdom tooth 7 months previously. She had recently developed trismus, with one finger breadth of maximal incisal opening. Biopsy showed adenoid cystic carcinoma. **B,** Axial MRI shows tumor involving left palate and pterygoids. **C,** Coronal MRI shows extension to the floor of the maxillary sinus. **D,** Specimen after left hemimaxillectomy via a Weber Fergusson approach. A cribriform pattern adenocystic carcinoma with perineural infiltration and surgical margins negative for involvement was found. Postoperative irradiation was given, and the patient is alive and well 5 years after surgery.

Malignant tumors are proportionately more common in children than in adults. The pleomorphic adenoma is virtually the only benign epithelial salivary tumor. Mucoepidermoid carcinoma is the most common malignant epithelial salivary malignancy at all sites, with acinic cell tumors also reported. Epithelial salivary tumors in children are managed by resection in the same manner as their adult counterparts.

REFERENCES

1. Bhaskar SN: Oral tumors of infancy and childhood, *J Pediatr* 63:195, 1963.
2. Byars LT, Ackerman LV, Peacock E: Tumors of salivary origin in children, *Ann Surg* 146:40, 1957.
3. Kaufman SL, Stout AP: Tumors of the major salivary glands in children, *Cancer* 16:1317, 1963.
4. Krolls SO, Trodahl JN, Boyers RC: Salivary gland lesions in children. A survey of 430 cases, *Cancer* 30:459, 1972.
5. Jacques DA, Krolls SO, Chambers RG: Parotid tumors in children, *Am J Surg* 132:469, 1976.
6. Bhaskar SN, Lilley GS: Salivary gland tumors of infancy: report of twenty-seven cases, *J Oral Surg* 21:306, 1963.
7. Ellis GL, Auclair PL, Gnepp DR: Salivary gland neoplasms: general considerations. In Ellis GL, Auclair, PL, Gnepp DR, editors: *Surgical pathology of the salivary glands,* Philadelphia, 1991, WB Saunders.
8. Lack EE, Upton MP: Histopathologic review of salivary gland tumors in childhood, *Arch Otolaryngol Head Neck Surg* 114:898, 1988.
9. Wawro NW, Frederickson RW, Tennant R: Hemangioma of the parotid gland in infants, *Cancer* 8:595, 1955.
10. Mulliken JB, Glowacki J: Hemangiomas and vascular malformations in infants and children: a classification based on endothelial characteristics, *Plast Reconstr Surg* 69(3):412-422, 1982.
11. Scarcella JV, Dykes ER, Anderson R: Hemangiomas of the parotid gland, *Plast Reconstr Surg* 36:38, 1965.
12. Drolet BA, Esterly NB, Friden IJ: Hemangiomas in children, *N Engl J Med* 341:3, 173, 1999.
13. Campbell JS: Congenital capillary hemangiomas of the parotid gland, *N Engl J Med* 254:56, 1956.
14. Roebuck DJ, Ahuja AT: Hemangioendothelioma of the parotid gland in infants: sonography and correlative MR imaging, *Am J Neuroradiol* 21:219, 2000.
15. Huchzermeyer P, Birchall MA, Kendall B, et al: Parotid hemangiomas in childhood: a case for MRI, *J Laryngol Otol* 108:892, 1994.
16. Conway H: Cavernous hemangioma of the parotid gland treated by x-radiation at the time of operation, *Plast Reconstr Surg* 8:237, 1951.
17. Campbell JS: Congenital capillary hemangiomas of the parotid gland, *N Engl J Med* 254:56, 1956.
18. Howard JM, Rawson AJ, Koop CE, et al: Parotid tumors in children, *Surg Gynecol Obstet* 90:307, 1950.
19. Takato T, Komuro Y, Yonehara Y: Giant hemangioma of the parotid associated with Kasabach-Merritt syndrome, *J Oral Maxillofac Surg* 51:425, 1993.
20. Robertson JS, Winegard DA, Schaitkin BM: Life threatening hemangioma arising from the parotid gland, *Otolaryngol Head Neck Surg* 104:858, 1991.
21. Frieden IJ, Eichenfield LF, Esterly NB, et al: Guidelines outcomes committee. Guidelines of care for hemangiomas of infancy, *J Am Acad Dermatol* 37:631, 1997.
22. Gangopadhyay AN, Sinha CK, Gopal SC, et al: Role of steroids in childhood hemangioma: a 10-year review, *Int Surg* 82:49, 1997.
23. Enjolras O, Riche MC, Merland JJ, Escarde JP: Management of alarming hemangiomas in infants: a review of 25 cases, *Pediatrics* 85:491, 1990.
24. Ezekowitz RAB, Mulliken JB, Folkman J: Interferon alfa-2a therapy for life-threatening hemangiomas of infancy, *N Engl J Med* 326:1456, 1992.
25. Soumekh B, Adams GL, Shapiro RS: Treatment of head and neck hemangiomas with recombinant interferon alpha-2b, *Ann Otol Rhinol Laryngol* 105:201, 1994.
26. Blei F, Isakoff M, Deb G: The response of parotid hemangiomas to the use of systemic interferon alpha-2a or corticosteroids, *Arch Otolaryngol Head Neck Surg* 123:841, 1997.
27. Lingeman RE: Cystic lymphangioma of the parotid region, *Laryngoscope* 70:983, 1960.
28. Callender DL, Frankenthaler RA, Luna MA, et al: Salivary neoplasms in children, *Arch Otolaryngol Head Neck Surg* 118:472, 1992.
29. Seifert G, Okabe H, Caselitz J: Epithelial salivary gland tumors in children and adolescents: analysis of 80 cases (Salivary Gland Register 1965-1984), *ORL J Otorhinolaryngol Relat Spec* 48:137, 1986.
30. Ogata H, Satoshi E, Kiyoshi M: Salivary gland neoplasms in children, *Japan J Clin Oncol* 24:88, 1994.
31. Castro EB, Hvvos AG, Strong EW, Foote FW: Tumors of the major salivary glands in children, *Cancer* 29:312, 1972.
32. Hicks J, Flaitz C: Mucoepidermoid carcinoma of salivary glands in children and adolescents: assessment of proliferation markers, *Oral Oncol* 36:454, 2000.
33. Shikhani AH, Johns ME: Tumors of the major salivary glands in children, *Head Neck Surg* 10:257, 1988.
34. Dahlqvist Å, Österberg Y: Malignant salivary tumors in children, *Acta Otolaryngol* 94:175, 1982.
35. Galich R: Salivary gland neoplasms in childhood, *Arch Otolaryngol* 89:100, 1969.
36. Ord RA: Management of parotid tumors, *Oral Maxillofac Surg Clin North Am* 73:529, 1995.
37. Lederman M: Adenolymphoma of the parotid salivary gland, *Br J Radiol* 16:383-385, 1943.
38. Baker SR, Malone B: Salivary malignancies in children, *Cancer* 55:1730, 1985.
39. Donath K, Seifert G, Lentrodt J: The embryonal carcinoma of the parotid gland. A rare example of an embryonal tumor, *Virchows Arch A Pathol Anat Histopathol* 403:425, 1984.
40. Som PM, Brandwein M, Silvers AR, Rothschild MA: Sialoblastoma embryoma: MR findings of a rare pediatric salivary gland tumor, *Am J Neuororadiol* 18:847, 1997.
41. Ord RA: Management of intra-oral salivary gland tumors, *Oral Maxillofac Surg Clin North Am* 6:499, 1994.
42. Waldron CA, El-Mofty SK, Gnepp DR: Tumors of the intra-oral minor salivary glands: a demographic and histologic study of 426 cases, *Oral Surg Oral Med Oral Pathol* 66:323, 1988.
43. Jansisyanont P, Blanchaert RB, Ord RA: Intra-oral minor salivary gland neoplasm: a single institution experience of 80 cases, *Int J Oral Maxillofac Surg* 31:257-261, 2002.
44. Pogrel MA: Tumors of the "minor" salivary glands: A histological and clinical review, *Br J Oral Surg* 17:47, 1979.
45. Gustaffson H, Dahlqvist Å, Anniko M, Carlsöö B: Muco-epidermoid carcinoma in a minor salivary gland in childhood, *J Laryngol Otol* 101:1320, 1987.
46. Caccamese JF, Ord RA: Pediatric mucoepidermoid carcinoma of the palate, *Int J Oral Maxillofac Surg* 31:136, 2002.

CHAPTER 15

Jaw Tumors in Children

Maria J. Troulis, W. Bradford Williams, and Leonard B. Kaban

Central jaw tumors in children occur infrequently, and few surgeons have extensive experience in treating these lesions. There are few comprehensive papers in the literature specifically dealing with jaw tumors in children.[1-4] This chapter is based mostly on the senior author's experience with pediatric jaw tumors over a 30-year period. The major principle learned from this experience is that treatment of primary jaw tumors must be determined by a combination of clinical characteristics, histologic appearance, and, most importantly, biologic behavior of the tumor.[4] A "benign" histologic diagnosis should not be the sole determining factor in deciding treatment.

CLASSIFICATION

Primary jaw tumors are classified into odontogenic and nonodontogenic groups.[4] Odontogenic tumors are common in childhood. However, for the most part, they are odontomas, treated simply by curettage and with no tendency to recur. Ameloblastomas and ameloblastic fibromas occur in children, although the former are extremely rare and the latter are well known but less common than odontomas. Nonodontogenic tumors are grouped by cell line of origin, if known, histologic appearance, and clinical behavior: (1) benign mesenchymal tumors, (2) hematopoietic and reticuloendothelial tumors, (3) neurogenic tumors, (4) vascular lesions, (5) malignant mesenchymal tumors, and (6) malignant epithelial tumors (Box 15-1). In this chapter we discuss odontogenic, benign mesenchymal, hematopoietic, and reticuloendothelial tumors, and tumors of neurogenic origin. Malignant tumors are presented in Chapter 16 and vascular lesions in Chapter 17.

ODONTOGENIC TUMORS

Given the complexity of the process of odontogenesis, the germ layers involved, and the total number of teeth, it is remarkable that odontogenic tumors are not more common. When the complex cellular inductive process of odontogenesis does become disturbed, cysts and tumors result. Odontogenic tumors are classified according to the cell layer of origin: ectoderm, mesoderm, or mixed[4,5] (Box 15-2).

Odontoma

Diagnosis. Odontogenic tumors derived from mesenchymal elements of the dental follicle are common in childhood. Complex and compound odontomas occur most often in the mandible. They usually are detected as asymptomatic radiopaque lesions on routine diagnostic radiographs. In other cases, they prevent eruption of, or

BOX 15-1   Classification of Nonodontogenic Jaw Tumors in Children

Benign Mesenchymal Tumors
Giant cell lesions
Fibro-osseous lesions
Myxoma

Hematopoietic and Reticuloendothelial Tumors
Langerhans cell histiocytosis
Burkitt's lymphoma
Lymphoma

Neurogenic Tumors
Neurofibroma
Neurilemoma
Neuroma
Ganglioneuroma
Neuroblastoma
Melanotic neuroectodermal tumor

Vascular Lesions
Vascular malformation (capillary, lymphatic, venous, arterial, combined)
Hemangioma
Aneurysmal bone cyst

Malignant Mesenchymal Tumors
Osteogenic sarcoma
Chondrosarcoma
Fibrosarcoma
Ewing's sarcoma

Malignant Epithelial Tumors
Squamous cell carcinoma
Mucoepidermoid carcinoma
Adenoid cystic carcinoma
Adenocarcinoma

Modified from Choung R, Kaban LB: *J Oral Maxillofac Surg* 43:323-332, 1985.

BOX 15-2   Classification of Odontogenic Tumors in Children

Epithelial Tumors
Ameloblastoma
Peripheral
Unicystic
Solid, multicystic

Adenomatoid odontogenic tumor
Calcifying epithelial odontogenic tumor (Pindborg tumor)

Mesodermal Tumors
Cementoma
Periapical cemental dysplasia
Cementifying fibroma
Cementoblastoma

Odontogenic fibroma

Mixed Tumors
Ameloblastic fibroma
Odontoma

Modified from Gorlin R, Meskin LH, Brodwy R: *Ann N Y Acad Sci* 108:722-771, 1963.

appear to be primitive teeth, while complex odontomas have dental elements without being organized into a recognizable tooth.

Treatment. Odontomas are treated by enucleation or curettage and have no tendency to recur. Skeletal reconstruction is usually not necessary because the resultant defect is small enough to permit spontaneous bone regeneration.

form in place of, a normal tooth that failed to develop. They rarely appear with intraoral or extraoral swelling, and there is usually no pain and no paresthesia. Radiographically, there is no root resorption of adjacent teeth and no cortical perforation, although occasionally there will be cortical thinning. The lesions may look like abnormal teeth or simply a disorganized calcified mass (see Chapter 10, Figures 10-23 and 10-24). Histologically, odontomas have a variety of pulpal and dentin-like elements (Figure 15-1). The degree of organization into recognizable toothlike configurations determines the label placed on the tumor. Compound odontomas

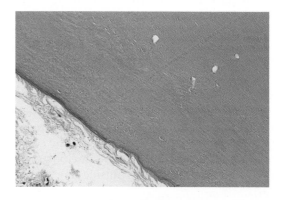

Figure 15-1

Histologic slide of an odontoma at original magnification (×100). Note the normal-appearing tooth structures (dentin and cementum). (Courtesy Dr. Bill Faquin.)

Ameloblastoma

Ameloblastoma is a tumor of the odontogenic epithelium,[6] first described by Cusick in 1827.[7] It accounts for less than 1% of all odontogenic cysts and tumors. Although all ameloblastomas have the same cell of origin, there are several biologically distinct forms. The differences are especially important in pediatric cases.[8-10] Central ameloblastomas occur as unicystic,[8] multicystic, or solid lesions.[10] The unicystic ameloblastoma resembles a dentigerous or primordial cyst clinically and radiographically and often occurs in teenage patients (Figure 15-2). Multicystic or solid ameloblastomas occur most commonly in patients 30 to 50 years of age and are extremely rare in childhood.[11] Chuong and Kaban's review[4] of pediatric jaw tumors found only one case in 10 years. Bhaskar[12] and Blackwood[13] reviewed odontogenic tumors in pediatric patients under 15 and found no ameloblastomas.

Diagnosis. In the pediatric population, ameloblastoma must be considered in the differential diagnosis of radiolucent lesions of the jaws. In the vast majority of pediatric cases, however, these turn out to be either odontogenic or nonodontogenic cysts or nonodontogenic primary jaw tumors. The two ameloblastic lesions that are found in childhood are the ameloblastic fibroma and the unicystic ameloblastoma.

The ameloblastic fibroma appears as an asymptomatic radiolucent lesion, often associated with an impacted tooth and indistinguishable from an odontogenic cyst. The patients are usually under 12 years of age (Figure 15-3; see also Chapter 10, Figure 10-25).

The unicystic ameloblastoma occurs in teenagers, most commonly in the mandible. Robinson and Martinez[8] reported 14 patients with this lesion, and 10 were below the age of 20. Leider et al.[14] reported on 33 patients whose average age was 26.9, with 75% of patients diagnosed during the second decade. The patient exhibits a painless facial swelling or a radiolucency, usually associated with an impacted third molar. The lesion is most commonly uniloculated and may produce cortical expansion or perforation. Roots of adjacent teeth may be displaced or resorbed. Aspiration reveals clear serous fluid from a cystic mass (see Figure 15-2).

Histologically, the unicystic ameloblastoma may demonstrate one of three patterns. Most commonly, there is an epithelium-lined cyst with ameloblastic tissue located in its wall (luminal). A second pattern consists of ameloblastic elements free-floating in the cyst cavity (intraluminal). Occasionally, an ameloblastoma is found in the cyst wall but outside the cyst cavity (mural).[8,15,16]

Treatment. Treatment of both unicystic ameloblastomas and ameloblastic fibromas consists of enucleation. The specimen must be examined in multiple serial sections to determine the extent of the tumor.

Although initial treatment is the same for a dentigerous cyst and a unicystic ameloblastoma, close follow-up of the patient with ameloblastoma is important because of the potential for recurrence.[8,15] In unicystic ameloblastomas, if there is evidence of extension through the fibrous capsule, marginal resection with 1-cm margins should be performed (see Figure 15-2).

Treatment of solid or multicystic ameloblastoma in adults is not the subject of this chapter. In contrast to ameloblastic fibroma and unicystic lesions, however, the standard treatment for ameloblastoma is resection with 1.5-cm margins, because curettage is inadequate.[1] Recurrence of multicystic or solid ameloblastomas in adults after conservative surgical excision occurs in 50% to 60% of cases,[17,18] as compared with 4.5% after wide resection.[17] Recurrence may occur as late as 10 years after resection; therefore, long-term follow-up is essential.[11,14,19]

Ameloblastic fibromas (see Figure 15-3) are more common than ameloblastomas in children. They most commonly arise in the mandibular parasymphysis region and have a low recurrence rate after enucleation and curettage. For a more detailed discussion of this lesion, see Chapter 10.

Cementoma

The term *cementoma* refers to a variety of odontogenic lesions derived from the periodontal membrane. The most common is periapical cemental dysplasia. This is an asymptomatic radiographic finding at the dental root apices. The mandibular anterior teeth are the most frequently affected. An initial radiolucent phase appears identical to a periapical abscess radiographically. With time, the lesion progressively calcifies and becomes radiopaque. Cementomas may be multiple. The teeth are asymptomatic and test vital to the electrical pulp tester.

A cementifying fibroma may be indistinguishable from fibrous dysplasia, although cementum may be calcified more densely and the tumor may have a more intimate relationship to the root apices. Cementifying fibroma occurs most commonly in the molar-premolar region. The tumor may display rapid expansion and growth like other fibro-osseous lesions. This biologic behavior is not explainable by the histologic characteristics of the tumor. Treatment must, therefore, be determined by clinical behavior.

NONODONTOGENIC TUMORS
Benign Mesenchymal Tumors

Benign mesenchymal lesions are the most common nonodontogenic tumors in childhood[4] (Box 15-3). Included in this group are (1) giant cell lesions, (2) fibro-osseous lesions, (3) myxomas, and (4) aggressive

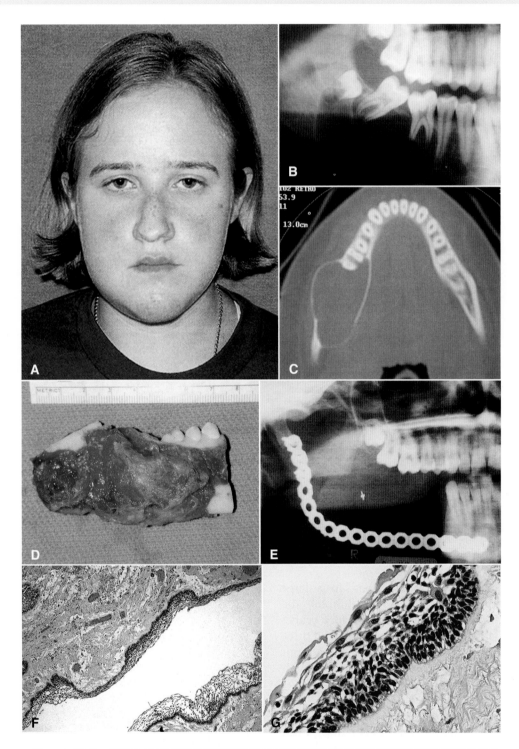

Figure 15-2

A, Frontal photograph of a 15-year-old girl with swelling in the right mandible. Panoramic radiograph **(B)** and axial CT image **(C)** reveal a unicystic, radiolucent lesion in the right mandible that by incisional biopsy was confirmed to be ameloblastoma. Because of the large size of the lesion, thinned cortical rim, and evidence of cortical perforation into the soft tissue, en bloc resection **(D)** and immediate reconstruction **(E)** were performed using a 2.7-mm reconstruction plate. **F** and **G,** Hematoxylin and eosin–stained histologic slides (original magnification ×100 and ×400, respectively) show typical appearance of unicystic ameloblastoma. Note the polarization of the basal layer. (**F** and **G** courtesy Dr. Bill Faquin.)

Continued.

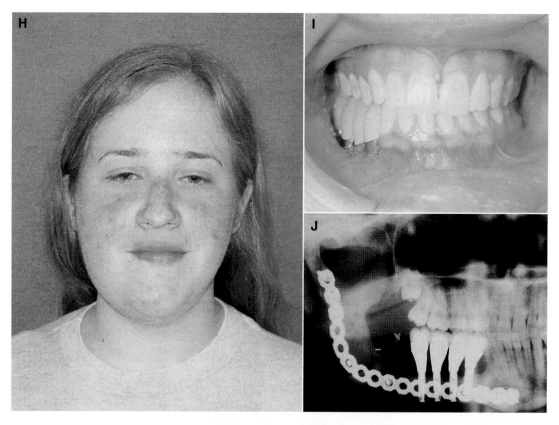

Figure 15-2—continued
Frontal **(H)** and intraoral **(I)** photographs and panoramic radiograph **(J)** 1 year later. The patient has undergone bone graft and implants for complete rehabilitation.

fibromatosis and desmoplastic fibromas. In a large series of nonodontogenic tumors in childhood, the average age at the time of diagnosis was 10.4 years.[4] Swelling was a characteristic initial symptom of all three types of tumors. Pain, loose or displaced teeth, and root resorption occurred most frequently in patients with giant cell lesions.

Giant Cell Lesions

Diagnosis. Giant cell lesions traditionally have been classified into three groups: brown tumor of hyperparathyroidism, central giant cell granuloma (CGCG), and giant cell tumor. Brown tumor of hyperparathyroidism occurs in children in association with chronic renal failure and secondary hyperparathyroidism (Figure 15-4). Primary hyperparathyroidism is rare in children. The bone lesion is a result of osteoclastic bone resorption in response to an elevated parathyroid hormone level. Serum calcium and alkaline phosphatase values are elevated and serum phosphorus level is low.

BOX 15-3	Benign Mesenchymal Tumors

Giant Cell Lesions
Nonaggressive giant cell lesions (Giant cell reparative granuloma)
Aggressive giant cell lesions (Giant cell tumor)
Brown tumor (Hyperparathyroidism)

Fibro-osseous Lesions
Fibrous dysplasia
Cherubism
Cementifying fibroma
Ossifying fibroma
Osteoblastoma

Myxoma

Modified from Chuong R, Kaban LB: *J Oral Maxillofac Surg* 43: 323-332, 1985.

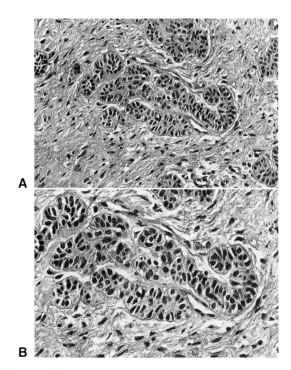

Figure 15-3

A and **B**, Hematoxylin and eosin–stained histologic slides (original magnification ×100 and ×400, respectively) of ameloblastic fibroma. Note the typical strands of odontogenic epithelium, two to three layers wide. Despite its name, this lesion is not a subtype of ameloblastoma. (Courtesy Dr. Bill Faquin.)

The diagnosis is confirmed by an elevated parathyroid hormone level. Serum creatinine and blood urea nitrogen values are abnormally elevated in patients with chronic renal failure. Panoramic and dental radiographs demonstrate loss or thinning of the lamina dura around the teeth, and hand radiographs show resorption lacunae in the phalanges of the fingers.[4,20] Brown tumor must be considered in the differential diagnosis of all giant cell lesions, particularly when there has been a recurrence or multiple lesions.

The term *central giant cell granuloma* implies a reactive, inflammatory process, which is usually not the case, particularly in children. A more rational way to classify these lesions is to call them giant cell lesions and then further categorize them as (1) brown tumor, (2) nonaggressive giant cell lesions, and (3) aggressive giant cell lesions.

The three lesions (brown tumor, nonaggressive giant cell lesions, and aggressive giant cell lesions) appear indistinguishable by standard histologic techniques, even though they display a wide range of clinical behavior and aggressiveness. The giant cells found in these tumors are present in a variety of benign and malignant jaw tumors, which includes aneurysmal bone cyst, fibrous dysplasia, cherubism, ossifying fibroma, and osteogenic sarcoma. However, their significance is poorly understood.

The diagnosis and classification of giant cell lesions is based on clinical behavior and radiographic charac-

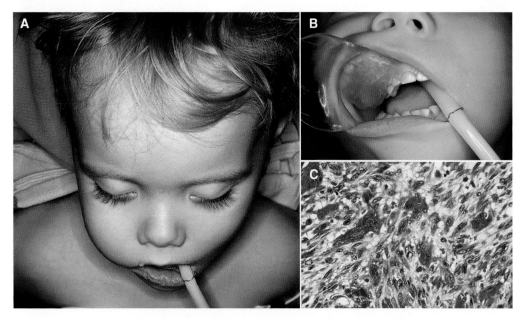

Figure 15-4

A, A 3-year-old patient with chronic renal failure and progressive right facial swelling. **B,** Intraoral view shows mass in right maxilla. The diagnosis of secondary hyperparathyroidism was made on the basis of the patient's chronic renal failure and elevated serum calcium and parathyroid hormone levels. The giant cell lesion was enucleated and parathyroidectomy performed. **C,** Histologic appearance of brown tumor (hematoxylin and eosin, original magnification ×400) is indistinguishable from that of other giant cell lesions (see Figures 15-5, *G,* and 15-6, *E*).

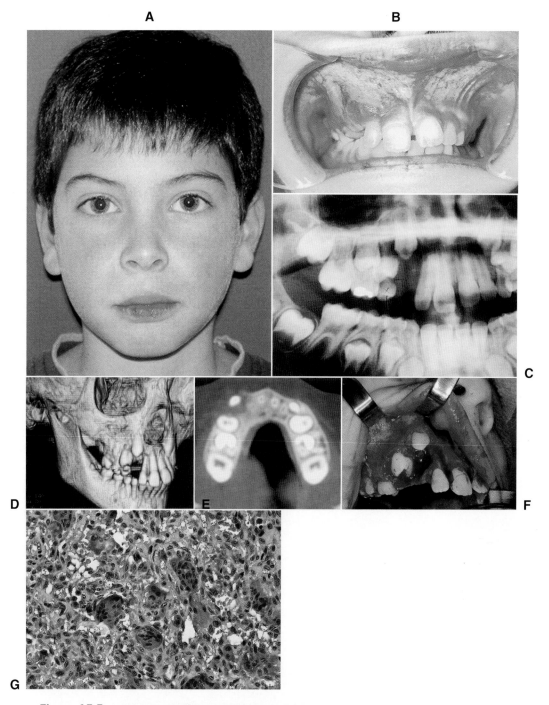

Figure 15-5

Frontal **(A)** and intraoral **(B)** photographs of a 9-year-old boy with a right maxillary giant cell lesion. Panoramic radiograph **(C)** and 3D **(D)** and axial **(E)** CT images show a small lesion (<5 cm), minimal to no tooth displacement (both right and left canines appear at same level), and no root resorption. The lesion was classified as a nonaggressive giant cell lesion. **F,** The child underwent curettage. **G,** Histologic appearance (hematoxylin and eosin, original magnification ×400) of this nonaggressive giant cell lesion. Histologically, it is indistinguishable from the brown tumor (see Figure 15-4, *C*) and an aggressive giant cell lesion (see Figure 15-6, *E*).

teristics. A giant cell lesion is classified as aggressive by the following characteristics: (1) size greater than 5 cm, (2) rapid growth, (3) tooth loosening or displacement, (4) radiographic evidence of root resorption or tooth displacement, (5) radiographic evidence of cortical bone thinning or perforation, and (6) recurrence after treatment. If the lesion is larger than 5 cm or if it recurs after treatment, it is considered to be an aggressive giant cell lesion on the basis of one or both of these characteristics. Otherwise, the lesion must exhibit at least three of the six features. All other lesions are considered nonaggressive. This is significant, because the recurrence rate for nonaggressive lesions is low when treated by simple enucleation or curettage, whereas the recurrence rate for aggressive lesions is high.

The peak incidence of giant cell lesions is between 10 and 20 years of age. The female-to-male ratio is 2:1, and the lesion occurs more often in the mandible than in the maxilla. The giant cell lesion is the most common central jaw tumor that occurs in the anterior body and symphysis of the mandible, with the canine-premolar region being the most common location. The lesion rarely is located posterior to the 6-year molar. Patients with nonaggressive giant cell lesions are usually asymptomatic, and the lesions are discovered as an incidental finding on routine diagnostic radiographs. Symptoms may include local swelling, most commonly without pain or paresthesia. The initial finding may be a mild facial asymmetry noticed by a family member who has not seen the child for awhile. Radiographically, there is a radiolucent lesion which may be uniloculated or multiloculated.

The existence of a true "giant cell tumor" of the jaws was controversial in the past. More recently, however, clinicians have recognized a locally aggressive and destructive giant cell lesion of the jaws that has a high rate of recurrence with little tendency to metastasize.[4,21-25]

Giant cell tumors of the long bones occur in an older age group (greater than 20 years) than do the aggressive giant cell lesions of the jaws. The long bone tumors are also locally aggressive and recur frequently. The occurrence of metastasis (to the lung) from long bone lesions, although uncommon, is well known. The two tumors, therefore, are at least related if not identical.[4,21,22]

To provide more evidence for this concept, Chuong et al.[21] and Ficarro et al.[22] investigated cytometric and histopathologic predictors of clinical behavior of giant cell lesions. Both studies demonstrated a greater fractional surface area occupied by giant cells in clinically aggressive lesions, and Ficarro[22] showed a statistically significant increase in the size of giant cells in aggressive lesions. However, in the clinical setting there are no readily available biologic markers to predict clinical behavior. For this reason the management of giant lesions of bone remains challenging for oral and maxillofacial and orthopedic surgeons, alike.

Attempts have therefore been made to classify giant cell lesions, by clinical, radiographic, and cytometric techniques[21,22] into aggressive and nonaggressive categories. Aggressive giant cell lesions tend to occur in younger patients (mean age = 6.3 years), cause pain, exhibit rapid growth, and characteristically demonstrate root resorption and perforation of the cortex radiographically.[21] The nonaggressive giant cell lesions (mean age = 9.3 years) appear as asymptomatic radiolucencies without pain, root resorption, or cortical perforation.[23] Unfortunately, aggressive lesions have a high recurrence rate unless treated by en bloc resection. Chuong and Kaban[4] reported no recurrences in a group of five patients with nonaggressive lesions treated by curettage and followed for a mean of 36 months. However, three patients with aggressive lesions had nine separate recurrences beginning an average of 2 years after curettage. These three patients and three others with aggressive lesions had no recurrences after en bloc resection and primary reconstruction, with a mean follow-up of 3 years.

Treatment. Treatment of giant cell lesions is determined by a combination of clinical and histologic characteristics and, most importantly, by the biologic behavior of the tumor.

Brown Tumors of Hyperparathyroidism. Brown tumors of hyperparathyroidism regress when the endocrine abnormality is treated, usually by parathyroidectomy or by control of the renal failure. The tumor may be treated by curettage when necessary (e.g., bleeding, pain, convenience). The lesions have no tendency to recur as long as the primary disease is controlled (see Figure 15-4).

Nonaggressive Giant Cell Lesions. Enucleation or curettage is the appropriate primary treatment for nonaggressive lesions (Figure 15-5).

Aggressive Giant Cell Lesions. En bloc resection to achieve 1.0 cm histologically clear margins is the standard treatment of choice for aggressive giant cell lesions even when the pathologist labels the tumor as *benign CGCG*[4,21,26,27] (Figure 15-6).

In the search for minimally invasive surgical and pharmacologic therapies for this disease, a number of alternatives to en bloc resection (for the treatment of the aggressive giant cell lesions) have been proposed. These therapies include enucleation with adjuvant therapy such as cryotherapy or peripheral ostectomy or Carnoy's solution,[4,21,28-32] intralesional steroid injections,[29] embolization,[33,34] calcitonin,[28,30] or debulking followed by interferon therapy.[31,32,35]

Intralesional steroid injection, calcitonin therapy, and enucleation with adjuvant interferon therapy have all been reported to achieve cure of aggressive giant cell lesions in case series.[4,21,28-35] However, there have been reported failures with both intralesional steroid injections and calcitonin[26] (Figure 15-7). The mechanism of action of these therapies appears to be related to either their anti-angiogenic effect (steroids and interferon) or to their inhibition of osteoclastic mediated bone resorption (calcitonin and interferon).[26] Interferon, in addition, appears to stimulate osteoblast activity, which, in combination with osteoclast inhibition, acts to rapidly obliterate the bone cavity after enucleation.[26,27,31]

In a recent case series by Kaban et al.,[27] patients with aggressive giant cell lesions were treated successfully with enucleation (with preservation of teeth and nerves) and

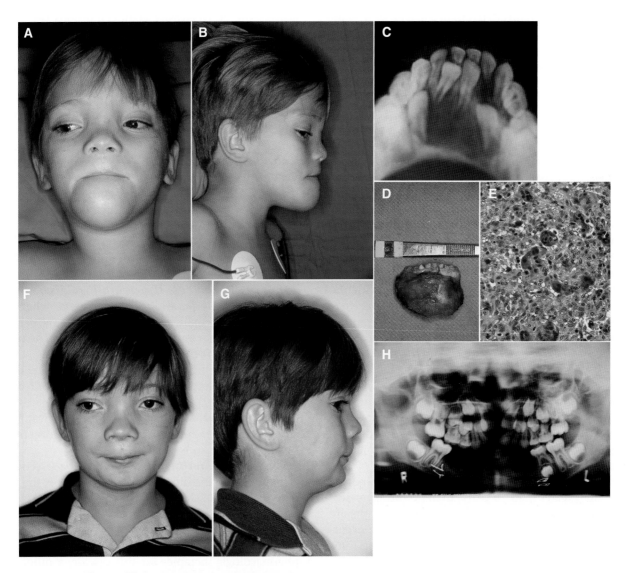

Figure 15-6

Frontal **(A)** and lateral **(B)** photographs of a 6-year-old patient with a rapidly growing mass over the chin that had developed during a period of 2 weeks. The lesion extended from the first deciduous molar on the right to the first deciduous molar on the left and was greater than 5 cm. **C,** Occlusal radiograph demonstrates a radiolucent lesion with cortical thinning, tooth displacement, and root resorption. The CT image demonstrated cortical perforation and cortical thinning. The lesion was classified as aggressive, based on the size, rapid growth, and radiographic findings despite the pathologic diagnosis: benign central giant cell granuloma. **D,** Operative photograph of the specimen after en bloc resection. **E,** Photomicrograph shows a typical giant cell lesion with giant cells interspersed in a fibrous stroma and a generous vascular network (hematoxylin and eosin, original magnification ×400). Frontal **(F)** and lateral **(G)** photographs of the patient 5 years later, along with his panoramic radiograph **(H)**. There was no recurrence.

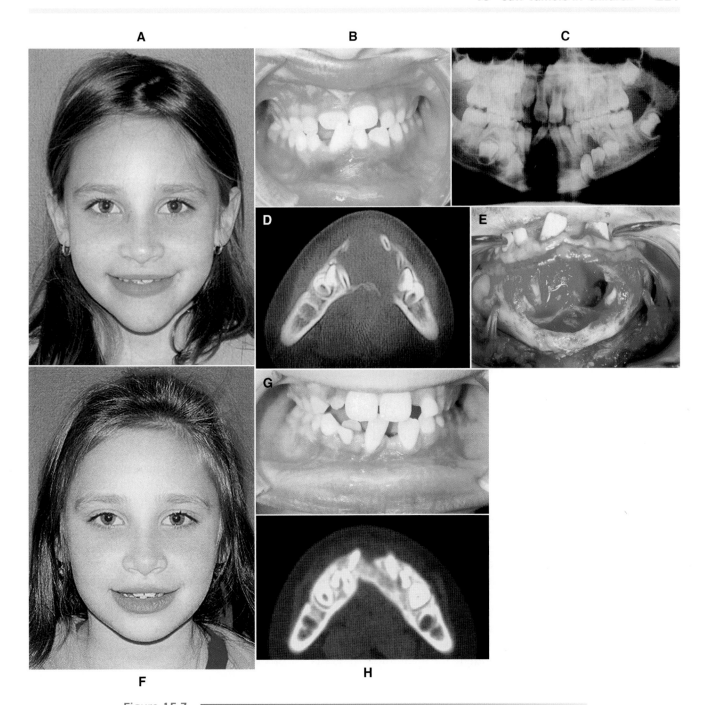

Figure 15-7

Frontal (A) and intraoral (B) photographs of 6-year-old child with rapidly expanding swelling of the chin. Panoramic radiograph (C) and axial CT image (D) show the large radiolucent lesion, with cortical thinning, root resorption, and tooth displacement. During intralesion steroid injection the lesion continued to grow. Based on these findings the lesion was classified as an aggressive giant cell lesion. E, Curettage with preservation of vital anatomic structures (teeth and nerve) was performed, and a 7-month course of interferon therapy started. Frontal (F) and intraoral (G) photographs and axial CT image (H) 1 year after the completion of therapy. Note the bone fill on the CT image.

interferon therapy. Although the case series was small (N = 8), at a mean follow-up of 1.9 years no recurrences have been observed (see Figure 15-7).

Fibro-osseous Lesions. Fibro-osseous lesions include fibrous dysplasia, cherubism, ossifying fibroma, and osteoblastoma (see Boxes 15-1 and 15-3). In this group of tumors, normal bone is replaced by fibrous and mineralized tissue, new blood vessels, and giant cells in varying proportions.[36,37] Chuong and Kaban[4] reported the average age at diagnosis was 9.5 years. Slowly enlarging, painless swelling was the most common initial symptom. Pain and paresthesia occurred in only one case, a patient with rapidly expanding maxillary fibrous dysplasia. Other complaints reflected the location of the tumor, such as trismus associated with an osteoblastoma involving the glenoid fossa and proptosis in cases of fibrous dysplasia involving the orbit and maxilla.

Fibrous Dysplasia

Diagnosis. Fibrous dysplasia of the jaws is more often monostotic than polyostotic. However, the child may have multiple foci of disease, with or without endocrine abnormalities (precocious puberty) and café-au-lait spots (McCune-Albright syndrome). The patient complains of painless swelling appearing during the first or second decade of life.[36-38] Growth is cyclic, with the greatest active change occurring during childhood or coinciding with onset of puberty or pregnancy. During periods of rapid growth, the patient may experience pain, with or without paresthesia, or functional deficits such as impairment of vision, depending on the location of the disease (Figures 15-8 and 15-9). The tumor usually becomes quiescent and "burns out" by age 20 to 25, although females may experience further growth with pregnancy or birth control pills. After age 25, it is rare for a patient to experience major changes in fibrous dysplasia.[38]

The maxilla is involved more often than the mandible, and extension into the orbital floor may produce proptosis or infraorbital paresthesia or both. In the mandible, fibrous dysplasia often occurs at the angle and must be differentiated from osteomyelitis, masseter hypertrophy, myositis ossificans, and other primary jaw tumors. Radiographically, fibrous dysplasia may appear as a multilocular radiolucency with cortical bone thinning. The teeth may spread apart, and there may be delayed dental eruption. In clinically quiescent lesions, there may be a mixed radiolucent to radiopaque, or simply a radiopaque, mass on a radiograph. Indicators of metabolic bone disease such as serum calcium, phosphorus, and alkaline phosphatase are at normal levels. Microscopic examination reveals a mixture of fibrous tissue, bone, giant cells, and blood vessels. Smith[38] noted a correlation between cellularity of the connective tissue matrix and rate of tumor growth. Kaban et al.[39] noted a correlation

between number of mast cells and osteoclasts at the periphery of the lesion and clinical growth activity of the tumor.

McCune-Albright syndrome (MAS) is a sporadic disease consisting of polyostotic fibrous dysplasia, café-au-lait spots, precocious puberty, and other hyperfunctional endocrine disorders with normal or decreased hormone levels.[40,41] The pathogenesis of MAS has been discovered only recently to result from a gene mutation leading to prolonged or inappropriate activation of the intracellular second messenger cyclic adenosine monophosphate in the presence of little or no hormone.[42-44] Cells containing this mutation are distributed in a mosaic pattern, with the greatest number present in the most affected tissues.[45,46] Most patients with MAS have polyostotic fibrous dysplasia, which appears during the first decade of life.[42] Patients also exhibit at least one pigmented macule (café-au-lait spot) with irregular borders ("coast of Maine").[42] Café-au-lait spots tend not to cross the midline, and most are distributed on the same side as the osseous lesions[42,45] (Figure 15-10). Endocrine abnormalities may involve any endocrine tissue, with the most common abnormality being gonadal hyperfunction resulting in precocious puberty.[42]

Treatment. In most instances, the indication for operation is to confirm the diagnosis histologically or to improve appearance. Rapid increase in the size of the tumor or onset of pain, paresthesia, or a functional deficit are additional indications for an operation (see Figures 15-8, 15-10, and 15-11). In some children, enlargement of the mandible and obliteration of the nasal passage(s) can produce airway obstruction. Orbital tumor growth can cause optic nerve compression and impair vision (Figure 15-10). In adult patients, the tumor is treated with contour excision when it has been stable for at least 1 year (Figure 15-12). More recently, Munro and Chan[47] described complete excision of the bony mass and replacement with bone grafts. Most of the patients in this series had frontal orbital-zygomatic fibrous dysplasia. Other authors have reported osteotomy of the maxilla or mandible or both, in combination with contour excision in patients who have malocclusion secondary to fibrous dysplasia.[48] The functional problems most frequently requiring operative treatment are proptosis, vision impairment, trismus, and paresthesia. In these cases, an operation is performed despite the risk for recurrence.

Malignant transformation has been reported after radiation therapy. Therefore, radiation therapy should not be considered as a treatment of fibrous dysplasia. Sudden, rapid expansion and the onset of paresthesia should be viewed as suspicious for malignant transformation despite the rare occurrence of sarcomatous change.

A

B

C

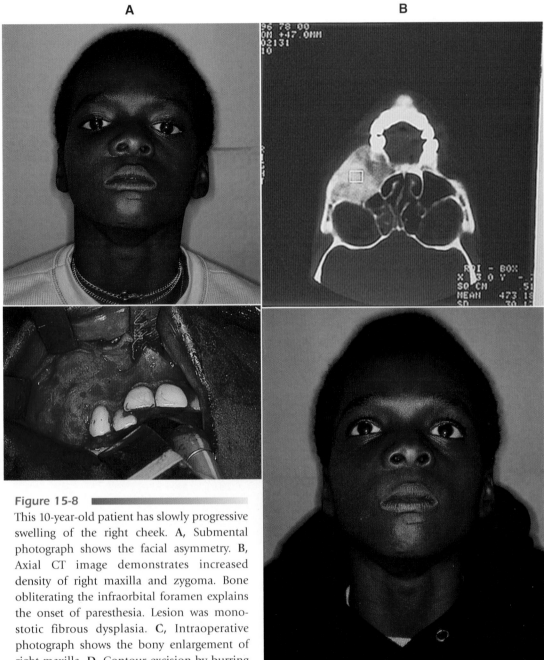

Figure 15-8

This 10-year-old patient has slowly progressive swelling of the right cheek. **A,** Submental photograph shows the facial asymmetry. **B,** Axial CT image demonstrates increased density of right maxilla and zygoma. Bone obliterating the infraorbital foramen explains the onset of paresthesia. Lesion was monostotic fibrous dysplasia. **C,** Intraoperative photograph shows the bony enlargement of right maxilla. **D,** Contour excision by burring and decompression of the infraorbital nerve was carried out (2 year postoperative photograph).

D

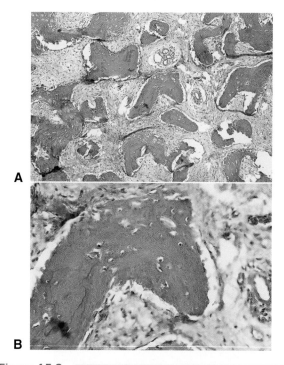

Figure 15-9

Hemotoxylin and eosin–stained histology slides at original magnification of ×100 (**A**) and ×400 (**B**) show typical pattern of fibrous dysplasia.

Ossifying Fibroma

Diagnosis. Ossifying fibroma is a variant of fibrous dysplasia, which appears as a localized, painless swelling. It occurs in the mandible more frequently than in the maxilla and grows slowly over an average of a year before detection. Although it most commonly occurs during the third and fourth decades of life, it does occur in children (Figure 15-13), especially teenagers (Figure 15-14). Pain is usually absent but displacement of teeth may occur.[1,49,50]

Radiographically, these lesions are seen as a well-defined radiolucency (see Figures 15-13 and 15-14). They may become more radiopaque with less distinct borders as they undergo maturation. Histologically, ossifying fibroma appears to be well circumscribed, with more distinct margins than fibrous dysplasia.

Treatment. Ossifying fibromas are usually well encapsulated and easily dissected from adjacent bone. Treatment, therefore, consists of local enucleation or excision. There have been reports of aggressive ossifying fibromas that have recurred after enucleation.[4,51] These lesions occur most often in the maxillas of young children (see Figure 15-13). The histologic appearance does not correlate with the aggressive clinical behavior. In addition, it is not possible to distinguish this rapidly growing tumor histologically from fibrous dysplasia in

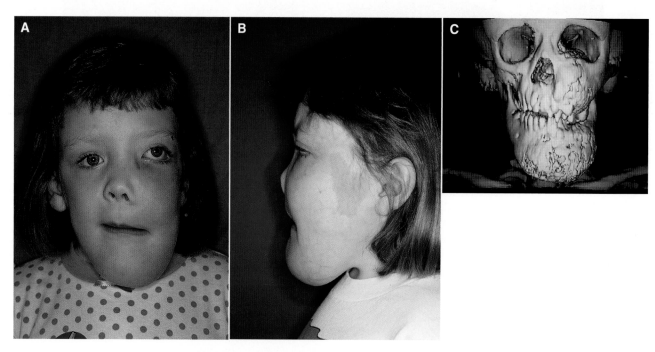

Figure 15-10

Frontal (**A**) and lateral (**B**) photographs of a 9-year-old girl with McCune-Albright syndrome. She had airway obstruction and failure to thrive because of massive growth of fibrous dysplasia in the symphysis region, displacing the tongue posteriorly into the oropharynx. She also had nasal airway obstruction due to obliteration of the left nasal passage and impaired vision due to left optic nerve compression. **C,** Three-dimensional CT image illustrates the enlargement of the mandible, left zygoma, maxilla, and orbital floor.

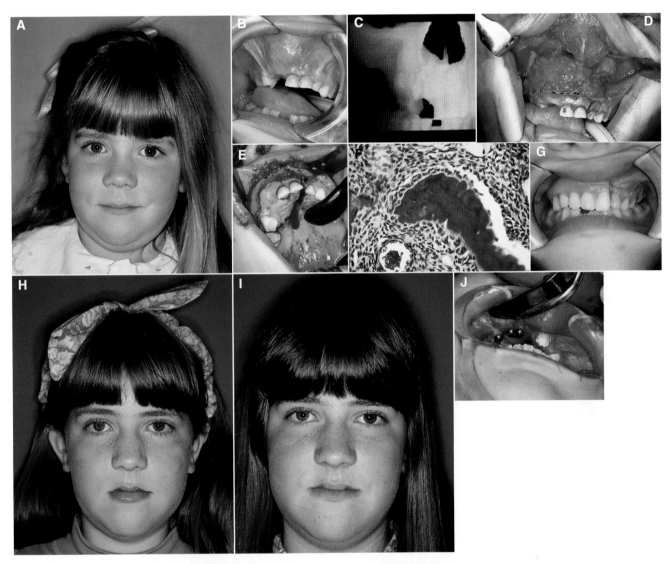

Figure 15-11

A, A 3-year-old patient with rapid onset of swelling in the anterior maxilla. The lesion had been treated with curettage several weeks previously but had recurred and increased in size. **B,** Intraoral view at time of presentation at the clinic. Note the swelling and the missing right lateral incisor and canine. These were removed as part of the previous surgery because they were loose and involved with the mass, **C,** 3D CT image shows the lesion and its relationship to the floor of the nose. **D** and **E,** Intraoperative views show en bloc resection (wide margins) dictated by the aggressive biologic behavior of this tumor. **F,** Histology slide of specimen. The tumor was labeled as an aggressive fibro-osseous lesion. Intraoral **(G)** and frontal **(H)** views 2 years later. The child has an obturator-prosthesis. **I,** Frontal view 5 years postoperatively, after having undergone bone graft reconstruction of right maxilla and subsequent implant placement **(J).** There has been no recurrence.

an active growth phase. We, therefore, classify these tumors simply as aggressive fibro-osseous lesions. In these cases, the tumor is treated by en bloc resection.

Cherubism
Diagnosis. This is an autosomal dominant trait, with 50% to 70% penetrance in females and 100% pene-

trance in males, that was first described by Jones in 1933.[52] The jaw bones are replaced by fibro-osseous tissue with a variable number of giant cells. The lesion is usually bilateral and symmetric.[53]

Age at onset is usually 3 to 4 years, and the patient has a slowly progressive, painless swelling of the jaws, more commonly in the mandible than in the maxilla

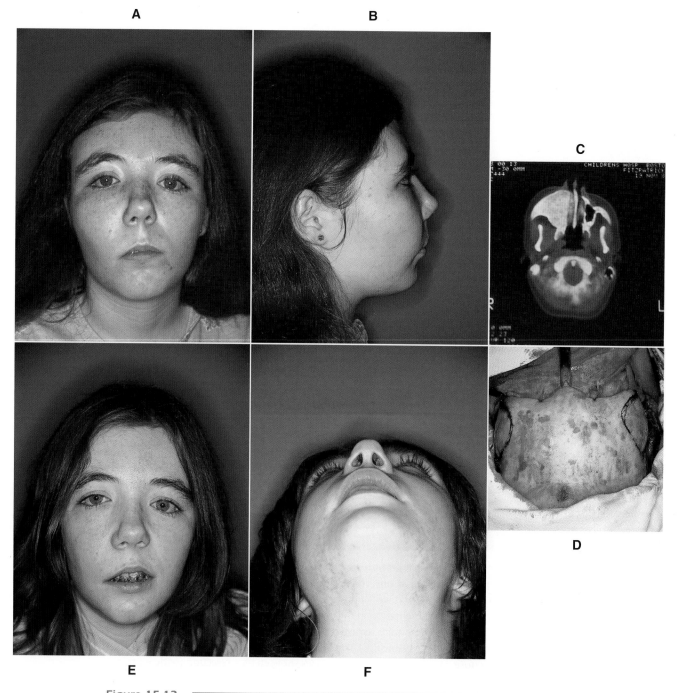

Figure 15-12

Frontal (**A**) and lateral (**B**) photographs and axial CT image (**C**) of a teenage patient with fibrous dysplasia of the maxilla, zygoma, orbit, and frontal bone bilaterally. The right zygoma and maxilla are larger than the left. **D,** Intraoperative view from the top of the head illustrates bulging of both temporal regions. The skull was exposed through a coronal incision and craniofacial dissection. The regions to be excised are drawn on the skull. Frontal (**E**) and submental (**F**) views 1 year after contour excision of both temporal regions and right zygoma and maxilla. Note the more normal contour of temporal regions and symmetry of the cheeks.

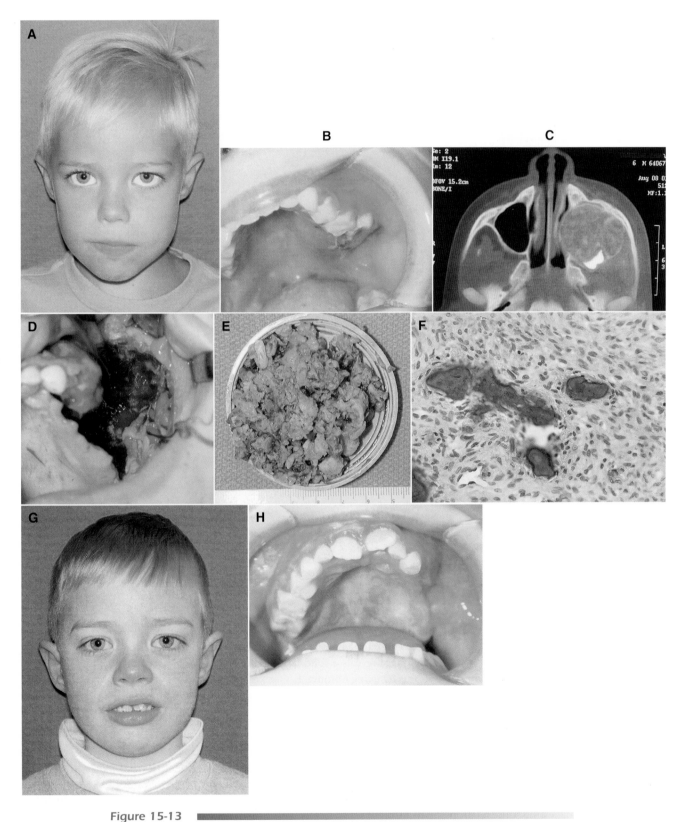

Figure 15-13

Frontal (**A**) and intraoral (**B**) photographs of a 6-year-old boy with a rapidly expanding lesion of the left maxilla. **C,** Axial CT image confirms a large tumor. Urine basic fibroblast growth factor (bFGF) was three times normal. **D** and **E,** Intraoperative views show the thorough curettage. **F,** Histology confirmed juvenile ossifying fibroma (hematoxylin and eosin, original magnification ×400). Adjuvant interferon therapy followed for 1 year. Frontal (**G**) and intraoral (**H**) photographs 2 years postoperatively. The child remains tumor free, and urine bFGF is normal. (**F** courtesy Dr. Bill Faquin.)

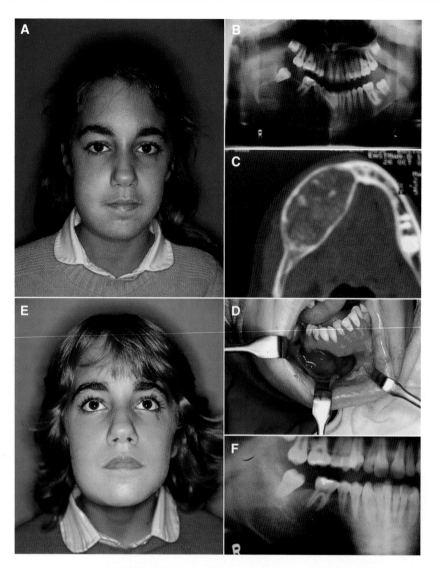

Figure 15-14

A, Teenage patient with right mandibular swelling, which was noted by a relative who had not seen her for more than a year. **B,** Panoramic radiograph shows large radiolucency and displaced second molar. **C,** Axial CT image reveals a solid lesion. **D,** Intraoperative view of enucleation of lesion. Biopsy report was ossifying fibroma. **E,** One year after enucleation, the mandible is symmetric. **F,** The defect is almost completely filled in with bone. No graft was placed.

(Figure 15-15). Swelling is most rapid during the first 2 years after onset and then gradually slows down and ceases by age 10. The disease usually is confined to the facial bones. Skin pigmentation occurs in about one third of patients, suggesting some relationship to Albright's syndrome. The patients may also have cervical adenopathy. The deciduous teeth usually are shed early, and there are often missing permanent teeth and delayed eruption.

The radiographic findings consist of bilateral symmetric radiolucencies with cortical expansion and thinning (see Figures 15-15 and 15-16). The posterior mandible is affected most commonly, and the teeth

appear to be floating in empty space. The condyles usually are spared and appear normal. When the lesions regress, the bone regains a more radiodense appearance.

There is no systemic metabolic disease and, histologically, cherubism may be indistinguishable from CGCG. Diagnosis is based on the family history, characteristic clinical picture, and location of the lesions. Recently, the gene for cherubism has been discovered, making definitive genetic diagnosis possible (see Chapter 2).

Treatment. Treatment consists of observation. When the disease becomes quiescent, the jaw can be recontoured for esthetic purposes. Surgical contouring

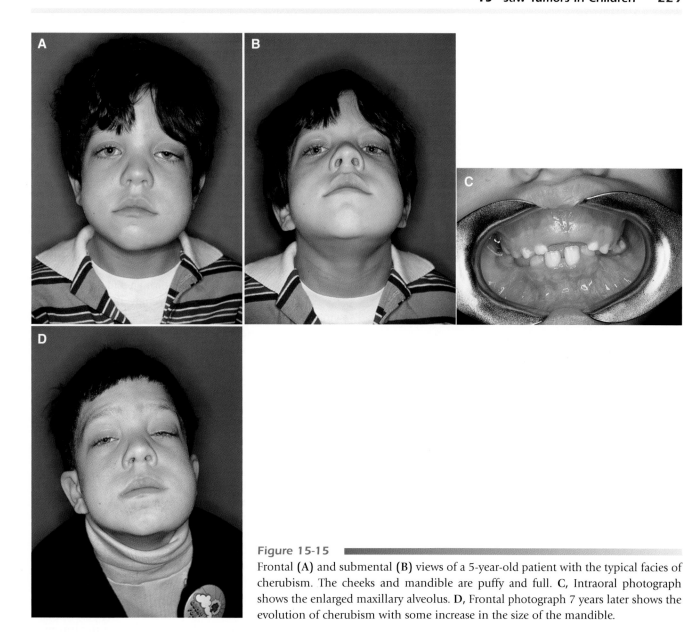

Figure 15-15
Frontal (**A**) and submental (**B**) views of a 5-year-old patient with the typical facies of cherubism. The cheeks and mandible are puffy and full. **C,** Intraoral photograph shows the enlarged maxillary alveolus. **D,** Frontal photograph 7 years later shows the evolution of cherubism with some increase in the size of the mandible.

during the growth phase is usually not necessary. The problem of early loss of deciduous teeth and delayed development and eruption of the permanent teeth is difficult, and no good treatment is available. Space maintainers are used while waiting for the permanent teeth to erupt. Surgical exposure is sometimes necessary.

There are reported cases of rapid growth and airway obstruction necessitating resection as a lifesaving maneuver.[53] In these cases, the histologic appearance of the tumor is typical of cherubism and is not predictive of the aggressive biologic behavior.

Osteoblastoma
Diagnosis. Osteoblastoma occurs most commonly in the vertebrae and long bones (80% of cases), rarely in the jaws. The tumor affects children and young adults,

with an age range of 5 to 22 years.[4,49,54] The patients experience swelling and, commonly, chronic dull pain. The calvarium is the second most common site, and the patients may have trismus if the temporal bone (glenoid fossa) and zygomatic arch are involved (Figure 15-17). Radiographically, the osteoblastoma is usually a solitary radiolucent lesion.

Treatment. En bloc resection is the required treatment for osteoblastoma because of the tendency for recurrence.

Myxoma
Diagnosis. This tumor, in our experience, occurs most commonly in the non-tooth-bearing region of the mandibular angle and ramus.[4,49] We, therefore, have classified it in the group of nonodontogenic benign

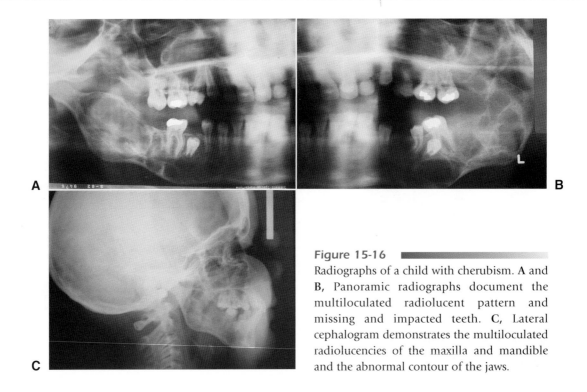

Figure 15-16
Radiographs of a child with cherubism. **A** and **B,** Panoramic radiographs document the multiloculated radiolucent pattern and missing and impacted teeth. **C,** Lateral cephalogram demonstrates the multiloculated radiolucencies of the maxilla and mandible and the abnormal contour of the jaws.

mesenchymal lesions. Other authors, however, consider myxomas to be of odontogenic origin because they rarely occur outside the mandible or maxilla. One series of 11,000 bone tumors had only three myxomas that did not occur in the mandible or maxilla.[55] Myxoma usually occurs between 20 and 40 years of age, with a mean age at diagnosis of 30 years.[56] However, the tumor also occurs frequently in children under age 10 years.[4,49,57] Children exhibit a rapidly growing, painful jaw mass. Because of the rapid onset of swelling and pain, the tumor may be diagnosed incorrectly as an acute infection such as Garre's osteomyelitis. Paresthesia is uncommon. The angle of the mandible is the most common location (Figure 15-18).

Radiographically, myxoma appears as a multiloculated radiolucency that appears to be growing out from within the bone (see Figure 15-18). Cortical perforation is common, and the lesion may be visible primarily in the soft tissue. When the maxilla is involved, the tumor may invade the antrum.

Grossly, the tumor is rubbery in consistency with a shiny, gelatinous cut surface. There is usually a fibrous capsule that may be incomplete. Histologically, there are mesenchymal cells and fibroblasts in a myxomatous stroma. The delicate reticulin fibers in the stroma may resemble the stellate reticulum of developing teeth. The tumor appears innocuous histologically, which is incon-sistent with its clinical behavior. Treatment, therefore, must not be governed by the "benign" histology report.

Treatment. Myxomas have a 25% recurrence rate partly explainable by the finger-like extensions of the multiloculated tumor into the surrounding bone.[58] Inadequate excision by curettage and expansion out of the fibrous capsule are other causes of the high recur-rence rate.[4,49] Treatment must consist of en bloc resec-tion with at least 5- to 10-mm margins. Marginal resection may be adequate for small tumors. Reconstruction may be carried out as soon as the margins are confirmed. Early reconstruction is psychologically beneficial for the child and allows continued symmetric growth of the mandible and adjacent structures (see Figure 15-18).

Aggressive Fibromatosis

Diagnosis. Aggressive fibromatosis is another "benign" but locally aggressive neoplasm of childhood.[59-62] Clini-cally, children exhibit a firm, painless swelling. Diagnosis usually occurs between the ages of 8 and 15 years.[63,64] The abdomen is the most commonly affected region, and head and neck lesions represent a large percentage of the extraabdominal lesions.[59,65,66] In the head and neck region, the mandible is affected more often than the maxilla.[62]

Radiographic findings usually show a radiolucent lesion with erosion of the adjacent cortexes.[60,63] Com-

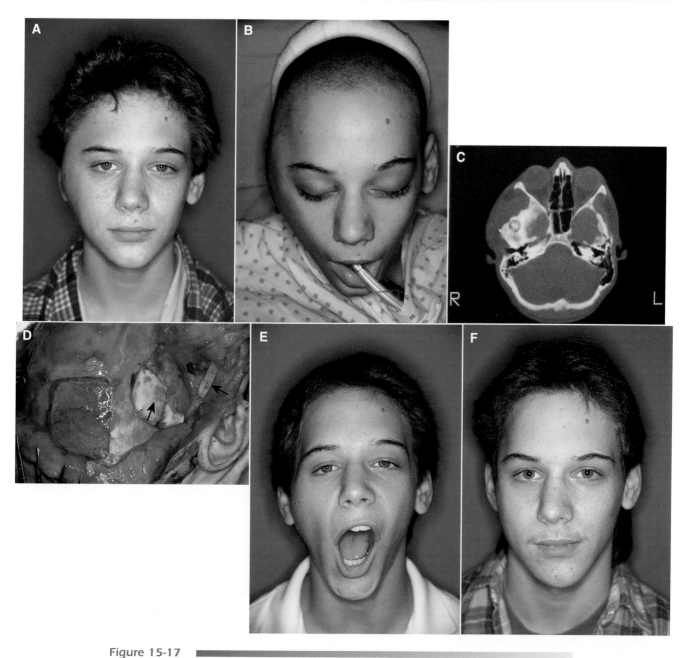

Figure 15-17

Preoperative (**A**) and intraoperative (**B**) photographs of a teenager with swelling over the right temporomandibular joint (TMJ). The patient complained of swelling, pain, and decreased motion. Maximal incisal opening was 18 mm. **C,** Axial CT image shows a bone lesion (osteoblastoma) involving the right TMJ and the floor of the middle cranial fossa. **D,** Intraoperative view, from the top, demonstrating exposure with coronal incision. The tumor has been removed, and the temporal bone, zygomatic arch, and glenoid fossa reconstructed with calvarial bone *(arrows)*. **E,** One year postoperatively the patient has a normal range of motion. **F,** Frontal photograph shows better facial symmetry.

puted tomography is helpful in determining the extent and anatomic relationships of the lesion.[61,67]

Microscopic evaluation of these lesions reveals a benign appearance consisting of mature fibroblasts within a collagen bed. The degree of cellularity is highly variable even

within the same lesion. Usually only a few mitotic figures are seen. Examination of the periphery of the lesion usually demonstrates the infiltrative nature of these lesions.[59,60,68]

Treatment. En bloc resection is the required treatment for aggressive fibromatosis because of this lesion's locally aggressive behavior and tendency for recurrence. Lesions in the head and neck have up to a 50% recurrence rate.[60,63] Wide surgical excision is the most important factor in decreasing the recurrence rate. Neither chemotherapy nor radiotherapy has been shown to be curative, although both have been effective in controlling inoperable lesions.[60]

Desmoplastic Fibroma

Diagnosis. Desmoplastic fibroma is considered by many to be the osseous counterpart of the soft tissue fibromatosis.[69-75] It is a benign lesion known to exhibit locally aggressive behavior and a high recurrence rate, with no metastatic potential. It most commonly occurs

in the metaphysis of long bones, the pelvis, and mandible, respectively, with rare cases having been reported in the maxilla.[69,71,76] Within the mandible, the posterior molar region, angle, and ascending ramus are affected most often[71,76,77] (Figure 15-19). Desmoplastic fibroma typically is seen in the first three decades of life with no sex predilection.[78-80] The clinical picture is typically a slowly enlarging mass that may be associated with pain.[71,76-78]

Radiographically, this lesion causes either a unilocular or multilocular radiolucency.[69,76,79] Cortical expansion is common, as is cortical thinning and perforation associated with soft tissue infiltration[71,76-78] (see Figure 15-19). Histologically, desmoplastic fibroma

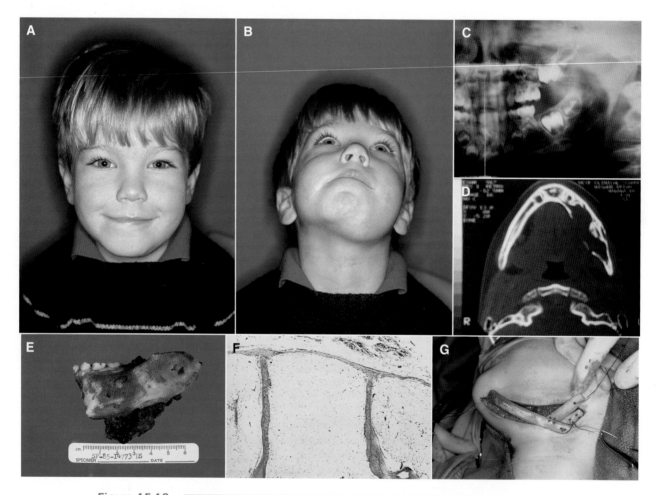

Figure 15-18

Frontal (**A**) and submental (**B**) views of a 3-year-old patient with a 3-week history of rapidly progressive swelling of the left mandible. **C,** Panoramic radiograph shows the multiloculated radiolucency mostly below the teeth and at the angle. **D,** Axial CT scan shows the tumor in the body and the ramus with perforation of lingual cortex. **E,** Lateral view of specimen. Resection was from midramus to left lateral incisor. Note tumor projecting from the inferior border. **F,** Histologic slide showing typical appearance of myxoma (hematoxylin and eosin, original magnification ×10). **G,** Reconstruction with rib grafts was performed several weeks later, when clear margins were confirmed pathologically.

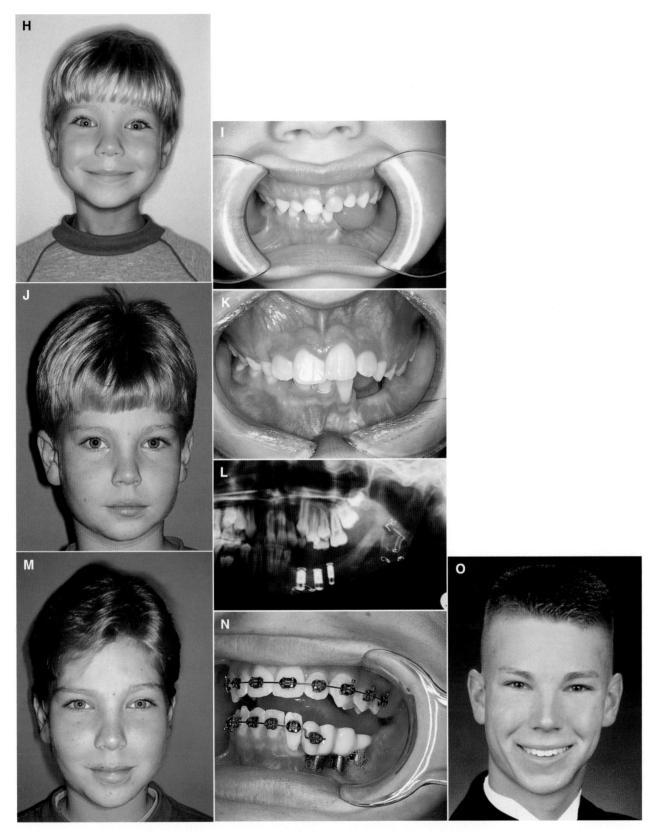

Figure 15-2—continued

Frontal (**H**) and intraoral (**I**) photographs of the patient 3 years postoperatively. Frontal (**J**) and intraoral (**K**) photographs 5 years postoperatively. Child has a symmetric face and stable occlusal relationship. The mandibular dental midline is only slightly off to the left. **L,** Panoramic radiograph shows the placement of implants 5 years after the initial surgery. Frontal (**M**) and intraoral (**N**) view of the patient 8 years after initial resection with completed reconstruction. Note the implant-borne prosthesis. **O,** High school graduation photograph.

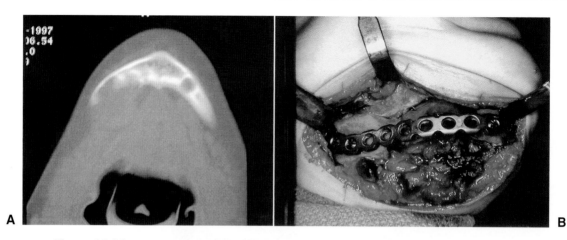

Figure 15-19

A, Axial CT image of the mandible of a 3-year-old child (same child as in Figure 10-22) with desmoplastic fibroma. Note that the lesion starts in the bone and expands into the soft tissue. **B,** En bloc resection with immediate plate reconstruction. Child underwent a staged protocol with complete reconstruction, as shown in Figure 10-22.

is identical to its soft tissue counterpart, fibromatosis. It is characterized by regions of fibroblasts of varying cellularity within an abundant matrix of collagenized fibrous connective tissue, lacking cellular pleomorphisms, mitotic figures, and hyperchromasia.[69,73,74,77,78] The absence of atypical cells is important in the distinction between desmoplastic fibroma and low-grade fibrosarcoma or intraosseous osteosarcoma, which have similar clinical and radiographic appearances[69,71,77,81] (see Figure 15-19).

Hematopoietic and Reticuloendothelial Tumors

A complete discussion of hematopoietic reticuloendothelial tumors is beyond the scope of this book. The purpose of this section is to present the relevant considerations when a pediatric patient is being evaluated for a jaw tumor that turns out to be Langerhans cell histiocytosis or Burkitt's lymphoma.

Langerhans Cell Histiocytosis

Diagnosis. The most common hematopoietic reticuloendothelial tumor in childhood is Langerhans cell histiocytosis. There are three recognized forms of this disease of unknown etiology: (1) eosinophilic granuloma, a localized bone lesion, (2) generalized or disseminated histiocytosis (previously called Hand-Schüller-Christian disease), a chronic systemic form with exophthalmos, diabetes insipidus, and bone lesions, and (3) Letterer-Siwe disease, an acute malignant form of histiocytosis with a poor prognosis.

The onset of disease is usually in early or late childhood. These children may first have oral symptoms. Chuong and Kaban[4] reported that in five (of six) of their patients, the diagnosis was made as a result of symptoms in the maxillofacial region: swelling of the jaw, pain, nonhealing gingival swelling, ulcers, and loose teeth (Figures 15-20 to 15-22). Other symptoms include malaise, fever, weight loss, and a skin rash. Children with multiple bone lesions may have exophthalmos and diabetes insipidus. Those with Letterer-Siwe disease have bone marrow involvement with a leukemia-like initial clinical picture. Patients with eosinophilic granuloma develop isolated bone lesions.

Central lytic lesions of the jaws occur in all three forms of histiocytosis. They are localized, "punched out" radiolucencies with no calcification and no sign of sclerosis or reaction at the borders. There may be severe alveolar bone resorption producing the appearance of teeth "floating" in space (see Figure 15-21).

Diagnostic workup includes biopsy of the jaw mass and skeletal survey to detect other bone lesions. A complete blood count, urinalysis, urine and serum osmolality, electrolyte levels, and bone marrow biopsy are also obtained (Figure 15-23).

Treatment. Patients with generalized Langerhans cell histiocytosis are treated with chemotherapy (alkylating agents, folate antagonists, steroids). Thymic humeral factor also has been used in a variety of clinical trials. Eosinophilic granuloma is cured by either enucleation or, in rare cases, local low-dose radiation (600 rads), depending on the location of the tumor. Although these lesions are very sensitive to radiation, most are treated

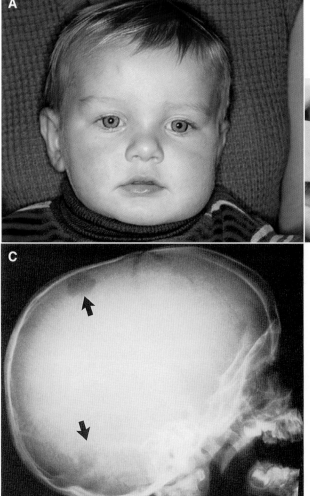

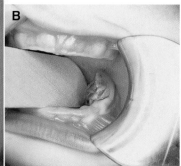

Figure 15-20
A, Photograph of an 18-month-old child with rapidly enlarging swelling of the left mandible. This was initially thought to be an infection, but lack of response to intravenous antibiotics led to referral to our clinic. **B,** Intraoral view shows exophytic mass of the left body of the mandible. Biopsy of this lesion led to the pathologic diagnosis of Langerhans cell histiocytosis. **C,** Lateral radiograph of the head shows lesions *(arrows)*.

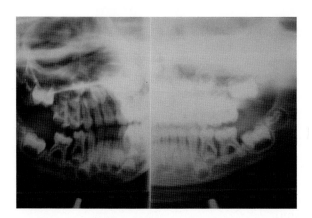

Figure 15-21
Panoramic radiograph of a child with bone resorption and loosening of teeth secondary to histiocytosis.

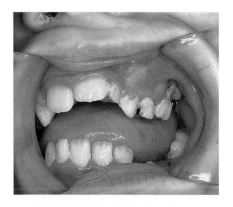

Figure 15-22
Intraoral view of a child with histiocytosis demonstrating gingival recession and bone resorption in the left maxillary molar region.

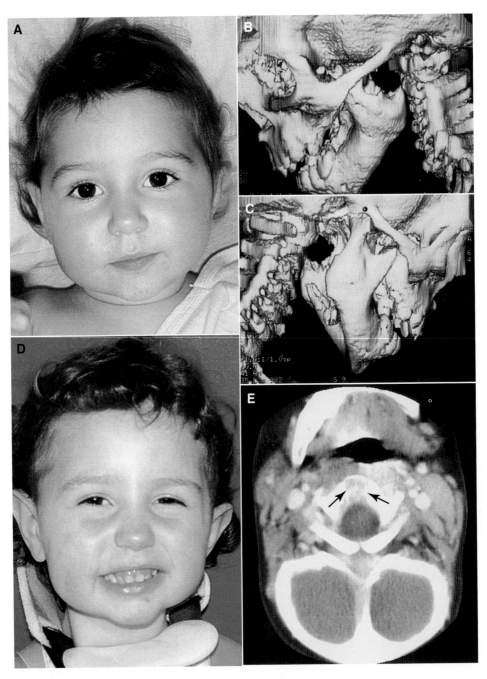

Figure 15-23

A, Frontal photograph of an 18-month-old child. **B** and **C,** 3D CT images demonstrate a lytic lesion of the left ramus and condyle. Excisional biopsy led to histologic diagnosis of eosinophilic granuloma. Initial body scan revealed no other lesions. Subsequent scans revealed multiple lesions of the cervical and thoracic vertebral bodies, leading to the diagnosis of Langerhans cell histiocytosis, disseminated form. **D,** Frontal photograph of the child wearing a stabilizing brace. **E,** Axial CT image showing lesion *(arrows)* within the C2 vertebral body. Child is currently on chemotherapy for disseminated disease.

by enucleation to avoid long-term growth complications and malignant transformations.

Burkitt's Lymphoma

Diagnosis. Burkitt's lymphoma, first reported in 1958, is an undifferentiated form of lymphoma that frequently produces extranodal disease.[82] The etiology is thought to be the Epstein-Barr virus, although this has not been established definitively.[83] The tumor most commonly affects children and involves abdominal or pelvic viscera, retroperitoneum, facial and long bones, central nervous system, and salivary glands[84] (Figure 15-24).

Jaw tumors occur more frequently in the African form than in the American form of Burkitt's lymphoma. The maxilla is involved twice as frequently as the mandible, although involvement of both jaws is not uncommon. The patient experiences swelling, premature loss of teeth, mild pain, and only rarely paresthesia. The posterior maxilla is the most common site, and invasion into the maxillary sinus may lead to proptosis. Radiographically, the lesion is radiolucent and the lamina dura around the teeth may be lost. Histologically, the tumor demonstrates the "starry sky" appearance of numerous small round cells in a fibrous stroma.

Treatment. Treatment of Burkitt's lymphoma consists of high-dose alkylating agents and selective surgical debulking. This results in remission in over 90% of cases. Relapse, when it occurs, may respond to further chemotherapy.[85] Untreated, this disease carries an extremely poor prognosis; death occurs within 6 months in most cases.

Neurogenic Tumors

Neurofibroma. Tumors of neurogenic origin are among the most rare primary jaw tumors in children. Chuong and Kaban[4] found six such cases in their series. The youngest patient had a melanotic neuroectodermal tumor appearing as an enlarging maxillary mass at age 7 weeks. A 10-year-old patient had a metastatic ganglioneuroma to the mandible. She experienced pain

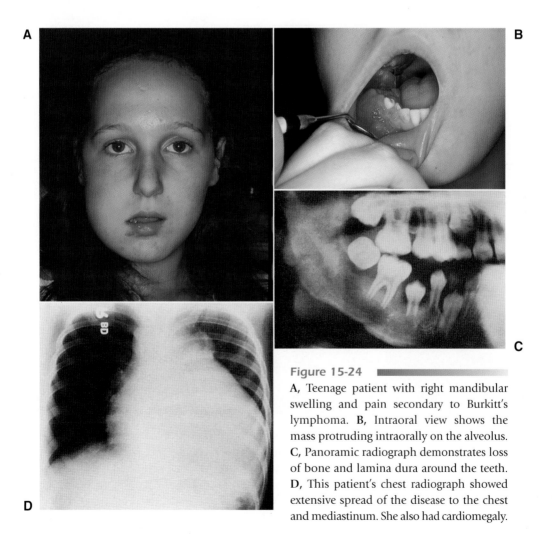

Figure 15-24

A, Teenage patient with right mandibular swelling and pain secondary to Burkitt's lymphoma. **B,** Intraoral view shows the mass protruding intraorally on the alveolus. **C,** Panoramic radiograph demonstrates loss of bone and lamina dura around the teeth. **D,** This patient's chest radiograph showed extensive spread of the disease to the chest and mediastinum. She also had cardiomegaly.

and swelling 7 years after a primary adrenal tumor had apparently been treated successfully by resection and chemotherapy. Neurofibromas were the most common jaw tumors of neurogenic origin. They involved the maxilla (n = 2), mandible (n = 1), and both jaws (n = 1). The patients exhibited multilocular radiolucencies and bony expansion. The neurofibroma of the jaw usually was associated with an overlying soft tissue neurofibroma (Figure 15-25). There was generally no pain or paresthesia. In three of the five cases, involvement was extensive, including the temporal bone and zygoma in addition to the maxilla (Figure 15-26). During the same 10-year period, 14 cases of extensive neurofibromatosis involving the face were encountered, but only the four mentioned showed direct involvement of the jaw bones.

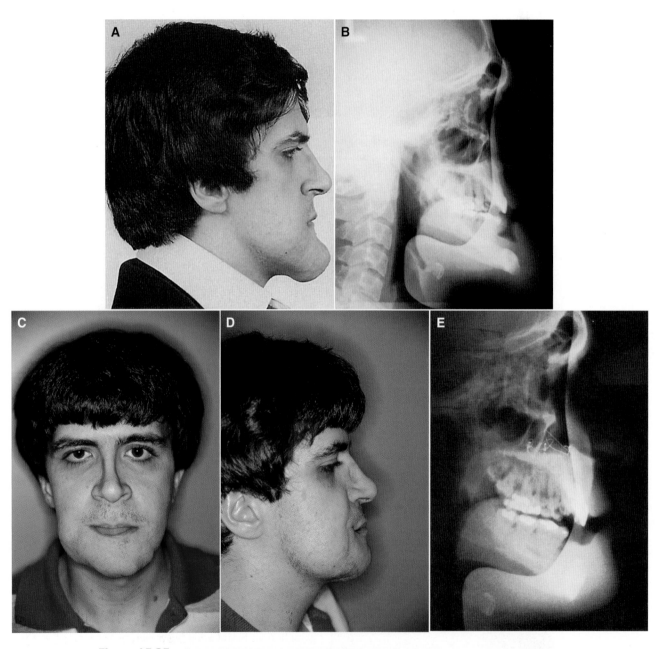

Figure 15-25

A, Lateral photograph shows a large neurofibroma of the mandible and overlying soft tissue. **B,** Lateral cephalogram shows an atrophic mandible deep to the neurofibroma. This lesion, including the mandibular alveolus, had been partially excised in the past. Frontal **(C)** and lateral **(D)** photographs several years after excision of the mass and bone graft to the mandible. **E,** Postoperative lateral cephalogram.

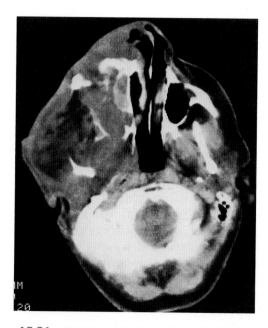

Figure 15-26

Axial CT image of a patient with extensive soft tissue and bony neurofibroma of the right maxilla, zygoma, and orbit.

Diagnosis. Central neurofibromas of the jaws occur more often as solitary lesions rather than as part of a generalized neurofibromatosis.[86] The bone adjacent to or directly involved is extremely vascular. The patients usually have dull pain and paresthesia. Most often, the lesions occur in the mandible,[87] appearing radiographically as a fusiform expansion of the mandibular canal. Bone adjacent to an overlying soft tissue neurofibroma may appear as a radiolucency with cortical thinning and irregular boundaries (see Figures 15-25 and 15-26).

Bone involvement in neurofibromatosis usually results from subperiosteal erosion.[86,88] Others report predominantly bony hypoplasia associated with facial neurofibromatosis.[89,90] Our cases were consistent with erosion and expansion of bone in areas contiguous with soft tissue neurofibromas.[4] The bone is extremely vascular and very much like a primary bony vascular malformation in character.

Histologically, the neurofibroma is composed of Schwann cells and neurites in an irregular pattern. Development of a sarcoma in neurofibromatosis occurs in approximately 15% of cases; no specific figure is available for central jaw lesions. It is known, however, that solitary neurofibromas rarely undergo malignant transformation.

Treatment. Treatment consists of close observation and surgical excision of lesions that exhibit progressive growth or produce pain or paresthesia. The purpose of the operation is to excise or debulk the soft tissue mass and recontour the underlying bone. Because neurofibromatosis is a systemic disease and present in all cells,

even when total gross excision of a bone lesion is achieved, the recurrence rate is high. The tumors are extremely vascular, and significant blood loss is a major problem. The patients have to be observed for life for recurrent and new lesions.

Melanotic Neuroectodermal Tumor of Infancy

Diagnosis. The melanotic neuroectodermal tumor of infancy was reported first in 1918. Since that time many other names have been applied to this tumor as a result of multiple theories on the tissue of origin.[49,91] Currently, it is believed that the tumor arises from neural crest tissue. This is supported by the elevated levels of urinary vanillylmandelic acid, a feature of other tumors derived from the neural crest (neuroblastoma and pheochromocytoma).[92]

Melanotic neuroectodermal tumor of infancy usually occurs within the first 6 months of life in the anterior maxilla. There is usually a swelling in the canine region with elevation of the upper lip. Mandibular involvement is rare, as are tumors in extraoral sites such as the scapula, mediastinum, epididymis, and cerebellum. There are no systemic signs or symptoms. Grossly, the lesion is brown or black in color. Radiographically, it is radiolucent and displaces the adjacent tooth buds.[91-93]

Histologically, the tumor is nonencapsulated, with infiltrating projections of tumor cells in alveolar-like arrangements within a vascular stroma. Cells have a pale cytoplasm and contain brown melanin granules.

Treatment. This tumor is best treated by conservative local en bloc excision or enucleation. The recurrence rate has been reported as 15%; none of the tumors has metastasized.[94]

Vascular Lesions

Primary vascular lesions of the jaws occur infrequently in children. The literature is replete with confusing terminology and concepts of diagnosis and treatment. Chapter 17 is devoted completely to diagnosis and treatment of vascular lesions. Most vascular lesions do not involve bone primarily. Hemangiomas very rarely occur in bone, and vascular malformations are present in bone in only 35% of cases.[95,96] In a review of pediatric jaw tumors, there were two primary vascular lesions of the jaws: (1) a central vascular malformation of the mandible in a patient with Rendu-Osler-Weber syndrome and (2) an aneurysmal bone cyst.[4]

Malignant Mesenchymal Tumors

Patients with these tumors experience progressive pain and swelling, often without paresthesia. A lack of sensory disturbance is not a reliable sign of benign versus malignant disease in children. Examination reveals a painful swelling, and radiographs reveal a radiolucency that may be multilocular. There may be a layered, "onion skin," peripheral periosteal reaction. The most common histologic pattern on biopsy is osteogenic sarcoma, followed by chondrosarcoma and then fibrosarcoma, malignant mesenchymoma, and Ewing's sarcoma.

Patients with osteosarcoma are most frequently teenagers, and the mandible is the most common site. They may seek treatment for a slow-growing mass with little pain and no paresthesia or with a painful mass with paresthesia. Any suspicious mandibular bone lesion, especially if it increases in size or displaces teeth, should be biopsied to rule out osteosarcoma (Figure 15-27). Treatment of osteosarcoma at the Massachusetts General Hospital for Children consists of biopsy to confirm diagnosis. In the pediatric patient, this is followed by an induction phase of chemotherapy (10 weeks). Between weeks 10 and 12, the tumor is resected with 1.5 cm of clear margins. The specimen is examined histologically for the percentage of tumor cells killed. If the number is greater than 95%, the chemotherapy is completed with a 20- to 25-week post-operative chemotherapy phase (also called the *continuation phase*), and the prognosis is 85% event free (Figure 15-28). If percentage is less than 95%, then the chemotherapy regimen is changed and the prognosis is reduced markedly.[97] For further details on osteosarcoma, see Chapter 16.

In our series, a Ewing's sarcoma (Figure 15-29) occurred in the mandible of a teenager, whereas the other sarcomas occurred in the maxilla[4] (Figure 15-30). Treat-ment consisted of radical surgical excision followed by radiation and chemotherapy. Radiation was the primary treatment for the patient with Ewing's sarcoma.

Malignant Epithelial Tumors

Malignant epithelial tumors of the jaws are the most rare pediatric jaw tumors. In the Children's Hospital series,[4] there was only one malignant mucoepidermoid carcinoma of the anterior maxilla in a 16-year-old girl. Initial symptoms were pain and swelling of the upper lip and maxillary alveolus. Apical curettage during surgical endodontic treatment of an upper incisor provided tissue for diagnosis. Recurrence occurred 6 months after partial maxillectomy. At that time, metastases to the cervical lymph nodes were also noted. Further local resection in combination with radical neck dissection was carried out. The patient was tumor free at 36 months' follow-up (see Chapter 14).

DISCUSSION

Benign mesenchymal tumors are the most common jaw tumors in the pediatric patient group. They all appear histologically "benign" and do not metastasize. However, giant cell lesions and myxomas, as well as some fibro-osseous lesions, may exhibit a locally aggressive growth pattern with a high recurrence rate. Treatment must, therefore, be planned with particular attention to the biologic behavior of the tumor and not its name. Tumors that exhibit a rapid growth pattern, pain, paresthesia, displacement of adjacent teeth, and root resorption should be treated with en bloc excision

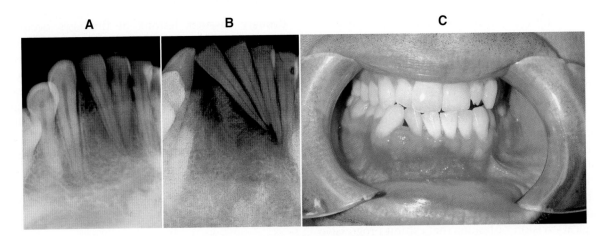

A   B   C

Figure 15-27

A, Periapical radiograph of a teenager 10 years before presentation. Note the displaced roots but no obvious lesion. **B** and **C,** As a young adult, the patient noted a rapidly expanding intraoral lesion. Biopsy confirmed osteogenic sarcoma.

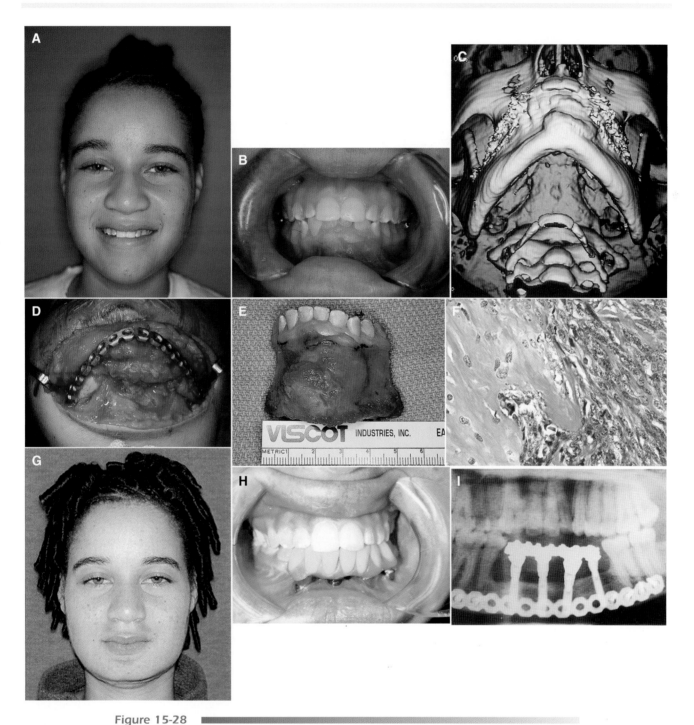

Figure 15-28
Frontal (A) and intraoral (B) photographs and 3D CT image (C) of a 14-year-old girl with a rapidly growing lesion of the anterior mandible. Incisional biopsy confirmed osteogenic sarcoma. The child underwent preoperative chemotherapy. D and E, En bloc resection was performed with immediate plate reconstruction. F, Histology of typical osteogenic sarcoma. The percentage of tumor kill was greater than 95%. Postoperative chemotherapy was completed. Frontal (G) and intraoral (H) photographs and panoramic radiograph (I) 3 years later after bone graft, implant placement, and prosthetic reconstruction. (F courtesy Dr. Bill Faquin.)

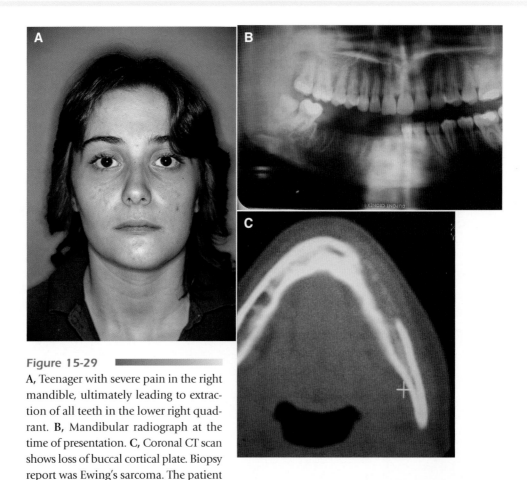

Figure 15-29

A, Teenager with severe pain in the right mandible, ultimately leading to extraction of all teeth in the lower right quadrant. **B,** Mandibular radiograph at the time of presentation. **C,** Coronal CT scan shows loss of buccal cortical plate. Biopsy report was Ewing's sarcoma. The patient had no metastatic disease at this time but eventually died of metastasis 2 years later.

regardless of the histologic diagnosis. Less biologically aggressive lesions may be treated by enucleation or curettage.

Giant cell lesions illustrate this point best. Aggressive and nonaggressive central giant cell lesions and brown tumors of hyperparathyroidism are indistinguishable histologically from each other and from some types of fibro-osseous lesions (e.g., cherubism). However, these tumors may have significantly different biologic behavior patterns. For example, the lesion of cherubism is generally slow growing and has a tendency to regress as a child approaches puberty. There are, however, instances of rapid expansion of this lesion causing airway compromise and gross disfigurement that cannot be explained histologically.[53] The brown tumor, on the other hand, develops secondary to an endocrine derangement and typically resolves after correction of the hyperparathyroidism. Finally, the aggressive giant cell lesion has a high recurrence rate if treated by enucleation alone.

Central jaw tumors in the pediatric age group are uncommon. When they occur, they usually are derived from nonodontogenic mesenchymal tissue.[1,4,49] In general, pain is a significant complaint in patients with malignant lesions such as osteogenic sarcoma, Burkitt's lymphoma, and biologically aggressive "benign" tumors such as giant cell lesions, myxomas, and rapidly growing fibroosseous lesions. Loose and displaced teeth with radiographic evidence of root resorption are also common in malignant and aggressive benign tumors. Paresthesia is a very uncommon finding, although subtle sensory changes may be difficult to document because of the young age of the patients. Systemic symptoms such as fever, malaise, weight loss, and decreased appetite are characteristic of the hematopoietic and reticuloendothelial lesions.

The surgeon may be confused by a variety of benign and malignant lesions that contain giant cells. Benign lesions include aneurysmal bone cyst, brown tumor of hyperparathyroidism, fibrous dysplasia, giant cell lesions,

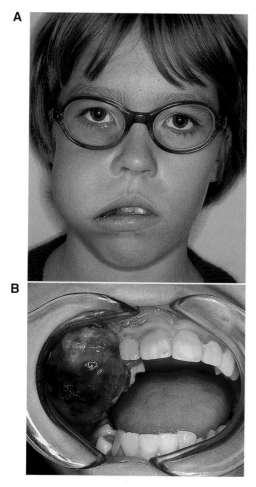

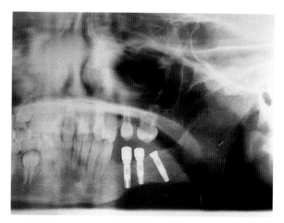

Figure 15-31

Panoramic radiograph of a 12-year-old child with implants in the mandible. Five years previously, at age 7, the child had an en bloc resection for a benign but locally aggressive tumor. No bone graft was placed. The mandible completely regenerated spontaneously.

Figure 15-30

A, This child presented with rapidly growing, painful swelling of the right cheek and maxilla. **B,** Intraoral view shows large tumor. There was no paresthesia. The mass was biopsied, and the pathologic diagnosis was rhabdomyosarcoma.

ossifying fibroma, and cherubism. Malignant lesions that contain giant cells include osteogenic sarcoma, fibrosarcoma, malignant fibrous histiocytoma, and malignant giant cell tumor. Histologically differentiation among these lesions may be difficult. For example, Waldron[98] reviewed 28 cases of giant cell tumors of the jaws and concluded that 9 had been misdiagnosed and represented fibrous dysplasia instead.

Comprehensive treatment of children with jaw tumors must also include rehabilitative surgery. We recently reported treatment of nine children with aggressive jaw lesions using a staged protocol consisting of (1) en bloc resection of the tumor and immediate placement of a rigid reconstruction plate across the mandibular defect (or an obturator for maxillary defects), (2) restoration of skeletal continuity with an autogenous bone graft approximately 6 months later, (3) placement of osseoin-tegrated implants (6 months after the bone graft, and (4) prosthetic restoration.[99]

In a staged protocol, the use of rigid internal fixation techniques without an immediate bone graft allows the surgeon to accomplish the resection and maintain the jaw segments, occlusion, and facial esthetics. The surgeon is then able to obtain definitive pathologic analysis of the resection margins. If an immediate bone graft is used, a positive margin may result in loss of the bone graft. Furthermore, in younger children the bone may regenerate spontaneously after resection (Figure 15-31). Maintenance of regenerated or grafted bone volume can be achieved using endosseous implants (see Chapter 10, Figure 10-22).[99]

CONCLUSION

A careful history and a complete physical examination are particularly important in the diagnosis of jaw tumors in children. When appropriate, intraoral or panoramic radiographs are obtained to screen rapidly for radiolytic or radiopaque lesions. Laboratory studies include serum calcium, phosphorus, total protein, and alkaline phosphatase determinations, and a complete blood count. Hand radiographs may help to support the diagnosis of hyperparathyroidism. In children, hyperparathyroidism associated with chronic renal failure is much more common than primary hyperparathyroidism. Computed tomography with selective use of intravenous contrast material may assist in distinguishing vascular from nonvascular lesions. Radionucleotide bone scans using technetium and gallium or indium or magnetic resonance imaging may help to differentiate osteomyelitis from noninflammatory lesions of the jaws.

Biopsy establishes the histologic diagnosis. In children, this is best done under general anesthesia. Although most jaw lesions are accessible intraorally, the surgeon should not hesitate to obtain tissue by an extraoral approach. Failure to obtain adequate tumor tissue was the most common reason for incorrect diagnosis reported by Chuong and Kaban.[4] If, after biopsy, there is uncertainty about the diagnosis, or if the diagnosis is not consistent with the clinical course, more tissue should be obtained. Communication between surgeon and pathologist is essential to establish the correct diagnosis and treatment. This is particularly true of pediatric jaw tumors, because histology and biologic behavior often do not correlate. The extent of resection should be determined by the latter. Concerns about interference with facial growth by resection are subordinate to control of the primary tumor and are not necessarily valid.[3,4,100,101] Children who undergo major resections of the maxilla or mandible appear to grow normally after early reconstruction with autogenous bone.

REFERENCES

1. Dehner LP: Tumors of the mandible and maxilla in children. I. Clinicopathologic study of 46 histologically benign lesions, *Cancer* 31:364, 1973.
2. Dehner LP: Tumors of the mandible and maxilla in children. II. A study of 14 primary and secondary malignant tumors, *Cancer* 32:112, 1973.
3. Lewin ML: Nonmalignant maxillofacial tumors in children, *Plast Reconstr Surg* 38:186, 1966.
4. Chuong R, Kaban LB: Diagnosis and treatment of jaw tumors in children, *J Oral Maxillofac Surg* 43:323, 1985.
5. Gorlin RI, Meskin LH, Brodwy R: Odontogenic tumors in man and animals—pathological classification and clinical behavior: a review, *Ann N Y Acad Sci* 108:722, 1963.
6. Sehdev MK, Huvos AG, Strong EW, et al: Ameloblastoma of maxilla and mandible, *Cancer* 33:324, 1974.
7. Cusak IW: Report of the amputations of portions of the lower jaw, *Dublin Hosp Rec* 4:1, 1827.
8. Robinson L, Martinez MG: Unicystic ameloblastoma: a prognostically distinct entity, *Cancer* 40:2278, 1977.
9. Gardner DG: Peripheral ameloblastoma: a study of 21 cases, including 5 reported as basal cell carcinoma of the gingival, *Cancer* 39:1625, 1977.
10. Gardner DG: A pathologist's approach to the treatment of ameloblastoma, *J Oral Maxillofac Surg* 42:161, 1984.
11. Ord RA, Blanchaert RH, Nikitakis NG, Sauk JJ: Ameloblastoma in children, *J Oral Maxillofac Surg* 60:762-770, 2002.
12. Bhaskar SN: Oral tumors of infancy and childhood, *J Pediatr* 63:204, 1963.
13. Blackwood HI: Odontogenic tumors in the child, *Br Dent J* 119:431, 1965.
14. Leider AS, Eversole LR, Barkin ME: Cystic ameloblastoma: a clinicopathologic analysis, *Oral Surg Oral Med Oral Pathol* 60:624, 1985.
15. Carr RF, Halperin V: Malignant ameloblastomas from 1953 to 1966: review of the literature and report of a case, *Oral Surg* 25:514, 1968.
16. Ackermann GL, Altini M, Shear M: The unicystic ameloblastoma: a clinicopathological study of 57 cases, *J Oral Pathol* 17:541, 1988.
17. Becker R, Pertl A: Zur therapie des ameloblastoma, *Dtsch Zahn Mund Kieferheilkd* 49:423, 1967.
18. Mehlisch DR, Dahlin DC, Masson IK: Ameloblastoma: a clinicopathologic report, *J Oral Surg* 30:9, 1972.
19. Fitzgerald GWN, Frenkiel S, Black MI, et al: Ameloblastoma of the jaws: a 12-year review of the McGill experience, *J Otolaryngol* 11:23, 1982.
20. Silverman S, Gordon G, Grant T, et al: The dental structures in hyperparathyroidism, *J Oral Surg* 15:426, 1962.
21. Chuong R, Kaban LB, Kozakewitch H, et al: Central giant cell lesions of the jaws: a clinicopathologic study, *J Oral Maxillofac Surg* 44:708, 1986.
22. Ficarro G, Kaban LB, Hansen L: Central giant cell lesions of the mandible and maxilla: a clinicopathologic and cytometric study, *J Oral Surg* 64:44, 1987.
23. Granite EL, Aronoff AK, Gold L: Central giant cell granuloma of the mandible: a case report, *J Oral Surg* 53:241, 1982.
24. Small GS, Rowe NH: A true giant cell tumor: in the mandible, *J Oral Surg* 33:296-301, 1975.
25. Leban SF, Lepore H, Stratigos GI, Chu F: The giant cell lesion of jaws: neoplastic or reparative? *J Oral Surg* 29:398, 1971.
26. Kaban LB, Dodson TD: Calcitonin therapy for central giant cell granuloma, *J Oral Maxillofac Surg* 61:653, 2003.
27. Kaban LB, Troulis MJ, Ebb D, et al: Antiangiogenic therapy with interferon-alpha for giant cell lesions of the jaws, *J Oral Maxillofac Surg* 60:1103, 2002.
28. Pogrel MA: Calcitonin therapy for central giant cell granuloma, *J Oral Maxillofac Surg* 61:649, 2003.
29. Terry BC, Jacoway JR: Management of central giant cell lesions: an alternative to surgical therapy, *Oral Maxillofac Clin North Am* 6:579, 1994.
30. Harris M: Central giant cell granulomas of the jaws regress with calcitonin therapy, *Br J Oral Maxillofac Surg* 31:89, 1993.
31. Kaban LB, Mulliken JB, Ezekowitz RA, et al: Antiangiogenic therapy of a recurrent giant cell tumor of the mandible with interferon alpha-2a, *Pediatrics* 103:1145, 1999.
32. Reference deleted in proofs.
33. Lin PP, Guzel VB, Moura MF, et al: Long-term follow-up of patients with giant cell tumor of the sacrum treated with selective arterial embolization, *Cancer* 95(6):1317, 2002.
34. Lackman RD, Khoury LD, Esmail A, Donthineni-Rao R: The treatment of sacral giant cell tumours by serial arterial embolisation, *J Bone Joint Surg Br* 84(6):873, 2002.
35. Folkman J: Discussion: antiangiogenic therapy with interferon alpha for giant cell lesions of the jaw, *J Oral Maxillofac Surg* 60(10):1111, 2002.
36. Zimmerman DC, Dahlin DC, Stafne EC: Fibrous dysplasia of the maxilla and mandible, *J Oral Surg* 11:55, 1958.
37. Houston WO: Fibrous dysplasia of maxilla and mandible: clinicopathologic study and comparison of facial bone lesions with lesions affecting general skeleton, *J Oral Surg* 23:17, 1965.
38. Smith JF: Fibrous dysplasia of the jaws, *AMA Arch Otolaryngol* 81:592, 1965.
39. Kaban LB, Pelletier R, Glowacki J: Relationship of mast cell count to clinical behavior of fibrous dysplasia. Unpublished data, 1984.
40. McCune DJ, Bruch H: Osteodystrophia fibrosa, *Am J Dis Child* 54:806, 1937.
41. Albright F, Butler AM, Hampton AO, Smith P: Syndrome characterized by osteitis fibrosa disseminata, areas of pigmentation and endocrine dysfunction, with precocious puberty in females, *N Engl J Med* 216:727, 1937.

42. Ringel MD, Schwindinger WF, Levine MA: Clinical implications of genetic defects in G proteins: the molecular basis of McCune-Albright syndrome and Albright hereditary osteodystrophy, *Medicine* 75(4):171, 1996.

43. Shenker A, Weinstein LS, Moran A, et al: Severe endocrine and non endocrine manifestations of the McCune-Albright syndrome associated with activating mutations of stimulatory G protein G$_s$, *J Pediatr* 123(4):509, 1993.

44. Foser CM, Ross JL, Shawker T, et al: Absence of pubertal gonadotropin secretion in girls with McCune-Albright syndrome, *J Clin Endocrinol Metab* 58(6):1161, 1984.

45. Schwindinger WF, Francomano CA, Levine MA: Identification of a mutation in the gene encoding the a subunit of the stimulatory G protein of adenylyl cyclase in McCune-Albright syndrome, *Proc Natl Acad Sci U S A* 89:5152, 1992.

46. Happle R: The McCune-Albright syndrome: a lethal gene surviving mosaicism, *Clin Genet* 29(4):321, 1986.

47. Munro IR, Chan Y: Radical treatment for frontoorbital fibrous dysplasia: the chain-link fence, *Plast Reconstr Surg* 67:719, 1981.

48. Sach SA, Kleiman M, Pasternak R: Surgical management of a facial deformity secondary to craniofacial fibrous dysplasia, *J Oral Maxillofac Surg* 42:192, 1984.

49. Kaban LB, Chuong R: Nonmucosal neoplasms of the maxillofacial region. In Peterson DE, Elias EG, Sonis ST, editors: *Head and neck management of the cancer patient*, Boston, 1986, Martinus Nijhoff.

50. Hamner JE, Scofield HH, Cornyn J: Benign fibro-osseous jaw lesions of periodontal membrane origin: an analysis of 249 cases, *Cancer* 22:861, 1968.

51. Kennett S, Curran JB: Giant cemento-ossifying fibroma: report of a case, *J Oral Surg* 30:513, 1972.

52. Jones WA: Familial multilocular cystic disease of the jaws, *Am J Cancer* 17:946, 1933.

53. Hamner JE, Ketcham AS: Cherubism: an analysis and treatment, *Cancer* 23:1133, 1969.

54. Farman AG, Nortje CJ, Grotepass F: Periosteal benign osteoblastoma of the mandible: report of a case and review of the literature pertaining to benign osteoblastic neoplasms of the jaws, *Br J Oral Surg* 14:12, 1976.

55. McClure DK, Dahlin DC: Myxoma of bone: report of 3 cases, *Mayo Clin Proc* 52:249, 1977.

56. Zimmerman DC, Dahlin DC: Myxomatous tumors of the jaws, *Oral Surg* 11:1069, 1958.

57. Smith GA, Konrad HR, Canalis RF: Childhood myxomas of the head and neck, *J Otolaryngol* 6:423, 1977.

58. Whitman RA, Stewart S, Stoopack JG, Jerrold TL: Myxoma of the mandible: report of a case, *J Oral Surg* 29:63, 1971.

59. Conley J, Healey WV, Stout AP: Fibromatosis of the head and neck, *Am J Surg* 112:609, 1996.

60. Fowler CB, Hartman KS, Brannon RB: Fibromatosis of the oral and paraoral region, *Oral Surg Oral Med Oral Pathol* 77:373, 1994.

61. Petchprapa CN, Haller JO, Schraft S: Imaging characteristics of aggressive fibromatosis in children, *Comput Med Imaging Graph* 20:153, 1996.

62. Donohue WB, Malexos D, Pham H: Aggressive fibromatosis of the maxilla. Report of a case and review of the literature, *Oral Surg Oral Med Oral Pathol* 69:420, 1990.

63. Vally IM, Altini M: Fibromatoses of the oral and paraoral soft tissues and jaws, *Oral Surg Oral Med Oral Pathol* 69:191, 1990.

64. Dehner LP, Askin FB: Tumors of fibrous origin in childhood, *Cancer* 38:888, 1976.

65. Kauffman SL, Stout AP: Congenital mesenchymal tumors, *Cancer* 18:460, 1965.

66. Das Gupta TK, Brasfield RD, O'Hara J: Extra-abdominal desmoids, *Ann Surg* 170:109, 1969.

67. Thompson DH, Kahn A, Gonzalez C, Auclair P: Juvenile aggressive fibromatosis: report of three cases and review of the literature, *Ear Nose Throat J* 70:462, 1991.

68. De Santis D: Fibromatosis of the mandible: case report and review of previous publications, *Br J Oral Maxillofac Surg* 36:384, 1998.

69. Inwards CY, Unni KK, Beabout JW, Sim FH: Desmoplastic fibroma of bone, *Cancer* 68:1978, 1991.

70. Miralbell R, Suit HD, Mankin HJ, et al: Fibromatoses: from postsurgical surveillance to combined surgery and radiation therapy, *Int J Radiat Oncol Biol Phys* 18:535, 1990.

71. Bertoni F, Present D, Marchetti C, et al: Desmoplastic fibroma of the jaw: the experience of the Istituto Beretta, *Oral Surg Oral Med Oral Pathol* 61:179, 1986.

72. Jaffe HL: Giant cell reparative granuloma, traumatic bone cyst and fibrous dysplasia of jaw bones, *J Oral Surg* 6:159, 1953.

73. Masson JK, Soule EH: Desmoid tumors of the head and neck, *Am J Surg* 112:615, 1996.

74. Rabhan WN, Rosai J: Desmoplastic fibroma, *J Bone Joint Surg* 50-A:487, 1968.

75. Sugiura I: Desmoplastic fibroma, *J Bone Joint Surg* 58-A:126, 1976.

76. Makek M, Lello GE: Desmoplastic fibroma of the mandible: literature review and a report of three cases, *J Oral Maxillofac Surg* 44:385, 1986.

77. Templeton K, Glass N, Young SK: Desmoplastic fibroma of the mandible in a child: report of a case, *Oral Surg Oral Med Oral Pathol* 84:620, 1997.

78. Cranin AN, Gallo L, Madan S: Desmoplastic fibroma. A rare oral tumor in children, *N Y State Dent J* 60:34, 1994.

79. Crim JR, Gold RH, Mirra JM, et al: Desmoplastic fibroma of bone: radiographic analysis, *Radiology* 172:827, 1989.

80. Addante RR, Laskin JL: Case 55: large right mandibular mass, *J Oral Maxillofac Surg* 43:531, 1985.

81. Kwong K: Aggressive fibromatosis of the tonsillar fossa: a case report, *J Laryngol Otol* 99:411, 1985.

82. Burkitt D: A sarcoma involving jaws in African children, *Br J Surg* 46:218, 1958.

83. Judson SC, Henle W, Henle G: A cluster of Epstein-Barr-virus–associated American Burkitt's lymphoma, *N Engl J Med* 297:464, 1977.

84. Ziegler JL: Burkitt's lymphoma, *Med Clin North Am* 61:1073, 1977.

85. Ziegler JL: Treatment results of 54 American patients with Burkitt's lymphoma are similar to the African experience, *N Engl J Med* 297:75, 1977.

86. Eversole LR: Central benign and malignant neural neoplasms of the jaws: a review, *J Oral Surg* 27:716, 1969.

87. Prescott GH, White RE: Solitary central neuro-fibroma of the mandible: report of a case and review of literature, *J Oral Surg* 28:305, 1970.

88. Lichtenstein L: *Bone tumors*, St Louis, 1965, Mosby, p 175.

89. Muller H, Slootweg PJ: Maxillofacial deformities in neurofibromatosis, *J Oral Maxillofac Surg* 9:89, 1981.

90. Koblin J, Reil B: Changes in the facial skeleton in cases of neurofibromatosis, *J Oral Surg* 3:23, 1975.

91. Lurie JI: Congenital melanocarcinoma, melanotic adamantinoma, retinal anlage tumor, progonoma and pigmented epulis of infancy, *Cancer* 14:1090, 1961.

92. Borello ED, Gorlin RJ: Melanotic neuroectodermal tumor of infancy—a neoplasm of neural crest origin: report of case associated with high excretion of vanilmandelic acid, *Cancer* 19:196, 1966.

93. Kerr DA, Pullon PA: A study of the pigmented tumors of jaws of infants (melanotic ameloblastoma, retinal anlage tumor, progonoma), *Oral Surg* 18:759, 1964.

94. Brekke JH, Gorlin RJ: Melanotic neuroectodermal tumor of infancy, *J Oral Surg* 33:858, 1975.

95. Kaban LB, Mulliken JB: Vascular anomalies of the maxillofacial region, *J Oral Maxillofac Surg* 44:203,1986.

96. Boyd JB, Mulliken JB, Kaban LB, et al: Skeletal changes associated with vascular malformations, *Plast Reconstr Surg* 74:789, 1984.

97. Bacci G, Ferrari S, Bertoni F, et al: Long-term outcome for patients with nonmetastatic osteosarcoma of the extremity treated at the Istituto Ortopedico Rizzoli according to the Istituto Ortopedico Rizzoli/osteosarcoma-2 protocol: an updated report, *J Clin Oncol* 18:4016, 2000.

98. Waldron CA: Giant cell tumors of the jaw bones, *J Oral Surg* 6:1055, 1953.

99. Troulis MJ, Williams WB, Kaban LB: Staged protocol for resection, skeletal reconstruction, and oral rehabilitation of children with jaw tumors, *J Oral Maxillofac Surg* 2003 (in press).

100. Perzik SL: Management of advanced odontogenic mandibular tumors in children, *AMA Arch Surg* 83:816, 1960.

101. Rappaport I, Fumas DW: Tumors of the facial skeleton in children: growth pattern after maxillectomy and mandibulectomy, *Am J Surg* 130:421, 1975.

CHAPTER 16

Head and Neck Malignancies in Children

Robert A. Ord

Cancer is the second leading cause of childhood mortality after accidents (trauma); however, it is a rare occurrence, with 129.5 cases per million in white and 104.1 cases per million in black children under 15 years of age.[1] Two to five percent of childhood malignancies arise as primary tumors in the head and neck.[2,3] However, approximately 25% of all malignancies in children, at some stage, affect the head and neck region.

Excluding retinoblastoma and brain tumors, the small blue round cell tumors are the most common cancers of the head and neck in children.[4] Jaffe and Jaffe[5] reviewed 178 pediatric head and neck malignant tumors and reported 55% lymphomas, 11% rhabdomyosarcomas, 10% other sarcomas, 5% malignant thyroid tumors, and 5% neuroblastomas. Cunningham et al.,[6] in 411 pediatric head and neck cancer cases, reported 60.5% lymphomas, 13% rhabdomyosarcomas, 9% thyroid cancers, 5% neuroblastomas, 4.5% other sarcomas, and 4.5% nasopharyngeal carcinomas. Robinson et al.,[3] in 147 cases, documented 37% lymphomas, 31% Langerhans cell histiocytosis, 18% rhabdomyosarcomas, and 10% neuroblastomas. Rapidis et al.[7] reviewed 1007 childhood tumors of the head and neck and found that 308 (31%) were malignant. These included 52% lymphomas, 22.3% rhabdomyosarcomas, 5.8% squamous cell carcinomas, 5.8% neuroblastomas, 4.2% other sarcomas, and 3.9% thyroid carcinomas. The results of all these studies are remarkably consistent, with lymphoma being the most common neoplasm followed by rhabdomyosarcoma. Differences probably reflect variations in the age mix reported. Below the age of 3 years, retinoblastoma is the most frequently diagnosed cancer, with rhabdomyosarcoma and neuroblastoma being second and third in incidence. Between 3 and 11 years of age, rhabdomyosarcomas predominate followed by lymphomas. From 12 through 21 years of age, lymphomas are the most common malignant neoplasm followed by rhabdomyosarcomas.[4]

The most common site for a head and neck malignancy in pediatric patients is the neck (58%[6-8] to 70%[6]), followed by the nasopharynx (11.4% to 17%[6,7]). Most authors stress that children with malignant tumors of the head and neck have nonspecific symptoms such as headache, earache, blocked nostrils, or enlarged lymph nodes. Because of the nonspecific nature of the symptoms, the diagnosis often is missed until the disease is at an advanced stage. A high index of suspicion must be maintained if early diagnoses are to be made.

There are no reports of large series of malignant tumors of the maxillofacial region in children. In most series, benign and malignant tumors of the oral and maxillofacial area are combined. Sato et al.,[9] in a review of 250 children under 15 years of age with oral and maxillofacial tumors, found that 18 (7%) had malignant tumors: 14 were sarcomas. Similarly, Koch[10] reported on 195 children under age 15 years, and 14 (7.8%) had malignancies: 12 were sarcomas. Bhaskar[11] surveyed 293 children under age 14 years with oral tumors: 9% were malignant. Kaban and Chuong[12] found 12 of 48 (25%) primary jaw tumors in children to be malignant: six hematopoietic reticuloepithelial, five mesenchymal, and one salivary gland in origin. In addition, Dehner[13] reviewed 60 pediatric patients (under 15 years of age) with jaw tumors and found that 14 (23%) tumors were primary or secondary malignancies. It would appear, therefore, that primary tumors of the jaws are more likely to be malignant than those at other oral and maxillofacial sites.

However, to appreciate the rarity of childhood malignancy in the oral and maxillofacial region, it is necessary to review large series of patients, evaluating all biopsies of these sites in children. Das and Das[14] reviewed 2370 biopsies (patients under 20 years of age), and only 288 (11.6%) specimens were neoplasms, of which 3 (0.13%) were malignant. Chen et al.[15] examined 534 oral biopsies in children under 15 years and reported that 11 (2.5%) were malignant.

Thus, malignant head and neck tumors are rare in children and even less frequent in the oral and maxillofacial region. Small blue round cell tumors (lymphomas, rhabdomyosarcomas, Ewing's sarcoma/primitive neuroectodermal tumors [PNET]) predominate.

GENERAL TREATMENT CONSIDERATIONS

The diagnosis of cancer in a child always has devastating psychosocial consequences for both the patient and family. In the treatment of head and neck cancer, the clinician is faced with many difficult decisions because the most common tumor types require combinations of chemotherapy, radiation therapy, and resection. The short-term and long-term functional, cosmetic, growth, and psychological consequences of therapy and its complications can have an impact as significant as the cancer itself.

Both chemotherapy and radiation can affect the oral soft tissues and development of the craniofacial skeleton and dentition. Mucositis, ulcers, gingivitis, and candida infections are seen more commonly in children than adults having chemotherapy or radiation because of a high mucosal turnover rate.[16] Chemotherapy, alone, causes enamel hypoplasia, discoloration, and tooth agenesis, especially when given to children during active dental development.[17] The addition of radiation therapy to the head and neck significantly increases the incidence and magnitude of dental and facial skeletal abnormalities. Even dosages as low as 0.72 to 1.22 Gy have caused abnormalities in root and enamel development.[18] Microdontia, agenesis, failure of eruption, premature apexification, and V-shaped roots are all common in patients who have received radiation during development of the dentition.[19] Dental abnormalities were diagnosed in 5 of 23 (24%) children receiving chemotherapy alone. However, in 45 children receiving maxillofacial

radiation (43 also had chemotherapy), 37 (82%) had dental and maxillofacial skeletal abnormalities.[20] In this series, the authors showed more severe abnormalities of growth and function in children treated at an earlier age and with higher dosages of radiation. They described root and enamel abnormalities with dosages of 20 to 40 Gy, but in patients with rhabdomyosarcoma receiving dosages of 45 to 65 Gy they also described trismus, nasal voice, caries, and maxillary and mandibular deformities (Figure 16-1).

Sonis et al.[21] examined children having chemotherapy or chemotherapy plus radiation for central nervous system (CNS) prophylaxis. They confirmed an increase in dental abnormalities in children treated while under 5 years of age and in those receiving radiation. Only the group of children under age 5 years who received 2400 cGy of radiation had craniofacial abnormalities. Deficient mandibular development was evident in 18 of 20 (90%) of these children. These authors also reviewed the evidence for growth hormone deficiency following head and neck irradiation as an etiologic factor in craniofacial deformity.

Dahllöf[22] demonstrated that dental development could be affected by chemotherapy or radiation if given to very young children. However, he also found that craniofacial development, especially mandibular growth deficiency, was related to cranial irradiation only before age 5 years. In bone marrow transplant patients receiving total body irradiation, the mandible is four times more sensitive than the maxilla. In children receiving high-dose cyclophosphamide and total body irradiation before a bone marrow transplant, treatment with recombinant growth hormone has allowed normal mandibular growth.[23,24]

There are few series examining the effect of radical surgery on subsequent facial growth in children. Rappaport and Furnas[25] reported growth patterns following maxillectomy or mandibulectomy in 13 children, most of whom had aggressive benign tumors. These authors reported little major effect on facial growth and noted that resection of tooth roots did not necessarily jeopardize vitality, eruption potential, or growth. They recommended reconstruction of the maxilla with an obturator modified at intervals and used free iliac crest and particulate bone for mandibular reconstruction.

More recently, authors have advocated the use of microvascular bone flaps for both the pediatric mandible[26,27] and maxilla[27] after tumor resection. Genden et al.[27] examined the donor site morbidity and craniofacial growth in seven children and concluded there were no problems with growth or function at the donor site following vascularized fibula or scapular flaps. Their longest follow-up was 4 years 2 months, and four of the seven patients had successful dental implants placed in the bone flaps. Implants can be used to restore occlusion in children over 7 years of age.[28]

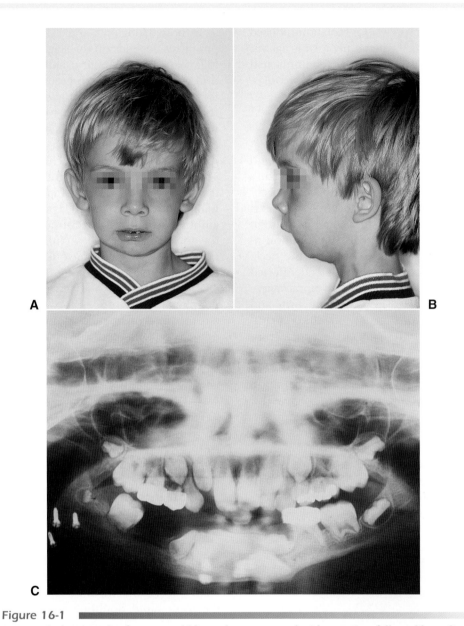

Figure 16-1

A, Frontal photograph of a 9-year-old boy who was treated with resection followed by radiation therapy for a malignant epithelioid hemangioma of the right mandible at age 4 years. **B,** Profile shows marked mandibular hypoplasia, despite growth hormone replacement and reconstruction of the mandible on the right side with rib grafts. **C,** Panorex film shows typical radiation effects on dental development. Note complete agenesis of maxillary and mandibular premolars, absent root formation of the mandibular and maxillary first molars, absent root formation and failed eruption of mandibular incisors and canines, premature apexification of maxillary incisors and canines, and hypoplastic developing maxillary and mandibular right second molars. Screws are seen in previous rib graft reconstruction.

In addition to the adverse effects on craniofacial growth, chemotherapy and radiation therapy can induce second primary tumors. In certain cases, such as patients with retinoblastoma, this may be due to the underlying genetic abnormality. In these patients, osteosarcomas may occur even when radiation is not given.

Sarcomas are the most commonly induced second cancer after irradiation. There is usually a latency period of at least 12 years. However, early radiation-induced sarcoma of the head and neck has been reported recently.[29] Other tumors induced by radiation include leukemias, lymphomas, thyroid cancer, skin cancer,[4,30] and salivary neoplasms.[31,32] The 5-year survival for radiation-induced sarcomas is less than 30%.[33] Chemotherapeutic agents, in particular the alkylating agents, have been implicated in inducing leukemia, lymphomas, and osteosarcomas.

SMALL BLUE ROUND CELL TUMORS

Lymphomas

Lymphomas account for over 50% of pediatric head and neck malignancies.[5-7] They may be divided into Hodgkin's and non-Hodgkin's lymphomas, which appear to occur with almost equal frequency.[5,6] Hodgkin's disease is found most often in adolescents and is rare in children younger than 5 years of age. It is twice as common in boys, and 80% to 90%[5,6] of cases occur in the neck. Seventy-five percent of these cases are unilateral. Affected submandibular nodes occur in 90% and supraclavicular nodes in 10% of cases. The nodes are firm and rubbery (Figure 16-2). Approximately one third of children have systemic symptoms that include night sweats, pruritus, and weight loss. Physical examination reveals firm, rubbery, enlarged lymph nodes.

Non-Hodgkin's lymphoma is also more common in boys but occurs at a younger age (2 to 12 years).[34] Involvement of extranodal sites is more common than in Hodgkin's disease. Tumors in the tonsils, Waldeyer's ring, scalp and forehead, jaw, nasopharynx, orbit, nose and sinuses, and parotid have all been reported. The supraclavicular nodes are a more common site than upper cervical nodes. Children may have CNS involvement, which carries a poor prognosis, and non-Hodgkin's lymphoma can undergo leukemic transformation.

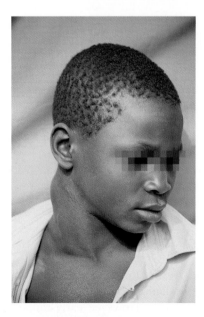

Figure 16-2
A 14-year-old boy with matted rubbery cervical nodes secondary to Hodgkin's lymphoma.

In both Hodgkin's and non-Hodgkin's lymphoma, prognosis depends on the stage of disease and its histologic pattern. Treatment usually consists of a combination of chemotherapy and radiation therapy. Prognosis for Hodgkin's disease is good, with 90% complete response and cure in stages I and II. The prognosis for non-Hodgkin's lymphoma is worse.

The oral and maxillofacial surgeon is asked not infrequently to examine a child with a cervical mass. The vast majority of these are inflammatory. However, it is important to retain a high degree of suspicion of malignancy for any chronic lymph node swelling. Some authors have advocated a trial of antibiotic therapy if the node is thought to be of inflammatory origin. Lymph node biopsy is performed to exclude malignancy if there is no resolution in 6 to 8 weeks.[35]

Knight et al.,[36] in a review of 239 children who had peripheral lymph node biopsy, found that duration of adenopathy, consistency, and the presence of more than one site were not specific in differentiating reactive hyperplasia from a serious disease process. They therefore advocated early biopsy for children with supraclavicular adenopathy accompanied by a fever of 1 week, weight loss of unknown cause, and skin fixation. Other authors have stressed rapid growth, a hard mass, matted nodes,[37] and a raised lactate dehydrogenase level as reasons for early biopsy. An alternative to an open procedure is fine-needle aspiration biopsy, which has been shown to have a high degree of accuracy in children.[38,39]

One of the non-Hodgkin's lymphomas is of particular interest to oral and maxillofacial surgeons: Burkitt's lymphoma. Endemic African Burkitt's lymphoma is strongly associated with Epstein-Barr virus and typically manifests as a jaw mass, with the maxilla the most common site. The disease is often advanced, with loose teeth, ptosis, and trismus. This lymphoma has one of the most rapid doubling times of all tumors and is exquisitely sensitive to chemotherapy but surprisingly radioresistant. In nonendemic (American) Burkitt's lymphoma, jaw involvement is less frequent at 7% to 16%.[40,41] The mandible is the most common site. In addition, other sites in the head and neck such as the tonsil, nasopharynx, and cervical nodes have been reported and rapid growth may cause airway compromise.[3]

Rhabdomyosarcoma

Rhabdomyosarcoma is the most common pediatric sarcoma, with 35% to 40% arising in the head and neck. Approximately 70% of patients are younger than 12 years of age. In one series, 80% of girls were younger than 4 years and 77% of boys were younger than 5 years of age.[42] Twenty-five percent of head and neck rhabdomyosarcomas occur in the orbit, 50% are parameningeal, and 25% occur at other sites (oral cavity, cheek, parotid, larynx, and scalp). Orbital tumors rarely metastasize and have the best prognosis, followed by tumors at other sites. The parameningeal rhabdomyosarcomas, which include infratemporal, nasal cavity and paranasal sinuses, nasopharynx, and middle ear tumors, have the worst prognosis. Symptoms from the parameningeal tumors are very nonspecific, such as earache, otitis media, stuffy nose, and headache. They are, therefore, frequently diagnosed late, when skull base invasion and involvement of the cranial nerves and meninges already have occurred (Figure 16-3).

Histologically, embryonal and botryoid osteosarcomas are the most frequent types in the head and neck. These occur in younger children, who have the best prognosis.[43] Alveolar rhabdomyosarcomas tend to occur in adolescents. The pleomorphic histologic type has the poorest prognosis and occurs in adults. In the Intergroup Rhabdomyosarcoma studies (IRS), three related tumors (extraosseous Ewing's sarcomas, sarcoma of undetermined histology, and undifferentiated sarcoma) also are included and these have very poor survival rates. Prognosis for rhabdomyosarcoma depends on histologic type, clinical stage, and site. Currently, a site-based TNM (tumor, nodes, metastasis) staging system is being evaluated against the traditional surgicopathologic clinical grouping system[44] (Table 16-1).

TABLE 16-1	Intergroup Rhabdomyosarcoma Study Tumor Staging
Stage I	Localized disease, completely resected; regional nodes not involved
Stage IIA	Grossly resected tumor with microscopic residual disease; no evidence of regional node involvement
Stage IIB	Regional disease (extension into adjacent organ or regional nodes); completely resected
Stage IIC	Regional disease with involved nodes; grossly resected, but with evidence of microscopic residual disease
Stage III	Gross residual disease after surgery
Stage IV	Metastatic disease at diagnosis

Treatment protocols include multiple modalities: resection, radiation, and chemotherapy. Before the IRS, survival with single-modality therapy was 8% to 20%. In IRS-I (trial number one), 3-year relapse-free survival was 91% for orbital, 75% for "other sites," and 46% for parameningeal rhabdomyosarcoma.[45] Improvements

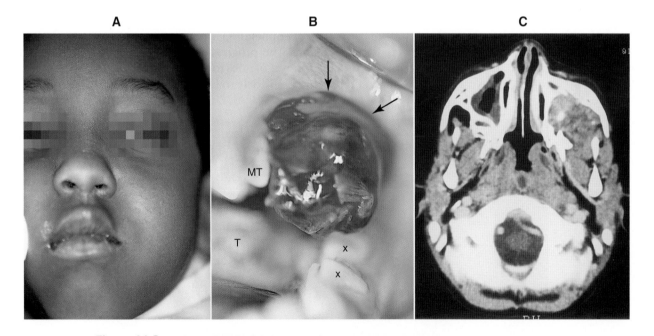

A, A 4-year-old boy with left facial swelling, elevated left eye, and ptosis. **B,** Intraoral view shows the fleshy left maxillary mass (rhabdomyosarcoma) where a loose second deciduous molar had been extracted, prolapsing from antrum (*arrows,* tumor; *MT,* maxillary teeth; *T,* tongue; *x,* mandibular teeth). **C,** CT scan shows mass in sinus with destruction of posterior wall and invasion of pterygoids. This patient is alive and well 5 years after chemoradiation.

have continued with IRS-I and IRS-II (trial number 2) patients, and overall survival rates are 60% to 70%.[44,46] In IRS-II, survival in parameningeal rhabdomyosarcoma was improved from 33% to 57% by treating the CNS axis with radiation and intrathecal chemotherapy.[47] Radiation therapy requires dosage schedules of 50 Gy or more with wide fields. Chemotherapy regimes have included vincristine, actinomycin D, and cyclophosphamide (VAC), as well as doxorubicin, etoposide, and ifosfamide. If complete resection of the tumor is possible, this gives the best overall survival when combined with chemotherapy (Figure 16-4). In parameningeal sites, however, complete resection is rarely possible due to functional and esthetic considerations (see Figure 16-3). In these cases, biopsy only is recommended.

Lyos et al.[48] reported 56 rhabdomyosarcomas of the head and neck in children. Complete resection was possible in only three (5.4%) patients, and incomplete resection with microscopic residual disease occurred in 13 (23.2%) patients. Forty patients (71.4%) had grossly positive margins, most having only incisional biopsy. Five-year disease-specific survival was 63% using protocols incorporating radiation and chemotherapy. However, the prognosis for patients with recurrent or metastatic disease was dreadful, with 95% mortality.[45]

Ewing's Sarcoma/Primitive Neuroectodermal Tumor

The Ewing's sarcoma/PNET group encompasses a group of tumors thought to arise from neuroectodermal tissue. The peripheral primitive neuroectodermal tumor (pPNET) group is complex and controversial, including such tumors as Ewing's sarcoma (osseous and extraosseous), peripheral neuroepithelioma, Askin's tumor, melanotic neuroectodermal tumors, ectomesenchymoma, and peripheral medulloepithelioma. The two most com-monly seen are Ewing's and peripheral neuroepithe-lioma (malignant PNET of bone and soft tissues). They are thought to be a spectrum of the same tumor, Ewing's being least differentiated and peripheral neuroepithe-lioma the most differentiated.[49]

Ewing's sarcoma accounts for 27% of malignant pediatric bone tumors[50] and is more common in males than females. It is rare in blacks. Approximately 7% of all Ewing's sarcomas occur in the mandible.[51] The patient seeks treatment for swelling and pain. Plain radiographs most commonly show a lytic lesion. Systemic symptoms of fever, anemia, leukocytosis, and increased sedimentation rate may lead to a diagnosis of odontogenic infection and thus delay the true diagnosis. It is thought that approximately 80% to 90% of patients have micrometastases, and diagnostic workup includes chest computed tomography (CT), bone scan, and bone marrow aspiration.

Treatment is with radiation plus chemotherapy, and the head and neck is regarded as a favorable site. In the jaws, resection has been advocated to reduce the effects of radiation on facial growth, and studies have shown little difference in survival rates between radiation and resection.[52,53] All patients receive chemotherapy and, in the head and neck, 72.8% long-term survival is reported.[4]

Peripheral neuroepithelioma (malignant PNET) is rare. The prognosis is poor, with a 5-year disease-free survival of 30% to 45%.[54] PNET is aggressive and metastasizes widely to lung, liver, and bone. In a review of the

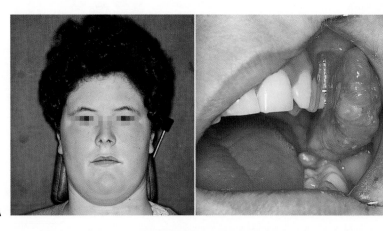

A

B

Figure 16-4

A, Frontal photograph of a 17-year-old girl with rapidly growing mass in the left cheek. **B,** Intraoral view shows the botryoid-like alveolar rhabdomyosarcoma of the left cheek. The tumor was managed by complete surgical resection and postoperative chemotherapy. (Patient treated under the care of Mr. Brian Avery, Consultant Maxillofacial Surgeon, Middlesborough General Hospital, England).

literature, 30 of 42 (71.5%) head and neck cases were found in children below 20 years of age; 18 of these (42.9%) patients were below 10 years.[55] The orbit was the most common site, followed by the neck, parotid, and temporal areas (Figure 16-5).

The recommended treatment is early resection, followed by radiation and dosage-intensive chemotherapy. Multimodality chemotherapy with alternating cycles using agents such as vincristine, doxorubicin (Adriamycin), cyclophosphamide (Cytoxan), VP16, and ifosfamide provides the best control. Because PNET-peripheral neuroepithelioma shares many of the histologic characteristics of Ewing's sarcoma, including occasionally the 11:22 chromosomal translocation, it may be difficult to differentiate the two lesions. It appears likely that many tumors originally diagnosed as Ewing's are PNET tumors, and this entity is not as rare as has been reported.[56,57] In view of the poor prognosis for PNET, it is important to make the distinction. Five new cases in the last 8 years were seen at the University of Maryland and reported.[55]

OSTEOSARCOMA

Osteosarcomas account for 2.6% of all pediatric malignant tumors, and 8% of these occur in the head and neck.[58] This is reflected in most large series of pediatric

malignancies: two of 411 patients,[6] two of 178 patients,[8] and none of 308 patients.[7] However, in reports specifically on the maxillofacial region, 5 of 14 pediatric head neck malignancies were osteosarcomas[10] and three of five primary jaw malignancies were osteosarcomas.[13] In children, bilateral hereditary retinoblastoma, postradiation retinoblastomas, radiation therapy for other tumors (Figure 16-6), and fibrous dysplasia may be associated with development of osteosarcoma. In general, the average age for primary osteosarcoma of the jaws is 35 years, much older than osteosarcoma of the long bones. In adults, jaw osteosarcoma has a much better prognosis than in children. They are more frequently low grade or chondroblastic, and distant metastasis is less common.

Osteosarcomas are best visualized on magnetic resonance imaging (MRI) to delineate involvement of the marrow and soft tissue. CT scans are useful to assess cortical bone. Staging is accomplished with chest CT and skeletal scintigraphy. The classic "sunburst" is less common on plain radiographs of the jaws, but widening of the periodontal ligament is an early sign.[59]

Management is primarily by jaw resection, with wide margins of 3 cm if possible (Figure 16-7). In Dehner's series, all 3 children were alive at 4½, 11, and 18 years after radical resection.[13] The role of chemotherapy is controversial. The authors of one retrospective report

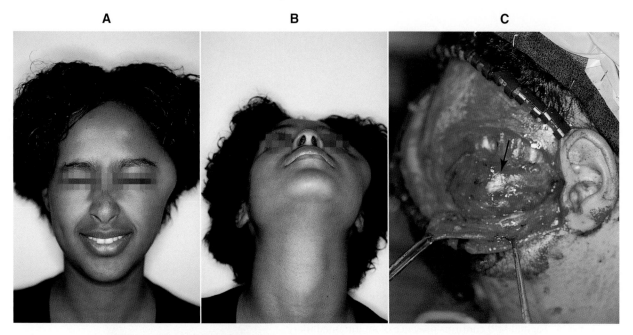

A **B** **C**

Figure 16-5

A, Frontal photograph of a 19-year-old woman with 3-month swelling of left temporalis. B, View from below. The tumor was found to be malignant pPNET (peripheral neuroepithelioma). C, Hemicoronal flap shows mass arising in temporalis muscle *(arrow)*. The patient was treated with excision followed by radiation and dose-intense chemotherapy. She is alive and well 2 years postoperatively.

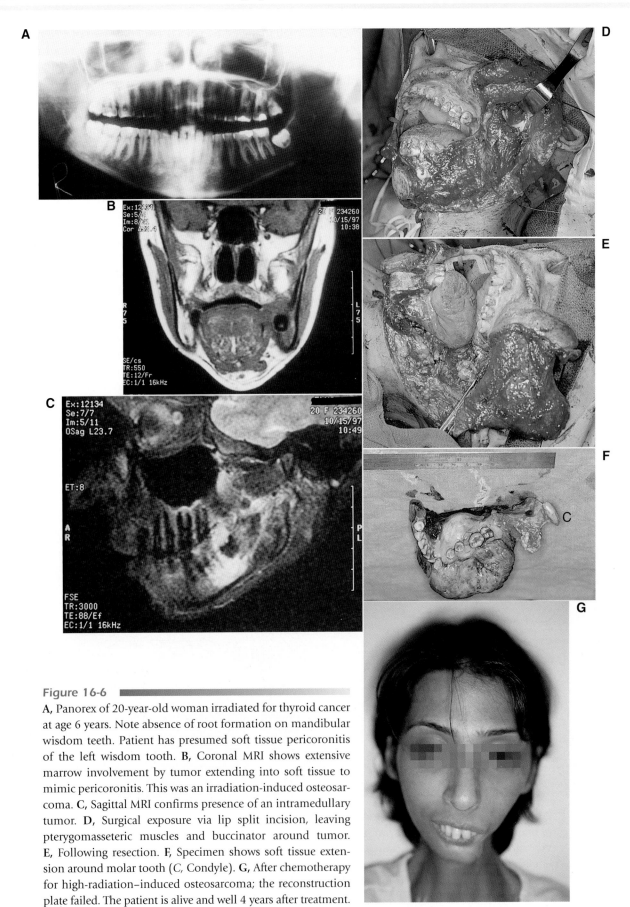

Figure 16-6

A, Panorex of 20-year-old woman irradiated for thyroid cancer at age 6 years. Note absence of root formation on mandibular wisdom teeth. Patient has presumed soft tissue pericoronitis of the left wisdom tooth. **B,** Coronal MRI shows extensive marrow involvement by tumor extending into soft tissue to mimic pericoronitis. This was an irradiation-induced osteosarcoma. **C,** Sagittal MRI confirms presence of an intramedullary tumor. **D,** Surgical exposure via lip split incision, leaving pterygomasseteric muscles and buccinator around tumor. **E,** Following resection. **F,** Specimen shows soft tissue extension around molar tooth (*C,* Condyle). **G,** After chemotherapy for high-radiation–induced osteosarcoma; the reconstruction plate failed. The patient is alive and well 4 years after treatment.

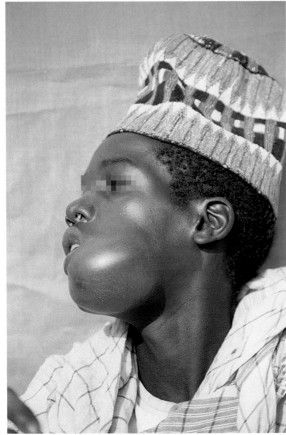

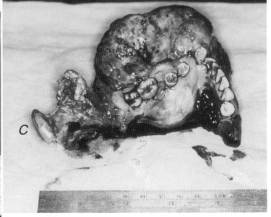

Figure 16-7

A, 16-year-old boy with osteosarcoma of the left mandible. **B,** Resection specimen shows 3 cm–plus margins. *C,* Condyle.

concluded that chemotherapy improved survival.[60] However, it is not clear whether the benefit was only in high-grade tumors. In patients with clear margins, disease-free survival of 68.8% has been reported at 5 years.[61] When tumor remains at the primary site and margins are not clear, survival rates are extremely low.[62]

LANGERHANS CELL HISTIOCYTOSIS

Although there is doubt whether histiocytosis is a true malignant neoplasm, in one series, nine of 10 cases of Langerhans cell histiocytosis in females were monoclonal.[63] Robinson et al.[3] pointed out that many large series of pediatric head and neck malignancies excluded Langerhans cell histiocytosis. However, they included these tumors because the mortality rate at their institution was 31%.[3] It was also the most common tumor found in children under 2 years of age. Kaban and Chuong[12] reported five cases of histiocytosis in a series of 47 nonodontogenic jaw tumors. The mean age was 2.2 years. Three forms of this disease are encountered commonly: eosinophilic granuloma, multifocal eosinophilic granuloma (includes Hand-Schüller-Christian disease), and Letterer-Siwe disease (Figure 16-8).

Approximately 10% of cases involve the oral cavity,[64,65] and the mandible is involved alone or with other sites in 73% of cases.

Eosinophilic granuloma usually affects one bone, causing pain and swelling. In the mandible, radiographs show a rounded radiolucency, which is usually well defined. Alternatively, a panoramic radiograph may show the "floating tooth sign." Teeth loosening occurs in 9% of children.[65] These lesions may regress spontaneously, but simple curettage is usually curative. Alternatively, intralesional steroid injections or low-dose irradiation may be used for recalcitrant lesions.

Multifocal eosinophilic granuloma usually affects the mandible, skull, axial skeleton, or femur (see Figure 16-8), but the skin, liver, and spleen may also be involved. Although said to be more common in children than infants, 17 of 21 patients reported by Robinson et al.[3] were under 2 years of age. These children may respond to simple localized treatment, but most require systemic chemotherapy. There was a 37% mortality rate from progressive disease in one series.[3]

Letterer-Siwe disease is the most severe form of Langerhans cell histiocytosis, mostly occurring in younger children. In children under 2 years of age, mortality may

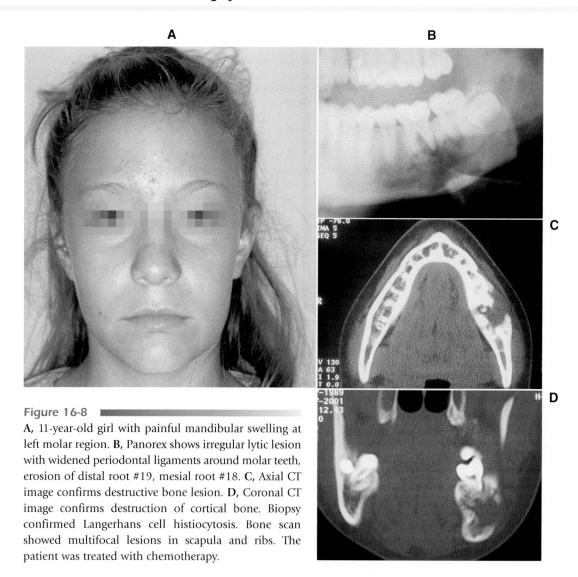

Figure 16-8

A, 11-year-old girl with painful mandibular swelling at left molar region. **B,** Panorex shows irregular lytic lesion with widened periodontal ligaments around molar teeth, erosion of distal root #19, mesial root #18. **C,** Axial CT image confirms destructive bone lesion. **D,** Coronal CT image confirms destruction of cortical bone. Biopsy confirmed Langerhans cell histiocytosis. Bone scan showed multifocal lesions in scapula and ribs. The patient was treated with chemotherapy.

be more than 50%. In this form of the disease, widespread involvement of bone and soft tissues occurs. Skin rash is a common finding. Lymphadenopathy, fever, and anemia are not uncommon. Thrombocytopenia is a poor prognostic sign.

Chemotherapy, with vincristine, vinblastine, and corticosteroids, and radiation for bone lesions is the usual management. Current trials of bone marrow transplantation and gene therapy are being assessed for resistant cases.

MISCELLANEOUS TUMORS

Nasopharyngeal carcinoma in children is rare. It is most common in adolescent black patients who have masses in the superior deep cervical nodes. Most of these cancers in children are of the undifferentiated (lymphoepithelial) type and there is a strong association with Epstein-Barr virus antibody titers. Using a combination of chemotherapy and radiation for locally advanced disease in children, disease-free survival was 61% at 75 months.[66]

Squamous cell carcinoma of the oral cavity is extremely rare, with occasional case reports in the literature. Immunosuppressive drugs, Fanconi's anemia,[67] and xeroderma pigmentosum are associated with oral squamous cell carcinoma in young patients.

Malignant melanoma accounts for approximately 1% to 3% of pediatric malignancies[68] and follows the same skin distribution as in adults. Mucosal melanoma is extremely unusual. Because the clinical and histopathologic features can be misleading, diagnosis can be delayed, but the natural history and prognosis appear the same as for adults.[69,70] Modern techniques for managing melanoma in adults, such as sentinel node biopsy, have been applied successfully to children.[71]

CONCLUSION

Because head and neck cancer is rare in children and symptoms nonspecific, the clinician must retain a high index of suspicion in order to make an early diagnosis. Small blue round cell tumors, lymphomas, and rhabdomyosarcomas account for most malignant maxillofacial tumors. Management frequently involves multimodality therapy with radiation and chemotherapy in addition to resection. Although this strategy has led to increased survival, this has come at the cost of increased morbidity, with facial growth deformities and induced second primary malignancies.

REFERENCES

1. Young JL, Ries LG, Silverberg E, et al: Cancer incidence survival and mortality for children younger than age 15 years, *Cancer* 58:598-602, 1986.
2. Cunningham MJ, Myers EN, Bluestone CD: Malignant tumors of the head and neck in children: a twenty year review, *Int J Pediatr Otolaryngol* 13:279, 1987.
3. Robinson LD, Rightmire J, Smith RJM, et al: Head and neck malignancies in children: an age incidence study, *Laryngoscope* 98:11, 1988.
4. Ord RA: Head and neck tumors. In Stringer MD, Oldham KT, Mouniquad PDE, Howard ER, editors: *Pediatric surgery and urology: long term outcomes,* Philadelphia, 1998, WB Saunders.
5. Jaffe BF, Jaffe N: Head and neck tumors in children, *Pediatrics* 51(4):731, 1973.
6. Cunningham MJ, McGuirt WF, Myers EN: Cancer of the head and neck in the pediatric population. In Myers EN, Suen JY, editors: *Cancer of the head and neck,* Philadelphia, 1996, WB Saunders.
7. Rapidis AD, Economidis J, Goumas PD, et al: Tumors of the head and neck in children: a clinico-pathological analysis of 1007 cases, *J Craniomaxillofac Surg* 16:279, 1988.
8. Jaffe BF: Pediatric head and neck tumors: a study of 178 cases, *Laryngoscope* 83:1644, 1973.
9. Sato M, Tanaka N, Sato T, et al: Oral and maxillofacial tumors in children: a review, *Brit J Oral Maxillofac Surg* 35(2):92, 1997.
10. Koch H: Statistical evaluation of tumors of the head and neck in infancy and childhood, *J Oral Maxillofac Surg* 2:26, 1974.
11. Bhaskar SN: Oral tumors of infancy and childhood, *Pediatrics* 63(2):195, 1963.
12. Chuong R, Kaban LB: Diagnosis and treatment of jaw tumors in children, *J Oral Maxillofac Surg* 43:323, 1985.
13. Dehner LP: Tumors of the mandible and maxilla in children: a study of 14 primary and secondary malignant tumors, *Cancer* 32:112, 1973.
14. Das S, Das AK: A review of pediatric oral biopsies from a surgical pathology service in a dental school, *Pediatr Dent* 15:208, 1993.
15. Chen YK, Lin LM, Huang HC, et al: A retrospective study of oral and maxillofacial biopsy lesions in a pediatric population from southern Taiwan, *Pediatr Dent* 20:7, 1998.
16. Childers NK, Stinnett EA, Wheeler P, et al: Oral complications in children with cancer, *Oral Surg Oral Med Oral Pathol* 75:41, 1993.
17. Alpaslan G, Alpaslan C, Göken M, et al: Disturbances in oral and dental structures in patients with pediatric lymphoma after chemotherapy, *Oral Surg Oral Med Oral Pathol* 87:317, 1999.
18. Rosenberg SW, Kolodney H, Wong GY, et al: Altered dental root development in long-term survivors of pediatric lymphoblastic leukemias: a review of 17 cases, *Cancer* 59:1640, 1987.
19. Dahllöf G, Barr M, Bolme P, et al: Disturbances in dental development after total body irradiation in bone marrow transplant recipients, *Oral Surg Oral Med Oral Pathol* 65:41, 1988.
20. Jaffe N, Toth BB, Hoar RE, et al: Dental and maxillofacial abnormalities in long-term survivors of childhood cancer: effects of treatment with chemotherapy and radiation to the head and neck, *Pediatrics* 73(6):816, 1984.
21. Sonis AL, Tarbell N, Valachovic RW, et al: Dentofacial development in long-term survivors of acute lymphoblastic leukemia: a comparison of three treatment modalities, *Cancer* 66(12):2645, 1990.
22. Dahllöf G: Craniofacial growth in children treated for malignant disease, *Acta Odontol Scand* 56:378, 1998.
23. Dahllöf G, Borgström B, Forsberg CM: The effect of growth hormone treatment in children treated with total body irradiation and bone marrow transplantation, *Acta Paediatr Scand* 83:1165, 1994.
24. Dahllöf G, Forsberg CM, Näsman M, et al: Craniofacial growth in children treated with growth hormone after total body irradiation, *Scand J Dent Res* 99:44, 1991.
25. Rappaport I, Furnas DW: Tumors of the facial skeleton in children: growth patterns after maxillectomy and mandibulectomy, *Am J Surg* 130:421, 1975.
26. Hildago DA, Shenaq SM, Larson DL: Mandibular reconstruction in the pediatric patient: controversies, *Head Neck* 18:354, 1996.
27. Genden EM, Buchinder D, Chaplin B, et al: Reconstruction of the pediatric maxilla and mandible, *Arch Otolaryngol Head Neck Surg* 126:293, 2000.
28. Perrott DH, Sharma AB, Vargervik K: Endosseous implants for pediatric patients: unknown factors indications contraindications and special considerations, *Oral Maxillofac Surg Clin North Am* 6:79, 1994.
29. Johns MM, Concus AP Beals TF, et al: Early-onset post irradiation sarcoma of the head and neck: report of three cases, *Ear Nose Throat J* 81(6):402, 2002.
30. Hazen RW, Pifer JW, Toyooka ET, et al: Neoplasms following irradiation of the head, *Cancer Res* 26:305, 1966.
31. Belsky JL, Takieichi N, Yamamoto T, et al: Salivary gland neoplasms following atomic radiation: additional cases and re-analysis of combined data in a fixed population 1957-1970, *Cancer* 35:555, 1975.
32. Shore-Freedman E, Abrahams C, Recant W, et al: Neurilemomas and salivary gland tumors of the head and neck following childhood irradiation, *Cancer* 51:2159, 1983.
33. Wiklund TA, Blomquist CP, Ray J, et al: Post-irradiation sarcoma: analysis of a nationwide cancer registry material, *Cancer* 68:524, 1991.
34. Armitage JO: Treatment of non-Hodgkin's lymphoma, *N Engl J Med* 328:1023, 1993.
35. Brown RL, Azizkhan G: Pediatric head and neck lesions, *Pediatr Clin North Am* 45(4):889, 1998.
36. Knight PJ, Mulne AF, Vassey LE: When is lymph node biopsy indicated in children with enlarged peripheral nodes? *Pediatrics* 69:391, 1982.
37. Zitelli BJ: Neck masses in children: adenopathy and malignant diseases, *Pediatr Clin North Am* 28(4):813, 1981.
38. Mobeley DL, Wakely PE, Frable MA: Fine needle aspiration biopsy: application to pediatric head and neck masses, *Laryngoscope* 101(5):469, 1991.
39. Ponder TB, Smith D, Ramzy I: Lymphadenopathy in children and adolescents: role of fine needle aspiration in management, *Cancer Detect Prev* 24(3):228, 2000.
40. Wang MB, Strasnik B, Zimmerman MC: Extranodal Burkitt's lymphoma of the head and neck, *Arch Otolaryngol Head Neck Surg* 118:193, 1992.
41. Sariban E, Donahue A, Magrath IT: Jaw involvement in American Burkitt's lymphoma, *Cancer* 53:1777, 1984.
42. Newton WA, Soule EH, Hamoudi AB, et al: Histopathology of childhood sarcomas: intergroup rhabdomyosarcoma studies I and II: clinicopathologic correlation, *J Clin Oncol* 6:67, 1988.

43. Bonilla JA, Healey GB: Management of malignant head and neck tumors in children, *Pediatr Clin North Am* 36(6):1443, 1989.

44. Dagher R, Helman L: Rhabdomyosarcoma: an overview, *Oncologist* 4(1):34, 1999.

45. Sutow WW, Lindberg R, Gehan E, et al: Three year relapse-free survival rates in childhood rhabdomyosarcoma of the head and neck, *Cancer* 49:221-227 1982.

46. Maurer MM, Betangody M, Gehan EA, et al: The intergroup rhabdomyosarcoma study: a final report, *Cancer* 61:209, 1988.

47. Raney R, Teft M, Maurer MM, et al: Improved prognosis with intensive treatment of children with cranial soft tissue sarcomas arising in non-orbital parameningeal sites: a report from the intergroup rhabdomyosarcoma study, *Cancer* 59:147, 1987.

48. Lyos AT, Goepfert H, Luna MA, et al: Soft tissue sarcoma of the head and neck in children and adolescents, *Cancer* 77(1):193, 1996.

49. Fletcher CDM: Peripheral neural tumors. In Fletcher CDM, editor: *Diagnostic histopathology of tumors*, Edinburgh, 1995, Churchill Livingstone.

50. Young JL, Miller RW: Incidence of malignant tumors in US children, *Pediatr* 86:254, 1975.

51. Bernstein PE, Bone RC, Feldman PS: Ewing's sarcoma of the mandible, *Ann Otol Rhinolaryngol* 88:105, 1979.

52. Duns J, Sauer R, Burgers JM, et al: Radiation therapy as local treatment in Ewing's sarcoma: results of the co-operative Ewing's sarcoma studies CESS81 and CESS86, *Cancer* 67:2828, 1991.

53. Sailer SJ, Harmon DC, Mankin HJ et al: Ewing's sarcoma: surgical resection as a prognostic factor, *Int J Radiat Oncol Biol Phys* 15:43, 1988.

54. Jurgens H, Bier V, Harms D, et al: Malignant peripheral neuroectodermal tumors: a retrospective analysis of 42 patients, *Cancer* 61:349, 1988.

55. Nikitakis NG, Salama AR, O'Malley BW, et al: Malignant peripheral primitive neuroectodermal tumor—peripheral neuroepithelioma of the head and neck: report of five cases and review of the literature, *Head Neck Surg* 25:488, 2003.

56. Kushner BH, Hajdu SI, Gulati SC, et al: Extracranial primitive neuroectodermal tumors, the Memorial Sloan-Kettering Cancer Center experience, 67:1825, 1991.

57. Jones JE, McGill T: Peripheral primitive neuroectodermal tumors of the head and neck, *Arch Otolaryngol Head Neck Surg* 121:1392, 1995.

58. Clark JL, Unni KK, Dhanlin DC, et al: Osteosarcoma of the jaw, *Cancer* 51:2311, 1983.

59. Gardener DG, Mills DM: The widened periodontal ligament of osteosarcoma of the jaws, *Oral Surg* 41:652, 1976.

60. Smeele LE, Kostense PJ, van der Waal I, et al: Effects of chemotherapy on survival of craniofacial osteosarcomas: a systematic review of 201 patients, *J Clin Oncol* 15:363, 1997.

61. Smeele LE, van der Waal JE, Van Diest PJ, et al: Radical surgical treatment in craniofacial osteosarcoma gives excellent survival; a retrospective cohort study of 14 patients, *Oral Oncol Eur J Cancer* 30B:374, 1994.

62. Goepfert H, Raymond AK, Spires JR, et al: Osteosarcoma of the head and neck, *Cancer Bull* 42:347, 1990.

63. Willman CI, Busque L, Griffith BB, et al: Langerhans-cell histiocytosis (histiocytosis X)—a clonal proliferative disease, *New Engl J Med* 331:154, 1994.

64. Hartman KS: Histiocytosis X: a review of 114 cases with oral involvement, *Oral Surg Oral Med Oral Pathol* 49:38, 1980.

65. Kilpatrick SE, Wenger DE, Gilchrist GS, et al: Langerhans cell histiocytosis (histiocytosis X) of bone: a clinicopathologic analysis of 263 pediatric and adult cases, *Cancer* 76:2471, 1995.

66. Zubizarreta PA, D'Antonio G, Raslawski E, et al: Nasopharyngeal carcinoma in childhood and adolescence: a single institution experience with combined therapy, *Cancer* 89(3):690, 2000.

67. Jansisyanont P, Pazoki A, Ord RA: Squamous cell carcinoma of the tongue in Fanconi's anemia, *J Oral Maxillofac Surg* 58(12):1454, 2000.

68. National Cancer Institute: Annual cancer statistics review including cancer trends 1950-1985, NIH pub no 88:2789, Washington, DC, 1988, US Dept of Health and Human Services.

69. Ruiz-Maldonado R, Orozco-Covarrubias MA, de lea Luz: Malignant melanoma in children, *Arch Dermatol* 133:363, 1997.

70. Gibbs P, Moore A, Robinson W, et al: Pediatric melanoma: are recent advances in the management of adult melanoma relevant to the pediatric population? *J Pediatr Hematol Oncol* 25(5):428, 2000.

71. Kogut KA, Flemming AM, Pappo AS, et al: Sentinel lymph node biopsy for melanoma in young children, *J Pediatr Surg* 35(6):965, 2000.

Vascular anomalies frequently occur in the pediatric age group. Oral and maxillofacial surgeons usually are called on to treat these children when there is an odontogenic infection or a skeletal abnormality associated with the vascular lesion.[1] The process of understanding and treating vascular anomalies in general, and facial vascular abnormalities in particular, has been hampered by a confusing and largely descriptive nomen-clature. The variety of terms traditionally used to describe vascular anomalies has failed to provide insight into their pathogenesis or into the mechanism of altered skeletal growth. The word *hemangioma* has been applied indiscriminately to both congenital and acquired lesions, including some that regress and others that do not. There is even more confusion about vascular anomalies that primarily involve bone and vascular anomalies of soft tissue with secondary skeletal changes. This confusion, which persists in the oral and maxillofacial surgical literature, continues to hamper rational and appropriate patient care.

This chapter focuses on maxillofacial vascular anomalies in an effort to improve understanding of these lesions and to aid in their diagnosis and treatment. Mulliken and Glowacki[2] analyzed the clinical behavior and endothelial cell characteristics of vascular lesions and proposed a biologic classification system in 1982. Vascular lesions were categorized as hemangiomas or vascular malformations. Hemangiomas are tumors of endothelial cell origin, and vascular malformations are structural abnormalities of blood vessels lined by normal endothelial cells. This elegantly simple biologic classification was the foundation of a textbook by Mulliken and Young,[3] and the system was accepted at the 1996 biennial meeting of the International Society for the Study of Vascular Anomalies in Rome[4,5] (Box 17-1).

Hemangioma of infancy is the most common vascular tumor; other neoplasms include hemangioendothelioma, tufted angioma, pyogenic granuloma, hemangiopericy-toma, and angiosarcoma.[4-7] Vascular malformations are subdivided by the type of vessels involved and their flow characteristics: slow-flow lesions (capillary malformation, lymphatic malformation, venous malformation) and fast-flow lesions (arterial malformation, arteriovenous malformation [AVM]). There are also complex-combined

BOX 17-1   Classification of Vascular Anomalies

Vascular Tumors
Hemangioma (infantile)
Hemangioendothelioma
Angiosarcoma

Malformations
Slow flow
Capillary (CM)
Lymphatic (LM)
Venous (VM)
Combined (CLM, CVM, LVM, CLVM)

Fast flow
Arterial (AM, AVM)

CLM, Capillary-lymphatic malformation; *CVM,* capillary venous malformation; *LVM,* lymphaticovenous malformation; *CLVM,* capillary lymphaticovenous malformation; *AM,* arterial malformation; *AVM,* arteriovenous malformation; *AVF,* arteriovenous fistula.

vascular malformations that often are associated with overgrowth of bone and soft tissue. The binary classification also serves as a guide for research into the etiology, pathogenesis, and molecular basis of vascular anomalies.[8,9] This nosologic system will be used to illustrate and discuss the variety of vascular anomalies in the maxillofacial region.

CLASSIFICATION OF VASCULAR ANOMALIES

Vascular anomalies are classified into two major categories: vascular tumors and malformations.[2-7]

Vascular Tumors

Vascular tumors arise by abnormal proliferation of endothelial cells. The term *hemangioma* usually refers to the most common vascular tumor of infancy. These infantile hemangiomas have a curious gender predilection for females (female-to-male ratio = 3:1 to 5:1) and are more common in white children than those of color.[2,7] Although these lesions may be present at birth (as a pale spot or a telangiectatic or macular stained

area), they typically appear during early infancy (2 weeks) and grow rapidly until the infant reaches the age of 10 to 12 months (proliferating phase). After 1 year of age, the tumor begins to regress slowly and predictably (involuting phase). The bright red color fades and becomes more dull and purplish. The skin becomes pale, particularly in the center of the lesion, and the tumor feels softer on palpation. The involution phase may last until 10 to 12 years of age.[3,7,10] After complete regression, normal skin is restored in 50% of children, while the remainder have some laxity, discoloration, scarring, telangiectasias, or a residual fibrofatty mass (involuted phase).[5,7]

Occasionally, hemangiomas can be identified in utero and are fully developed at birth. These are congenital hemangiomas. Some of these tumors do not undergo the usual postnatal proliferation and, instead, involute rapidly during the first year of life[11] (Figure 17-1). However, not all congenital hemangiomas involute rapidly; some do not regress and increased blood flow persists.[12]

Infantile hemangiomas generally do not involve bone. Unfortunately, the term *intraosseous hemangioma* has been used inaccurately in the literature to describe what are usually slow-flow type vascular malformations.[1,5,7,13] However, bony distortion, such as depression of the outer cortex, nasal deviation, orbital enlargement, and minor hypertrophy of the maxilla or mandible are occasionally noted in the presence of or after involution of a large cutaneous facial hemangioma. This skeletal overgrowth is presumably secondary to increased blood flow during the tumor's proliferating phase.[5,7,13]

Sixty percent of infantile hemangiomas occur in the head and neck region.[7,10] These cutaneous tumors can be deep or superficial, or they may extend through all layers of the skin and occasionally into muscles. About 20% of infantile hemangiomas are multifocal, and in these instances tumors can grow in the brain, liver, lung, spleen, or gastrointestinal tract.[14] Large cutaneous hemangiomas or multiple intrahepatic hemangiomas can cause life-threatening congestive heart failure and anemia.[10,14,15] Skin or mucosal breakdown over a hemangioma leads to ulceration and secondary infection.

Infantile hemangiomas are considered benign lesions. Other vascular tumors are classified as being intermediate or borderline malignant. The most well known is kaposiform hemangioendothelioma. In 1940, the term *Kasabach-Merritt syndrome* was introduced to describe a patient with thrombocytopenia, petechiae, and bleeding in association with a giant hemangioma.[7,16] This is not a syndrome, but rather a coagulopathic phenomenon. It occurs in association with kaposiform hemangioendothelioma and less frequently with tufted angioma.[3,17,18] The features of Kasabach-Merritt phenomenon are profound throm-

A

B

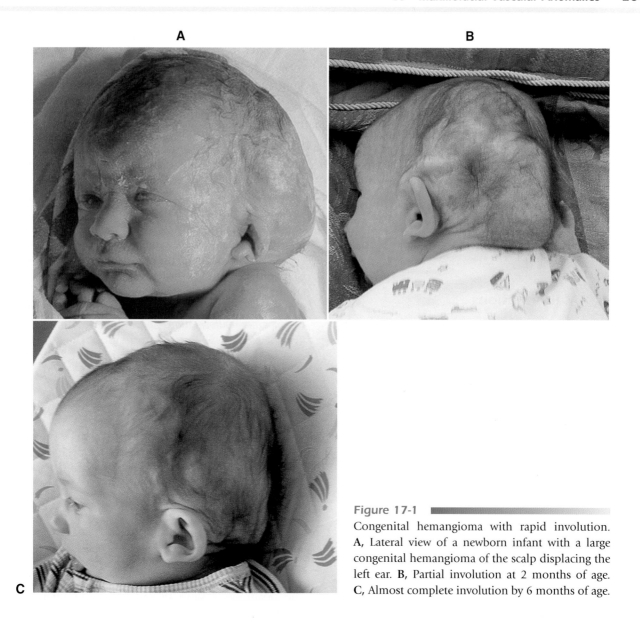

C

Figure 17-1

Congenital hemangioma with rapid involution. **A,** Lateral view of a newborn infant with a large congenital hemangioma of the scalp displacing the left ear. **B,** Partial involution at 2 months of age. **C,** Almost complete involution by 6 months of age.

bocytopenia (<10,000 mm³), low fibrinogen levels, and increased fibrin split prod-ucts. The prothrombin time and activated partial throm-boplastin time are visibly, but minimally, elevated. Proper hematologic terminology is important because the coagulopathy should *not* be treated with heparin, which may actually stimulate growth of the lesion.[3,7,17,18] The term *Kasabach-Merritt phenomenon* has been applied incorrectly to patients with extensive slow-flow vascular malformations who develop a *consumptive coagulopathy*. In these patients (who are often adults) the platelet count is depressed to

50,000 to 150,000 per mm³ and treatment with heparin improves the coagulopathy.[7]

Proliferating phase infantile hemangioma is characterized by increased endothelial cell turnover.[2,19] Capillary endothelium derived from these tumors grows easily in tissue culture and forms tubules.[19,20] During the proliferating phase, hemangiomas express endothelial markers such as CD31 and factor VIII–related antigen (von Willebrand factor), among others.[5,7-9,19,20] The angiogenic peptides, vascular endothelial growth factor (VEGF) and basic fibroblast growth factor (bFGF), proliferating cell nuclear antigen (PCNA), and type IV collagenase are upregulated during proliferation.[5,8,9,19]

As infantile hemangioma enters the involuting phase (approximately 1 year of age), mast cells, other monocytes, and fibroblasts become evident and deposit fibrous tissue around vessels and interstices.[21] Apoptosis begins and reaches an apogee by 2 years.[19,22] A suppressor of new blood vessel formation, tissue inhibitor of metalloproteinase (TIMP-1), is produced and regulated by an autocrine induction loop.[19] At the end of its life cycle, only a few vessels remain in the hemangioma, which is now lined by flat, mature endothelial cells and surrounded by variable fibrofatty tissue.[3,5,7,21]

Vascular Malformations

Malformations, the second major group of vascular anomalies, are the result of abnormalities of blood and lymphatic vessel morphogenesis. Vascular malformations are present at birth, although many do not become clinically obvious until late in infancy or childhood.[2,5-7] They usually grow proportionately with the patient; they never regress, and they persist throughout life. Vascular malformations expand or increase in size with trauma, infection, or endocrine changes (e.g., pregnancy and puberty).[1,2,5-7] Most vascular malformations were considered to be sporadic; however, some are inheritable in a classic mendelian autosomal dominant pattern.[3,7] Vikkula and colleagues[8] have written a review of the molecular basis of familial vascular anomalies.

Vascular malformations are associated with skeletal alterations in one third of cases.[1,5,10,13] There may be a primary intraosseous vascular malformation, or the bone adjacent to a malformation can exhibit a change in size, shape, or density.[1,5,10,13,23] The most common

abnormality is expansion or overgrowth of bone, deep to a slow-flow cutaneous vascular malformation. On a cellular level, these anomalies are characterized by a normal endothelial cell cycle, unless the lesion is perturbed by thrombosis, trauma, or endovascular or surgical intervention.[2,3,5,7]

Vascular malformations are classified anatomically by the vessels involved and flow characteristics. Most lesions are composed of a single type of anomalous vessel, but so-called *combined malformations* also occur (see Box 17-1). The malformation should be described according to the predominant type(s) of vessel(s) involved. For example, the port wine stain, once erroneously referred to as a *capillary hemangioma*, should be called a *capillary malformation*. This is a congenital dermal ectasia of capillaries and venules. Similarly, the nineteenth century terms *lymphangioma* and *cystic hygroma* connoted a tumor of lymphatic origin, but the more precise term is *lymphatic malformation*. The old designation *cavernous hemangioma* is a venous malformation. The term *hemangiolymphangioma* indicates a combined lymphaticovenous malformation. Arterial malformations are aneurysms, ectasias, or stenoses. Arteriovenous fistulas and arteriovenous malformations also occur in the maxillofacial region.

The type of channel anomaly can also be categorized by flow characteristics, in that capillary, venous, lymphatic, and most combined malformations are slow-flow lesions, whereas AVMs are fast-flow lesions. The lesions called "hemangiomas" in the oral surgical literature are most commonly venous malformations, or AVMs.[1,13,24,25]

CASE REPORTS

The nosologic system described in this chapter (see Box 17-1) is illustrated by the following case reports of vascular anomalies in the maxillofacial region.

CASE REPORT 1   INFANTILE HEMANGIOMA

This female infant, who was otherwise completely normal, had a slight discoloration of the skin in the region of the upper lip noted shortly after birth. The lesion grew rapidly during the following 10 months. Over the next 2 years, it slowly involuted and the residual tumor was excised partially to improve the lip contour

(Figure 17-2). This cutaneous vascular lesion represents the most common benign tumor in childhood, occurring in 5% to 10% of white infants. The rapid proliferation during the first months of life, followed by slow involution without involvement of the underlying bone, characterizes hemangiomas of infancy.

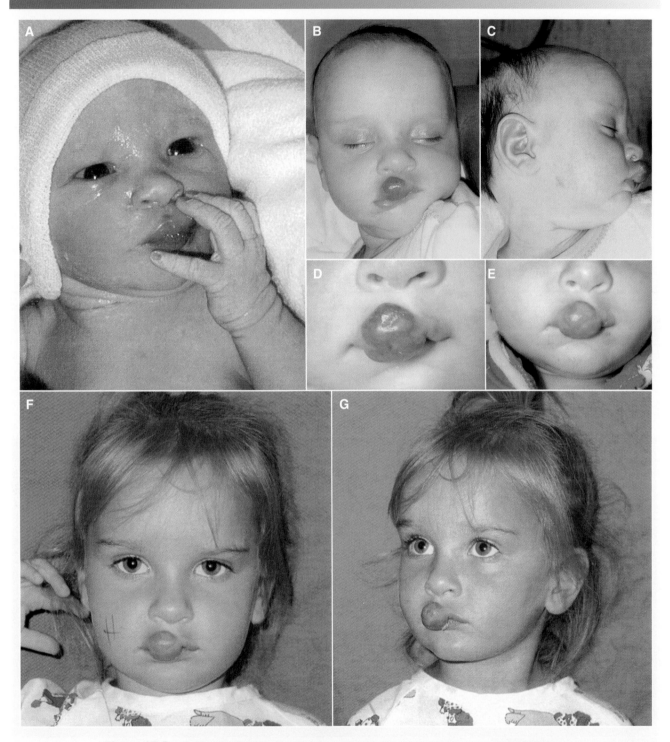

Figure 17-2

A, A newborn infant with normal facial appearance except for a small reddish discoloration at the lower end of the philtral column. Frontal **(B)** and lateral **(C)** photographs at 3 months of age show rapid growth of the lesion (proliferative phase hemangioma). **D,** Superficial ulceration is present 1 month later. **E,** Partial involution after a series of three intralesional triamcinolone injections (17 months of age). **F** and **G,** At 2½ years (30 months) of age, there has been further involution. The child is now left with a soft, hanging mass and residual hemangioma.

Continued

CASE REPORT 1   INFANTILE HEMANGIOMA—cont'd

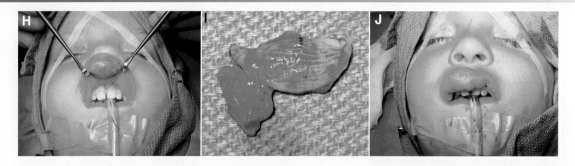

Figure 17-2—continued   ▐

H, Intraoperative view of the mucosal incision used for elliptical excision. I, Specimen showing mucosal excision and hemangioma. J, Wound closure demonstrating improved contour of the lip.

CASE REPORT 2   FACIAL CAPILLARY MALFORMATION

This teenage boy has a facial capillary malformation in the V2-V3 distribution. There was distortion of the adjacent underlying maxillary alveolar ridge, mandibular body, and symphysis, with resultant malocclusion (Figure 17-3). The bone was abnormal in size and shape, but there was no intraosseous vascular malformation. An orthognathic procedure was necessary to correct the malocclusion. As expected, bleeding was not excessive during the operation.

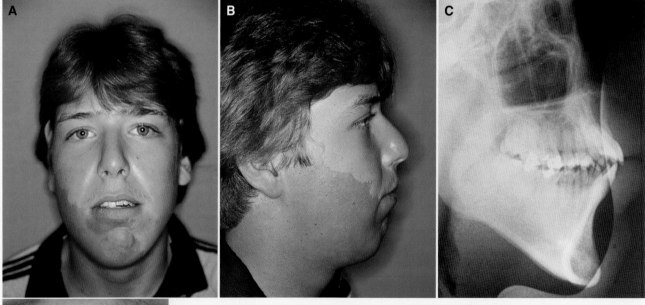

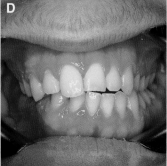

Figure 17-3   ▐

Capillary malformation (port wine stain) with hypertrophy of the underlying maxilla and mandible. Frontal (A) and lateral (B) photographs of a teenage boy with a capillary malformation in the right third division dermatome. Note the vertical maxillary excess and strain of mentalis muscles to close the lips. C, Lateral cephalogram shows the long lower face height and bimaxillary dentoalveolar protrusion. D, Intraoral photograph shows the step in the maxillary occlusal plane at the midline, indicating excessive vertical growth of the alveolus on the right side.

Continued

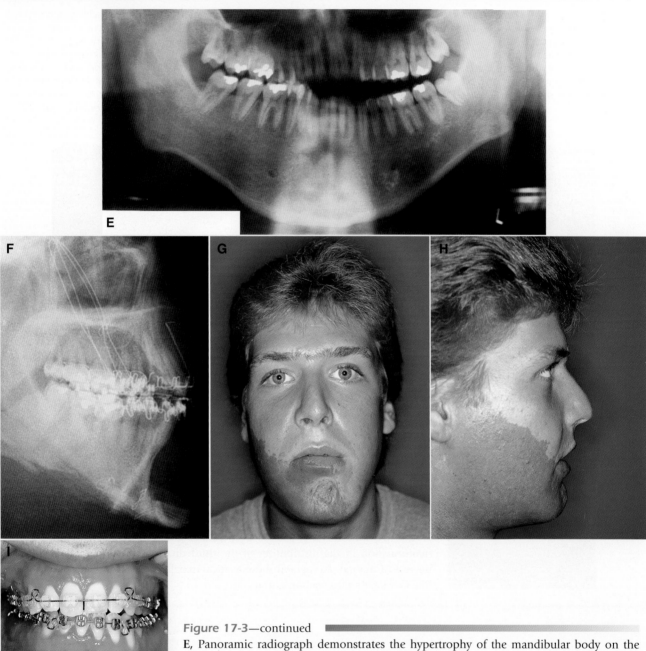

Figure 17-3—continued

E, Panoramic radiograph demonstrates the hypertrophy of the mandibular body on the right side. Since this malformation did not directly involve the bone, orthognathic surgery could be performed without risk of bleeding. **F,** Postoperative lateral cephalogram demonstrating the change in jaw relations. Frontal **(G),** lateral **(H),** and intraoral **(I)** views after multiple segment Le Fort I osteotomy, bilateral mandibular osteotomies, and a genioplasty.

CASE REPORT 3 DERMAL CAPILLARY MALFORMATION

This teenage girl has a typical dermal capillary malformation, also called port wine stain (Figure 17-4). The lesion was present at birth and grew proportionately with the patient. Distribution of these lesions often follows one, or a combination of, trigeminal nerve dermatomes, in this case the third (mandibular) division. The underlying cheek, lip, and alveolar mucosa, as well as the gingiva, often are involved.

This patient developed an open bite with vertical maxillary excess, probably unrelated to the vascular malformation. The adjacent bone was normal and not involved. However, distortion and overgrowth of the facial skeleton typically is seen in Sturge-Weber syndrome (facial port wine stain with choroidal and leptomeningeal vascular abnormalities).[10] Labial and gingival hypertrophy and chronic bleeding commonly occurs in older patients with this disorder (Figure 17-5).

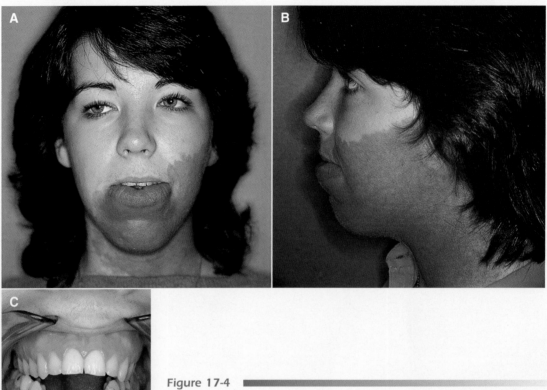

Figure 17-4

Frontal (**A**) and lateral (**B**) views of a teenage girl with dermal capillary malformation in the distribution of the third division of the trigeminal nerve. **C,** Intraoral photograph shows vertical maxillary excess and an open bite unrelated to the malformation.

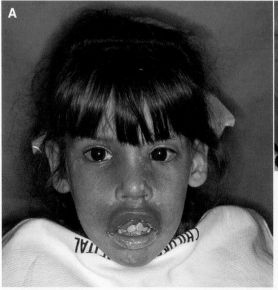

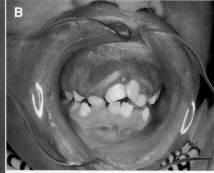

Figure 17-5

A girl with Sturge-Weber syndrome. Note the deep-red port wine stain of the midface and the deep reddish blue color and swelling of the anterior maxillary gingival and alveolar mucosa.

CASE REPORT 4   VENOUS MALFORMATION

This teenage girl has a small venous malformation of the lower lip (Figure 17-6). In the past, such a lesion was incorrectly labeled cavernous hemangioma. There was considerable distortion of the adjacent alveolar ridge, but radiographs did not show bony abnormalities. For this reason, a dentoalveolar procedure would not be expected to cause abnormal bleeding. In addition, this small lesion would be unlikely to be associated with a localized or generalized consumptive coagulopathy, a possibility with more extensive venous lesions (see Case Report 7).

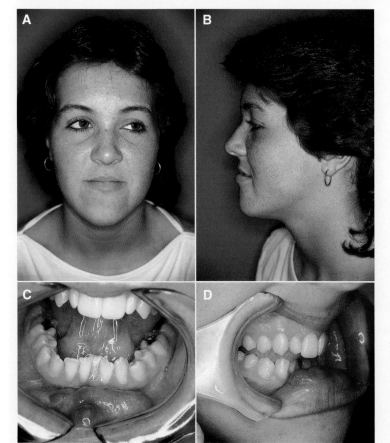

Figure 17-6

Frontal (**A**) and lateral (**B**) views of a teenage girl with swelling of the lower lip between the vermillion border and labiomental fold. This is a venous malformation of the lower labial mucosa. **C** and **D**, Intraoral photographs show the mucosal venous malformation and deformation of the adjacent alveolar ridge. The alveolar bone was abnormal in shape, but there was no intraosseous malformation.

This teenage girl has a combined slow-flow lesion of the capillary-lymphatic type (Figure 17-7). She had a long history of intermittent pain, swelling, trismus, and fever, accompanied by a darkening hue of the vascular malformation due to intermittent intralesional bleeding. It was difficult to differentiate clinically between cellulitis, thrombophlebitis, and phlebothrombosis in this patient.

Such lesions increase in size, not only in relation to viral illnesses, adjacent infection, and trauma, but also secondary to intralesional infection or clotting. Occasionally, the patients develop systemic sepsis related to local infection with hematogenous spread. In these cases, hospital admission and intravenous antibiotic therapy are necessary.

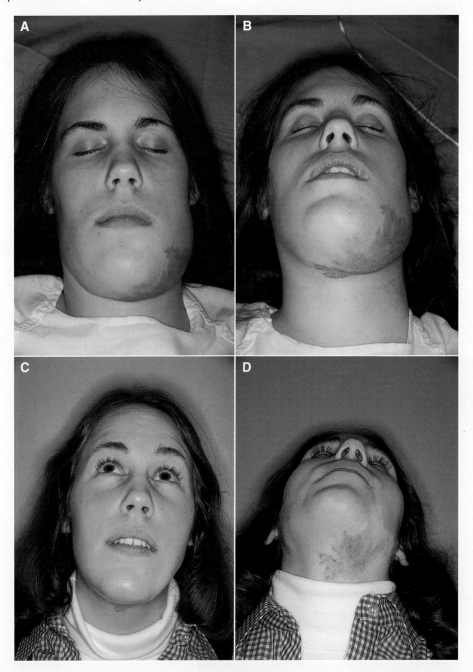

Figure 17-7

Combined capillary-lymphatic malformation (CLM). Frontal **(A)** and submental **(B)** views of a teenage patient with a CLM in the left third division dermatome. This malformation extended to the mucosa, but the mandible was not involved. The malformation is swollen, hot, tender, and very deep purple in color as a result of infection or thrombophlebitis. Frontal **(C)** and submental **(D)** views several months after the infection was controlled with intravenous antibiotics. Note the marked decrease in swelling and the loss of the deep purple color. The texture of the skin surface *(right)* is pebbly.

CASE REPORT 6   LYMPHATIC MALFORMATION

This 10-year-old patient was born with a large lymphatic malformation (previously called cystic hygroma) on the left side of the face, extending from the temporal region to the clavicle (Figure 17-8). The malformation also involved the skin, mucosa, tongue, and floor of the mouth. Overgrowth and distortion of the underlying maxilla and mandible, as well as adjacent auricular cartilage, are typical of the skeletal changes seen with lymphatic malforma-tions (see Figure 20-6). The lateral skull radiograph demonstrated decreased bone density with increased size of the mandible. There was also macrodontia and increased spacing between the teeth (overgrowth of the mandibular body), indicative of intraosseous malformation. In this patient, upper respiratory tract infections typically were accompanied by increased swelling of the malformation.

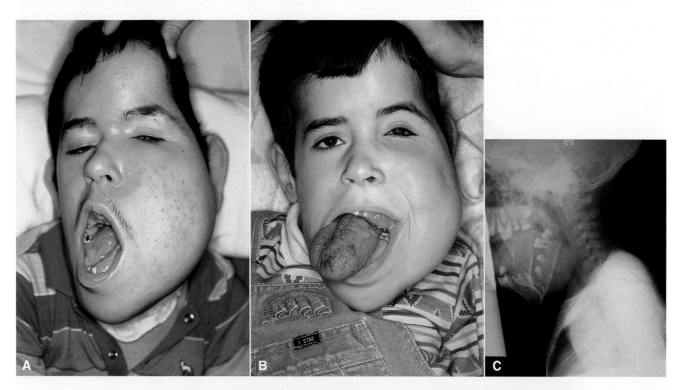

Figure 17-8
Lymphatic malformation (LM). **A** and **B**, Large LM of left face, floor of mouth, and tongue. Note the increase in the size of the left ear cartilage and craniomaxillary skeleton—a common finding adjacent to a lymphatic malformation. **C**, Lateral head radiograph shows decreased density of bone in mandible and separation and displacement of the teeth.

CASE REPORT 7   EXTENSIVE VENOUS MALFORMATION

This patient had an extensive venous malformation (Figure 17-9) and a long history of intermittent swelling and pain in both jaws. He had been denied dental care because of the fear of excessive bleeding. Physical examination demonstrated an extensive vascular malformation of the face, neck, thorax, and one upper extremity. The soft tissue over the mandible was deep purple, tender, and edematous. Intraorally, there was purulent drainage from around the remaining mandibular teeth and maxillary molars. The vascular malformation involved the buccal mucosa, alveolar ridge, palate, floor of the mouth, and tongue (Figure 17-9). The teeth were mobile and there was considerable osteolysis of the mandible, prima facie evidence of an intraosseous vascular malformation.

Panoramic and lateral cephalometric radiographs confirmed loss of mandibular bone mass and marked distortion of mandibular shape. An arteriogram showed a normal arterial phase with an internal maxillary artery of normal caliber. However, there was rapid onset of the venous phase, suggesting possible microarteriovenous

Continued

shunting. The late venous phase demonstrated pooling of contrast medium in large vascular "lakes," characteristic of venous malformation (Figure 17-9).

Hematologic evaluation revealed normal prothrombin (PT) and partial thromboplastin times (PTT), but a lengthened thrombin time. The hematocrit was 37.2%, the hemoglobin level 12.8 g/dl, the leukocyte count 5200/mm³, and the platelet count 112,000/mm³. The fibrinogen level was low (65 mg/dl with a normal range of 200 to 400). Fibrin split products were elevated (20 μg/ml with a normal value of less than 10 μg/ml). Thus the abnormal hematologic values were indicative of a low-grade disseminated intravascular coagulopathy, secondary to localized stasis, clotting, and consumption of coagulation factors within the venous malformation.

The coagulopathy was treated with aspirin 325 mg/day and intravenous heparin 1000 U/hr. After 7 days of anticoagulant therapy, PT, PTT, fibrinogen levels, and fibrin split product values were normal. Both internal maxillary arteries were embolized with Gelfoam. Forty-eight hours later, the remaining mandibular teeth and several infected maxillary molars were removed in the operating room. Hemostasis was achieved by packing with microfibrillar collagen (Avitene) wrapped in surgical sheets held in place with figure-of-eight sutures across the sockets. Intraoperative blood loss was 300 ml. The administration of heparin (1000 U/hr) to control the levels of fibrinogen and fibrin split products was continued for 1 week following the procedure. By that time, the patient had no further oozing from the extraction sites, and he was discharged 3 days later (11 days after operation).

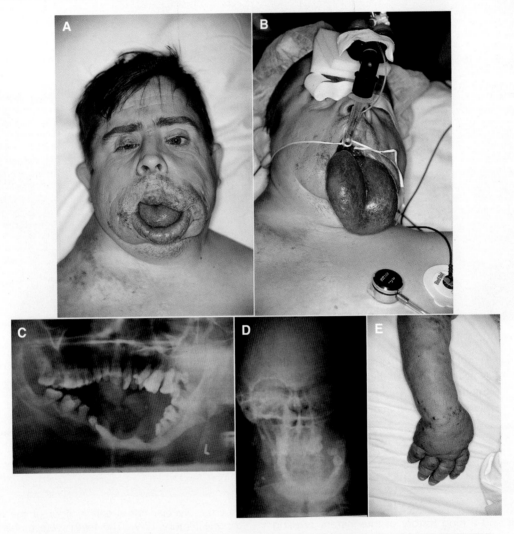

Figure 17-9

Extensive soft tissue and intraosseous venous malformation (VM) with microshunting and coexisting acute infection. **A,** Frontal view of a patient with onset of acute odontogenic infection related to the mandibular teeth. The infection produced increased swelling of the VM of the tongue and the floor of the mouth. **B,** Progressive swelling of the tongue occurred with the patient on antibiotics. Intubation was necessary to alleviate the airway obstruction. **C,** Panoramic radiograph documents extensive bone resorption in the mandible. There was purulent drainage around all these periodontally infected teeth. **D,** Anteroposterior cephalogram shows loss of bone in the anterior mandible. Calcifications in the soft tissues over the right mandible are phleboliths. **E,** Right arm illustrates extremity VM in this patient.

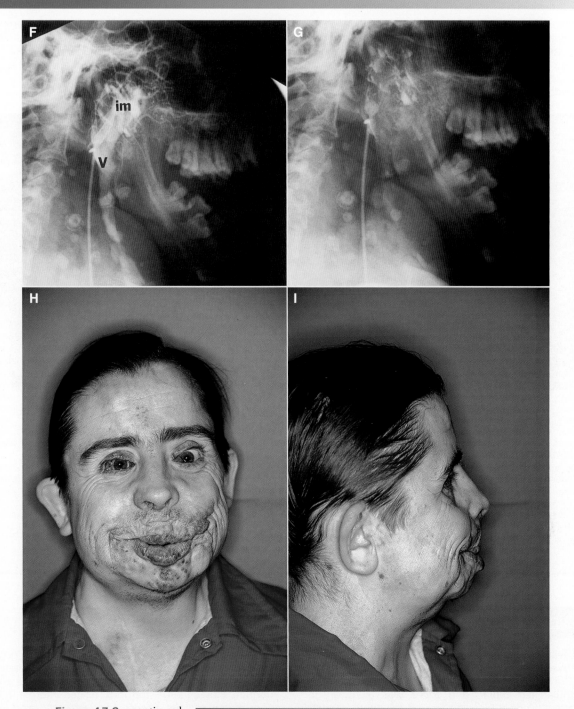

Figure 17-9—continued

F, Arterial phase of arteriogram shows normal-caliber internal maxillary *(im)* artery with slightly increased tortuosity. There is rapid filling of the venous system. Note dilated internal jugular *(V)*. **G,** Late venous phase of arteriogram shows venous lakes in the area of the ramus and phleboliths in the neck. Frontal **(H)** and lateral **(I)** views after the infection was cured. Note that the facial and tongue swelling decreased markedly.

CASE REPORT 8   EXTENSIVE VENOUS MALFORMATION[26]

This patient has an extensive venous malformation. The malformation involved the maxilla, mandible, floor of the mouth, tongue, neck, thorax, and right upper extremity. Complete removal of this vascular malformation was impossible. Partial resection was performed as a life-saving maneuver under cardiopulmonary bypass and deep hypothermic arrest.[26] Follow-up photographs illustrate the residual malformation that continued to expand, involving the neck, mediastinum, and anterior chest (Figure 17-10). The patient died of a massive hemorrhage into his airway below a permanent tracheostomy.

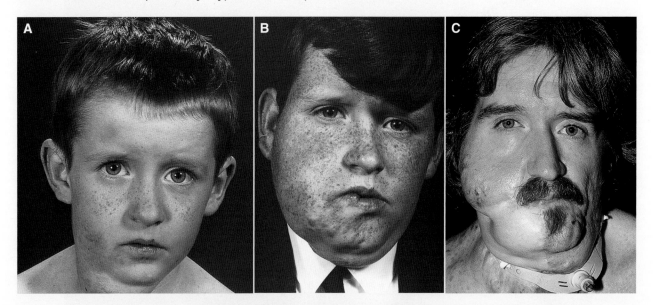

Figure 17-10

Extensive venous malformation with microscopic arteriovenous shunting. **A,** An 8-year-old boy with venous malformation of the right face, submandibular region, and neck. **B,** The patient at age 14 years, showing an increase in the size of the malformation despite attempted subtotal resection. **C,** At age 24 years the patient is shown 7 years after massive resection of the tongue, floor of the mouth, and cheek—under cardiopulmonary bypass and deep hypothermic arrest. This was done as a life-saving procedure for massive, sudden bleeding of the tongue. Note expansion of the malformation at the borders of the resection. The tracheostomy tube became progressively deviated to the left, with expansion of the malformation within the neck and mediastinum.

CASE REPORT 9   ARTERIOVENOUS MALFORMATION

This 8-year-old boy had a painful, tender, warm vascular lesion over the left mandible that had been present since birth (Figure 17-11). He had a toothache related to a loose mandibular left molar, and there was a history of intermittent gingival bleeding around this tooth. Physical examination revealed a deep capillary stain over the left mandible and submandibular region. The area was warm, edematous, and tender to palpation; there was a palpable thrill and an audible bruit. Intraorally, the malformation involved the buccal and alveolar mucosa, as well as the gingiva and floor of the mouth. The 6-year molar was loose and tender to percussion, and there was slow oozing around the gingival margin. Radiographs revealed an increase in the size of the left mandible, decreased bone density, and widened spaces between the teeth, indicative of intraosseous high-flow malformation.

Hematologic and coagulative findings were negative. Axial computed tomography demonstrated AVM in the soft tissue and involvement of the underlying mandible. An arteriogram showed large, tortuous, dilated internal maxillary and inferior alveolar arteries and extremely rapid venous filling (Figure 17-11). The dense contrast in the bone was indicative of intraosseous malformation. Skeletal scintigraphy with technetium-99m–methylene diphosphonate revealed increased uptake in the bone and vascular phases, confirming an intraosseous vascular malformation. The intralesional infection was controlled with clindamycin, administered intravenously for 5 days, and the tooth was extracted. There was a rapid blood loss of 750 ml; the socket was packed with microfibrillar collagen (Avitene) wrapped in surgical sheets and sutured with a 2-0 chromic catgut figure-of-eight stitch. There were no postoperative problems with hemostasis.

Continued

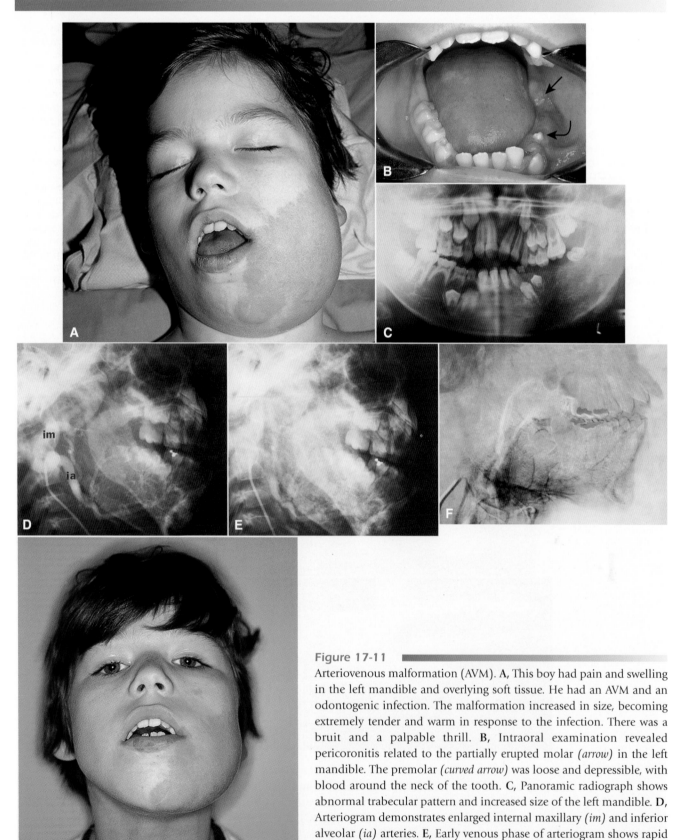

Figure 17-11

Arteriovenous malformation (AVM). **A,** This boy had pain and swelling in the left mandible and overlying soft tissue. He had an AVM and an odontogenic infection. The malformation increased in size, becoming extremely tender and warm in response to the infection. There was a bruit and a palpable thrill. **B,** Intraoral examination revealed pericoronitis related to the partially erupted molar *(arrow)* in the left mandible. The premolar *(curved arrow)* was loose and depressible, with blood around the neck of the tooth. **C,** Panoramic radiograph shows abnormal trabecular pattern and increased size of the left mandible. **D,** Arteriogram demonstrates enlarged internal maxillary *(im)* and inferior alveolar *(ia)* arteries. **E,** Early venous phase of arteriogram shows rapid venous filling indicative of arteriovenous shunts. **F,** Subtraction film of bone phase shows dense blush in mandible, indicating intraosseous malformation. **G,** Full face view after the infection was controlled, as described in text. The swelling is decreased, and the color is lighter.

This young boy has a fast-flow AVM involving the left maxilla, mandible, and surrounding soft tissues. The lesion was present at birth and the patient was asymptomatic until approximately 6 years before admission to the oral maxillofacial surgery service. At that time, he began to have recurrent episodes of bleeding and expansion of the malformation. The bleeding episodes increased in severity and frequency, necessitating endovascular embolization every 4 to 6 months. Just before hospital admission, a massive bleeding episode occurred around the left maxillary teeth. The patient's hemoglobin decreased to 8 g/dl and a transfusion was required.

Physical examination revealed a large, soft, bluish red cutaneous mass and an obvious facial asymmetry (Figure 17-12, A). The area was warm and pulsatile and exhibited a bruit on auscultation. All teeth in the posterior maxilla and mandible were mobile, and the gingiva and mucosa were deep blue in color (Figure 17-12, B and C).

There were large multilocular radiolucencies in the left maxilla and mandible on the panoramic radiograph (Figure

17-12, D), and there was bone resorption (osteolysis) around the teeth. Angiograms demonstrated a fast-flow AVM involving the left maxilla, mandible, and soft tissues of the cheek. There were four major arterial sources: right and left facial and internal maxillary arteries, along with multiple small arteries, as well as large lytic lesions (varices) of the left posterior maxilla and mandible (Figure 17-12, E). The patient was treated eventually with direct puncture platinum coil embolization for the maxillary and mandibular varices and extraction of the posterior teeth. The osteolytic areas of the maxilla and mandible filled in with bone and the patient has been free of bleeding episodes for 5 years.

In this case, complete excision of the extensive AVM involving the external carotid system, after multiple previous embolization procedures, would not have been possible. The goal of treatment was to diminish inflow to the lesion to allow extraction of the teeth. Once extraction was accomplished and the wounds healed, the risk of bleeding would diminish. An added benefit was obliteration of the large intraosseous vascular cavities, with bone formation in response to the platinum coils.

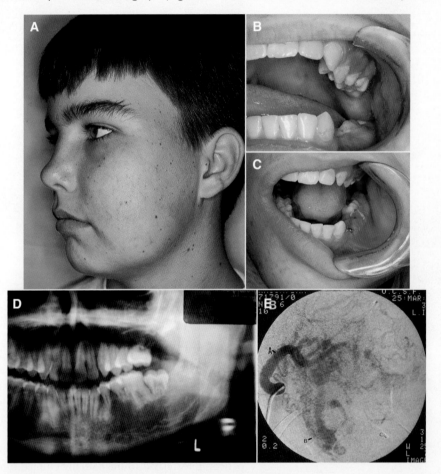

Figure 17-12

Arteriovenous malformation (AVM) of the maxilla and mandible. **A,** Lateral view demonstrating swelling of facial soft tissue over the left maxilla and mandible. The cheek was soft but warm in relation to the surrounding soft tissue. **B,** Intraoral view of the left maxilla. Note the deep red color of the gingiva and alveolar mucosa. The teeth were mobile and compressible. **C,** Intraoral view of the left mandible demonstrates similar findings. The teeth were mobile and compressible. **D,** Panoramic radiograph demonstrating diffuse lytic changes in the left mandibular body and left maxilla. **E,** Lateral view angiogram showing catheter in the enlarged and tortuous left internal maxillary artery *(A),* and large varix of the mandible *(B)* and surrounding soft tissue.   *Continued*

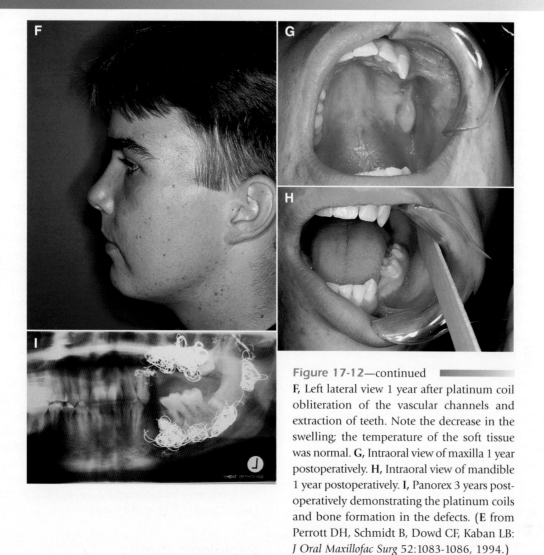

Figure 17-12—continued F, Left lateral view 1 year after platinum coil obliteration of the vascular channels and extraction of teeth. Note the decrease in the swelling; the temperature of the soft tissue was normal. G, Intraoral view of maxilla 1 year postoperatively. H, Intraoral view of mandible 1 year postoperatively. I, Panorex 3 years postoperatively demonstrating the platinum coils and bone formation in the defects. (E from Perrott DH, Schmidt B, Dowd CF, Kaban LB: *J Oral Maxillofac Surg* 52:1083-1086, 1994.)

A CONCEPTUAL APPROACH TO MAXILLOFACIAL VASCULAR ANOMALIES

The first, and most crucial, step in evaluating a patient with a maxillofacial vascular anomaly is to determine whether the vascular lesion is a tumor (hemangioma, hemangioendothelioma, or angiosarcoma) or a malformation. Accurate historical data are obtained from the patient and family; it is critical to review the newborn, infant, and childhood photographs whenever possible. History and physical examination provide an accurate diagnosis in more than 90% of infants and children with vascular lesions involving skin or mucosa.[3,7,28]

Although infantile hemangioma may be present during the infant's stay in the nursery, as a tiny or macular telangiectasia or a pale spot, most tumors appear within 2 to 4 weeks after birth and grow rapidly. Vascular malformations, unlike hemangiomas, are almost always noticed at birth and grow proportionately with the patient.[1,2,5-7,10] Spontaneous expansion of a vascular malformation, or bleeding secondary to trauma or infection, can cause an acute painful swelling. Some vascular malformations do not become clinically evident until the patient is older; this is particularly true of intraosseous lesions. Vascular malformations frequently cause bony distortion, destruction, or hypertrophy, whereas intraosseous hemangiomas are extremely rare, if they occur at all.[1,2,10,13] *Consequently, a vascular lesion involving bone is almost certain to be a malformation (lymphatic, venous, or arterial) rather than a tumor.* Nevertheless, there are primary vascular tumors that occur in bone, such as epithelioid hemangioendothelioma and hemangiopericytoma.[4-7,29]

The distinction between a vascular tumor (hemangioma, hemangioendothelioma, or angiosarcoma) versus vascular malformation is extremely important because of the major implications for prognosis and treatment. Vascular malformations do not grow by cellular proliferation, but rather expand by dilation of abnormal channels and formation of collateral vessels. Complete resection is not possible in most cases, hence the possibility of uncontrollable bleeding during operation and the likelihood of persistence after resection (see Case Report 8, Figure 17-10). Occasionally, a well-localized, low-flow venous malformation of the jaw is resectable (Figures 17-13 to 17-15).

Clinical Examination

Infantile Hemangiomas. Infantile hemangiomas have distinct margins, whereas others are diffuse lesions throughout the upper dermis. Early superficial infantile hemangiomas are bright red, whereas deep lesions may not exhibit cutaneous or mucosal discoloration. Infantile hemangioma is firm to palpation, and there are no pulsations, although a prominent Doppler signal is present. Infantile hemangiomas are fast-flow lesions during the proliferating phase and slow-flow during regression. Frequently, dilated cutaneous veins are visible in the area of the tumor. By the time the patient is 1 year of age, infantile hemangioma begins to exhibit the first signs of involution. The bright red color of a superficial lesion deepens, small central areas on the surface become gray, and the lesion is less tense on palpation (see Figure 17-1). Deep hemangiomas, with intact overlying skin, soften and gradually involute, just as do the bright red superficial lesions.[7] Involution is usually complete by age 5 to 8 years. In some patients, complete involution may not occur until 10 to 12 years of age. The skin color typically fades to a normal hue, but often there is minor telangiectasia and lost elasticity. There may be a fibro-fatty residuum, particularly in the submucosa.[1,2,5-7]

Vascular Malformations. Vascular malformations vary in color and configuration, depending on the vessels involved. Capillary malformations are pink during infancy, darken during childhood, and become deep purple in older patients. They are smooth in children, with the texture of normal skin, whereas in adults the surface often becomes pebbly and slightly raised. Venous malformations are bluish, soft, and easily compressible; phleboliths are often palpated. Venous malformations occur in a spectrum, from isolated skin or mucosal varicosities or ectasias, to localized spongy masses, to complex lesions permeated throughout tissue planes. Venous abnormalities expand with the Valsalva maneuver or dependency. Enlargement can follow injury or partial resection or can occur coincident with puberty, pregnancy, or medication to suppress ovulation.

Lymphatic Lesions. Lymphatic lesions are usually colorless, whereas combined lymphatic-venous malformations (called *hemolymphangiomas* in the past) are deep purple-blue in color. Expansion often occurs coincident with any upper respiratory tract infection. This anomalous lymphatic tissue seems unable to control the periodic seeding with oral microorganisms. Macrocystic lesions of the head and neck (called *cystic hygroma* in the past) usually can be transilluminated. Lymphatic malformations also can expand suddenly secondary to bacterial infection (cellulitis) or intralesional bleeding.[1,3,7,10] Intraorally, pure (lymphatic malformation) or combined capillary-lymphatic malformations often have very irregular surfaces, with clear or dark hemorrhagic bullae and vesicles that have been described as resembling salmon eggs (Figure 17-16). The patient may notice bleeding from these areas in the morning upon awakening, possibly due to the increased venous pressure of sleeping supine.

Arteriovenous Lesions. Arteriovenous lesions (AVM) are warm and sometimes tender and, if there is macroshunting, pulsations and a bruit can be appreciated. Schobinger introduced a clinical staging system for AVMs that is helpful in predicting the natural history.[7] Stage I lesions are quiescent; stage II are expansile and exhibit enlargement, pulsations, and a bruit; stage III lesions are destructive; and stage IV lesions are associated with decompensatory cardiac failure (Table 17-1). Intraorally, the mucosa is stained and often there is gingival hypertrophy. There may be bleeding around the necks of the teeth in the area of the malformation, and the teeth may be loose and depressible into the alveolus (see Figures 17-11 and 17-12).

Radiologic Studies

Magnetic resonance imaging (MRI) with gadolinium enhancement is the standard technique for studying vascular lesions. Infantile hemangiomas appear as a soft tissue mass of intermediate intensity on T1-weighted images and hyperintensity on T2-weighted images. There are flow voids around and within the tumor mass indicating high flow and shunting between arteries and veins[7] (Figure 17-17). Involuting hemangiomas demonstrate less flow and increasing lobularity and fatty tissue. MRI is useful in differentiating a deep hemangioma from a lymphatic or venous malformation.[7] Angiography is never indicated in the evaluation of hemangiomas[5,7,28,30] and is rarely used for diagnosis or to determine the hemodynamic nature and extent of a vascular malformation.[28,30] Angiography usually is done before endovascular treatment of a vascular malformation (Figure 17-16). Plain radiography and CT demonstrate bony changes in relation to vascular lesions. Rarely, a

A
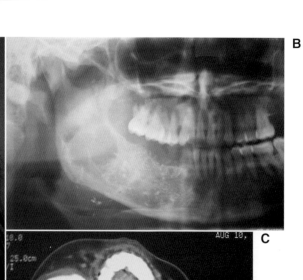
B

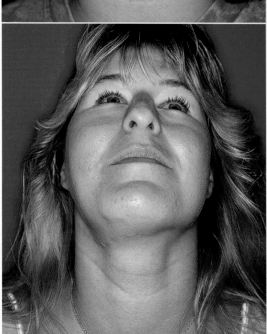
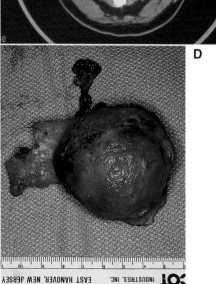
C

D

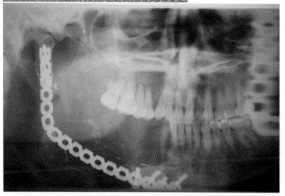
F

E

Figure 17-13

Low-flow venous malformation of the mandible. **A,** Submental view of an adult patient with a low-flow venous malformation present since birth. Because of increasing pain, increasing size, and concern for bleeding and esthetics, she requested resection, if possible. **B,** Panorex demonstrates lytic changes in the bone, evidence of intraosseous malformation. **C,** Axial CT image, with contrast, confirms large malformation of the mandible extending into the soft tissue. **D,** Resected specimen demonstrates the ability to remove well-localized low-flow malformations. **E,** Submental view 1 year postoperatively. **F,** Panoramic radiograph 1 year postoperatively shows bone plate and condylar prosthesis. The patient elected to delay skeletal reconstruction.

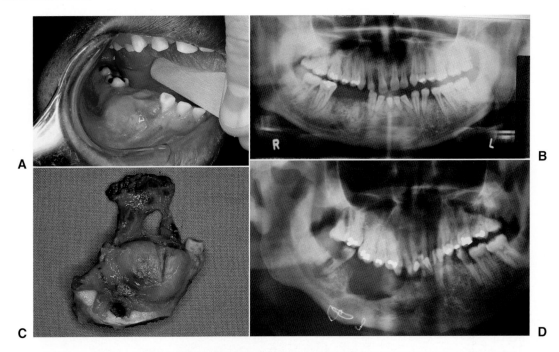

Figure 17-14

Intraosseous venous malformation (VM) of the mandible. **A,** Intraoral view of a patient with VM of the gingiva and bone of right mandible. **B,** Panoramic radiograph shows abnormal bone configuration in the canine-premolar region. These teeth were previously extremely mobile and were shed spontaneously without major bleeding. **C,** The patient underwent marginal resection for intermittent bleeding of the alveolar ridge. The specimen shows lesion and normal bone margins. **D,** The mandible was reconstructed with an iliac bone graft.

large infantile hemangioma can produce skeletal change by a mass effect or hypertrophy secondary to increased blood flow during the proliferating phase. In contrast, one third of vascular malformations of the head and neck area show skeletal aberrations.[13] Typical skeletal changes include increased size of the underlying bone, hypertrophy, distortion in shape (seen with venous, lymphatic, or combined lesions), or decreased skeletal density, such as bony destruction (seen with arteriovenous lesions).[1,13,23]

The evolution of skeletal changes associated with vascular malformations has been difficult to document because radiographs at birth are not available or have not been taken. In a study by Boyd et al.,[13] two patients with lymphatic malformations had normal radiographs of the affected region at birth. The earliest recorded skeletal change was seen at 11 months in a patient with a lymphatic malformation and secondary orbital expansion. Fifteen of the 27 head and neck patients evaluated by Boyd and colleagues[13] had alterations in the skeleton by age 10 years. Seventy-seven percent of the patients with a lymphatic malformation had radiologic evidence of altered skeletal growth by age 10 years.

TABLE 17-1   Schobinger Clinical Staging System for Arteriovenous Malformation

Stage	Description
I (Quiescence)	Pink-bluish stain, warmth, and arteriovascular shunting by continuous Doppler scanning or 20-MHz color Doppler scanning
II (Expansion)	Same as stage I plus enlargement, pulsations, thrill, and bruit and tortuous, tense veins
III (Destruction)	Same as stage II plus either dystrophic skin changes, ulceration, bleeding, persistent pain, or tissue necrosis
IV (Decompensation)	Same as stage III plus cardiac failure

From Mulliken JB, Fishman SJ, Burrows PE: *Curr Probl Surg* 37(8):520-576, 2000.

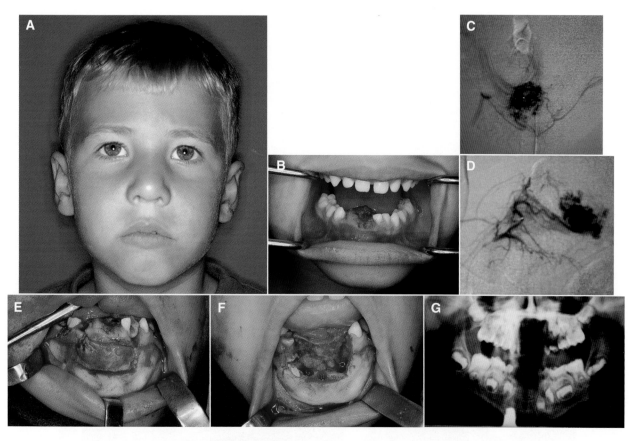

Figure 17-15

Low-flow venous malformation. **A,** A 6-year old boy with low-flow venous malformation of the mandibular symphysis region. Extraoral swelling below the lower lip is minimal. **B,** Intraoral view demonstrates bluish red lesion in the symphysis region with several missing deciduous incisors. Frontal **(C)** and lateral **(D)** subtraction arteriograms demonstrate the lesion. **E** and **F,** Intraoral views of the marginal resection illustrate the well-localized bone lesion and the defect after resection. **G,** Panorex 1 year later shows the bone fill in the defect. There was no recurrence.

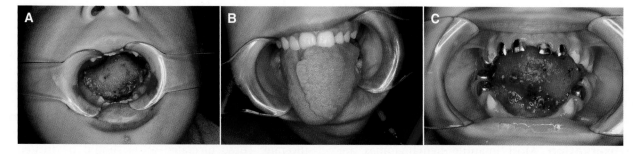

Figure 17-16

Intraoral low-flow malformations. **A,** Combined capillary-lymphatic malformation of the tongue with pebbly, "salmon eggs" appearance. **B,** Mixed lymphatic-venous malformation of the left side of the tongue. **C,** Combined capillary-lymphatic-venous malformation of the tongue and floor of the mouth. Note the pebbly texture, evidence of bleeding, and deformation of the mandible and maxilla, which produces an open bite.

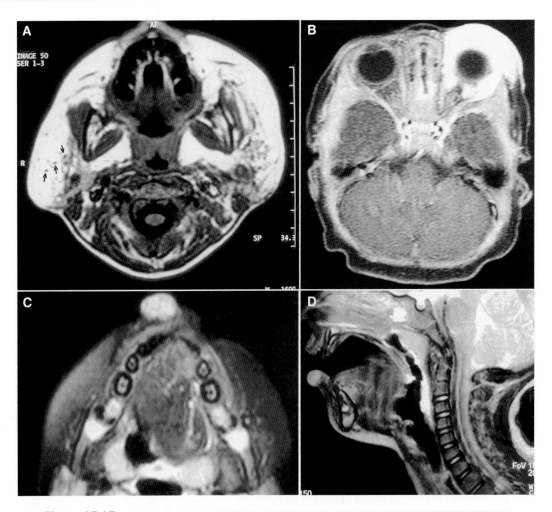

Figure 17-17

A, T-2 weighted axial MRI of a proliferative phase hemangioma of the right parotid gland demonstrates hyperintense signal and vascular flow voids *(arrows)*, indicating fast-flow in a proliferating lesion. **B,** T-2 weighted axial MRI of a periorbital proliferating phase hemangioma demonstrates hyperintense signal. Axial **(C)** and sagittal **(D)** MRI images of an involuting-phase hemangioma of the lower lip. There is contrast enhancement with gadolinium administration but significantly less than in the proliferating-phase tumors.

Management of Infantile Hemangioma

Oral and maxillofacial surgeons rarely are called on to evaluate and treat the common cutaneous infantile hemangioma. However, they are consulted frequently regarding lesions on the palate, gums, or lips. In many cases, these lesions are of little consequence; these should be allowed to undergo proliferation and spontaneous involution.

Observation. Most infantile hemangiomas are small and produce no functional or long-term problems for the patient. The child should be observed while the tumor proliferates and ultimately undergoes involution. Usually, the skin becomes normal in quality or only slightly blemished.[7,28,30] The pediatrician or surgeon should explain the natural history of infantile heman-

gioma and reassure the parents and family regarding the ultimate outcome. It may be helpful, in cases where there is family pressure for immediate operation, to show the parents photographs of a similar tumor during proliferation and involution.[7,28,30,31]

Local Treatment for Ulceration and Bleeding. It is common for infantile hemangioma of the lip to ulcerate. These ulcerated areas should be treated by frequent cleaning and application of topical antibiotic ointment. Occasionally, debridement is required, followed by dressing changes. If there is bleeding, this usually can be controlled by local pressure.[7,28,30] If the ulcer fails to heal with local measures, pharmacologic treatment is indicated.

Pharmacologic Treatment. Rapidly growing, locally destructive hemangiomas that produce necrosis, distortion of adjacent structures, and obstruction of vision or airway are treated pharmacologically. For small hemangiomas (less than 2 cm in diameter), intralesional injection of up to 3 to 5 mg/kg triamcinolone (10 to 15 mg/ml) is given through a 25-gauge needle. Several injections (usually 3 to 5) are required at 6- to 8-week intervals to accelerate involution.

Systemic corticosteroids are used for larger, destructive, problematic, or life-endangering lesions. Prednisolone, at a dosage of 2 to 3 mg/kg/day, is administered each morning for 2 weeks. If there is a response, the drug is continued and slowly tapered and withdrawn at about 10 to 11 months of age.

Boon et al.[32] evaluated the short-term and long-term complications of systemic corticosteroid treatment of proliferating infantile hemangiomas in a series of 80 patients who received a full course of therapy. Sixty-two of the eighty patients were available for follow-up ranging from 6 months to 15 years after cessation of treatment. The dosage range was 2 to 3 mg/kg/day for a mean duration of 7.9 months (range, 2 to 21 months). Short-term complications included cushingoid facies (71% of patients), personality changes (29%), gastric irritation (21%), oral or perineal fungal infection (6%), and diminished gain of height (35%) and weight (42%). Ninety-one percent of children who exhibited decreasing growth returned to their normal curves by 24 months of age. There were no significant long-term complications. The authors concluded that systemic corticosteroids, given at an initial dosage between 2 to 3 mg/kg/ day, then tapered and discontinued by 1 year of age, is safe for treatment of problematic or endangering hemangiomas.[32]

For life-endangering hemangiomas, particularly those unresponsive to corticosteroids, interferon alfa-2a or alfa-2b or vincristine are the second-line drugs. Interferon is administered daily, at a dosage of 3 million units/m² subcutaneously.[7,33] Transient side effects of interferon therapy in infants include fever and a flulike syndrome at the start of treatment (most patients), neutropenia, skin necrosis, and skin rash.[33] Interferon can adversely affect the central nervous system in infants, producing spastic diplegia. This is potentially reversible upon cessation of therapy; careful clinical observation and assessment is required during treatment.[34] Vincristine has been used successfully to treat intrahepatic hemangiomas causing congestive heart failure and kaposiform hemangioma causing Kasabach-Merritt phenomenon.[7]

Surgical Management. Excision of an infantile hemangioma is indicated for a well-localized tumor that is ulcerated, bleeding, producing airway obstruction (subglottic), or interfering with vision.[7,28,30] Otherwise, the standard is close observation, reassurance of the parents, and delay of excision until the involuting phase or until after complete involution.[7,28,30,31,33] Excision is indicated to remove abnormal skin and fibrofatty tissue and to correct any distortion of the soft tissue. If possible, this usually is done before the child starts school.

Infantile hemangioma produces an effect on the skin similar to that of a tissue expander. Based on this observation, Mulliken et al.[35] introduced the strategy of circular excision and purse-string closure for hemangioma in all three phases of its life cycle. A circular or ovoid incision is planned to include all the altered skin. In the proliferating phase, this includes damaged and ulcerated skin. In the involuted phase it includes atrophic, irregular skin and fibrofatty residuum. Minimal subcutaneous undermining is required and the wound edge is drawn together with a running, intradermal purse-string suture (4-0 or 5-0 polydioxanone). The suture is tightened to gather the edges and appose the wound margin. A gauze wick is placed if a small opening remains, and the wound is covered with an absorbent dressing. Alternatively, the edges may be closed with percutaneous sutures in the axis of relaxed skin tension. After several months of healing and remodeling, a decision is made to accept a small circular scar or to revise it (Figure 17-18). Staged resection is often necessary for labial hemangiomas because they cause distortion in three dimensions. The mass is debulked by excising involved mucosal and submucosal tissue, usually in a transverse axis. Excision at the vermilion-cutaneous junction should be delayed, and vertical incisions on the skin should be avoided (see Figure 17-2).[35]

Management of Vascular Malformations

Capillary Malformations. The first step in the care of a patient with a vascular malformation is to determine whether it is a fast-flow or slow-flow lesion. Capillary malformations and telangiectasias rarely present major problems for the oral and maxillofacial surgeon. Often there is vascular staining of the oral mucosa and skin. Histologically, there is ectasia of the upper dermalvascular plexuses. There is slow, progressive dilation of the anomalous dermal vessels, often in association with gradual hypertrophy of the involved cheek and lip. This is also a frequent finding in the Sturge-Weber syndrome that includes a capillary malformation of the V1 or V1-V2 trigeminal areas, choroidal vascular ectasia, and leptomeningeal vascular anomalies (see Figure 17-5). Pyogenic granulomas commonly develop in an area of capillary stain, particularly in the mouth.[1,7,28,36]

The underlying bone may not be affected in pure dermal and submucosal vascular anomalies. However, maxillary and mandibular overgrowth is common when there is staining of the overlying facial skin and mucosal lining. In patients with dentoalveolar distortion,

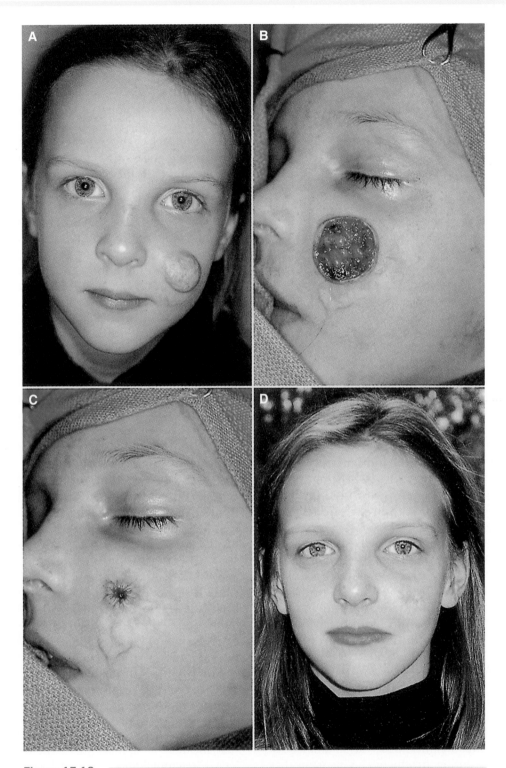

Figure 17-18

Circular excision of a hemangioma. **A,** A 7-year-old girl with involuting-phase hemangioma of the left cheek measuring 2.5 cm in diameter. **B,** Intraoperative view of the circular excision. **C,** The wound is closed with a purse-string suture. **D,** Patient at 10 years of age, after two circular excisions and subsequent lenticular excision. (From Mulliken JB, Rogers GF, Marler JJ: *Plast Reconstr Surg* 109:1544-1554, 2002.)

osteotomies can be performed without fear of excessive bleeding (see Figure 17-3). The teeth can be moved orthodontically when there is mucosal capillary staining. Capillary malformations also occur in association with lymphatic, venous, or arterial malformations. In such combined vascular anomalies, management is based on the characteristics of the predominant, deeper malformation.

A rare, hereditary form of vascular malformation occurring intraorally is hereditary hemorrhagic telangiectasia. (The historic, triple-eponymous term is *Rendu-Osler-Weber syndrome*.) It is a familial disorder, inherited in an autosomal dominant pattern, and two causative genes have been identified.[5] The intraoral lesions exhibit a characteristic ectasia of the mucosal vessels, usually less than 1 to 3 mm in diameter. The lesions often do not appear until puberty or later and increase in number with age. The structural abnormality is localized to small arteries and arterioles leading to the formation of minute arteriovenous shunts.[5]

Lymphatic Malformations. Lymphatic and venous malformations are the anomalies most likely to affect bony size and shape (see Figures 17-6, 17-8, and 20-6), whereas arterial malformations are most commonly the basis for bony destruction.[1,3,13] Lymphatic and venous malformations do not involve increased blood flow in the affected bone, as demonstrated by skeletal scintigraphy, nor can a local pressure phenomenon explain the bony changes, because they do not correlate with the size or extent of the vascular malformation.[1,3,13]

Lymphatic malformation commonly involves the tongue, floor of mouth, mandible, and submandibular and neck soft tissues. Padwa and colleagues[37] reviewed the clinical course and long-term soft tissue and skeletal problems in 17 patients with cervicofacial lymphatic malformations. The patients experienced considerable morbidity, including airway obstruction and feeding difficulties in infants and bleeding, infections, bone hypertrophy, and malocclusion in older children. Patients with macroglossia were especially prone to develop mandibular prognathism and open bite secondary to the progressive mandibular distortion. Histologic examination of bone removed to contour the mandible has shown intraosseous lymphatic malformation.[37]

All patients in this series required multiple soft tissue or bone operations or both. Subtotal cervical excision was performed an average of four times per patient. Lingual reduction was also commonly needed. Malocclusion and distortion of the maxillofacial skeleton was managed by a variety of orthognathic surgical procedures (see Chapter 20, Figure 20-6). The authors concluded that patients with large cervicofacial lymphatic malformations require serial, staged surgical excisions of the floor of the mouth and submandibular tissues. Soft tissue excisions should be carried out in anatomic regions and should be as extensive as possible, without damaging nerves. Orthognathic correction usually is carried out after the completion of growth, and only if the lingual size and position will permit (i.e., mandibular setback).

Venous Malformations. Venous malformations are the most common vascular anomaly. They vary in size, from small, well-localized lesions to diffuse lesions that also can involve bones. They are associated most commonly with distortion of shape and increase in size of the underlying skeleton, as illustrated by Case Report 4 (see Figure 17-6). There are also rare cases of venous malformation within craniofacial bones; the most common intraosseous location is the mandible and, less often, the maxilla. Unfortunately, these lesions often are referred to incorrectly as *central hemangioma* in the oral and maxillofacial surgery literature.[1,24,25,38]

When venous or combined lymphatic-venous malformations cause secondary bony distortion, without direct intraosseous involvement, orthodontic treatment and orthognathic procedures can be carried out safely, without fear of excessive bleeding. Patients (see Case Reports 7 and 8, Figures 17-9 and 17-10) with an intraosseous venous malformation, with microshunting, may exhibit major hemorrhage spontaneously or during an operation. In these instances, hemorrhage secondary to intraosseous vascular malformation, as well as bleeding from localized or systemic coagulopathy, must be considered.

Stasis and turbulence associated with the venous malformation leads to localized intravascular coagulation and sometimes disseminated intravascular coagulopathy. Hematologic evaluation shows that PT and PTT are often normal; levels of fibrin split products and fibrinopeptide may be elevated, with decreased fibrinogen and platelet levels. Heparin treatment is instituted when indicated; only when the coagulopathy is corrected are surgical procedures feasible. Another approach is to begin giving heparin, followed by antifibrinolytic therapy with ε-aminocaproic acid. Failure to address this chronic consumptive coagulopathy can cause problems with hemostasis during a procedure.

For large venous malformations with localized venous "lakes," direct injection of absolute (100%) ethanol (sclerosing agent of choice in the United States) is indicated. This requires general anesthesia with real-time fluoroscopic guidance. Usually several sessions are necessary to shrink a large venous malformation; recanalization is a recognized occurrence. Sclerotherapy in this situation can be dangerous and should be performed by an experienced interventional radiologist. Complications include local blistering, full-thickness skin necrosis, and nerve damage. Systemic complications include hemolysis and potential for renal toxicity and cardiac arrest.[7] Small oral mucosal venous malformations can be sclerosed with injection of 1% sodium tetradecyl sulfate.

A common problem encountered in venous and combined lymphatico-venous lesions is intermittent swelling, pain, and fever (see Case Reports 5 and 7 and Figures 17-7 and 17-9). In these patients, it is difficult to distinguish between cellulitis, intralesional abscess, thrombophlebitis, and phlebothrombosis. In some cases, high fever develops and blood culture results are positive. There may be a local source for infection, such as carious teeth or periapical abscess. Administration of the appropriate antibiotic (usually penicillin or clindamycin in the maxillofacial region) is begun. A drainage procedure is carried out only for an obvious abscess. Aspirin anticoagulation therapy may be useful if there are no local or systemic sources of infection and when there are tender phleboliths. In patients who respond to aspirin, the administration of this antiplatelet drug is continued indefinitely (325 mg per day).

Arteriovenous Malformations. Arteriovenous malformations in the head and neck area are far less common than intracranial arterial anomalies. In the maxillofacial region, they involve the dentoalveolar segment and are associated with loose teeth, bleeding around the gingival margins, and massive hemorrhage, either spontaneous or intraoperative (see Case Reports 9 and 10, Figures 17-11 and 17-12). AVMs are slightly more frequent in females than males (male-to-female ratio = 1:1.5) and are more common in the head and neck than in the extremities or trunk. They often are noticed at birth but may be overlooked because they seem innocuous. Fast flow becomes evident later in childhood when the patient and family note a deepening of the color and warmth. A bruit and thrill confirm the diagnosis. Later the patient may develop pain and intermittent bleeding. In the maxillofacial region this often is manifested as loosening of the teeth, ability to depress the teeth into the socket, and bleeding in the gingival cuff. The natural history of AVMs is documented by the Schobinger classification[7] (see Table 17-1). Kohout and colleagues[38] found that most (69%) head and neck malformations occur in the midface (ear, cheek, nose, maxilla, and upper lip) with the cheek being the most common site. In contrast, 14% and 17% of AVMs were present in the upper and lower face, respectively. In this series of 81 head and neck AVMs, involvement of midfacial bones or mandible was noted in 22 patients. In 4 of 8 (50%) mandibular AVMs, there was no involvement of the overlying soft tissue.

Patients with AVMs seek evaluation and treatment when the lesion expands and causes symptoms. This most commonly occurs with trauma (fall or local injury), puberty, or pregnancy.

Ultrasonography and color Doppler examination are inexpensive and noninvasive imaging techniques and are used most commonly to confirm the diagnosis. The extent of the AVM in the soft tissue is documented by MRI and magnetic resonance angiography. Bony involvement can be visualized best by CT scans. Super-selective angiography usually is not undertaken until therapeutic intervention is done.[7]

The ability to reduce inflow to AVMs by superselective arterial embolization is a major advance in the management of these lesions.[7,26] This technology does not provide definitive treatment but can be lifesaving in the presence of acute bleeding; together with extensive excision it may control these anomalies. In Case Report 7, the combination of heparin therapy and embolization made it possible to extract the infected teeth safely, without major coagulopathic problems.

Management of Arteriovenous Malformations. Super-selective arterial or retrograde venous embolization is used for palliation of pain, bleeding, or congestive heart failure. Relief is only temporary. Ligation or proximal embolization is contraindicated because of the rapid development of collateral flow to the nidus of the malformation.

The current strategy for management of AVMs is arterial embolization for occlusion of the nidus, followed 24 to 72 hours later by surgical excision. Sclerotherapy or insertion of platinum coils placed by direct puncture of the nidus, in conjunction with local arterial and venous occlusion, may be used if there are tortuous vessels or if the feeding arteries have been ligated.[7,26,37] The surgical goal is complete resection of the AVM nidus and involved overlying tissue.

Unfortunately, AVMs usually are not well localized, and recurrence of the AVM with expansion of vessels deep or at the periphery of the resection occurs in a high percentage of patients. Kohout et al.[38] reported an overall success rate of 60% with 88% for stage I, 67% for stage II, and 48% for stage III lesions. For these patients embolization is palliative and reoperation may not be feasible.

CONCLUSION

A classification system is justified only if it serves as an intellectual framework to guide in the understanding of the problem, aid in diagnosis and treatment, and stimulate future research. Vascular anomalies have been understood poorly in the past because of an illogical descriptive nomenclature. This nosologic confusion has led to inaccurate diagnosis and incorrect treatment. The classification system employed in this chapter provides a framework for rational management of vascular anomalies in the maxillofacial region.

Patients with extensive or complex vascular anomalies should be managed by a vascular anomalies team. These multidisciplinary teams provide the most up-to-date treatment and serve as a focus for clinical and basic research.

REFERENCES

1. Kaban LB, Mulliken JB: Vascular anomalies of the maxillofacial region, *J Oral Maxillofac Surg* 44:203, 1986.
2. Mulliken JB, Glowacki J: Hemangiomas and vascular malformations in infants and children: a classification based on endothelial characteristics, *Plast Reconstr Surg* 69:412, 1982.
3. Mulliken JB, Young AE: *Vascular birthmarks: hemangiomas and malformations*, Philadelphia, 1988, WB Saunders.
4. Enjolras O, Mulliken JB: Vascular tumors and vascular malformations (new issues), *Adv Dermatol* 13:375-423, 1997.
5. Cohen MM Jr: Vasculogenesis, angiogenesis, hemangiomas and vascular malformations, *Am J Med Genet* 108:265-274, 2002.
6. Hand JL, Frieden IJ: Vascular birthmarks of infancy: resolving nosologic confusion, *Am J Med Genet* 108:257-264, 2002.
7. Mulliken JB, Fishman SJ, Burrows PE: Vascular anomalies, *Curr Probl Surg* 37(8):520-576, 2000.
8. Vikkula M, Boon LM, Mulliken JB, Olsen BR: Molecular basis of vascular anomalies, *Trends Cardiovasc Med* 8:281-292, 1998.
9. Vikkula M, Boon LM, Mulliken JB: Molecular genetics of vascular malformations, *Matrix Biol* 20:327-335, 2001.
10. Finn MC, Mulliken JB, Glowacki J: Congenital vascular lesions: clinical application of a new classification, *J Pediatr Surg* 18:894, 1983.
11. Boon LM, Enjolras O, Mulliken JB: Congenital hemangioma: evidence of accelerated involution, *J Pediatr* 128:329-335, 1996.
12. Enjolras O, Mulliken JB, Boon LM, et al: Non-involuting congenital hemangioma: a rare cutaneous vascular anomaly, *Plast Reconstr Surg* 107:1647-1654, 2001.
13. Boyd JB, Mulliken JB, Kaban LB, et al: Skeletal changes associated with vascular malformations, *Plast Reconstr Surg* 74:789, 1984.
14. Burke EC, Winkelman RK, Strickland MK: Disseminated hemangiomatosis, *Am J Dis Child* 108:418, 1964.
15. Cooper AG, Bolande RP: Multiple hemangiomas in an infant with cardiac hypertrophy, *Pediatrics* 35:27, 1965.
16. Kasabach HH, Merritt KK: Capillary hemangioma with extensive purpura: report of a case, *Am J Dis Child* 59:1063-1070, 1940.
17. Enjolras O, Wassef M, Mazoyer E, et al: Infants with Kasabach-Merritt syndrome do not have true hemangiomas, *J Pediatr* 130:631-640, 1997.
18. Sarkar M, Mulliken JB, Kozakewich HPW, et al: Thrombocytopenic coagulopathy (Kasabach-Merritt phenomenon) is associated with kaposiform hemangioendothelioma and not with common hemangioma, *Plast Reconstr Surg* 100:1377-1386, 1997.
19. Takahashi K, Mulliken JB, Kozakowich HP: Cellular markers that distinguish the phases of hemangioma during infancy and childhood, *J Clin Invest* 93:2357-2364, 1994.
20. Mulliken JB, Zetter BR, Folkman J: In vitro characteristics of endothelium from hemangiomas and vascular malformations, *Surgery* 92:348, 1982.
21. Glowacki J, Mulliken JB: Mast cells in hemangiomas and vascular malformations, *Pediatrics* 70:48, 1982.
22. Razon MJ, Kräling BM, Mulliken JB, Bischoff J: Increased apoptosis coincides with onset of involution in infantile hemangioma, *Microcirculation* 5:189-195, 1998.
23. Williams HB: Facial bone changes with vascular tumors in children, *Plast Reconstr Surg* 63:309, 1979.
24. Haywood JR: Central cavernous hemangioma of the mandible: report of 4 cases, *J Oral Surg* 39:526, 1981.
25. Lamberg M, Transanen A, Jaakelainen J: Fatality from central hemangioma of the mandible, *J Oral Surg* 37:578, 1979.
26. Mulliken JB, Murray JE, Castaneda A, Kaban LB: Management of vascular malformation of the face using total circulatory arrest, *Surg Gynecol Obstet* 146:168-172, 1978.
27. Perrott DH, Schmidt B, Dowd CF, Kaban LB: Treatment of a high-flow arteriovenous malformation by direct puncture and coil embolization, *J Oral Maxillofac Surg* 52:1083-1086, 1994.
28. Mulliken JB: Vascular anomalies. In Aston SJ, Beasley RW, Thorne CH, editors: *Grubb and Smith's plastic surgery*, ed 5. Philadelphia, 1997, Lippincott Raven.
29. Unni KK, Ivins JC, Beaubout JW, Dahlin DC: Hemangioma, hemangiopericytoma and hemangioendothelioma of bone, *Cancer* 27:1403, 1971.
30. Mulliken JB, Frieden IJ: Special symposium: management of hemangiomas, *Pediatr Dermatol* 14:57-83, 1997.
31. Margileth AM, Museles M: Cutaneous hemangiomas in children: diagnosis and conservative management, *JAMA* 194:523, 1965.
32. Boon LM, MacDonald DM, Mulliken JB: Complications of systemic corticosteroid therapy for problematic hemangioma, *Plast Reconstr Surg* 104:1617-1623, 1999.
33. Ezekowitz RA, Mulliken JB, Folkman J: Interferon alfa 2a therapy for life-threatening hemangiomas of infancy, *N Engl J Med* 326:1456-1463, 1992.
34. Barlow CF, Priebe CJ, Mulliken JB: Spastic diplegia as a complication of interferon alfa-2a treatment of hemangiomas of infancy, *J Pediatr* 134:527-530, 1998.
35. Mulliken JB, Rogers GF, Marler JJ: Circular excision of hemangioma and purse-string closure: the smallest possible scar, *Plast Reconstr Surg* 109:1544-1554, 2002.
36. Watson WL, McCarthy WD: Blood and lymphatic vessel tumors: report of 1056 cases, *Surg Gynecol Obstet* 71:569, 1940.
37. Padwa BL, Hayward PG, Ferraro NF, Mulliken JB: Cervicofacial lymphatic malformation: clinical course, surgical intervention, and pathogenesis of skeletal hypertrophy, *Plast Reconstr Surg* 95:951-960, 1997.
38. Kohout MP, Hansen M, Pribaz JJ, Mulliken JB: Arteriovenous malformations of the head and neck: natural history and management, *Plast Reconstr Surg* 102:643-654, 1998.

CHAPTER 18

Facial Pain in Children

Jeffry Shaefer

CHAPTER OUTLINE

Orofacial pain is a confusing problem for the clinician and a frightening one for the child. It includes pain conditions associated with the hard and soft tissues of the head, face, neck, and all the intraoral structures. Routine daily activities such as talking, chewing, swallowing, washing the face, or brushing teeth may trigger pain. The diagnoses range from headache to musculoskeletal pain, such as arthritis and fibromyalgia, to neurogenic pain, psychogenic pain, and pain from diseases such as cancer. The clinician must be aware of the anatomy and physiology of the craniofacial region, the multiple etiologies of pain, differential diagnosis, and treatment options.

EPIDEMIOLOGY OF FACIAL PAIN IN CHILDREN

More than 80% of the population reports at least one significant pain experience, with a high percentage of this pain located in the facial region.[1] Lipton et al.,[2] in a survey of 45,711 American households, found that 22% of Americans had experienced one of five types of face pain during the prior 6 months. The most common type of orofacial pain was toothache (12.2%), while temporomandibular joint (TMJ) pain was reported by 5.3% and face or cheek pain by 1.4% of the population. Facial pain commonly is associated with temporomandibular disorders (TMD).

The prevalence of signs and symptoms of TMD in children is lower than in adults and gradually increases with age.[3] The incidence of TMJ sounds in adolescents has been reported to be as high as 17.5%.[4] In comparison, Mintz's survey[5] of adults and children found both groups to have equal prevalence (38% to 40.6%) of signs and symptoms of jaw dysfunction. Jaw pain severity also is reported to be equal across all age groups, while the presence of TMJ anatomic changes increases with age.[6] Based on available data, the clinician can expect that approximately 10% of children might have a problem with jaw function that could manifest as facial pain.[7,8]

In children, the incidence of vascular headaches, like migraine, is low (3% to 10%) when compared with adults (20%), but it gradually increases with age and verbalization skills.[9,10] The prevalence of headache in association with facial pain can be much higher and should be expected in the child with a facial pain complaint.[8,11]

EVALUATION OF THE PEDIATRIC PATIENT WITH FACIAL PAIN

The complexity of the diagnosis and treatment of facial pain in children requires a multidisciplinary approach. A comprehensive workup includes assessment of all contributing factors: behavioral, social, emotional, cognitive, biologic, and environmental. Other factors may be predisposing and indirect, such as joint laxity; direct or initiating, such as trauma; or perpetuating factors, such as anxiety or depression. Belfer and Kaban[12] found that 35% of children arriving at a hospital-based oral surgery clinic with facial pain had a diagnosis of co-morbid depression. In these cases, the child's physical diagnosis might be clear while successful management of the patient would be compromised by addressing inadequately a psychiatric initiating or perpetuating factor.

Children may be poor historians; therefore, a clinician is forced to depend primarily on clinical examination to make the diagnosis. When evaluating a pediatric facial pain complaint, the diagnostician must be aware of the epidemiology of facial pain in children so that the most frequent problems will be recognized. The most common pain complaints in children are otalgia, headaches, tooth pain, and jaw pain associated with jaw function. Accordingly, in this chapter we concentrate on the etiology and management of these common facial pain complaints in children.

History

In children, as in adults, the history is the most important component of the evaluation. The clinician must document the chronologic order of the onset of symptoms and their frequency and duration.

From a detailed history, the clinician determines if the symptoms are acute or chronic, static or progressive, recurrent, intermittent or continuous, short or prolonged. The child's description of his or her symptoms provides clues as to the anatomic localization and possible etiology. The history should also include what precipitates, relieves, or changes the symptoms.

Similarly, the family and social history frequently provide clues for underlying genetic, hereditary, environmental, or psychological conditions that are the basis of the patient's complaints.[13] The history also provides insight into how the symptoms affect the child's day-to-day life, school performance, and quality of life.

Talking with Children

There are special considerations the provider should take into account when interviewing children[13] (Box 18-1; see Chapter 3). Children respond to nonverbal communication before they understand the meaning of words. Clinicians should be aware of how their own facial expressions, voices, and gestures influence a child's reactions. The child's emotional state is revealed by observation of facial expression, body posture, gestures, and voice tone and inflection. Children may be unresponsive to questions because of pain or uncertainty or because they are frightened of unfamiliar settings and people they consider strangers.

Too often, conversation involves only the clinician and a parent, with limited interaction with the child. Children can and will respond to seriously posed questions about themselves. Some children as young as 3 to 4 years of age and most children by the age of 8 years can participate verbally in providing a history.[13] By the age of 13 years, young people should be interviewed directly. Parents may be present, but explanations of diagnostic and treatment procedures should be made to the child. When evaluating the level of pain, consider a picture survey, such as the faces pain scale, for children of ages 4 to 8 years. This tool allows the child to match the severity of the symptoms to a series of faces from a frowning one to a smiley face (Figure 18-1). Children 9 years of age and above can reliably report their pain on a visual analog scale or a 0 to 10 number scale.

Understanding the Pain Process

Children who suffer from diseases with no definitive cure, such as rheumatoid arthritis, certain malignancies, migraines, and fibromyalgia, are at risk for chronic pain.[14] There may be perpetuating factors that persist after the disease has resolved. An example would be a painful

---

BOX 18-1	Talking with Children

1. Don't be condescending, but talk as you would with any patient.
2. Take what they say seriously.
3. Don't laugh at what children say unless you know they are joking.
4. Don't be flippant or joke continuously with children. Some humor is okay, but not continuously.
5. Consider whispering to very young children at the first visit to get their attention.
6. One can discuss symptoms and treatment in simple terms with children of 4 to 5 years.
7. Never discuss the illness or treatment of hospitalized children in their presence unless you are discussing it with them, as well.
8. When children fail to cooperate, assume that they are frightened. Then practice the technique "tell, show, do" to dispel their fears.

See Chapter 3.

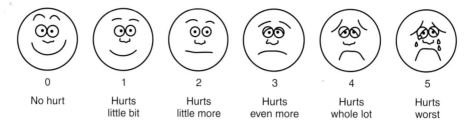

0	1	2	3	4	5
No hurt	Hurts little bit	Hurts little more	Hurts even more	Hurts whole lot	Hurts worst

Figure 18-1

The faces pain scale is recommended to monitor pain intensity in children. In contrast to a visual analog scale (commonly used for adults), it uses a progression of faces from smiling to crying. Children can relate to the faces more readily than to the numbers. (From Hockenberry MJ: *Wong's nursing care of infants and children*, ed 7, St Louis, 2003, Mosby.)

reflex muscle contraction occurring in the muscles of mastication about a painful TMJ with capsulitis. As the capsulitis resolves, the muscle nociceptors, which are prone to sensitization, remain symptomatic.[8,15] The initial acute muscle spasm from the painful joint leads to myofascial pain characterized by a dull, constant ache, limited range of motion, and painful jaw function. Clearly, psychological conditions are secondary contributing factors that can amplify and perpetuate chronic pain.[16] It is imperative that the clinician recognize psychosocial factors, such as learned behavior, that can influence the child's response to a chronic pain condition.

The clinician should follow a diagnostic process that begins with screening for disorders of extracranial and intracranial structures.[17-19] These should be addressed first, because they can be serious and require immediate attention. Extracranial conditions affect structures such as the sinuses, eyes, ears, and teeth. Intracranial disorders include those of the brain. One should then characterize the pain (Table 18-1) as muscular (steady ache), joint (preauricular ache), vascular (throbbing), neuralgia (sharp shooting), or causalgia (burning hyperesthesia).[18] If the clinician is unable to correlate physical findings with the pain complaint, a psychogenic (descriptive) etiology should be considered. Once the category of pain is determined, the clinician should go through a diagnostic process in which the most common disorders of each diagnostic group are considered.

Physical Examination of the Child with Facial Pain

Physical examination includes observation and evaluation of mandibular and head and neck range of motion.

Next, palpation of head and neck structures, such as the muscles of mastication and TMJs, should be carried out. Neurologic examination should include an assessment of cranial nerves II through XII, including eye movements, and pupillary light reflexes and visual acuity. Responses to light touch and mildly painful stimulation can be assessed by tickling or touching the child or lightly pinching fingers and observing facial expression, and withdrawal and avoidance movements.[13] It is imperative, during the maneuvers of the physical examination, that the clinician is able to reproduce, alleviate, or change the child's chief pain complaint. This helps to confirm the diagnosis. Finally, psychological assessment of the child is also imperative because of the high incidence of psychogenic pain presenting as TMD in children[12] (see Chapter 3).

TABLE 18-1	Characteristics of Facial Pain[18]
Diagnostic Group	**Pain Quality**
Extracranial and intracranial	Varies
Muscular	Steady ache increased with function
Joint	Preauricular ache increased with function
Neuralgia	Sharp shooting pain along nerve distribution
Causalgia	Burning hyperesthesia
Vascular	Throbbing
Psychiatric	Descriptive

Differential Diagnosis of Facial Pain

EXTRACRANIAL DISORDERS

Disorders of the Eye

Primary ophthalmic disorders rarely refer pain away from the eye toward other craniofacial structures. On the other hand, it is common to see patients with pain around the eye—related to sinus disease, headache (especially tension), TMD, dental disease, and intracranial tumor.[8] Optic neuritis may produce pain with eye movement. Ocular problems that produce pain are often of an acute nature such as a foreign body, uveitis, scleritis, closed-angle glaucoma, or an increase in ocular pressure. Chronic open-angle glaucoma has been associated with a low-grade headache.[8] Children with pain of ocular origin do not present a diagnostic dilemma, and a referral to a pediatric ophthalmologist is made.

Sinusitis

Children with acute sinusitis often have headache, nasal drainage, facial pain, and congestion, whereas those with chronic sinusitis have more subtle signs.[20] Infection, allergic reactions, anatomic obstruction, and underlying disease are among the causes that must be differentiated.[21] Acute sinusitis frequently follows upper respiratory tract infections. Children with chronic sinusitis can complain of nasal obstruction, postnasal drip, and intermittent facial pain, with symptoms persisting for 3 months or more.[22] Predisposition to the condition may be caused by rhinitis (allergic or nonallergic) or aberrant anatomy resulting in poor drainage and chronic infection of the sinuses. Quite often sinus disease can cause pain referred to other areas, confusing the diagnosis (Figure 18-2).[18] Palpation and percussion over the affected sinus can help localize the source of pain. Generally, plain radiographic views and sinus transillumination are of little value in young children. Computed tomography is much more sensitive, but the relevance of its findings for treatment decisions in children is controversial.[23]

Otalgia

Otalgia often is related to referred pain from nonotologic sources. In fact, 50% of chronic ear pain complaints are related to referred pain and not associated with any ear pathology.[8] Possible sources of pain include intracranial pathology, the TMJ, the muscles of mastication and neck, and dental pathology. In children, local ear pathology must be ruled out. When preauricular pain is related to a primary ear problem, infection is the most common etiology.[24] Infections of the ear represent a spectrum of diseases involving the outer (otitis externa), middle (otitis media), or inner ear (labyrinthitis) or the mastoid (mastoiditis).[25] Clinicians treating facial pain in children must recognize the symptoms of the two most common ear problems, otitis externa and otitis media.[26]

Otitis Externa

Otitis externa is defined as *inflammation of the skin lining the ear canal and surrounding soft tissue*. The most common causes are loss of the protective function of cerumen, self-trauma to the ear canal from overzealous cleaning, chronic drainage from a perforated tympanic membrane, and possibly infections from *Staphylococcus aureus* or *Pseudomonas aeruginosa*.[27] Symptoms include pain and itching in the ear, especially with chewing or pressure on the tragus.[28] Tugging on the pinna or tragus causes considerable pain. Drainage may be minimal and debris may be noticeable in the canal. Hearing is usually normal.

Otitis Media

Otitis media (inflammation of the middle ear) is an infection associated with middle ear fluid (effusion) or discharge due to a perforation in the tympanic membrane (otorrhea). Otitis media is primarily a disease of early childhood because of the lack of antibody to pathogens that colonize the nasopharynx.[29,30] The anatomy of the eustachian tube also plays a crucial role. For this reason, otitis media is common in patients with cleft palate.

Otitis media can be classified as acute or chronic (with and without complications). It is described further by frequency and duration. Acute otitis media is distinguished by pain and inflammation of the tympanic membrane and can be associated with a recent viral infection of the upper respiratory tract.[27] Management of acute otitis media commonly involves an antibiotic regimen, although if the problem is chronic, a definitive diagnosis should be made before antibiotics are prescribed.[20,31-34] One should consider mastoiditis when there is associated postauricular pain, fever, and an outwardly displaced pinna.[29,35]

An effusion of the middle ear is termed *otitis media with complications* when there is structural damage to the ear. Chronic suppurative otitis media is defined as *persistent otorrhea lasting longer than 6 weeks*.[36] Most often it occurs in children with tympanostomy tubes or tympanic membrane perforations. Occasionally, it can be an accompanying sign of an epidermal inclusion cyst (cholesteatoma).[28] A cholesteatoma appears as a grayish mass of tissue in the middle ear caused by an overgrowth of epithelium.

Factors associated with chronic or frequent otitis media are nasal obstruction, eustachian tube dysfunction, immunosuppression, and respiratory infections.[27] There have been reports of an association between chronic otitis media and TMD.[37]

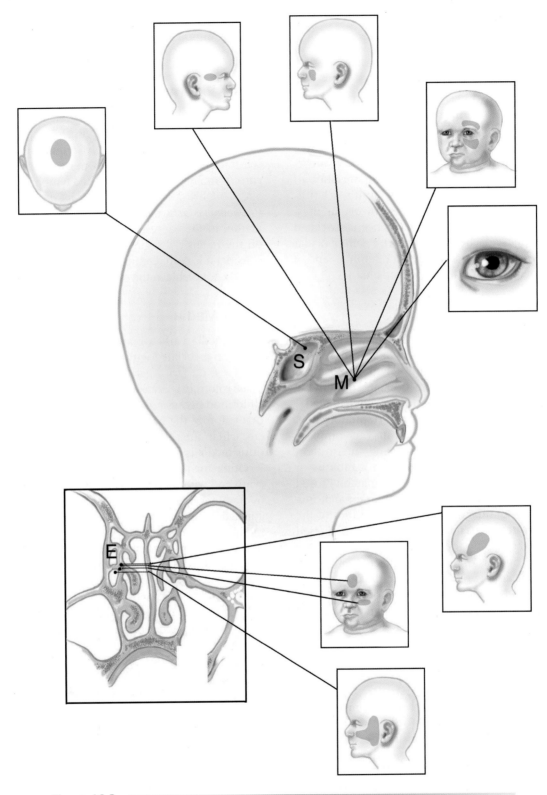

Figure 18-2
Facial pain referral patterns from the sphenoid *(S)*, ethmoid *(E)*, and maxillary *(M)* sinuses. Pain from the maxillary sinus may also be referred to the teeth. (Redrawn from Fricton JR, Kroening RJ, Hathaway KM: *TMJ and craniofacial pain: diagnosis and management*, St Louis, 1988, Ishiyaku EuroAmerica.)

Dental Disorders

A tooth problem will usually appear as such and not confuse the clinician. However, pulpalgia can create a confusing pattern of pain referral (Figure 18-3). When the child complains of toothache, the pain must be reproduced or altered clinically to ensure a definitive diagnosis. The appropriate dental radiographs should also be obtained. Temperature tests, electrical pulp tests, and palpation tests cannot always delineate an offending tooth. A diagnostic local anesthetic block will often rule out a tooth as the source of pain. If the pain remains after the block is administered, a source other than a tooth is probably the cause of the problem.[38,39]

When a child complains of tooth pain upon biting, three specific problems should be considered:

1. A periapical abscess requiring pulpotomy or extraction. This problem, if left to progress, can be quite painful and associated with cellulitis (see Chapter 12).

2. Gingivitis with overlying tissue swelling related to tooth eruption. Analgesics, with observation or tissue removal (operculectomy), should be considered.

3. A periodontal abscess characterized by localized tissue swelling at the gingival sulcus. This condition is associated with mild-to-moderate pain intensity compared with the severe pain of pulpal inflammation or necrosis. In children, food impaction into the gingival sulcus is the most likely cause and can be managed easily by tooth scaling with anesthesia.

If the clinician is unable to duplicate the child's tooth pain, referral from another source should be considered. Otalgia, TMJ pain, and myofascial pain from a masticatory muscle trigger point are the most likely referral sources.

INTRACRANIAL DISORDERS

Children do not always complain specifically of a headache. Often the parents will say that there has been a change in behavior. The clinician, when evaluating a child with facial and head pain, must decide if a neurologic cause is likely. If so, the patient should be referred for neurologic evaluation.

In children, primary brain neoplasms are far more prevalent than they are in adults. They account for almost 20% of all cancer in children but only 1% in adults.[40] Central nervous system tumors are the second leading cause of cancer-related deaths in children under 15 years of age.[40] The diagnosis sometimes can be elusive, and brain tumors often are misdiagnosed initially as a viral syndrome, gastroenteritis, or allergy.[19] Although headache or face pain is often a late symptom of brain tumor, the high prevalence of childhood headache (75%) forces one to rule out a brain lesion in each child with facial and head pain. A study of the spectrum of headache diagnoses from an emergency room revealed that the most common etiologies were viral illness, sinusitis, migraine, and posttraumatic headache. Tumors or other life-threatening conditions were uncommon. If the neurologic examination findings are normal, neuroimaging is not necessarily recommended.[40-43]

SYSTEMIC DISORDERS

In adolescents with chronic facial pain, three systemic disorders should be ruled out: multiple sclerosis, myasthenia gravis, and fibromyalgia.

Multiple sclerosis has a tendency to affect young adults and is second only to trauma as a cause of neurologic disability arising in early to middle adulthood.[44] The initial symptoms, relative to the orofacial region, include neuralgias, facial weakness resembling Bell's palsy (except

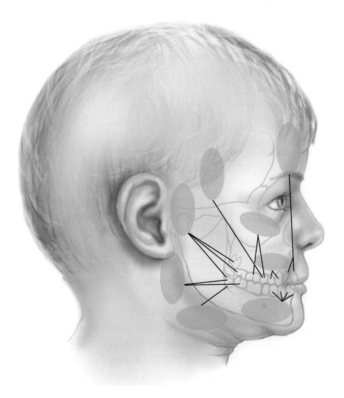

Figure 18-3 Dental pain (tooth pulpalgia) typically can refer pain to other facial areas as depicted in this diagram. (Redrawn from Fricton JR, Kroening RJ, Hathaway KM: *TMJ and craniofacial pain: diagnosis and management*, St Louis, 1988, Ishiyaku EuroAmerica.)

no taste changes), and chronic flickering contractions (myokymia) of the facial musculature.[44]

Juvenile myasthenia gravis is characterized by muscle fatigue, particularly in the extraocular muscles and muscles of mastication, swallowing, and respiration.[45] The patient may first be seen by an otolaryngologist or psychiatrist. The more prominent signs are difficulty in chewing, dysphagia, a nasal voice, ptosis, and ophthalmoplegia. Associated disorders include autoimmune conditions, especially thyroid disease. Girls are affected more frequently than boys. The age at onset is over 10 years in 75% of patients. In females, this often begins shortly after menarche. The etiology is a circulating antibody that binds to the acetylcholine receptor protein and thus reduces the number of motor end plates for binding by acetylcholine.[45]

Fibromyalgia is a chronic pain syndrome characterized by multiple tender sites and symptoms related to fatigue. It is a generalized muscle pain problem present in all four body quadrants, as compared with myofascial pain, which is a regional complaint. There is generalized pain of varying intensity at rest and increased pain with function. Pharmacologic therapy usually is not helpful, while aerobic conditioning and sleep management are reported to be beneficial.[46] Patients with fibromyalgia who have facial myofascial pain symptoms respond to specific exercise programs that increase the use of the masticatory muscles.

NEUROLOGIC DISORDERS
Neuralgia

Trigeminal neuralgia is a frequent cause of paroxysmal facial pain and headache in adults, but only 1% of the cases occur in children.[47] Glossopharyngeal neuralgia is even less common but can cause severe episodic pain in the ear and throat. There are case reports of only three children with documented neurovascular compression causing severe neuralgic pain and disability.[48] In contrast to trigeminal neuralgia, idiopathic trigeminal sensory neuropathy is rare in adults but has been reported in children.[19,49,50]

Trigeminal neuralgia is a neuropathic pain syndrome characterized by excruciating pain occurring in the distribution of the branches of the trigeminal nerve. The pain occurs suddenly, is brief, and is described as lancinating or stabbing or like an electric shock. The etiology is unknown, but compression, distortion, or stretching of the trigeminal nerve root by arteries, vascular malformations, or tumors can be identified in some patients. Patients with the demyelinating condition, multiple sclerosis, can also develop trigeminal neuralgia at a young age, and sometimes bilaterally.

The location of pain depends on the nerve involved: posterior tongue, larynx, tonsillar pillar (glossopharyn-

geal); throat, submandibular region, or under the ear (superior laryngeal); occipital region (greater or lesser occipital nerves); or the ear and posterior pharynx (geniculate-nervus intermedius).

Pharmacologic treatment should be the initial approach (gabapentin [Neurontin], carbamazepine [Tegretol]). Surgical intervention (radiofrequency lesion, alcohol blocks, decompression, gamma knife) is considered for those refractory to or who cannot tolerate medical treatment. In children, open surgical treatment is advocated if pain is refractory to medication.[48] Neurovascular compression of the affected cranial nerve, as it leaves the brain stem, is usually responsible for the neuralgias in children.[31,48,51-54] Some neurosurgeons consider decompression the best choice for young patients, even though it is more invasive than neuroablative techniques such as radiofrequency lesioning, glycerin blocks, and gamma knife procedures. These all have higher recurrence rates and a greater incidence of dysesthesia than operative decompression.[52]

Other atypical neuralgias are rare in children. Eagle's syndrome (pain on turning the head and pain with tonsillar palpation from a calcified stylohyoid ligament) has been reported in one child.[55] Atypical facial pain is characterized by a persistent burning or aching in contrast to the paroxysmal pain of trigeminal neuralgia.[8,38,39] This has not been reported in children. Postherpetic neuralgia refers to a neuropathic pain which persists after viral (Herpes zoster) lesions heal. This is rare in children.

HEADACHES
Epidemiology

Many authors have tried to estimate the frequency of headaches in the pediatric population.[11,56,67] Bille[11] studied 9000 children in Sweden; 40% by the age of 7 years and 75% by the age of 15 years already had significant headaches. There has been a weak correlation between TMD symptoms and headache as an initial symptom.[8] In a 20-year longitudinal study of children with symptomatic TMD, Egenmark et al.[56] found that 85% stated they had had a headache at some time: 12% reported frequent headaches, 7% had severe headaches, and 9% had headaches in the morning. On the other hand, Liljestrom[57] reported no correlation between TMD tension-type headaches in children.

Migraine diagnosis in children can be confusing.[58] Classic migraine headaches begin abruptly with a visual aura and progress rapidly to throbbing or pulsating pain.[59] Migraines without aura are similar to classic migraine but proceed to a headache without prodrome (feeling of impending headache). Migraines seem to affect females more than males in a 2:1 ratio. These headaches are usually unilateral, pulsating, and throbbing. Other symptoms include nausea, photophobia, and phonophobia. There is usually a family history of migraine. The headache is often aborted by going to sleep, and when the child awakens it is gone. The child would have had similar headaches in the past and the headache cannot be explained by an organic disorder.[60]

Tension headaches are referred to as *muscle tension headaches* and cause a dull ache of moderate severity. They are bilateral, usually intermittent, and occur in the temporal or occipital areas. Tension-type headaches are thought to be part of a headache continuum that includes migraine.[49,61-63] They are bilateral and last from 30 minutes to 72 hours. They are called *episodic* if occurring less than 15 times per month and *chronic* when more frequent.[64,65]

Chronic paroxysmal hemicrania is a painful, unilateral, severe headache that can occur episodically 10 to 30 times each day with a duration of 5 to 30 minutes.[66] Autonomic signs can occur on the ipsilateral side, as in cluster headache. It is strictly a unilateral, severe, sharp, and jolting pain located around the eye, temple, forehead, ear, and occiput.

Children with headache should be referred to a neurologist for diagnosis and management.[67] The surgeon should determine if the child has an effective headache abortive agent and, if the headaches occur more than 2 to 3 times per week, an effective preventative agent.[68]

TEMPOROMANDIBULAR DISORDERS

TMDs consist of a spectrum of signs and symptoms related to the jaw muscles and joints or both.[8] The most common diagnosis is myofascial pain, which accounts for roughly 55% of TMD cases.[18] Pain in and around the TMJ may arise from structural abnormalities of the bones or the meniscus (internal derangement) or muscular dysfunction (myofascial pain).[18] Trauma, degenerative changes, disk displacement, and inflammatory arthritis may also affect the joint. In Skeppar's retrospective analysis[69] of 99 children with facial pain evaluated at an oral health center, 50% had headaches, 49% jaw clicking, and 48% pain with jaw function. The diagnoses included disk displacement (32% of patients) and a muscle problem (16%). Parafunctional habits such as day and nighttime clenching or tooth grinding may lead to acute and chronic muscle soreness and joint inflammation.[70-72] These habits are common in children; 70% of preschool children reported a parafunctional habit, with 41% nail biting and 20% bruxing the teeth at night.[73] Thirty-five to sixty-two percent of adolescents have some sign or symptom of TMD, although mostly mild and fluctuating.[4,74] In an epidemiologic study of children and adolescents, 33% had muscle tenderness on palpation and 8% to 14% had moderate or severe signs of dysfunction.[75] Twenty

years later, the progression to severe symptoms was rare but so was recovery from mild to moderate symptoms.[56] In this group, parafunctions gradually decreased over time except for nighttime bruxism, for which prevalence increased with age.

The role of occlusion in the etiology of TMD is controversial. Many authors have claimed an association between occlusal factors and the initiation of TMD, but epidemiologic studies have not demonstrated a clear correlation between the two. There is no scientific evidence to support the concept that early treatment of malocclusion will prevent TMD.[3]

Management of pain conditions of the TMJ requires an understanding of normal TMJ function and an understanding of the capacity of the TMJ complex to adapt to structural changes.

Clinical Examination

Physical examination in children with TMD consists of inspection for the pattern and the presence of noise or deviation on opening. Range of motion is assessed initially with the examiner facing the patient while he or she is opening the jaw as far as possible. Normal vertical opening is equal to the width of three fingers from the child's dominant hand. The difference between maximal pain-free opening and maximal opening with pain should be determined. The child is asked to point to the area of pain on opening. This often helps to distinguish between a joint or a muscle problem. The muscles of mastication should be palpated for tenderness, hypertrophy, and spasm and the joints palpated (tenderness, noise) and auscultated (noise).

The magnitude of opening is also a helpful guide to localizing the source of pain. Maximal incisal opening of less than 20 to 25 mm points to a muscle problem, while preauricular pain beginning at 25 to 30 mm indicates a diagnosis of TMJ capsulitis. Assessment of lateral range of motion can also help discern a muscle from a joint problem. A lateral movement, greater than 5 mm, is normal for a child and indicates a well-functioning TMJ with normal rotation and translation. Therefore the child with normal right and left lateral movement but painful limited vertical opening most likely has a muscle problem.

Palpation of the masseter muscle should be carried out along its insertion on the mandible to its origin on the zygoma, and from its anterior to posterior border, being careful to distinguish the superficial from the deep masseter. The temporalis, medial pterygoid, and posterior digastric muscles should be palpated extraorally. The lateral and medial pterygoids and the temporalis tendon can also be palpated intraorally. However, the diagnostic validity of intraoral palpation is hampered by the discomfort generated when placing a hand in the mouth of any pediatric patient. If the child complains of neck soreness or pain, the trapezius, sternocleidomastoid, and splenius capitis muscles should be palpated. Masticatory pain or headaches can be referred from the cervical area, although this is an unusual occurrence in children.

A 1-minute clench test should be considered. Positive responses and the location of such responses help localize the pain to the TMJ versus the muscles. The child clenches on a tongue blade placed unilaterally on the posterior teeth. When the problem is related to muscle hyperactivity, this maneuver will produce ipsilateral pain. In the case of TMJ capsulitis, it will cause pain of the contralateral joint. Then place tongue blades bilaterally on the posterior teeth and have the child clench down. If the child's pain from clenching is relieved when biting on the tongue blades, splint therapy often will improve the symptoms.

TMJ tenderness is evaluated by having the patient open slightly, bringing the condyle and disk from under the zygomatic arch. The retrodiskal area is then palpated by having the patient open wide. The clinician then presses on the surface posterior to the condyle. Alternatively, the little fingers can be placed in the external auditory canal to press on the condylar head. Lateral or posterior palpation sensitivity indicates either capsulitis or synovitis or both.

TMJ noise during range of motion measurements should be noted. However, prospective studies on the outcome of joint noise in children over time have demonstrated no correlation with jaw dysfunction or pain.[5] A reproducible click in two of three trials indicates disk displacement. The type of disk displacement can be determined by noting when the noise occurs during vertical and lateral range of motion.[76] For instance, a change in the articular surface of the condyle, eminence, or disk could create a noise that occurs at the same vertical measurement on opening and closing. In contrast, the noise from disk displacement with reduction occurs at greater vertical during opening than the noise heard during closing. The Research Diagnostic Criteria to determine the diagnosis of disk displacement with reduction includes clicking during vertical and either lateral or protrusive motion.[76] Alternatively, have the child protrude the jaw and then open. In disk displacement with reduction, the click will disappear during this protrusive opening.

The panoramic radiograph is the standard screening image for all patients with facial pain. This is particularly important in children when the clinical examination implicates a primary joint problem, progressive open bite development (suggestive of a condylar resorption), or a suspicion that the disorder may be linked to prior trauma. Additional magnetic resonance imaging is warranted if the child does not respond to therapy as anticipated or if the patient is being evaluated for a TMJ operation. If bony changes are suspected, documentation of the state of the disease via tomograms or computed tomography scans should be considered. One needs to keep in mind that these images may not differentiate between developmental and pathologic changes.

Joint Inflammation

Inflammation of the synovial, capsular, or retrodiskal tissues of the TMJ is termed *synovitis* or *capsulitis*. The inflammatory condition may be a result of infection, trauma, systemic disease (autoimmune disorder), articular surface degeneration, or disk displacement. Olson[77] evaluated 70 patients with juvenile chronic arthritis (called juvenile rheumatoid arthritis in the United States) and found 41% with TMJ radiographic findings, 26% with crepitus, and 32% with limited jaw motion.

The diagnostic criteria for TMJ inflammation include localized TMJ pain (preauricular) aggravated by function, sensitivity to joint palpation, and TMJ pain when distalizing (upward and backward) pressure is placed on the mandible (joint loading). Episodic swelling with associated occlusal changes (inability to occlude the teeth on the involved side) can occur. All these symptoms can be associated with osteoarthritic changes when the joints are imaged.

Disk Dysfunction

Disk displacement is defined as an alteration in the disk-condyle structural relationship. The articular disk is anteriorly or anteromedially displaced. Posterior displacement of the disk rarely occurs. Most children with disk displacement have normal jaw function and do not require treatment.

Disk displacement with reduction refers to a displaced disk in the closed mouth position and reduction during opening movements (the disk attains a normal relationship to the condyle). Clinical characteristics include reproducible joint noise (clicking) that occurs at variable positions during mandibular opening, closing, and in lateral or protrusive jaw movement. During opening, the jaw deviates to the affected side prior to clicking with a return toward midline following the click. Masticatory muscles may be sore and tender as a result of splinting in response to the painful joint.

Disk displacement without reduction (fixed dislocated disk or closed lock) is an altered or misaligned disk-condyle structural relationship that does not change during mandibular translation. The patient often relates a history of chronic jaw clicking and then a sudden onset of limited opening with disappearance of the click.

Clinical characteristics include mandibular deviation to the affected side on opening with marked limited lateral movement to the opposite side. Hard tissue imaging may reveal osteoarthritic changes of the condyle or the articular eminence.

Osteoarthritis and Osteoarthrosis

Osteoarthritis is defined as a degenerative disease of the joint characterized by deterioration and abrasion of the articular tissue with remodeling of the underlying subchondral bone. This condition is usually the result of mechanical overload of the joint beyond the adaptive capacity of the remodeling mechanism.[78,79] The term *secondary arthritis* is used when the condition is associated with a history of trauma, infection, or systemic disease. Clinical characteristics include pain and crepitus with jaw function, joint tenderness with palpation, and jaw pain with joint loading. When skeletal changes (without pain) are evident radiographically, the appropriate term is *osteoarthrosis*.[80] Wiberg[81] used TMJ tomography to demonstrate a 66% prevalence of bony changes in the TMJs of subjects aged 12 to 30 years with jaw pain. Researchers have been unable to draw a conclusion about the role of these radiographic findings in the development of facial pain symptoms.[69,80,82]

Generalized Arthritis

Children with juvenile rheumatoid arthritis (Still's disease) may have major disturbances in oral and maxillofacial growth, especially when the TMJ is involved. In addition, they may experience a significant decrease in oral opening. Bakke et al.[83] investigated the development of TMJ capsulitis in adults with a history of juvenile rheumatoid arthritis. She found 67% of these women had TMJ involvement and their symptoms were correlated to the chronicity of the disease as a child. Aspirin, nonsteroidal antiinflammatory agents and, in severe cases, steroids with or without methotrexate are used to manage these patients.

Treatment of Joint Disorders

Management of intracapsular disorders should start with patient education. The patient and parents should be instructed as to the nature of the problem. These are musculoskeletal injuries that have a strong potential to become chronic because of ever-present jaw function and contributing factors such as parafunction, anxiety, and depression. It is very important that the patient and parents understand the role of limiting function (a pain-free diet) to allow healing. They must also understand the importance of doing therapeutic exercises to rehabilitate the joint. Nonsteroidal antiinflammatory drugs and muscle relaxants occasionally are used to control symptoms, and the parents should be instructed in their use for children.

Physical therapy is used to reduce inflammation and to increase pain-free range of motion. This may consist of heat, sometimes ice, massage, and ultrasound. Gentle range-of-motion exercises, within the pain tolerance, should be done by the patient. (The joint(s) should not hurt more than 10 minutes after the exercise period.) Exercises are done frequently for short periods (6 times a day for 30 to 60 seconds). The physical therapist can do gentle distraction and mobilization to increase pain-free range of motion.

Nighttime splint therapy has been shown to have a long-term benefit in reducing symptoms of capsulitis and myalgia in children.[69] An orthotic (acrylic nightguard) can be very effective in reducing forces on the joint to promote healing. It can control parafunctional behavior at night, temporarily stabilize an uneven occlusion, and allow the joint to rest. The nightguard should be constructed as a flat plane that opens the bite several millimeters. A soft nightguard is most appropriate for children with a developing occlusion (mixed dentition).

In children with a painful click that is reduced with forward movement of the mandible, a mandibular orthopedic repositioning appliance can be considered (Figure 18-4). The criteria for its use include a painful click, elimination of the click when placing the jaw forward, and resolution of pain with the mandible forward. The appliance should be used only at night (part-time repositioning) to prevent the development of any permanent occlusal changes.

A surgical procedure such as arthrocentesis, lysis, and lavage can be considered based on the patient's response to nonsurgical management. Surgical management should be considered only if the patient's complaints are localized to the joint.[82]

Temporomandibular Joint Dislocation

TMJ dislocation (open lock) occurs when the condyle achieves a position anterior and superior to the crest of the articular eminence during jaw motion. The patient is unable to close the mandible, because the closing muscles do not allow the condyle to drop below the crest of the eminence. This is required to provide the condyle an unobstructed path back into the articular fossa. Joint dislocation is referred to as *subluxation* when the condyle is only momentarily out of the joint and relocates spontaneously. Dislocation is often very painful and there may be persistent or residual pain (from joint sprain) following relocation.

Jaw manipulation is required to reposition the condyle. Stand in front of the patient and grasp the mandible between the thumb and fingers. Push the mandible inferiorly (to clear the eminence) and then posteriorly and superiorly into the glenoid fossa. This

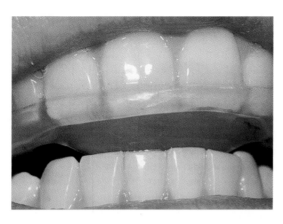

Figure 18-4

The mandibular orthopedic repositioning appliance depicted here is helpful in eliminating temporomandibular joint arthralgia. When the mouth is closed, the mandible comes forward along the ramp and the condyle moves away from inflamed retrodiskal tissue. This appliance is also effective in patients with anterior disk displacement with reduction. The mandible is in a forward position, which allows reduction of the disk and, eventually, there is fibrous adaptation of the retrodiskal tissues. The ramp shown here is designed to passively guide the mandible forward into an end-to-end anterior occlusion. The occlusal surface of this maxillary appliance has an indexed occlusion with 0.5-mm indentations for the mandibular teeth cusp tips, thereby dictating a specific mandibular position. The occlusion should be monitored carefully when this appliance is used, and it should be used only for short periods.

maneuver may be difficult, particularly if the dislocation has lasted a long time or if the child is anxious and in pain.

If pain is intolerable and the mandible is resistant to manipulation, pain reduction and muscle relaxation can be accomplished with an auriculotemporal nerve block to alleviate TMJ pain and reduce muscle splinting. Nitrous oxide sedation can also be helpful. However, in most children, general anesthesia is required if the relocation procedure cannot be accomplished quickly without medication. In children with recurring episodes of dislocation after reduction, a short period of treatment with muscle relaxants or maxillomandibular fixation or both may be required.

In children with chronic, intermittent open locking, isometric exercises can be used to help the patient identify the jaw opening position where the locking occurs. They can then be trained to limit their opening to prevent dislocation. Hinge axis–opening exercises, with pressure on the chin to prevent protrusion, are very helpful in cooperative children.

EXTRACAPSULAR DISORDERS

Acute Disorders: Myositis, Protective Muscle Splinting, Myospasm

Myositis is related to inflammation of a muscle by local causes such as infection or injury. There is tenderness over the entire muscle, with moderate to severe pain during a limited range of motion. Myositis from infection should resolve once the source of the infection is treated.

Myositis can also be the result of delayed onset muscle soreness. These children exhibit increased pain with mandibular movement. This occurs after prolonged or unaccustomed use, such as nighttime parafunction.

Protective muscle splinting is manifest by restricted or guarded mandibular movement. This is caused by contraction of muscles as a means of avoiding pain caused by movement. There is severe pain with function, but no pain at rest. The limited range of motion cannot be increased during passive stretch because the patient guards against opening further. The "hard end feel" of resistance to passive stretch can be confused with the limited range of motion seen in disk displacement without reduction.

Myospasm (acute trismus) is an involuntary, sudden, tonic contraction of a muscle with acute pain and severely limited range of motion. The muscle exhibits continuous muscle contraction. Treatment involves breaking the spasm with ice or heat and stretch, anesthesia, electrostimulation, or muscle relaxants.

Chronic Disorders: Myofascial Pain, Contracture, Fibromyalgia

The most common chronic facial pain disorder in children is myofascial pain. In contrast to fibromyalgia, this is a localized regional pain disorder with a dull, aching quality as compared with the burning allodynia which occurs when sympathetic nerves are involved (Complex Regional Pain Syndrome I and II). It is quite common for a child to have myofascial pain with a clinical picture of a tension-type headache. In pediatric patients, especially those in whom jaw function aggravates a headache, the myofascial pain etiology for tension-type headache seems clear.

Myofascial pain has been called myofascial pain dysfunction syndrome, temporomandibular dysfunction, muscle contraction headache, and numerous other terms that reflect local muscular pain. There are localized tender spots (trigger points) in muscle, tendons, or fascia that reproduce pain when palpated. These tender spots may produce a characteristic pattern of referred pain. Active trigger points exhibit continuous pain which often is aggravated by jaw function. In contrast, passive trigger points are painful only when palpated. Myofascial pain can be caused by postural problems, oral parafunctional habits, psychological disorders, stress, and trauma. Myofascial pain characteristically is reduced or eliminated with anesthetic injection into an active trigger point, or a spray-and-stretch procedure with fluormethane spray. The key to long-term successful management is the elimination of contributing factors such as parafunction, poor sleep, anxiety, depression, occlusal instability, headaches, and posture problems.

Treatment of Muscle Disorders

In children, the initial use of analgesics and muscle relaxants is recommended only to decrease acute severe pain. There is no scientific support for the long-term use of these medications for muscle pain. The patient and parents should be educated and encouraged to comply with a home rehabilitation program. A stabilization dental appliance (occlusal orthotic) should be used to reduce the influence of occlusal factors and bruxism when they are present (Figure 18-5).[69] Ingerslev[84] reported a 60% success rate when treating 366 adolescents with a soft bite splint; 34% of her patients became pain free.

Behavior modification should include stress management, relaxation training, coping skill development, and implementation of habit control regimens to decrease aggravating habits such as nail biting and daytime clenching. A referral to a psychologist with biofeedback training should be encouraged.

Physical therapy initially should involve modalities to decrease pain and gentle stretching exercises to mobilize and gradually increase jaw opening. The physical therapist or clinician should help the patient develop a home rehabilitation program with stretch and spray, postural reeducation, ergonomic awareness, aerobic exercise, and gentle mobilization. The goal of therapy is a gradual increase of pain-free range of motion with home rehabilitation and control of contributing factors. Generally, range of motion with muscle problems can be increased aggressively, whereas the program must be more gradual and slower when rehabilitating a joint problem.

CHRONIC PAIN IN CHILDREN

Children with persistent pain of longer than 3 months duration are considered chronic pain patients. They are complex and difficult to manage because of the history of multiple medical providers, multiple medications, and pain severity. The pain often influences daily activities and there is often a history of mental health or developmental problems, or presence of multiple painful sites (number of pain complaints). Reports on adults with chronic pain correlate poor response to treatment to an increased number of pain symptoms at the start of treatment. It is imperative that the complexity of the case be recognized at the start of therapy to facilitate the multidisciplinary treatment necessary to ensure success.[85]

Success in managing the pediatric patient with facial pain also depends on matching the complexity of the treatment to the complexity of the case. Vanderas[71] reported a correlation between the severity of facial pain

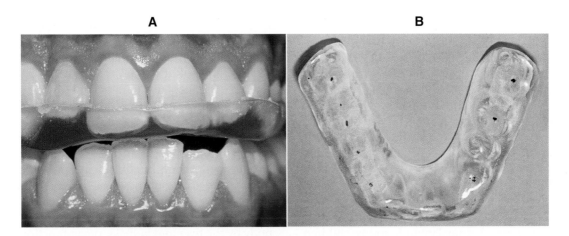

A   **B**

Figure 18-5

A, Stabilization appliance. The flat-plane stabilization appliance is designed to keep the mandible from completely closing, thereby decreasing intraarticular pressure at the temporomandibular joint. **B,** Point contact on the posterior teeth (dark marks) should be present bilaterally and can be assessed by using thin articulating paper, such as Acu-film.

and a child's emotional state. One must ensure that all the contributing factors that perpetuate the chronic pain problem are identified and treated.[86] As noted above, patients with multiple pain complaints have a poor prognosis for pain control. Review of the literature in adults and children reveals a common etiology in chronic somatic disorders such as migraine, myofascial pain, irritable bowel syndrome, chronic fatigue syndrome, fibromyalgia, and tension-type headaches. Wessely et al.[87] expressed this concept well and recommended a standard behavior-based treatment regimen for management of these chronic problems. This approach is reversible and makes sense especially for pediatric cases.

Song et al.[88] evaluated 73 children with chronic or recurrent musculoskeletal pain of greater than or equal to 6 weeks' duration. In 36 children, followed for 2 years, there was no identifiable organic etiology for the pain. The other 37 patients had an organic etiology for the pain. Use of an Inappropriate Symptom Checklist was helpful in distinguishing between these two groups of children with chronic pain. Seventy-seven percent of children with no inappropriate symptoms ultimately had an organic diagnosis. Conversely, in 79% of children with two or more inappropriate symptoms, no organic diagnosis was identified. Clearly the prognosis of children with identifiable organic pathology is more predictable and the treatment more straightforward. Song's study supported the use of a symptom checklist when evaluating patients with facial pain.

A single, common etiology for facial pain in children with multiple pain complaints might exist. Australian investigators compared children with typical migraine and those with abdominal migraine. Similar symptoms, triggers, and alleviating factors were found for both groups.[89] Buskila[90] suggested a common pathophysiology for children with chronic fatigue, fibromyalgia, or myofascial pain. He proposed that in these disorders, autonomic dysfunction within the hypothalamic-pituitary-adrenal axis and the sympathetic-adrenal system leads to a reduced corticotropin and epinephrine response to hypoglycemia. He recommended behavioral and cognitive behavioral therapy for children suffering from these disorders. In further support of behavioral therapy for pediatric facial pain, Pillemer and Kaban[91] found that 35% of their pediatric patients with facial pain had a contributing diagnosis of psychiatric impairment. This compared with just 6% of adults.

Physical exercise regimens seem to be the only therapeutic strategy to achieve consistent long-term successful results.[8] In a study from Finland, young children with widespread or regional pain (neck pain) had much higher emotional and behavioral scores than controls. Subjects with fibromyalgia had the highest depression scores.[92] The authors concluded that pain and depressive symptoms must be recognized and

managed together to prevent development of a chronic pain problem.

Children with complex regional pain syndrome present a considerable challenge for the clinician. They generally have burning, aching pain of long-standing duration from sympathetic nerve dysfunction after trauma. Sherry et al.[93] reported a series of 107 children with complex regional pain syndrome. They underwent an intensive exercise therapy program as the primary treatment (no medications) and 95 of 107 patients (92%) were symptom free during the initial follow-up period. More encouraging was that 88% of the 47 patients followed for 2 years remained pain free.

CRANIOFACIAL PAIN DISORDERS OF PSYCHOLOGICAL ORIGIN

Psychogenic or somatoform pain disorders can manifest as craniofacial pain in children. Somatization disorder, body dysmorphic disorder, hypochondriasis, conversion disorder, vocal cord dysfunction, pain disorder, and recurrent abdominal pain have all been described in children and adolescents.[17] The presence of a psychiatric disturbance does not preclude the existence of physical pathology. However, psychiatric disorders frequently complicate the diagnosis and management of patients with facial pain; 65% of chronic orofacial pain patients have a defined Diagnostic and Statistical Manual of Mental Disorders (DSM) IV diagnosis.[8] Collaboration with or referral to a mental health professional is the best strategy for long-term management of the chronic pediatric patient with facial pain.

DEVELOPING A PEDIATRIC DRUG REGIMEN

In general, pharmacologic management of children with facial pain should represent a last resort after failure of modalities such as counseling, biofeedback, physical therapy, and splint therapy. The patient's age is one of the most important parameters to consider when developing a drug therapy regimen. Both physiologic and psychological age should influence the choice of drug, the route of administration, the dosing regimen, and the monitoring parameters.[52,95] Psychological issues are most important in adolescents and older children, because the ability of these patients to accurately use a drug therapy can affect its efficacy and safety.

Because nearly all drugs are eliminated from the body by the liver and kidneys, organ function should be assessed before selecting drug therapy and during the treatment course. Many of the metabolites of drugs that are primarily degraded by liver enzyme systems are ultimately excreted by the kidneys and can accumulate in patients with renal dysfunction. Renal function can be assessed by using serum creatinine concentrations to estimate glomerular filtration rate.[94]

Close monitoring for drug toxicity is necessary when decreased liver function is suspected in children receiving hepatically metabolized drugs. Nearly every drug that has been used safely in pediatric patients has an established milligram-per-kilogram dosing range. Drug dosing based on a child's weight in kilograms is simple, convenient, and widely accepted (Table 18-2).[94]

The therapeutic index is the ratio of the maximum tolerated dosage to the minimum curative dosage. It is a measure of the relative benefits and risks of a selected drug regimen. A drug with a wide therapeutic index has a greater margin of safety than one with a narrow index. Box 18-2 lists commonly used drugs in children and their therapeutic indexes. Drugs with narrow therapeutic indexes should be dosed based on the specific milligram-per-kilogram guidelines and adjusted during therapy with serum drug level monitoring.[92] Drug dosing based on body surface area (BSA) may be more accurate. Many pediatric drugs with narrow therapeutic indexes, such as chemotherapeutic and antiviral agents, have dosing guidelines based on patient BSA (acyclovir can be based on mg/kg or BSA).[94]

Drug dosing based on age is the least accurate method. Dosages for over-the-counter medications most commonly are based on the age method.

BOX 18-2 Therapeutic Indexes of Selected Drugs

Wide
Acetaminophen
Benzodiazepines
Cephalosporins
Decongestants
Antihistamines
Ibuprofen
Penicillins
Cimetidine
Sucralfate

Narrow
Anticonvulsants
Heparin and warfarin
Lidocaine
Opiate narcotics (morphine, codeine)
Theophylline
Vancomycin

Data from Lessel S: *Surv Ophthalmol* 37(3):155, 1992.

TABLE 18-2 Recommended Dosages of Common Analgesics

Drug	Dosage (mg/kg)	Route	Frequency
Morphine	0.3	PO	q 3-4 hours
	0.1	IV	q 3-4 hours
Codeine	1.0	PO	q 3-4 hours
Hydromorphone	0.06	PO	q 3-4 hours
	0.015	IV	q 3-4 hours
Meperidine: not recommended			
Oxycodone	0.2	PO	q 3-4 hours
Acetaminophen	10-15	PO	q 3-4 hours
Aspirin	10-15	PO	q 3-4 hours
Ibuprofen	10	PO	q 3-4 hours
Naproxen	5	PO	q 3-4 hours

CONCLUSION

In this chapter the epidemiology of facial pain in children was reviewed. Differential diagnosis of pediatric pain conditions and a management philosophy consisting of careful diagnosis, patient education and counseling, physical therapy, and splint therapy, when indicated, were presented. The overriding concept is to avoid irreversible therapies in children.

REFERENCES

1. James FR, Large RG, Bushnell JA, Wells J: Epidemiology of pain in New Zealand, *Pain* 44:279, 1992.
2. Lipton JA, Ship JA, Larasch-Robinson D: Estimated prevalence and distribution of orofacial pain in the United States, *J Am Dent Assoc* 124:115, 1993.
3. Okesan J: Temporomandibular disorders in children, *Pediatr Dent* 11:4, 325, 1989.
4. Wanman A, Agorburg G: Mandibular dysfunction in adolescents 1. Prevalence of symptoms, *Acta Odontol Scand* 44:47, 1986.
5. Mintz SS: Craniomandibular dysfunction in children and adolescents: a review, *Cranio* 11(3):224, 1993.
6. Pereira F, Lundh H, Westesson P: Clinical findings related to morphological changes in TMJ autopsy specimens, *Oral Surg Oral Med Oral Pathol* 78:288, 1994.
7. List J: Temporomandibular disorders in children and adolescents; prevalence of pain, gender differences, and perceived treatment need, *J Orofac Pain* 13(1):9, 1999.
8. Okesan J: *Orofacial pain: guidelines for assessment, diagnosis, and management. the American Academy of Orofacial Pain*, ed 3. Chicago, 1994, Quintessence Publishing.
9. Linder S, Winner P: Pediatric headache, *Med Clin North Am* 85(4):1037, 2001.
10. Turner D, Stone A: Headache and its treatment: a random sample survey, *Headache* 19:74, 1979.
11. Bille B: Migraine in school children, *Acta Paediatr* 51(Suppl 136):151, 1962.
12. Belfer ML, Kaban LB: Temporomandibular joint dysfunction with facial pain in children, *Pediatrics* 69(5):564, 1982.

13. Behrman RE, Kliegman RM, Jenson HB: *Nelson textbook of pediatrics*, ed 16. Philadelphia, 2000, WB Saunders.

14. Fields HL: *Pain*, ed 5. New York, 1987, McGraw-Hill.

15. Woolf CJ, Mannion RJ: Neuropathic pain: aetiology, symptoms, mechanisms, and management, *Lancet* 353:1959, 1999.

16. Fields HL, Martin JB: Pain: pathophysiology and management. In Braunwald E, Fauci AS, Isselbacher KJ, et al, editors: *Harrison's online*, 2001-2002, New York, 2002, McGraw-Hill.

17. Fritz GK, Fritsch S, Hagino O: Somatoform disorders in children and adolescents: a review of the past 10 years, *J Am Acad Child Adolesc Psychiatry* 36(10):1329, 1997.

18. Fricton JR, Kroening RJ, Hathaway KM: *TMJ and craniofacial pain: diagnosis and management*, St Louis, 1988, Ishiyaku EuroAmerica.

19. May M, Fria TJ, Blumenthal F, Curtin H: Facial paralysis in children: differential diagnosis, *Otolaryngol Head Neck Surg* 89(5):841, 1981.

20. Berman S, Johnson C, Chan K, Kelley P: Ear, nose, and throat. In May W, editor: *Current pediatric diagnosis and treatment*, ed 16, Philadelphia, 2000, WB Saunders.

21. Wald ER: Diagnosis and management of sinusitis in children, *Adv Pediatr Infect Dis* 12:1, 1996.

22. Evans KL: Recognition and management of sinusitis, *Drugs* 56(1):59, 1998.

23. Ferguson BJ: Acute and chronic sinusitis. How to ease symptoms and locate the cause, *Postgrad Med* 97(5):45, 1995.

24. Stool S, Johnson CE, Stark A: Diagnosis and management of otitis media, *Pediatr Rev* 19:12, 1998.

25. Marchant CD, Carlin SA, Johnson CE, Shurin PA: Measuring the comparative efficacy of antibacterial agents for acute otitis media: the "Pollyanna phenomenon," *J Pediatr* 120:72, 1992.

26. Schwartz RH, Bahadore RS: What to do for runny ears, *Contemp Pediatr* 16:121, 1999.

27. Heikkinen T, Thint M, Chonmaitree T: Prevalence of various respiratory viruses in the middle ear during acute otitis media, *N Engl J Med* 340:260, 1999.

28. Leung AKC, Fong JHS, Leong A: Otalgia in children, *J Natl Med Assoc* 92:254, 2000.

29. Dagan R, Leibovitz E, Greenberg D, et al: Early eradication of pathogens from middle ear fluid during antibiotic treatment of acute otitis media is associated with improved clinical outcome, *Pediatr Infect Dis J* 17:776, 1998.

30. Dowell SF, Butler JC, Giebink GS, et al: Acute otitis media: management and surveillance in an era of pneumococcal resistance—a report from the Drug-Resistant *Streptococcus pneumoniae* Therapeutic Working Group, *Pediatr Infect Dis J* 18:1, 1999.

31. Canafax DM, Yuan Z, Chonmaitree T, et al: Amoxicillin middle ear fluid penetration and pharmacokinetics in children with acute otitis media, *Pediatr Infect Dis J* 17:149, 1998.

32. Roark R, Berman S: Continuous twice daily or once daily amoxicillin prophylaxis compared with placebo for children with recurrent otitis media, *Pediatr Infect Dis J* 16:376, 1997.

33. Rosenfeld RM: An evidence based approach to healing otitis media, *Pediatr Clin North Am* 43:1165, 1996.

34. Rosenfeld RM, Vertrees JE, Carr J, et al: Clinical efficacy of antimicrobial drugs for acute otitis media: meta-analysis of 5400 children from 33 randomized trials, *J Pediatr* 124:355, 1994.

35. Harley EH, Sdralis T, Berkowitz RG: Acute mastoiditis in children: a 12-year retrospective study, *Otolaryngol Head Neck Surg* 116:26, 1997.

36. Craig WA, Andes D: Pharmacokinetics and pharmacodynamics of antibiotics in otitis media, *Pediatr Infect Dis J* 15:944, 1996.

37. Youssis S: The relationship between craniomandibular disorders and otitis media in children, *Cranio* 9(2):169, 1991.

38. Marbach JJ: Phantom tooth pain, *Endo* 4:362, 1978.

39. Rees RT, Harris M: Atypical odontalgia, *Oral Surg* 49:196, 1980.

40. Lewis D, Dorbad D: The utility of neuroimaging in the evaluation of children with migraine or chronic daily headache who have normal neurological examinations, *Headache* 40:629-632, 2000.

41. Field AG, Wang E: Evaluation of the patient with non traumatic headache: an evidenced based approach, *Emerg Med Clin North Am* 17(1):127-138, 1999.

42. Dooley JM, Camfield PR, O'Neill M, Vohra A: The value of CT scans for children with headaches, *Can J Neurol Sci* 17:309-310, 1990.

43. Maytal J, Bienkowski RS, Patel M, Eviatar L: The value of brain imaging in children with headaches, *Pediatrics* 96:413, 1995.

44. Hauser SL, Goodkin DE: MS and other demyelinating diseases. In Braunwald E, Fauci AS, Isselbacher KJ, et al, editors: *Harrison's online*, 2001-2002, New York, 2002, McGraw-Hill.

45. Linduer A, Schalke B, Toyka KV: Outcome in juvenile onset myasthenia gravis: a retrospective study with long-term follow-up of 79 patients, *J Neurol* 244:515, 1997.

46. Reid GJ, Lang BA, McGrath PJ: Primary juvenile fibromyalgia: psychological adjustment, family functioning, coping, and functional disability, *Arthritis Rheum* 40(4):752, 1997.

47. Mason WE, Kollros P, Jannetta PJ: Trigeminal neuralgia and its treatment in a 13-month-old child: a review and case report, *J Craniomandib Disord* 5:213, 1991.

48. Childs M, Meaney JF, Ferrie CD, Holland PC: Neurovascular compression of the trigeminal and glossopharyngeal nerve: three case reports, *Arch Dis Child* 82(4):311, 2000.

49. Mathew NT, Stubits E, Nigam MP: Transformation of episodic migraine into daily headache: analysis of factors, *Headache* 22:66, 1982.

50. Matoth I, Taustein I, Shapiro Y: Idiopathic trigeminal sensory neuropathy in childhood, *J Child Neurol* 16(7):623, 2001.

51. Barker FG II, Jannetta PJ, Bissonnette DJ, et al: The long term outcome of microvascular decompression for trigeminal neuralgia, *N Engl J Med* 334:1077, 1996.

52. Koren G: Special aspects of perinatal and pediatric pharmacology. In Katzburg B, editor: *Basic and clinical pharmacology*, New York, 2001, McGraw-Hill.

53. Love S, Hilton DA, Coakham HB: Central demyelination of the fifth nerve root in trigeminal neuralgia associated with vascular compression, *Brain Pathol* 8:1, 1998.

54. Meaney JF, Eldridge PR, Dunn LT, Nixon TE, et al: Demonstration of neurovascular compression in trigeminal neuralgia with magnetic resonance imaging. Comparison with surgical findings in 52 consecutive operative cases, *J Neurosurg* 83:799-805, 1995.

55. Queresby FA, Gold ES, Arnold J, Powers MP: Eagle's syndrome in an 11-year-old patient, *J Maxillofac Surg* 59:94-97, 2001.

56. Egenmark I, Carlsson GE, Magnusson T: A 20-year longitudinal study of subjective symptoms of temporomandibular disorders from childhood to adulthood, *Acta Odontol Scand* 59:40, 2001.

57. Liljestrom MR, Jamsa A, Le Bell Y, et al: Signs and symptoms of temporomandibular disorders in children with different types of headache, *Acta Odontol Scand* 59:413, 2001.

58. Maytel J, Young M, Schechter A, et al: Pediatric migraine and the International Headache Society (IHS) criteria, *Neurology* 48:602, 1997.

59. Headache Classification Committee of the International Headache Society: Classification and diagnostic criteria for headache disorders, cranial neuralgias and facial pain, *Cephalalgia* 8(Suppl 7):1096, 1988.

60. Winner P, Wasieswski W, Gladstein J, et al: Multicenter prospective evaluation of proposed pediatric migraine revisions to the ISH criteria, *Headache* 37:545, 1997.

61. Guidetti V, Galli F: Evolution of headache in childhood and adolescence: an 8-year follow-up, *Cephalalgia* 22:66, 1982.

62. Olness KN, McDonald JT: Recurrent headaches in children: diagnosis and treatment, *Pediatr Rev* 8:307, 1987.

63. Rothner AD: Management of headaches in children and adolescents, *J Pain Symptom Manage* 8:81, 1993.
64. Lessell S: Pediatric pseudotumor cerebri (idiopathic intracranial hypertension), *Surv Ophthalmol* 37(3):155, 1992.
65. Spierings ELH, Schoeversa M, Honkoop PC, et al: Development of chronic daily headache: a clinical study, *Headache* 38:529, 1998.
66. Biondi DM: Cervicogenic headache: mechanisms, evaluation, treatment strategies, *J Am Osteopath Assoc* 100(Suppl 9):S7, 2000.
67. Kolar KR, Fisher W, Gordon V: "Nurse, my head hurts:" a review of childhood headaches, *J Sch Nurs* 17(3):120, 2001.
68. Levinstein B: A comparison study of cyproheptadine, amitriptyline and propranolol in the treatment of pre-adolescent migraine, *Cephalalgia* 4:11, 1991.
69. Skeppar J, Nilner M: Treatment of craniomandibular disorders in children and young adults, *J Orofacial Pain* 7(4):362, 1993.
70. Vanderas AP: Prevalence of craniomandibular dysfunction in children and adolescents: a review, *Pediatr Dent* 9(4):312, 1987.
71. Vanderas AP: Prevalence of craniomandibular dysfunction in white children with different emotional states: part III, a comparative study, *J Dent Child* 59(1):23, 1992.
72. Vanderas AP: Relationship between oral parafunctions and craniomandibular dysfunction in children and adolescents: a review, *J Dent Child* 61(5-6):378, 1994.
73. Widmalm SE, Christiansen RL, Gunn SM: Oral parafunctions as temporomandibular disorder risk factors in children, *Cranio* 13(4):242, 1995.
74. Nilner M: Prevalence of functional disturbances and diseases of the stomatognathic system in 15-18 year-olds, *Swed Dent J* vol 189, 1999.
75. Egaramrk-Eriksson I, Carlsson GE, Ingervall B: Prevalence of mandibular function and oral parafunction in 7, 11 and 15 year old Swedish children, *Eur J Orthod* 3:163, 1981.
76. Dworkin S, LeResche L: Research diagnostic criteria for temporomandibular disorders: review of criteria, examinations, and specifications, critique, *J Craniomandib Disord Facial Oral Pain* 6:301, 1992.
77. Olson L, Eckerdal O, Hallonsten AL, et al: Craniomandibular function in juvenile chronic arthritis. A clinical and radiographic study, *Swed Dent J* 15(2):71, 1991.
78. Hunt A, Joel S, Dick G, Goldman A: Population pharmacokinetics of oral morphine and its glucuronides in children receiving morphine as immediate-release liquid or sustained-release tablets for cancer pain, *J Pediatr* 135(1):47-55, 1999.
79. Stegenga B, de Bont LGM, Boering G: Osteoarthrosis as the cause of craniomandibular pain and dysfunction, *J Oral Maxillofac Surg* 47:249-256, 1989.
80. Westesson PL, Rohlin M: Internal derangement related to osteoarthrosis in temporomandibular joint autopsy specimens, *J Oral Surg* 57:17-22, 1984.
81. Wiberg B, Wanman A: Signs of osteoarthrosis of the temporomandibular joints in young patients, *Oral Surg Oral Med Oral Pathol* 86:158-164, 1998.
82. Dolwick FM: Intra-articular disc displacement: its questionable role in temporomandibular joint pathology, *J Oral Maxillofac Surg* 53:1069, 1995.
83. Bakke M, Zak M, Jensen BL, et al: Orofacial pain, jaw function, and temporomandibular disorders in women with a history of juvenile chronic arthritis or persistent juvenile chronic arthritis, *Oral Surg Oral Med Oral Pathol* 92:406, 2001.
84. Ingerslev H: Functional disturbances of the masticatory system in school children, *J Dent Child* 50(6):445-450, 1983.
85. Klass ES, Degotardi P, Ilowite NT, et al: Developing an assessment and treatment protocol for children with pain amplification syndromes, *Arthritis Rheum* 41(Suppl):S249, 1998.
86. Mikkelsson M, Sourander A, et al: Psychiatric symptoms in preadolescents with musculoskeletal pain and fibromyalgia, *Pediatrics* 100(2):220, 1997.
87. Wessely S, Nimnuan C, Sharpe M: Functional somatic syndromes: one or many? *Lancet* 354:936, 1999.
88. Song KM, Morton AA, Koch KD, et al: Chronic musculoskeletal pain in childhood, *J Pediatr Orthop* 18(5):576, 1998.
89. Abu-Arafeh I, Russell G: Prevalence and clinical features of abdominal migraine compared with those of migraine headache, *Arch Dis Child* 72(5):413, 1995.
90. Buskila D: Fibromyalgia, chronic fatigue syndrome, and myofascial pain syndrome, *Curr Opin Rheumatol* 12(2):113, 2000.
91. Pillemer FG, Masek BJ, Kaban LB: Temporomandibular joint dysfunction and facial pain in children: an approach to diagnosis and treatment, *Pediatrics* 80(4):565, 1987.
92. Miller S, Orma P, Fish DH: Drug therapy. In Jay WW, editor: *Current pediatric diagnosis and treatment*, ed 16. New York, 2002, McGraw-Hill.
93. Sherry DD, Wallace CA, Kelley C, et al: Short- and long-term outcomes of children with complex regional pain syndrome, *Clin J Pain* 15(3):218-223, 1999.
94. Reed ML, Gal P: Principles of drug therapy. In Behrman RE, Kliegman RM, Jensen HB: *Nelson textbook of pediatrics*, ed 16. Philadelphia, 2000, WB Saunders.
95. Romsing J, Walther-Larsen S: Peri-operative use of nonsteroidal anti-inflammatory drugs in children: analgesic efficacy and bleeding, *Anaesthesia* 52(7):673, 1997.

CHAPTER 19

Congenital Abnormalities of the Temporomandibular Joint

Leonard B. Kaban

Congenital and acquired growth deformities of the temporomandibular joint (TMJ) are particularly interesting because they require not only three-dimensional analysis of complex morphologic abnormalities but also consideration of a fourth dimension: time or growth. The anatomic deformity and the progressive secondary distortion of contiguous and contralateral facial skeletal structures are considered and analyzed together. The effects of an early operation on facial growth and body image must also be considered in pediatric patients.

This chapter discusses hemifacial microsomia and bilateral first and second pharyngeal arch defects (bilateral craniofacial microsomia and Treacher Collins syndrome). In Chapter 20, the focus is on acquired growth abnormalities secondary to condylar hyperplasia, condylar resorption, trauma, ankylosis, infection, and radiation therapy for neoplasm.

Hemifacial Microsomia

GENERAL CONSIDERATIONS

Hemifacial microsomia (HFM) is a variable, progressive, and asymmetric craniofacial deformity.[1] It involves the skeletal, soft tissue, and neuromuscular components of the first and second pharyngeal arches, and it is the second most common (1 in 5600 live births) congenital facial anomaly after cleft lip and palate.[2,3] The mechanism by which HFM develops in humans is unknown, but Poswillo[4] has described an animal phenocopy in mice. Hemorrhage from the developing stapedial artery produces a hematoma in the area of the first and second pharyngeal arches. The size of the hematoma and resultant tissue destruction explains the morphology and variability of HFM in the experimental model. This sequence may be applicable to the human condition. More recently, Johnston and Bronsky[5] produced deformities similar to HFM in the offspring of animals exposed to retinoic acid. This drug kills neural crest cells and interferes with their movement and dispersal. The resultant variable neural crest cell deficiency is also consistent with the spectrum of phenotypic expression of human HFM and with the potential for improved growth after early treatment.[6]

Treatment of HFM requires an integrated plan that takes into account all aspects of this complex deformity.

In the past, individual specialists who became interested in treating these patients had a tendency to concentrate on their own area of expertise. Plastic surgeons worked on the external ear or subcutaneous contour deficiency, while otolaryngologists focused on the hearing disorders and middle ear anatomy. Oral and maxillofacial surgeons concentrated on the jaw anomalies and orthodontists on malalignment of the teeth. Most of these patients are now cared for in centers for craniomaxillofacial anomalies staffed by multidisciplinary professional groups. This chapter presents an integrated approach to analysis and treatment of HFM.

FACIAL GROWTH IN HEMIFACIAL MICROSOMIA

Asymmetric mandibular growth is the earliest skeletal manifestation of HFM and plays an important role in progressive deformity of the ipsilateral and contralateral facial skeleton. The deficiency in soft tissue bulk, hypoplasia of the first and second pharyngeal arch muscles, and facial nerve palsy also play a role in the progressive skeletal distortion.[2]

The normal mandible grows downward and forward in relation to the cranial base by programmed bone deposition and resorption on periosteal and endosteal surfaces.[7] This pattern of growth determines the eventual size and shape of the mandible, as well as its three-dimensional spatial relationship to the maxilla, midface, and cranial base. An increase in the vertical height of the ramus is the result of bone deposition on the posteroinferior surface and resorption on the anterior surface. Resorption along the anterior border of the ramus also contributes to the length of the mandibular body. Resorption on the medial surface and deposition on the lateral surface account for the shape and width of the mandible in the transverse plane.[7] In patients with HFM, mandibular growth on the affected side is impaired and the resultant mandible is short, retrusive, and narrow.

The maxilla normally grows inferiorly (downward) and anteriorly (forward) as a result of bone resorption on the superior (nasal) and anterior surfaces and deposition of bone on the inferior (palatal) surface.[7] The nasomaxillary region, therefore, grows downward and forward, away from the cranial base. There is a complex, incompletely understood interaction between facial skeletal growth, growth of the brain, and expansion of the soft tissue and overlying muscle.[8]

In patients with HFM, mandibular hypoplasia inhibits normal downward (vertical) growth of the maxilla and midface. It prevents progressive separation of the orbit from the piriform apertures and maxillary alveolus. The result is a short maxilla with an occlusal plane that is canted upward on the abnormal side; the orbit may be displaced inferiorly.[1-3,9]

CLASSIFICATION
Skeletal Defects

The skeletal defect of HFM is classified by the anatomy of the mandibular ramus and TMJ[3,9,10] (Figure 19-1). A type I skeletal deformity consists of a mini-mandible and TMJ. All structures are present, normal in shape and location, but small. A type II skeletal deformity consists of a small and abnormally shaped mandibular ramus with a hypoplastic TMJ. This group is further subdivided into IIA and IIB based on the location and degree of hypoplasia of the TMJ.[11-15] In type IIA the degree of TMJ hypoplasia is mild, and the location of the TMJ is acceptable for symmetric function. The native TMJ does not have to be replaced with a constructed joint. In patients with a type IIB defect, the TMJ is so hypoplastic and so far medially, anteriorly, and inferiorly displaced (in relation to the normal side) that a new joint should be constructed. These patients are functionally similar to those with a type III deformity. Type III HFM is characterized by complete absence of the mandibular ramus and TMJ.[2,3,12-15]

Jaw motion and development of the muscles of mastication are consistent with the degree of skeletal deformity. In patients with type I HFM, the muscles of mastication and the articular disk are present. Jaw motion (i.e., opening, translation, and lateral excursions) are present. In type IIA and IIB deformities, the muscles of mastication and articular disk are progressively more hypoplastic, and translatory and lateral movements are restricted. In type III HFM, the lateral pterygoid muscle and articular disk are absent and the temporalis, masseter, and medial pterygoid are moderately to severely hypoplastic. The jaw does not translate on the affected side and does not move medially toward the normal side.[16]

The end-stage skeletal deformity of HFM consists of a short, medially displaced mandibular ramus and TMJ. The abnormal mandible is flat in contour and the chin point is deviated toward the affected side (Figure 19-2). A plane drawn between the mandibular dental and skeletal midlines is rotated so that the upper end (dental) is deviated toward the normal side and the lower end (skeletal) toward the affected side (see Figure 19-2). The midface is short, resulting in a canted occlusal plane (decreased distance between the infraorbital rim, piriform aperture, and maxillary alveolus). The zygomatic bone is flat, and the orbit is sometimes inferiorly displaced.[2,3]

Soft Tissue Defects

The soft tissue defect is analyzed by physical examination and review of frontal, lateral, oblique, and submental photographs. Components to consider include bulk of

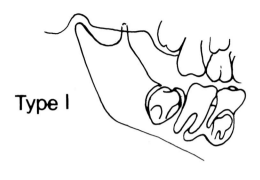

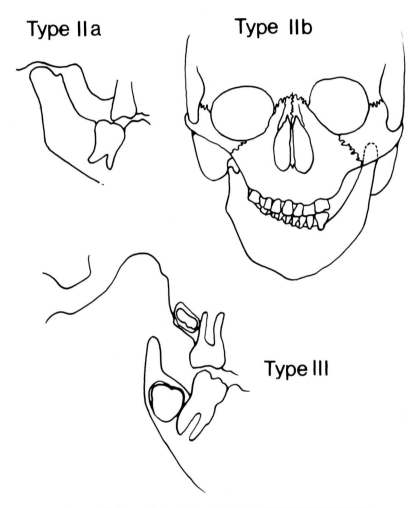

Figure 19-1
Tracings of radiographs representing the skeletal types of hemifacial microsomia. Note the medial and inferior displacement of the ramus and TMJ in type IIB.

subcutaneous soft tissue, muscles of mastication and facial expression, presence or absence of macrostomia, skin tags and facial clefts, cranial nerve function (particularly seventh nerve), and soft palate function.[3,9,11]

The deformity consists of a decrease in mass of subcutaneous tissue ranging from mild to severe (Figures 19-2 to 19-4); the degree of soft tissue hypoplasia usually, although not always, correlates with the severity of the skeletal defect. The muscles of mastication and of facial expression are hypoplastic. The patient may have macrostomia, and there may be skin tags along a line from the tragus to the commissure of the lips.

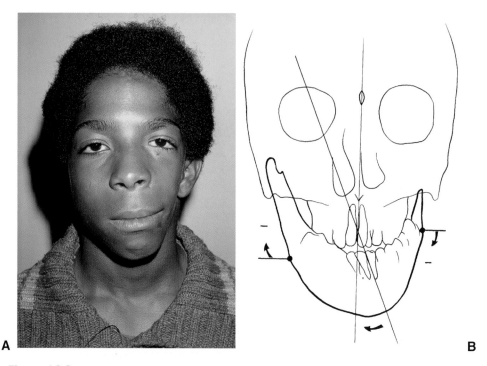

Figure 19-2

Teenage patient with left skeletal type IIB hemifacial microsomia (HFM). **A,** Frontal view demonstrating the typical physical findings of end-stage HFM: marked contour asymmetry resulting from soft tissue deficiency on the left side; left epibulbar dermoid; macrostomia; canting of the alar base and labial commissures upward toward the left; marked deviation of the chin to the left; low-set ear that is normal morphologically. **B,** Anteroposterior cephalometric tracing showing the medial, inferior displacement of the TMJ and ramus, deviation of the chin point, cant of the occlusal plane, and the orientation of a plane formed by the mandibular dental and skeletal midlines. Arrows show the direction of movement necessary to correct the deformity.

In patients with minimal subcutaneous and muscle hypoplasia, absence of or slight macrostomia, and a normal or mild auricular deformity (preauricular tags may be present), the disorder is classified as *mild*. Those with severe subcutaneous and muscle hypoplasia, facial clefts, macrostomia, and neuromuscular weakness are classified as having *severe* deformities. If the defects are in between, the classification is *moderate*.[3,9,11]

The external ear anomaly is documented using the system described by Meurman: (1) grade I: mild hypoplasia, mild cupping but all structures present, (2) grade II: absence of the external auditory canal and variable hypoplasia of the concha, and (3) grade III: absent auricle, anteriorly and inferiorly displaced lobule.[17] There is a conductive hearing loss due to hypoplasia of the ear ossicles, which are first and second pharyngeal arch derivatives (see Chapter 22).[3,11]

Analysis of the neuromuscular defect is included in the soft tissue evaluation. More than 25% of the patients have cranial nerve abnormalities, usually consisting of facial nerve palsy, with or without deviation of the palate toward the affected side with motion. Palatal deviation is due to a combination of muscle hypoplasia and cranial nerve weakness. The presence or absence of seventh cranial nerve palsy correlates with severity of the ear and not the skeletal defect (i.e., those patients with more severe ear abnormality are more likely to have seventh cranial nerve deficit) (see Figure 19-3). The most common facial nerve weakness involves the marginal mandibular branch, followed by the branch to the frontalis muscle. Rarely, a patient will have total seventh nerve weakness or a sensory deficit in the fifth nerve distribution.[18,19] Hypoplasia of the lateral pterygoid muscle ranges from mild in patients with type I skeletal defect to complete absence in those with type III defect. This muscle hypoplasia, the short ramus, and the abnormal location of the TMJ result in deviation of the mandible toward the abnormal side on opening.

Text continued on p. 309.

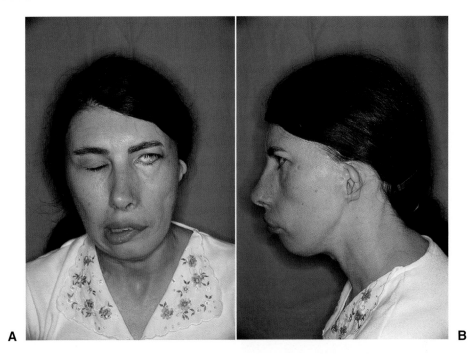

A   B

Figure 19-3

Frontal **(A)** and lateral **(B)** photographs of a patient with type I skeletal anatomy, mild soft tissue defect on the left side, grade III ear defect, and total facial nerve palsy. (Several reconstructive procedures had been done on the left ear before this photograph was taken.)

TABLE 19-1 Progression of Facial Asymmetry in Hemifacial Microsomia		
	Group I (n = 38) (Types I, IIA) Cant	Group II (n = 29) (Types IIB, III) Cant
Deciduous Dentition (≤6 years)		
Piriform rim	7.0 +/- 3.6 degrees	9.5 +/- 3.5 degrees
Maxillary occlusal plane	4.3 +/- 3.0 degrees	6.2 +/- 4.3 degrees
Intergonial angle	4.4 +/- 2.4 degrees	5.3 +/- 3.8 degrees
Mean age	4.1 +/- 0.9 years	3.4 +/- 1.4 years
Mixed Dentition (>6 to ≤13 years)		
Piriform rim	7.7 +/- 3.8 degrees	11.7 +/- 4.7 degrees
Maxillary occlusal plane	5.0 +/- 3.5 degrees	7.6 +/- 3.8 degrees
Intergonial angle	4.3 +/- 2.8 degrees	8.0 +/- 3.4 degrees
Mean age	8.6 +/- 2.3 years	8.0 +/- 1.7 years
Permanant Dentition (>13 years)		
Piriform rim	8.4 +/- 3.0 degrees	*
Maxillary occlusal plane	6.6 +/- 4.5 degrees	*
Intergonial angle	6.1 +/- 3.6 degrees	*
Mean age	21 +/- 8.9 years	*

From Kearns GJ, Padwa BL, Mulliken JB, Kaban LB: *Plast Reconstr Surg* 105:492-498, 2000.
*In this study, no unoperated patients were in this group.

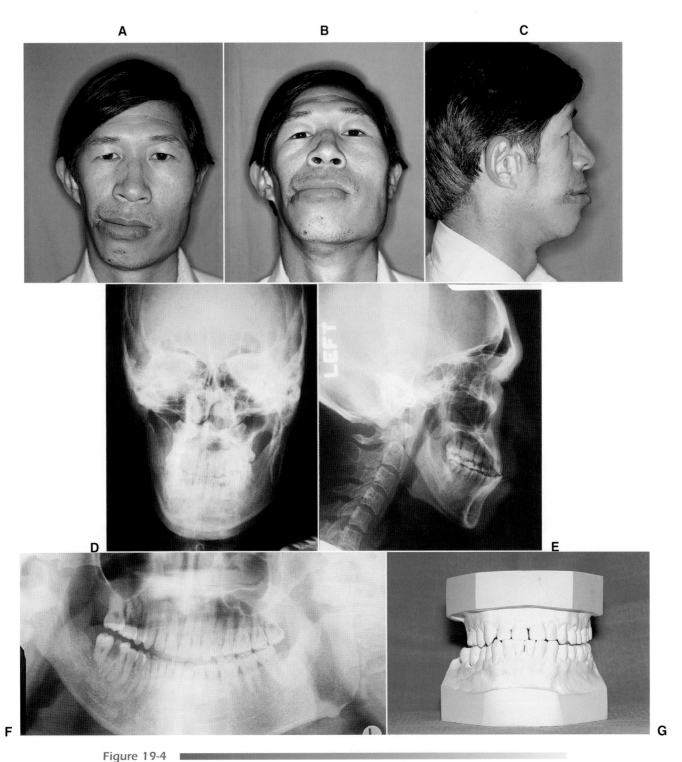

Figure 19-4

Adult end-stage hemifacial microsomia. Frontal **(A)**, submental **(B)**, and right lateral **(C)** views of a patient with end-stage type IIA skeletal and severe soft tissue contour defects. Patient has a grade I ear deformity and a repaired macrostomia. Note the bimaxillary dentoalveolar protrusion and a retruded chin. **D,** Anteroposterior cephalogram demonstrates the upward cant of the piriform aperture and occlusal plane on the right side. The chin point is deviated to the right. The right TMJ appears to be in a symmetric location in relation to the left TMJ. **E,** Lateral cephalogram shows the bimaxillary dentoalveolar protrusion, retruded chin, and double contour of the mandible resulting from the difference in ramus length. **F,** Panoramic radiograph shows the type II mandible (small in size, abnormal in shape). **G,** Articulated dental models show the deviation of mandibular dental midline to the right and a cross bite on the right side.

Continued.

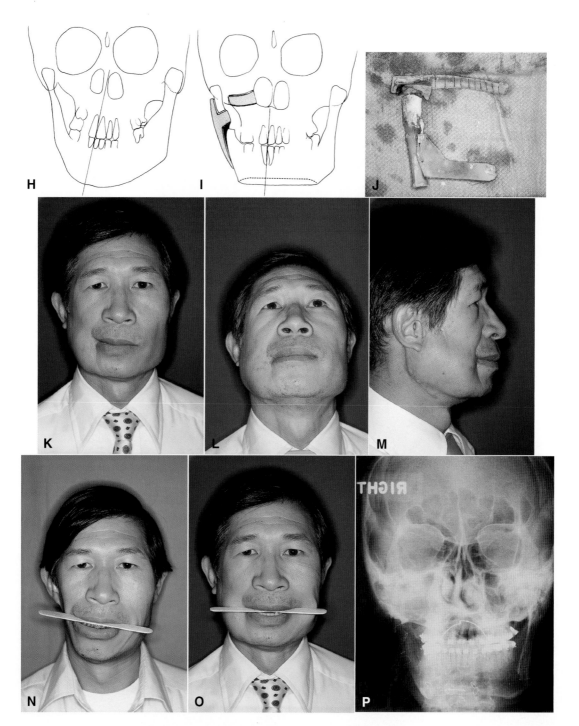

Figure 19-4—continued

H, Tracing of the anteroposterior cephalometric radiograph. A plane is drawn through the mandibular dental and skeletal midlines. This demonstrates the rotation of the skeleton as a result of the mandibular and midface growth deficiency on the right side. The TMJ was in good position. **I,** The correction included a Le Fort I osteotomy to correct the maxillary midline and level the occlusal plane. The fulcrum was at the molars on the normal side, so the midface was lengthened maximally on the affected side. Bilateral mandibular osteotomies and an asymmetric advancement genioplasty were planned. Iliac bone grafts were used for the maxillary and mandibular osteotomies and to augment the contour of the right cheek and mandible. **J,** In patients who require TMJ construction as adults, the iliac crest is used for the body, angle, and inferior ramus. A costochondral graft can be used for the condylar head. The size of the cartilage cap demonstrated here is too large. The cartilage is trimmed to approximately 1 to 2 mm thickness to prevent motion at the junction and overgrowth. The zygomatic arch is constructed with full-thickness rib or calvarial bone. The glenoid fossa is constructed medial to the arch and lined with perichondrium or temporalis fascia when present. Frontal **(K),** submental **(L),** and right lateral **(M)** views of the patient 3 years after skeletal correction and 2 years after free vascularized, de-epithelialized scapula flap for soft tissue augmentation. Note the facial symmetry in a patient who had a severe soft tissue contour deficit. **N,** Preoperative photograph illustrating occlusal cant. **O,** Photograph 3 years after the operation documenting level occlusal plane. **P,** Postoperative anteroposterior cephalogram shows skeletal symmetry.

OMENS Classification

Vento and colleagues[20,21] described a classification analogous to the TNM (tumor, node, metastasis) system for tumors. The OMENS classification of HFM is an acronym for the structures involved: orbit, mandible (and TMJ), ear, nerves, soft tissues. The orbit is normal (score 0) or abnormal in size (1), position (2), or both (3). The mandible may be normal (score 0), type I (1), type IIA (2A), IIB (2B), or type III (3). The ear anomaly is classified to correspond to Meurman's system and is designated E0-3. The facial nerve defect is described as N0-3 to correspond to no facial nerve involvement: upper, lower, or all branches involved. The soft tissue is classified as normal (0), mild (1), moderate (2), or severe (3). This is a rigorous system that forces the clinician to evaluate and document all aspects of the HFM anomaly in each patient. In addition, there is some evidence that a summation of the OMENS score in the different categories has some predictive value for the presence of additional anomalies, including skeletal, renal, and cardiac defects. Patients who have an OMENS score greater than 7 should have an abdominal ultrasonogram, skeletal survey, and cardiac evaluation.[22]

TREATMENT

Accurate classification of the skeletal defect is critical in developing a treatment plan. The skeletal type predicts the rate of progression of asymmetry and the end-stage distortion of contiguous and contralateral skeletal structures. Table 19-1 provides a summary of the progression of the clinical findings, which have implications for treatment.[6,16,23]

Skeletal Defects

Patients Who Are Not Growing. Surgical correction in a patient who is not growing begins by accurate three-dimensional analysis and classification of the end-stage deformity. Results of clinical examination, plain radiographs, and computed tomography (CT) scans form the data base for this analysis.

Assessment of orbital, midface, and mandibular asymmetry is made by examination of the patient in the frontal (coronal) view. The adolescent bites on a tongue depressor to help the examiner assess the relationship between the maxillary-mandibular occlusal plane and the interpupillary, alar base, and intergonial planes and the true horizontal (the cant). Frequently the supraorbital rims and interpupillary plane are parallel to the true horizontal. The alar bases, piriform rims, and occlusal and intergonial planes are canted upward on the affected side. This documents the abnormally short vertical height of the affected side of the face. In the sagittal plane, the surgeon must assess whether or not the maxilla and

mandible are retrognathic, and deficiency in width (horizontal plane) is facilitated by analysis of the dental models.

Radiographic studies include anteroposterior (AP) and lateral cephalograms, and a panoramic view. On the AP cephalogram, the piriform cant, occlusal cant, and intergonial cant can be assessed in relation to the true horizontal. The lateral cephalogram and panoramic radiographs are used to assess the sagittal position of the jaws and ramus height discrepancy, respectively. The skeletal type is determined from the panoramic radiograph.[2,6,9,17,23,24] More recently, CT scans have been used as the basis for three-dimensional diagnosis and treatment planning systems.[25,26]

The overall treatment strategy for three-dimensional correction of the end-stage deformity of HFM depends on the skeletal type. The first step is to level the midface (below the infraorbital rims), piriform apertures (floor of the nose), and alveolar portion of the maxilla in the coronal plane; to correct the position of the maxilla in the sagittal plane (advancement as required); and to correct any residual width deficiency and the maxillary dental midline (horizontal or transverse plane). This usually is accomplished with a Le Fort I osteotomy, although occasionally a higher midface or orbital osteotomy is required (Figures 19-4 to 19-6).

The surgeon must choose the correct fulcrum for leveling the maxilla in relation to the true horizontal. If there is vertical maxillary excess (with excessive maxillary incisor tooth show), the fulcrum of rotation of the maxilla is on the abnormal (short) side, leveling the occlusal plane completely by shortening the long (unaffected) side without any midface elongation. If the vertical length of the midface is normal, then the fulcrum of rotation is in the midline. Leveling of the maxillary occlusal plane is accomplished by a combination of lengthening the short (affected) side and shortening the long side. The relationship of the maxillary anterior teeth to the upper lip remains the same. This is the most common correction in patients with end-stage deformity. If the midface is short, the fulcrum is on the normal side, correcting the deformity completely by lengthening the short side. This produces maximal midface lengthening while leveling the occlusal plane. Once the maxilla is repositioned, bilateral mandibular osteotomies or TMJ and ramus-condyle unit (RCU) construction are required to rotate the lower jaw into its correct relationship with the maxilla. Then, a genioplasty is performed, if necessary, to achieve further advancement and/or correction of the location of the chin point. Contour defects in the skeleton are managed with onlay bone grafts or nonresorbable bone substitute implants such as Medpor (Porex Surgical Products, Newnan, GA.); the soft tissue and ear defects usually are corrected after skeletal symmetry has been achieved (see Figures 19-4 to 19-6).

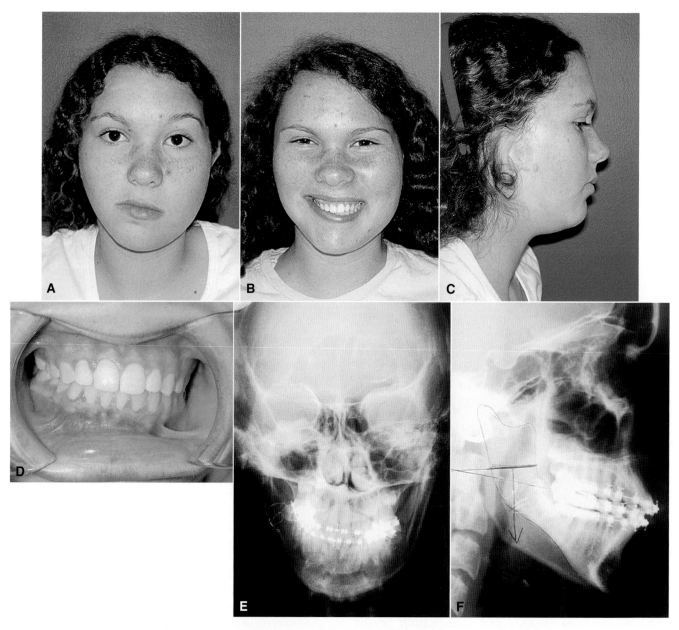

Figure 19-5

Frontal **(A)**, frontal smiling **(B)**, right lateral **(C)**, and intraoral **(D)** views of a teenage girl with end-stage type IIB hemifacial microsomia (HFM) (right side). The patient previously had mandibular ramus lengthening by costochondral graft at another institution. With growth, progressive asymmetry redeveloped. Her teeth were well interdigitated as a result of orthodontic treatment. Note the upward canting (on the right side) of the alar base and commissures. The chin is deviated toward the right, and there is an occlusal cant upward on the right. She has weakness of the right marginal mandibular branch, and the right ear—grade III in severity—has been constructed (at another institution) from rib cartilage. Preoperative anteroposterior **(E)** and lateral **(F)** cephalograms corroborate the clinical findings. Note the canting upward on the right of the piriform apertures, occlusal plane, and intergonial plane and deviation of the chin on the anteroposterior cephalogram. The double projection of the asymmetric mandible is evident on the lateral cephalogram.

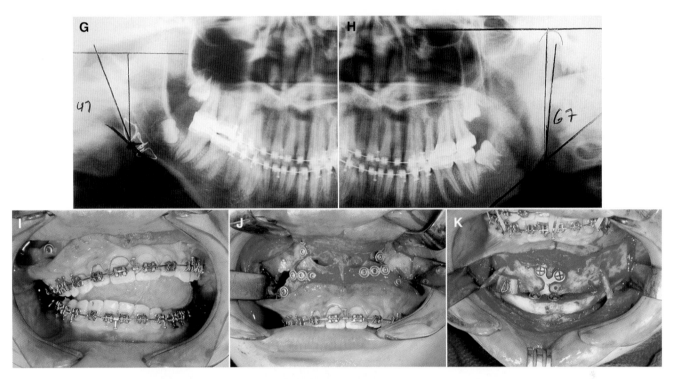

Figure 19-5—continued

G and **H,** Panoramic radiographs corroborate the clinical findings. The panoramic radiograph shows the short right mandibular ramus, which had been previously bone grafted. **I,** Intraoperative view of the maxilla with the occlusal plane leveled by lengthening the short side and shortening the long side, which was determined by the relationship of the upper anterior teeth to the upper lip. Note the premature contact on the right (lengthened) side and the open bite on the left (shortened) side. This demonstrates the extent of the vertical asymmetry. **J,** Maxilla bone grafted on the right and plated. **K,** Intraoperative view of the genioplasty. Note the dissected mental nerves.

Continued.

In patients with types IIB and III HFM, a new TMJ and RCU are constructed in the correct location. In the case of patients with a type IIB defect, the existing RCU and TMJ are so hypoplastic and abnormally positioned that they are not useful and must be excised and replaced. Patients with type III deformity are congenitally missing the RCU and TMJ; the temporal lobe of the brain is visible radiographically where the TMJ would normally be located.[3,9,11,13,19]

The proper location for the TMJ is first determined on a coronal or AP cephalogram. The true midline (vertical) is drawn from the crista galli through the upper part of the nasal septum (see Figures 19-2 and 19-4 to 19-6). The true horizontal line is drawn as a perpendicular to the true midline at the level of the supraorbital rims. The distances from the normal and abnormal TMJs to the midline are measured perpendicular to the true vertical. The vertical distances from the normal and abnormal TMJs to the true horizontal, at the level of the supraorbital rims, are measured. From these measurements, it is possible to determine the inferior and medial displacement of the abnormal TMJ.

At operation, the facial midline is drawn from the middle of the forehead through the glabella and dorsum of the nose. The distance from the true midline at the glabella to the tragus of the ear is measured on the normal and abnormal sides of the face. The distance from the lateral canthus, on the normal and abnormal sides, to the tragus is also documented. The location of the constructed TMJ is determined by these measure-

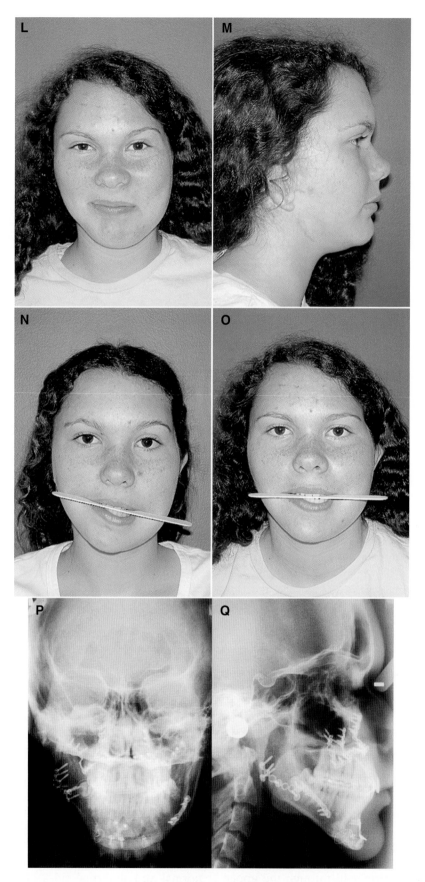

Figure 19-5—continued

Frontal (**L**) and right lateral (**M**) views 1 year postoperatively demonstrate correction of the asymmetry, especially the level alar bases, commissures, and occlusal plane. The chin point is in the midline. Preoperative (**N**) and 1 year postoperative (**O**) views of the patient biting on a tongue depressor and demonstrating the correction of the occlusal plane. Anteroposterior (**P**) and lateral (**Q**) cephalograms 1 year postoperatively demonstrate the achieved skeletal symmetry.

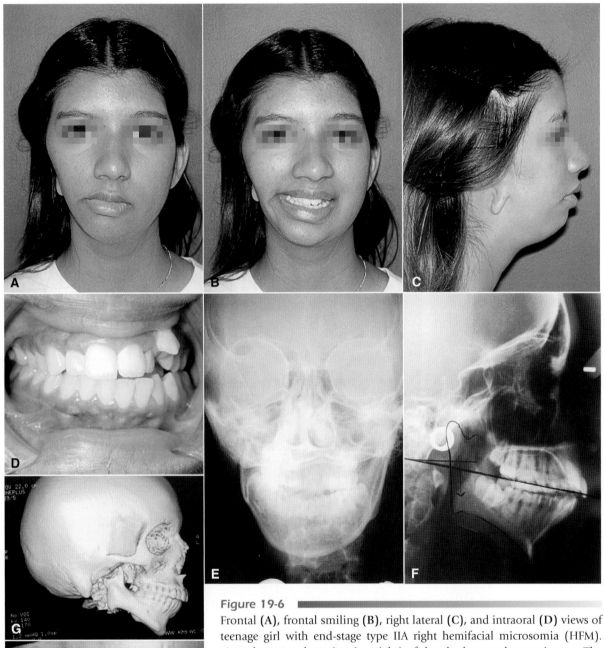

Figure 19-6

Frontal **(A)**, frontal smiling **(B)**, right lateral **(C)**, and intraoral **(D)** views of teenage girl with end-stage type IIA right hemifacial microsomia (HFM). Note the upward canting (on right) of the alar base and commissures. The chin is deviated to the right, and the occlusal cant is upward on the right. The grade III right ear has not been constructed. Preoperative anteroposterior **(E)** and lateral **(F)** cephalograms and 3D CT images **(G and H)** corroborate the clinical findings. Note the canting upward on the right of the piriform apertures, occlusal plane, and intergonial plane and deviation of the chin on the anteroposterior cephalogram. The double projection of the asymmetric mandible is evident on the lateral cephalogram. The CT images show the small, abnormally shaped right mandibular ramus. In this case, the upper lip is long, and the overall vertical midfacial height is short relative to the lip; therefore the correction of the occlusal cant is carried out by lengthening the short side without any shortening of the long side, allowing the use of bimaxillary distraction osteogenesis.

Continued.

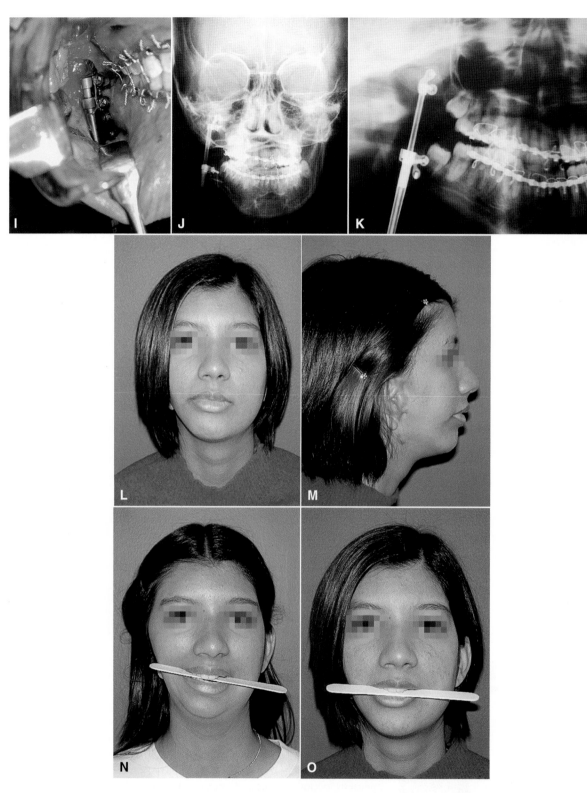

Figure 19-6—continued

I, Intraoperative view showing the right mandibular horizontal corticotomy. A Synthes (Paoli, PA) semiburied, unidirectional distraction device is fixed to the bone. The patient is placed in wire maxillomandibular fixation, and the distractor is activated after 48 hours. **Note: the patient had a simultaneous LFI osteotomy with the maxilla mobilized but not downfractured.** The intermaxillary fixation ensures that the maxilla and mandible will move as a unit. Anteroposterior cephalogram **(J)** and Panorex **(K)** at end distraction demonstrating the right facial lengthening. Frontal **(L)** and right lateral **(M)** views 1 year after treatment. Note the level alar bases, commissures, and occlusal plane, as well as the symmetry of the mandible. The chin point is in the midline. Preoperative **(N)** and 1 year postoperative **(O)** views of the patient showing the level of the occlusal plane.

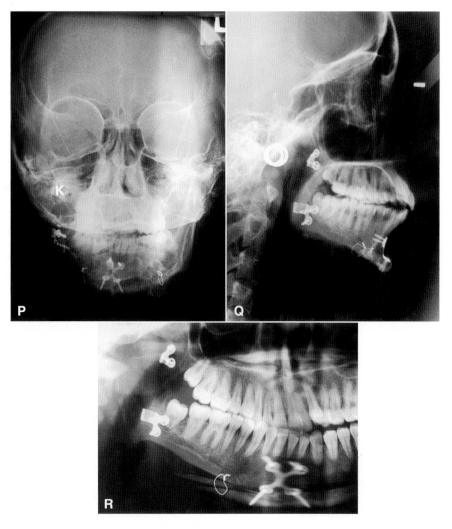

Figure 19-6—continued
Anteroposterior (**P**) and lateral (**Q**) cephalograms and panoramic radiograph (**R**) 1 year postoperatively. Note the retained detachable footplates from the distraction device.

ments. It should be realized that in some patients with type IIB or III deformity, although the TMJ is hypoplastic there is adequate development of the zygomatic arch and adequate bone in the skull base to provide an anatomic stop for the constructed RCU. In these cases, the TMJ does not have to be constructed.

The new RCU is constructed using a costochondral rib graft, with or without iliac crest. The location is guided by the cephalometric and intraoperative measurements described previously. The TMJ (glenoid fossa) is constructed from full-thickness rib, iliac crest, or calvarial bone. It is secured into place (with screws or plates and screws) lateral to the existing zygomatic arch or to the cranium if no zygomatic arch is present. A glenoid fossa is hollowed out of this graft and lined with perichondrium or temporalis fascia and muscle, if present[11,19] (see Figures 19-4 to 19-6). If the zygomatic

arch is hypoplastic or absent, this is constructed with rib or calvarial bone.[26a]

Correction of end-stage type I or IIA skeletal defects requires the same planning and operation on the maxilla. The mandible is repositioned with bilateral osteotomies with or without bone grafts, depending on the anatomy and degree of movement. The affected TMJ (glenoid fossa) is left intact (see Figures 19-4 to 19-6).

Growing Patients
Rationale and Goals of Early Correction. The overall goals of early correction of HFM are to achieve and maintain optimal facial symmetry and improved function (Figures 19-7 to 19-14). Thus, treatment is directed toward (1) increasing the size of the underdeveloped and malformed mandible and associated soft tissues, (2) creating an articulation between mandible and tem-

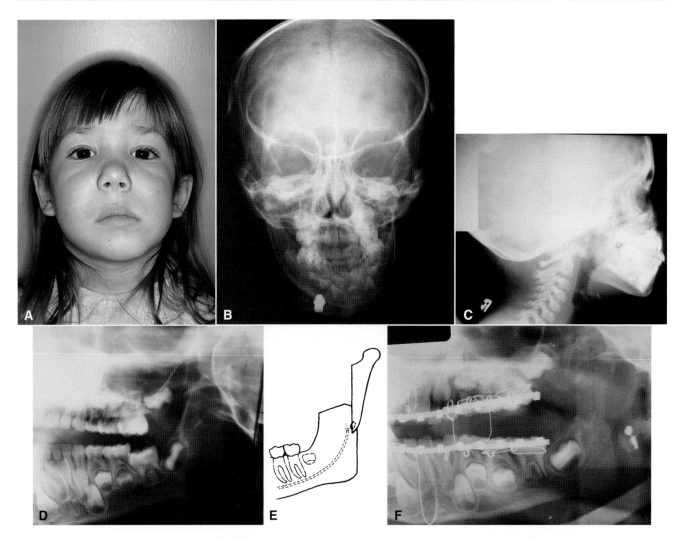

Figure 19-7

A 5-year-old girl with left type IIa hemifacial microsomia. **A,** Frontal photograph shows deviation of the chin point. **B,** Anteroposterior cephalogram shows deviation of the chin point, short ramus, and deviation of the mandibular dental midline. **C,** Lateral cephalogram demonstrates the double images of the short and long sides of the asymmetric mandible. **D,** Panoramic radiograph of the hypoplastic and abnormally shaped left ramus, type IIA. **E,** Diagram of elongation of the left ramus with vertical osteotomy. **F,** Immediate postoperative panoramic radiograph of the lengthened ramus and the surgically created open bite.

poral bone, when absent, (3) promoting vertical maxillary growth and therefore correcting secondary deformities of the maxilla, and (4) establishing a functional occlusion.

A child with HFM must be in the mixed dentition stage to benefit from early management. Success depends on potential for vertical growth of the midface as the deciduous teeth are shed and the permanent teeth erupt. The operation consists of elongation, rotation, and advancement of the hypoplastic mandible to bring the chin point to the midline and to create an open bite on the affected side. In type I and IIA and some type IIB deformities, this is achieved by mandibular osteotomy (with or without bone graft as indicated) or by distraction osteogenesis (DO). In most patients with type IIB and in all patients with type III HFM, the operation consists of costochondral construction of the RCU and building a glenoid fossa, if necessary. This treatment protocol is not applicable after the permanent teeth have erupted, because vertical midfacial growth is essentially complete by this time. Therefore, orthodontically controlled eruption of the permanent teeth into the

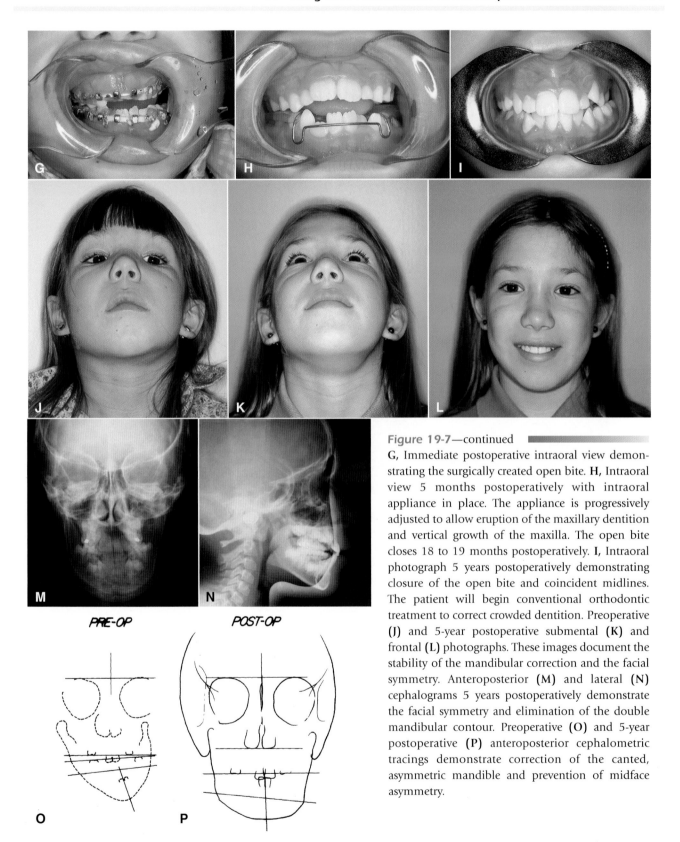

Figure 19-7—continued

G, Immediate postoperative intraoral view demonstrating the surgically created open bite. **H,** Intraoral view 5 months postoperatively with intraoral appliance in place. The appliance is progressively adjusted to allow eruption of the maxillary dentition and vertical growth of the maxilla. The open bite closes 18 to 19 months postoperatively. **I,** Intraoral photograph 5 years postoperatively demonstrating closure of the open bite and coincident midlines. The patient will begin conventional orthodontic treatment to correct crowded dentition. Preoperative **(J)** and 5-year postoperative submental **(K)** and frontal **(L)** photographs. These images document the stability of the mandibular correction and the facial symmetry. Anteroposterior **(M)** and lateral **(N)** cephalograms 5 years postoperatively demonstrate the facial symmetry and elimination of the double mandibular contour. Preoperative **(O)** and 5-year postoperative **(P)** anteroposterior cephalometric tracings demonstrate correction of the canted, asymmetric mandible and prevention of midface asymmetry.

PRE-OP   POST-OP

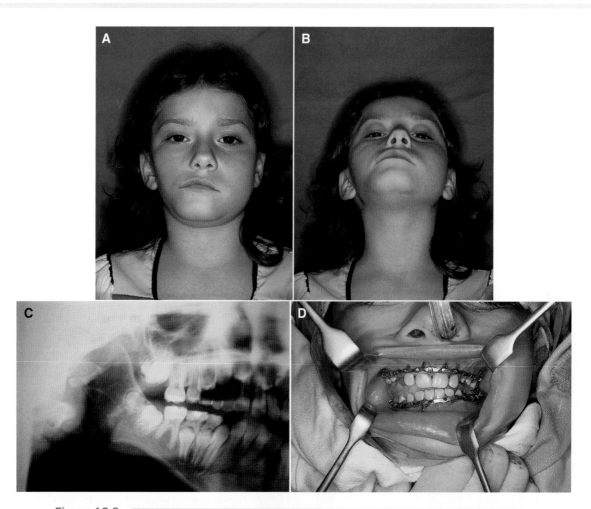

Figure 19-8

Frontal (**A**) and submental (**B**) views of a girl in mixed dentition with right type I skeletal defect and moderate soft tissue bulk asymmetry. **C,** Preoperative panoramic radiograph. The degree of lengthening was too large to accomplish with a vertical ramus osteotomy. **D,** Intraoperative occlusal view demonstrating the surgically created open bite accomplished by a horizontal osteotomy and interpositional bone graft. A compensatory osteotomy was not necessary on the left side.

open bite space will not be accompanied by adequate vertical midfacial growth. The teeth will simply extrude.

A major goal of early surgical correction of HFM is to achieve a symmetric maxilla and midface, with a level occlusal plane and level alar bases (piriform angle). An adequate open bite space must be created by the mandibular procedure, and it must be maintained and closed gradually over 18 to 24 months. Once closure is achieved, the maxillary occlusal plane is set. Secondary leveling of the maxilla is usually unnecessary[27-29] (see Figures 19-7 to 19-14).

Failure to understand this rationale leads to inadequate attention to creation and management of the open bite. The open bite space must be maintained by

an orthodontic appliance (occlusal bite block) for at least 3 to 6 months while the osteotomized or constructed ramus heals. Then the maxillary teeth can be allowed to erupt by a combination of passive movement and orthodontic forces, thereby leveling the occlusal plane. If the open bite space is not maintained adequately during this crucial period, it closes rapidly by a combination of supraeruption of the teeth and resorption and deformation of the lengthened ramus under the compressive forces of the occlusion. The desired effect of early treatment is lost.

Execution of the Treatment Protocol. Treatment must proceed stepwise, consisting of presurgical jaw orthopedic management (functional appliances in types

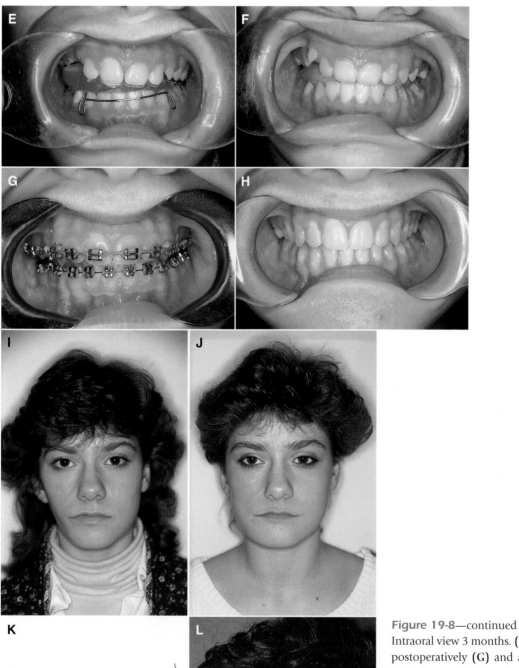

Figure 19-8—continued
Intraoral view 3 months. (**E**), 1 year (**F**), and 3 years postoperatively (**G**) and at end of treatment (**H**). Note the progressive closure of the open bite. At 3 years postoperatively, the open bite has been closed for 1 year. **I**, The patient 3 years postoperatively. The skeleton is symmetric in position, but there is a contour defect on the right side. **J**, One year after onlay iliac bone graft to the right mandible and 5 years after skeletal correction, the patient has a symmetric facial contour. **K**, Preoperative (*dotted line*) and 5-year postoperative (*solid line*) cephalometric tracings demonstrate the leveling of the piriform apertures and occlusal plane and the correct position of the chin point. **L**, Frontal photograph 10 years postoperatively demonstrating some recurrence of the contour asymmetry but overall acceptable facial and jaw symmetry.

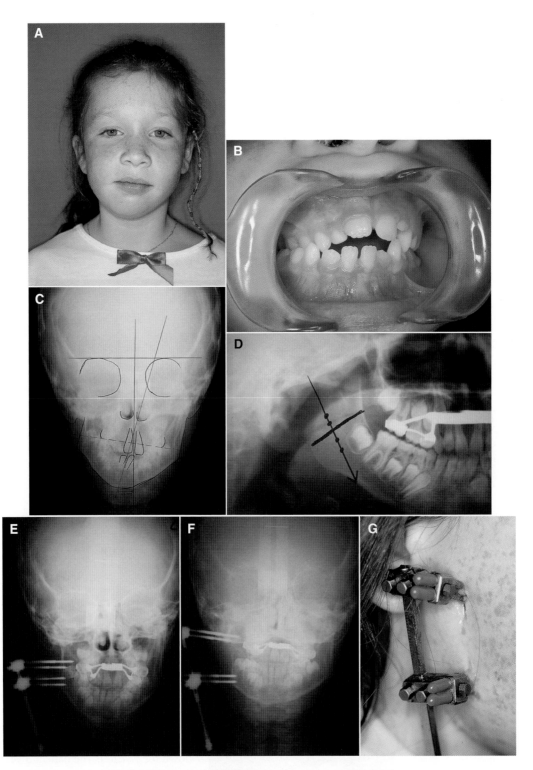

Figure 19-9

Type IIA hemifacial microsomia (right side). Frontal **(A)** and intraoral **(B)** photographs of a child demonstrates deviation of the chin point to the right and slight canting of the alar bases and commissures. Intraorally there is a unilateral cross bite treated by maxillary expansion with a removal device. **C,** Anteroposterior cephalogram and overlay tracing show deviation of the chin point, short ramus, and deviation of the mandibular dental midline. The piriform apertures and occlusal plane are canted upward to the right. **D,** Panoramic radiograph demonstrates type IIA mandible and location of proposed osteotomy. The arrow indicates the vector of movement of the jaw. **E,** Immediate postoperative anteroposterior cephalogram with distraction device in place. **F,** End DO anteroposterior cephalogram. **G,** End DO lateral photograph showing the separation of the proximal and distal mandibular segments (separation of the pins).

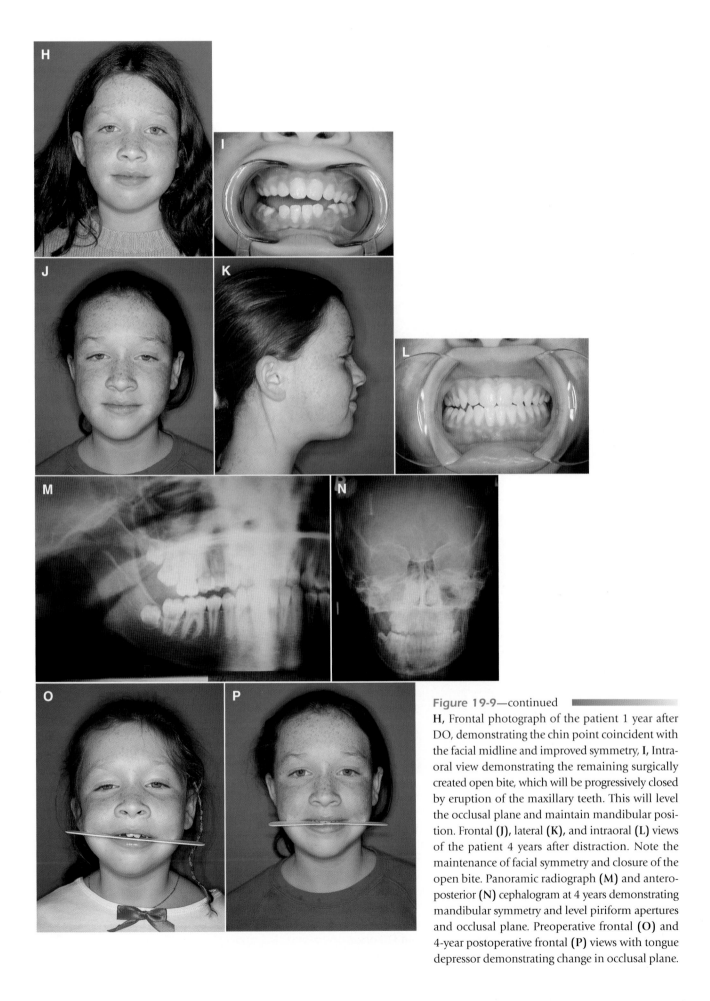

Figure 19-9—continued

H, Frontal photograph of the patient 1 year after DO, demonstrating the chin point coincident with the facial midline and improved symmetry, I, Intraoral view demonstrating the remaining surgically created open bite, which will be progressively closed by eruption of the maxillary teeth. This will level the occlusal plane and maintain mandibular position. Frontal (J), lateral (K), and intraoral (L) views of the patient 4 years after distraction. Note the maintenance of facial symmetry and closure of the open bite. Panoramic radiograph (M) and anteroposterior (N) cephalogram at 4 years demonstrating mandibular symmetry and level piriform apertures and occlusal plane. Preoperative frontal (O) and 4-year postoperative frontal (P) views with tongue depressor demonstrating change in occlusal plane.

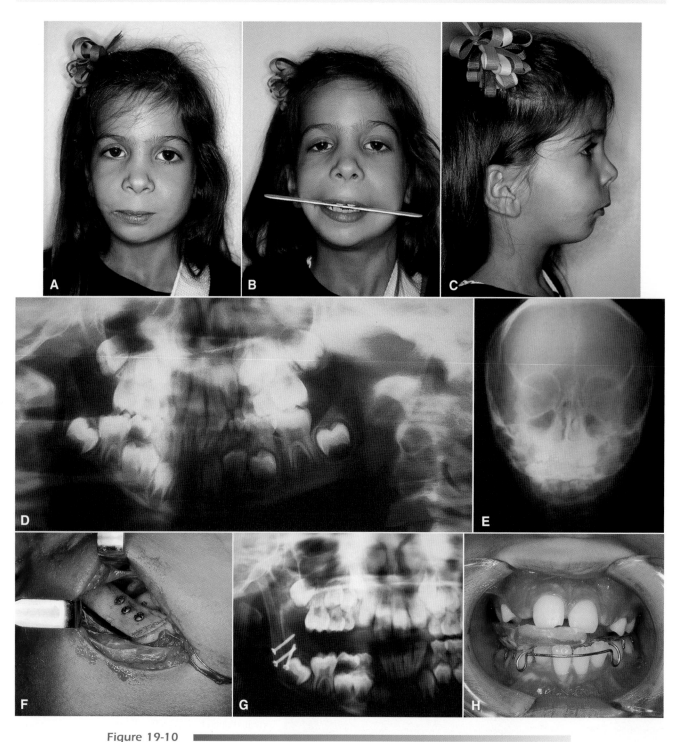

Figure 19-10

Frontal (**A**), frontal with tongue depressor (**B**), and right lateral (**C**) photographs of a child in early mixed dentition with type III right hemifacial microsomia. Note deviation of the chin to the right, upward cant of occlusal plane, and retrognathic mandible. Panoramic radiograph (**D**) and anteroposterior cephalogram (**E**) illustrating absent right mandibular ramus condyle unit and deviation of the symphysis to the right. **F,** Intraoperative view of costochondral graft in place and rigidly fixed. The glenoid fossa and zygomatic arch were present, and their construction was not necessary. **G,** Immediate postoperative panoramic radiograph demonstrates the graft in place and the surgically created open bite. **H,** Intraoral view immediately postoperatively with splint in place.

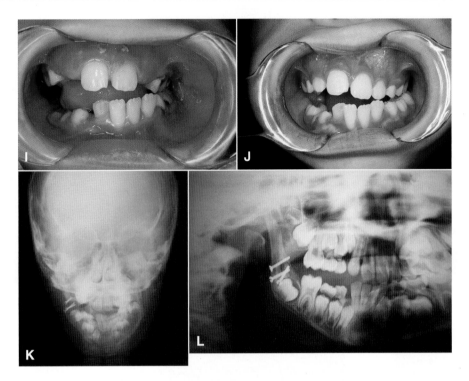

Figure 19-10—continued
Intraoral views immediately postoperatively without splint (**I**), demonstrating surgically created open bite, and 1 year postoperatively (**J**), demonstrating progressive closure of open bite. Anteroposterior cephalogram (**K**) and panoramic radiograph (**L**) 1 year postoperatively. (From Kaban LB, Padwa BL, Mulliken JB: *J Oral Maxillofac Surg* 56:628-638, 1998.)

I and IIA) when indicated, ramus-condyle and glenoid fossa construction if necessary, immediate postsurgical treatment to support graft remodeling, maxillary correction when necessary, final orthodontic treatment, and soft tissue augmentation.

Presurgical Orthopedic Treatment. A functional appliance is constructed to hold the affected side of the mandible in a lowered and forward position. The appliance stimulates bone apposition in the RCU by substituting for the normal translatory motion produced by the lateral pterygoid muscle. This treatment is applied routinely on our young patients during the presurgical growth management phase. Response to this "functional therapy" is beneficial, particularly for patients with type I and IIA deformity. A study of 15 patients with type I HFM showed that during treatment with a functional appliance, the affected side increased more than the contralateral side in four children, an amount equal to the contralateral side in another four, and slightly less in the remaining seven subjects. There was no significant group mean difference in growth of the two sides in this sample. All 15 patients ultimately had an operation, either during growth (n = 10) or after skeletal matura-

tion (n = 5).[30] A similar response to this type of treatment is documented by Melsen and co-workers.[31]

In a patient with type I or IIA who responds well to a functional appliance, surgical lengthening can be avoided, if the mandibular midline and chin point are acceptable and an occlusal cant is avoided. If the cant is severe, it is necessary to elongate the mandible on the affected side.

Orthodontic Treatment. Orthodontic treatment in childhood focuses on control of dental eruption and prevention or correction of dentoalveolar adaptations to the asymmetric position of the maxilla and mandible. There may be delayed tooth eruption and dental irregularities on the affected side, and crowding of teeth is common.[32] The orthodontist should be actively involved and coordinate the treatment for children with HFM throughout their growth periods.

Surgical Correction of Mandibular Deformity. Operative correction of the skeletal defect is indicated in selected children with HFM (see Figures 19-7 to 19-14). If mandibular lengthening and creation of an open bite is done early in the mixed dentition, vertical growth potential of the midface will minimize secondary defor-

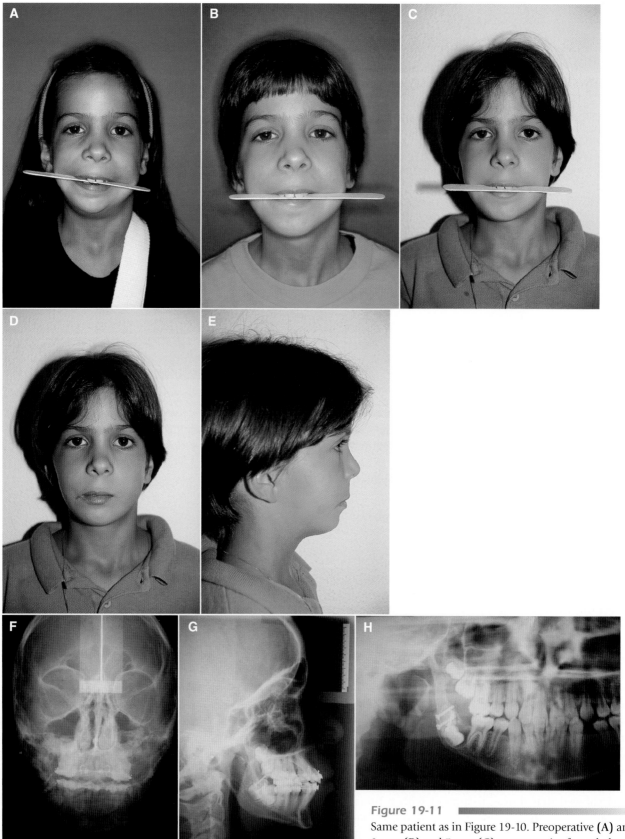

Figure 19-11

Same patient as in Figure 19-10. Preoperative (**A**) and 2-year (**B**) and 5-year (**C**) postoperative frontal photographs demonstrating stable correction of occlusal cant. **D**, Five-year postoperative frontal photograph illustrating excellent facial symmetry. **E**, Lateral photograph demonstrating slight retrognathism. Anteroposterior (**F**) and lateral (**G**) cephalograms 6 years and panoramic radiograph (**H**) 5 years postoperatively. (From Kaban LB, Padwa BL, Mulliken JB: *J Oral Maxillofac Surg* 56:628-638, 1998.)

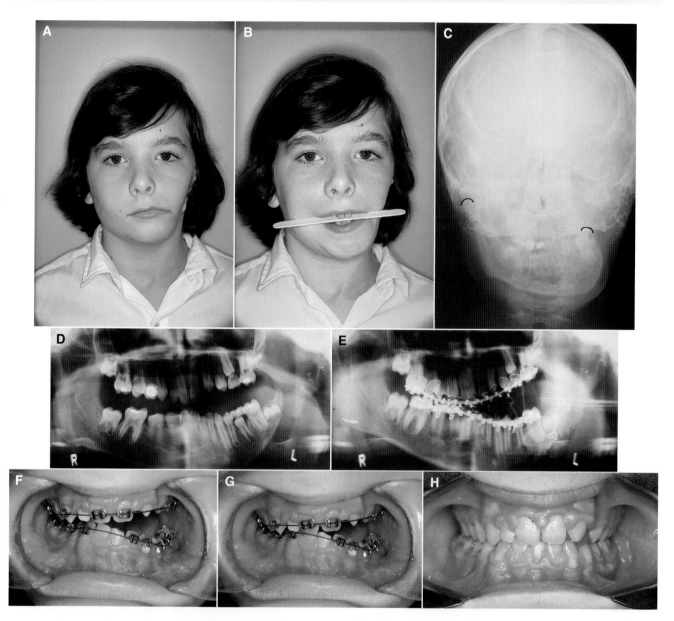

Figure 19-12

A, Frontal view of a patient with type III hemifacial microsomia (left side) showing contour defect, deviation of chin point, and cant of alar bases and commissures of the lips upward to the left. **B,** Frontal view demonstrating the occlusal cant. **C,** Anteroposterior cephalogram demonstrates the abnormal location of the rudimentary functioning articulating surface and cant of the piriform apertures. **D,** Panoramic radiograph shows the "forme-fruste" of a left mandibular ramus. **E,** Panoramic radiograph with the patient in intermaxillary fixation illustrates the 2.0 cm surgically created open bite. The patient underwent total construction of the ramus condyle unit, the zygomatic arch, and glenoid fossa with a combination of autogenous iliac bone and costochondral grafts. **F to H,** Intraoral photographs demonstrate progressive closure of the surgically created open bite during 18 months of postoperative orthodontic treatment (**F and G**) and at 3 years postoperatively (**H**).

Continued.

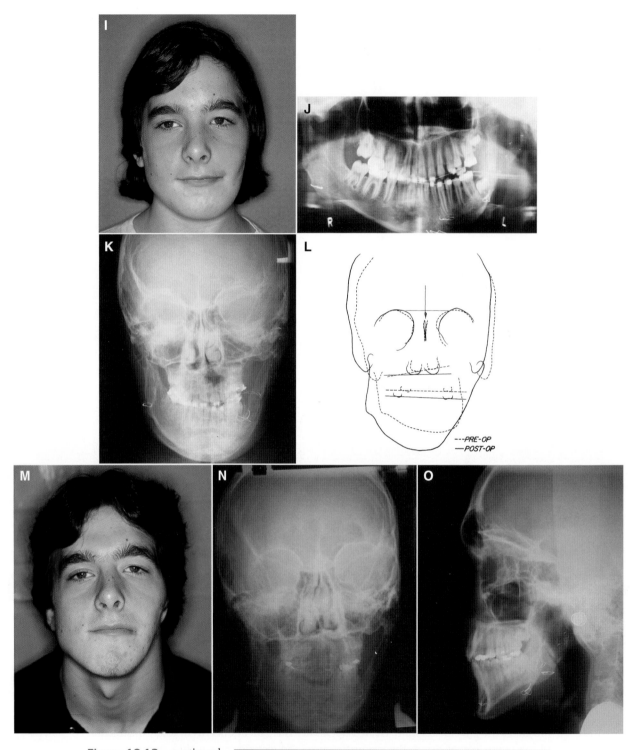

Figure 19-12—continued
I, Three years postoperatively, full face photograph demonstrates facial symmetry. Panoramic radiograph (J) and anteroposterior cephalogram (K) 3 years postoperatively show remodeling of the costochondral graft, closure of the open bite, a level occlusal plane, symmetric mandibular rami and TMJ locations, and chin point in the midline. L, Superimposed pretreatment and 3-year postoperative anteroposterior cephalometric tracings. Frontal photograph (M) and anteroposterior (N) and lateral (O) cephalograms 5 years postoperatively.

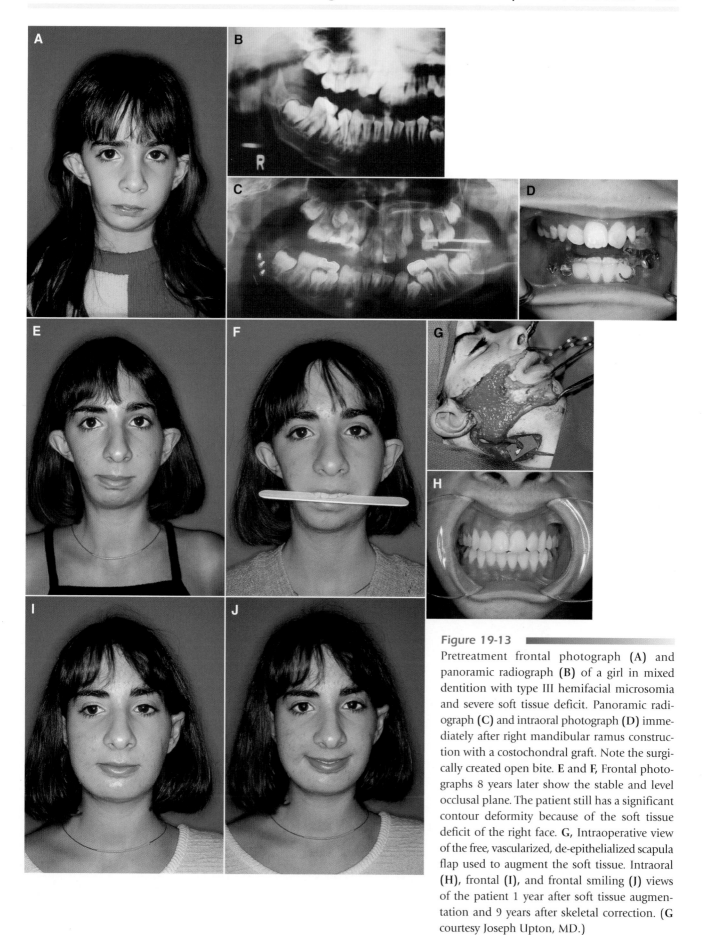

Figure 19-13

Pretreatment frontal photograph (**A**) and panoramic radiograph (**B**) of a girl in mixed dentition with type III hemifacial microsomia and severe soft tissue deficit. Panoramic radiograph (**C**) and intraoral photograph (**D**) immediately after right mandibular ramus construction with a costochondral graft. Note the surgically created open bite. **E** and **F**, Frontal photographs 8 years later show the stable and level occlusal plane. The patient still has a significant contour deformity because of the soft tissue deficit of the right face. **G**, Intraoperative view of the free, vascularized, de-epithelialized scapula flap used to augment the soft tissue. Intraoral (**H**), frontal (**I**), and frontal smiling (**J**) views of the patient 1 year after soft tissue augmentation and 9 years after skeletal correction. (**G** courtesy Joseph Upton, MD.)

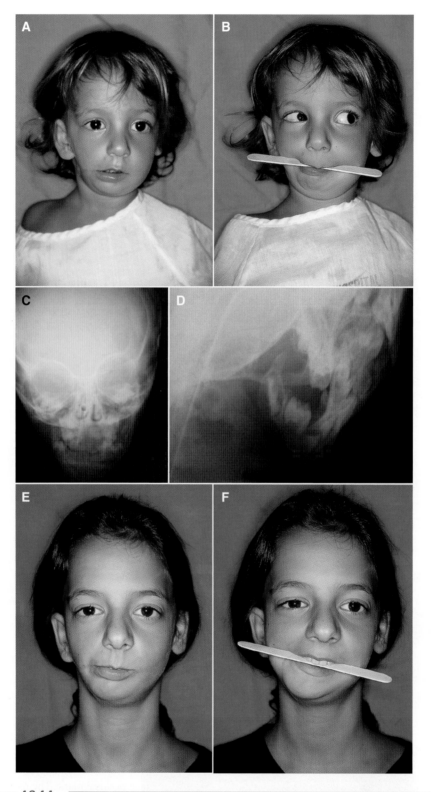

Figure 19-14
Frontal photographs (**A** and **B**) and anteroposterior (**C**) and lateral (**D**) radiographs of a girl in deciduous dentition with type III hemifacial microsomia. An operation to construct the ramus resulted in loss of the graft due to infection. **E** and **F**, Nine years later the deformity, as evidenced by the occlusal cant, has progressed significantly.

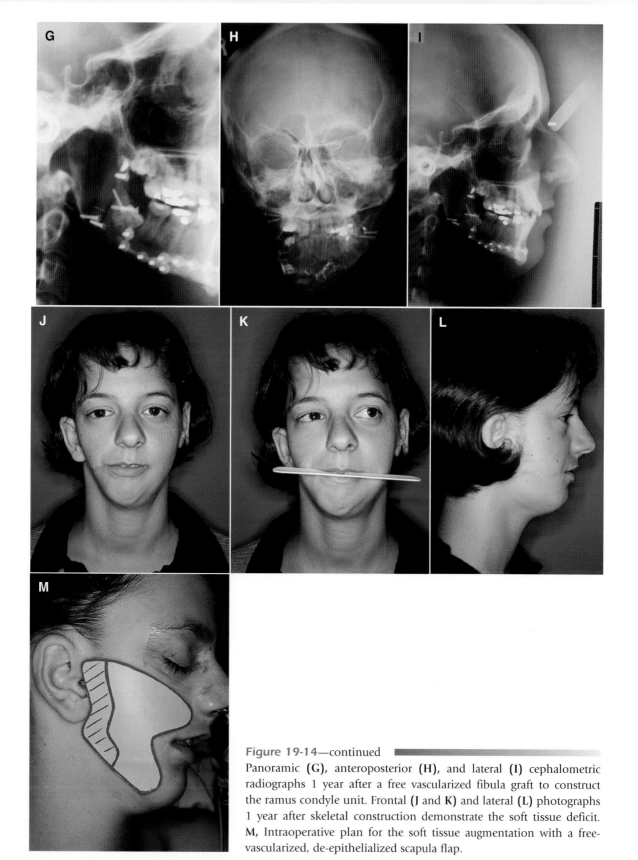

Figure 19-14—continued
Panoramic **(G)**, anteroposterior **(H)**, and lateral **(I)** cephalometric radiographs 1 year after a free vascularized fibula graft to construct the ramus condyle unit. Frontal **(J** and **K)** and lateral **(L)** photographs 1 year after skeletal construction demonstrate the soft tissue deficit. **M,** Intraoperative plan for the soft tissue augmentation with a free-vascularized, de-epithelialized scapula flap.

Continued.

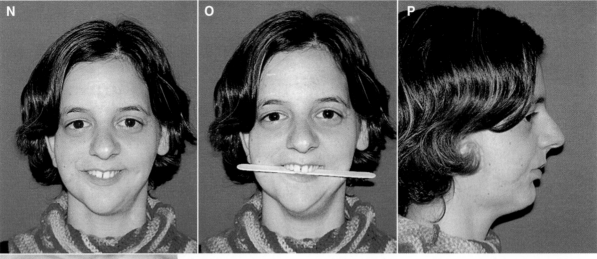

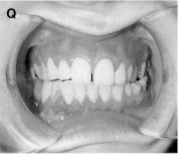

Figure 19-14—continued   ▬▬▬▬▬
Frontal (**N** and **O**), lateral (**P**), and intraoral (**Q**) photographs 1 year after soft tissue augmentation. Note the improved contour and stable skeletal and occlusal result. (**M** courtesy Joseph Upton, MD.)

mity. In patients with type I and IIA deformities (see Figures 19-7 to 19-9), the mandible is elongated and rotated to the proper midline. The native TMJ is accepted. A compensatory osteotomy of the normal side may be required to allow the mandible to sit passively in the new position. An open bite is created on the affected side, regulated by an orthodontic appliance to allow for eruption of teeth and vertical growth of the maxilla.[33-35] The open bite is maintained first by an occlusal bite block for 3 to 6 months. Then, eruption of the maxillary teeth is begun by gradually reducing the maxillary side of the bite block. Finally, open bite closure is completed by active orthodontic movement of the maxillary teeth. In patients with types IIB and III HFM (see Figures 19-10 to 19-14), the mandible is elongated and rotated by construction of a mandibular ramus and glenoid fossa using costochondral junction and rib, calvarial, or iliac crest bone grafts. The operation and orthodontic procedures are otherwise the same as for types I and IIA.

We have analyzed periodically the results of treatment of HFM in childhood at Boston Children's Hospital.[12,28] Kaban et al. evaluated 20 patients classified as type I or IIA (group I, n = 10) and type IIB or III (group II, n = 10). They were treated by the protocol described herein and

the mean follow-up time was 50.9 months (group I) and 45 months (group II). In all children, the midface grew vertically to close the surgically created open bite and the occlusal plane was leveled without maxillary osteotomy. In patients who had type I or IIA HFM followed to completion of growth (n = 9/10), none required a maxillary osteotomy or a second operation on the mandible. In patients with type IIB or III (n = 4), operated on during the deciduous dentition (below age 5 years), the affected mandible required a second elongation procedure in the late mixed dentition or early teen years. No patients needed midfacial osteotomy in this series. In a sense, the patients were converted from type IIB or III to type IIA HFM.

Padwa et al.[28] evaluated 33 children who underwent costochondral graft construction for types IIB (n = 19) and III (n = 14) HFM. Mean age at operation was 6.2 years, and the mean follow-up was 5.5 years. Stability of the results was judged on the basis of maintenance of the occlusal cant correction. Based on previously published data,[24] an occlusal cant of less than 5 degrees was considered a successful outcome (group I), more than 5 and less than 8 degrees acceptable (group II), and more than 8 degrees a failure (group III). The patients who had a successful result (group I) had a mean OMENS score significantly lower than those in groups II and III (6.3, 6.8, and 7.8, respectively) and were operated upon at an older age (6.7, 6.3 and 5.8 years, respectively). Furthermore, the occlusal cant in group I improved (decreased) with age, whereas the cants in group II remained stable and in group III worsened with time. The authors concluded that after construction of the RCU in types IIB and III HFM vertical midface lengthening occurred by a combination of midface and alveolar growth. The severity of the deformity, as reflected by OMENS score and the age at operation, affected the outcome.

The University of California, San Francisco Group[30] reported continual growth of the lengthened mandibular ramus in 7 of 10 patients operated on early and followed until growth was completed. In three patients, however, growth of the affected side did not keep pace with that of the contralateral side, and asymmetry recurred, requiring a second surgical procedure that also involved maxillary leveling. The maxilla was corrected orthodontically in all these patients.

The patient's ability to cooperate in using the initial occlusal appliance and to cooperate during orthodontic treatment must be considered in deciding whether to proceed with early surgical therapy. If this portion of the protocol cannot be carried out successfully, early treatment is likely to fail. Under these circumstances, it is prudent to delay intervention. If this window of opportunity closes, it is appropriate to wait until growth has completed and to correct the end-stage deformity.

HFM is the only major craniofacial anomaly in which early treatment has produced documented improvement in facial growth. We emphasize the important concept of progression of the deformity with time. The purpose of treatment in childhood is to enhance growth potential in the mandible, to decrease or prevent secondary deformity in contiguous and contralateral facial skeletal structures (especially the maxilla), and to improve body image development. The aesthetic and functional results of treatment in HFM are difficult to quantitate accurately because they involve many features, some of which are difficult to assess and some of which are not necessarily associated with the original anomaly.

Soft Tissue Defects

Treatment of the soft tissue abnormalities may begin during infancy. Skin tags are removed and significant macrostomia is repaired during the first year of life. If a hypoplastic ear is severely anteroinferiorly malpositioned, the lobule can be maneuvered surgically into a more normal position posteriorly and superiorly. This should be accomplished with minimal dissection and scarring so as not to compromise subsequent ear reconstruction. If the lobule is displaced minimally, it can be left alone until the definitive ear reconstruction[11] (see Chapter 22).

The external ear deformity usually is left untreated until after the skeletal correction is complete.[11] This is to ensure that the ear will be placed in its correct position. Too often, the patient comes in for skeletal correction with a constructed ear in an anteroinferior location. In these cases, the cartilaginous framework has to be removed and redone later. The ear reconstruction is carried out with autogenous tissue by the techniques described by Tanzer and refined by Brent and Byrd.[36-38] The principles and techniques of ear correction are presented in detail in Chapter 22.

The deficiency of subcutaneous fat is also corrected after the skeleton is symmetrical. Occasionally, the contour defect can be corrected with onlay bone grafts, but in patients with moderate and severe soft tissue deficiency, augmentation with soft tissue is necessary. The most common method involves the use of free vascularized tissue transfer. In the past, we have used free omentum placed into dissected subcutaneous pockets. The vascularized deepithelialized scapular flap is currently the favored technique, because it provides the most natural soft tissue texture without the disadvantage of gravitational sag. If the skin is hypoplastic, it can be expanded before completing the vascularized flap to avoid a cutaneous island patch with a less satisfactory color match (see Figures 19-13 and 19-14).[11]

Bilateral First and Second Pharyngeal Arch Defects

GENERAL CONSIDERATIONS

Patients with Treacher Collins syndrome (mandibulofacial dysostosis) and bilateral craniofacial microsomia have a characteristic constellation of anomalies that include hypoplastic TMJs, short mandibular rami, and decreased posterior face height. The importance of decreased posterior face height in the evolution of the end-stage deformity is often overlooked.[38] The joints in these conditions are often in the proper position, but they may have to be reconstructed if the glenoid fossa is too shallow to permit stability of a lengthened mandibular ramus.

Treacher Collins Syndrome

Treacher Collins syndrome (incidence 1:10,000 live births) is inherited as an autosomal dominant trait, with incomplete penetrance and variable expressivity.[39,40] The human deformity may be the result of an insult to the preotic neural crest cells during the first 4 to 6 weeks of embryogenesis. Poswillo[41] has produced an animal phenocopy of this deformity with vitamin A, in which he found focal necrosis of neural crest cells and a defi-

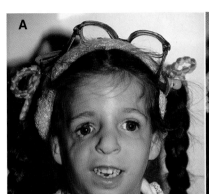
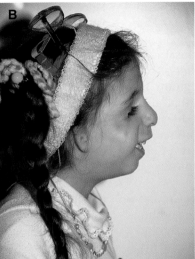
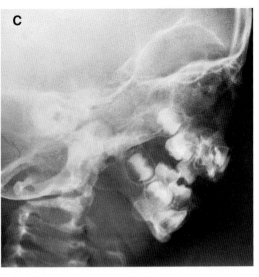

Figure 19-15

A, Frontal photograph of a 5-year-old girl with Treacher Collins syndrome. Note the downward cant of the lateral canthi, coloboma of the lower eyelids and soft tissue, bony deficit in the malar regions, and abnormal ears. **B,** Lateral photograph illustrates external ear abnormality (grade II) and mandibular retrognathism. The child wears conductive hearing aids attached to her hair band. **C,** Lateral cephalogram demonstrates the marked shortening of the posterior face height.

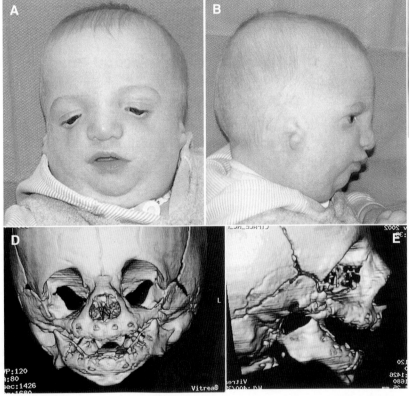
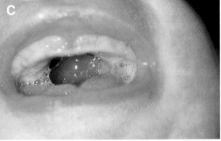

Figure 19-16

A, Frontal view of a 6-month-old infant with typical findings of Treacher Collins syndrome: coloboma of the lower eyelids, absence of eyelashes on the medial third of the lower eyelids, downward-slanting lateral canthi, bilateral grade III ear deformities, and micrognathia. **B,** Lateral photograph shows the ear anomaly, micrognathia, and the tracheostomy. **C,** Intraoral view of the cleft palate, present in 30% of patients with Treacher Collins syndrome. Frontal **(D)** and lateral **(E)** 3D CT images demonstrate the tear-drop-shaped orbits, zygomatic hypoplasia, absence of the zygomatic arches and mandibular ramus, TMJ hypoplasia, mandibular retrognathism, and markedly short posterior facial height.

Continued.

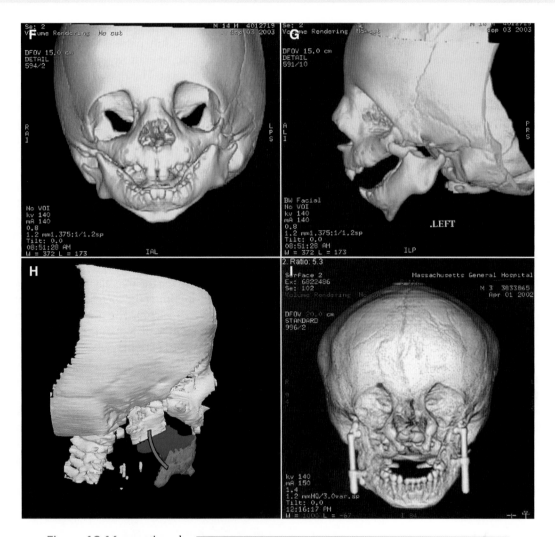

Figure 19-16—continued
Frontal (**F**) and lateral (**G**) 3D CT images at 18 months of age show similar findings but with a much better developed mandibular ramus. **H**, The CT data were imported into a three-dimensional treatment planning system (Osteoplan, Harvard Surgical Planning Laboratory, Boston) for the purposes of planning for mandibular advancement by distraction osteogenesis. The goal is to facilitate removal of the tracheostomy. The pink image represents the skull and the proximal mandible after DO. The blue image is the distal mandible in its native position. The red image is the desired new position of the distal mandible. Note the curvilinear path of movement (green arc) to achieve the final result. This movement can be accomplished with (1) a three-dimensional curvilinear distraction device, (2) a multidirectional external device, or (3) a unidirectional device followed by "molding" the regenerate. **I**, Three-dimensional CT image of another child with Treacher Collins syndrome who underwent distraction using a unidirectional, semiburied device (Synthes, Paoli, PA) to increase ramus length and posterior face height.

ciency of ectomesenchyme in the first and second pharyngeal arches. More recently, it has been discovered that the genetic basis for Treacher Collins syndrome resides in mutations in the *TCOF1* gene loci 5q32-q33.1[42] (see Chapter 2).

The clinical features of this syndrome were described by Thomson in 1847, Berry in 1889, and Treacher Collins in 1900.[43-45] Franchesetti and Klein[46] called it *mandibulofacial dysostosis*. Clinical findings are variable, with a wide spectrum of anomalies that are characteristically bilateral and symmetric.[47] There is an antimongoloid (downward) cant of the palpebral fissures, frequently a coloboma at the junction of the outer and middle third of the lower eyelids (sometimes the upper), and an absence of eyelashes along the medial third of the lower lids. The external ears are low set and hypoplastic. There is usually a conductive hearing loss in association with abnormalities of the external and middle ears. The inner ear, which is not a first or second pharyngeal arch derivative, develops normally. Skin tags may be present along a line from the tragus of the ear to the commissure of the mouth; there may be an extension of temporal hair onto the cheek. The nose is large, and the zygomatic bones and arches are hypoplastic or missing. As a result, the frontozygomatic suture is displaced inferiorly, and the orbital shape resembles that of a tear drop[43-48](Figures 19-15 and 19-16).

Bilateral Craniofacial Microsomia

Patients with bilateral craniofacial microsomia have skeletal deformities in the mandible, TMJ, and zygomatic regions that are similar to those common to Treacher Collins syndrome, but they do not have the characteristic soft tissue defects around the eyelids. In bilateral craniofacial microsomia, the skeletal and soft tissue defects are usually asymmetric, the patients have eyelashes on the medial one third of the lower eyelids, and they may have unilateral or bilateral facial nerve deficits and macrostomia, neither of which occurs in Treacher Collins syndrome. Finally, whereas Treacher Collins syndrome is inherited as an autosomal dominant trait, bilateral craniofacial microsomia is usually an isolated event without any known inheritance pattern[48,49] (Figure 19-17).

TREATMENT

This chapter does not discuss in detail correction of the orbital deformity of Treacher Collins syndrome. This is well described in the craniofacial literature, and the orbital deformity and its correction do not impact facial growth. The orbital defect is corrected with onlay bone grafts to the zygomas and orbital floors and recontouring of the supraorbital rims. In the early stages of craniofacial surgery, the choice of bone graft was rib, but this has been replaced almost universally by cranial bone because of its better contour and decreased resorption. The lateral canthi are elevated, and the soft tissue defects around the eyelids usually are corrected with local flaps. Secondary zygomatic augmentation as the child grows is now often accomplished with nonresorbable bone substitute materials such as Medpor (Porex Surgical Products, Newnan, Ga.).

We confine our remarks here to the TMJ anomaly and decreased posterior face height that occurs in both Treacher Collins syndrome and bilateral facial microsomia. Correction of the skeletal deformity of the TMJ in both syndromes consists of elongation of the mandibular rami and advancement of the mandible. The fundamental purpose of the operation is to increase the posterior face height. In the adult patient with end-stage deformity, this involves an operation on the maxilla, at either the Le Fort I or II level. The maxilla is rotated counterclockwise, with a center of rotation at the nasofrontal region or anterior nasal spine, to lengthen the posterior face. An interposition bone graft is placed in the gaps. The mandibular ramus is then lengthened with either a sagittal split osteotomy, an osteotomy and bone graft, or by construction of a new ramus and TMJ.[39]

In a growing child, the mandibular ramus is elongated, and the body is advanced and rotated counterclockwise to close any existing anterior open bite. The mandible is placed in a prognathic relationship to the maxilla and bilateral posterior open bite is created. The open bite is regulated and progressively reduced with an orthodontic appliance, allowing the maxilla and midface to grow vertically and maintaining the increase in posterior face height (Figures 19-7 to 19-17). The potential for vertical growth in this manner may be less in the Treacher Collins group (particularly the patients who have choanal atresia) than in patients with bilateral facial microsomia. However, in certain cases the mandible must be elongated and advanced for airway considerations at an age too early to do a Le Fort osteotomy. These patients will require a Le Fort l or II osteotomy at a later date. The maxillary procedure may possibly be avoided in the bilateral facial microsomia group as it is in the patients with HFM. Follow-up on this group of patients is too early to make a definitive statement about the results.

Roles of Computed Tomography–Based Three-Dimensional Treatment Planning and Distraction Osteogenesis

ROLE OF DISTRACTION OSTEOGENESIS

Since the original report of distraction osteogenesis (DO) by Codivilla[50] in 1905, there have been large numbers of studies published on skeletal expansion by this technique. These include the pioneering orthopedic work of Ilizarov[51-53] in the late 1950s and the clinical and experimental investigation of long bone and craniomaxillofacial DO.[54-63] DO is a technique of bone lengthening that uses the body's inherent healing mechanisms to form new bone. As described and popularized by Ilizarov[51-53] and then by McCarthy[54] for the mandible, a corticotomy is made in the bone, leaving the marrow and endosteal blood supply intact. A device is fixed to the bone across the gap and, after a latency period (4 to 7 days) to permit upregulation of bone metabolism, the device is activated at a rate of 1 mm per day. When the desired expansion is achieved, the bone is fixed rigidly for a period approximately 2 times the number of milli-

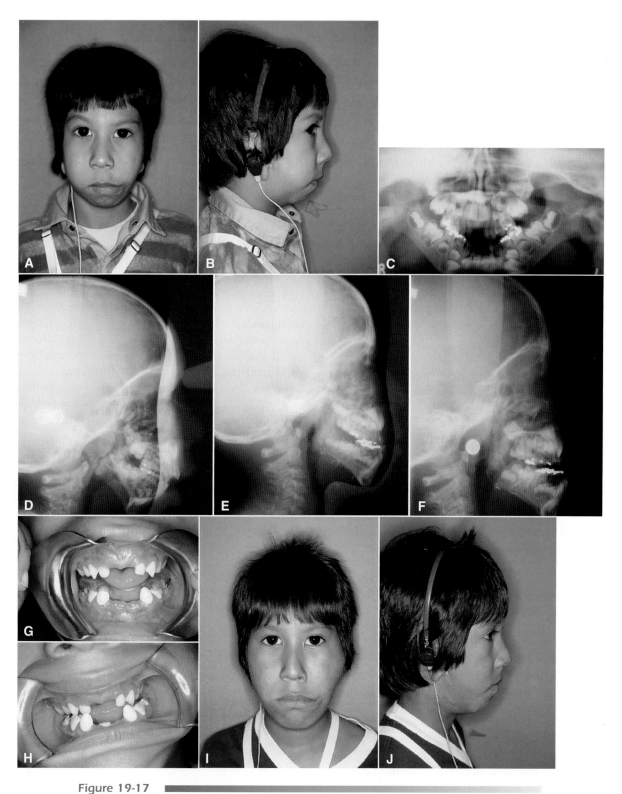

Figure 19-17

A 5-year-old boy with bilateral facial microsomia. **A,** Frontal view shows left macrostomia, retrognathism, long lower face height, and normal soft tissue around the eyes. Note the absence of external ears. **B,** Lateral view demonstrates the grade III ear defect and retrognathism. **C,** Panoramic radiograph documents a short mandibular rami and hypoplastic TMJs. **D,** Preoperative lateral cephalogram illustrates the retrognathism, open bite, and short posterior face height. Immediate **(E)** and 1-year postoperative **(F)** lateral cephalograms show the elongation and advancement of the mandible after construction of the rami and TMJs with costochondral grafts bilaterally. When bone stock is adequate, distraction osteogenesis using a multivector or curvilinear device can be used. The surgically created open bite (by either technique) is maintained and regulated with an acrylic appliance. Intraoral views 6 months **(G)** and 1 year **(H)** postoperatively demonstrate closure of the open bite. Frontal **(I)** and lateral **(J)** photographs of the child 1 year postoperatively.

meters of distraction. Bone fill is documented by plain radiographs or ultrasonography. The distraction protocols currently used in the craniomaxillofacial region are derived from clinical and experimental studies in the long bones[50-52] and from studies in the canine[53] and minipig.[64]

Although DO offers a promising alternative to conventional osteotomies and bone grafting procedures, there are some limitations. The cumbersome nature of distraction devices, the reliance on patient compliance, the necessity for cutaneous incisions, the resulting pin track scars, the lack of three-dimensional control of vectors of movement, and the lengthy treatment period have all been identified as problems.[64-66] In addition, DO is a method of skeletal expansion, and in complex, asymmetric craniomaxillofacial deformities the correct surgical procedure may include lengthening on one side and shortening on the other.

DO is a useful technique for bone lengthening in patients with HFM, bilateral craniofacial microsomia, and Treacher Collins syndrome. Surgeons using this technique must follow the treatment principles and guidelines described previously in this chapter, with DO substituted for the indicated osteotomies, acute movement, and bone grafts. However, the technique is applicable only for correction in patients who meet the following criteria: (1) enough bone stock exists in the mandibular RCU to allow for the corticotomy and placement of the distraction device and (2) the skeletal movements required to correct the deformity must be possible by DO. For example, most patients with HFM end-stage deformity require a combination of lengthening the short side and shortening the long side to correct the asymmetry. This type of three-dimensional, bilateral correction cannot be accomplished by DO, which can be used only to lengthen the skeleton (Tables 19-2 and 19-3). If, however, a patient with end-stage type I or IIA happens to have a long upper lip or normal vertical midface length on the unaffected side (with normal to inadequate tooth show), bimaxillary distraction of the short side is possible. For patients with type IIB or III, there is usually inadequate bone stock and the RCU must be constructed. In the growing child, with types I and IIA, DO of the short side using the guidelines for early treatment described above is feasible. Growing children with types IIB and III require construction of the RCU (see Table 19-2 and Figures 19-10 to 19-14).

DO is particularly useful in patients with Treacher Collins syndrome who have severe micrognathia, decreased posterior face height, and tracheostomy-dependent airway obstruction. It is the only technique that allows RCU lengthening and counterclockwise rotation of the mandible of the magnitude required in these children. Skeletal stability has been satisfactory, and prevention or elimination of tracheostomy has

been documented.[67-74] DO is used for the same reason in other syndromic and nonsyndromic cases of severe micrognathia (Figure 19-16).

THREE-DIMENSIONAL TREATMENT PLANNING

CT and magnetic resonance imaging of the human body have had an enormous impact on the practice of medicine and surgery during the past 20 years. Three-dimensional data acquisition allows visualization and analysis of complex craniomaxillofacial anomalies.[75,76] Application of three-dimensional imaging for surgical treatment planning and navigation[77,78] is critical for guiding minimally invasive reconstructive techniques such as DO. The success of most craniomaxillofacial surgical corrections depends on careful analysis and planning based on a variety of diagnostic information, such as clinical examination, photographs, radiographs, and articulated dental models. The lateral cephalogram has been a valuable tool for conventional planning and for outcomes evaluation. However, this radiograph has its limitations because it represents only a composite of

TABLE 19-2 Treatment Methods for Hemifacial Microsomia

Adult End-Stage Deformity	
Skeletal Types I and IIA	**Skeletal Types IIB and III**
Bimaxillary orthognathic surgery	Construction RCU +/- fossa
or	Bimaxillary orthognathic surgery
Bimaxillary DO	
Genioplasty	Genioplasty
Contour augmentation	Contour augmentation
Secondary bimaxillary DO in patients inadequately corrected in either group	

Correction in Growing Children	
Skeletal Types I and IIA	**Skeletal Types IIB and III**
Mandibular DO only	RCU construction +/- fossa
or	
Conventional osteotomy	
Orthodontic Rx to maintain open bite	Orthodontic Rx to maintain open bite
Secondary mandibular DO in patients inadequately corrected in either group	

DO, Distraction osteogenesis; *RCU,* ramus-condyle unit.

TABLE 19-3 Hemifacial Microsomia Treatment Plan by Age and Skeletal Type

Skeletal Type	Deciduous Dentition Age 0–5 Years	Mixed Dentition Age 6–12 Years	Adult Age > 12 Years
I	Observation. Activator appliance in cooperative patient, if asymmetry progresses to produce occlusal cant.	Mandibular advancement elongation, and rotation to create open bite when occlusal cant and mandibular asymmetry progress.	Maxillary and mandibular osteotomies to correct end-stage asymmetry.
IIA	Same as for type I. Activator less likely to be effective than in type I.	Same as for type I.	Same as for type I.
IIB	Existing TMJ and ramus cannot be used. Construction of glenoid fossa, condyle, and ramus. Surgically created open bite maintained with appliance to permit vertical midface growth.	Same as for ages 0–5.	Total TMJ construction plus maxillary and mandibular osteotomies to correct end-stage asymmetry.
III	TMJ and ramus absent. Construction of glenoid fossa, condyle, and ramus. Surgically created open bite maintained with appliance to permit vertical midface growth.	Same as for ages 0–5.	Same as for type IIB.

the sagittal plane and does not account for asymmetry, which is often present.[66,79] Advances in minimally invasive surgical techniques (including and especially DO) further heighten the need for accurate treatment planning.[66,80-82]

In collaboration with the Harvard Surgical Planning Laboratory, we have developed a three-dimensional treatment planning system called *Osteoplan*. The software uses CT data to produce three-dimensional images for visualization of the craniomaxillofacial skeleton and allows the operator to simulate osteotomies and to move the resultant bony fragments. The software also allows insertion of landmarks, measurement of angles and distances between landmarks, simulation of osteotomies, repositioning of bones and bone fragments, detection of virtual bone collisions, superposition and comparison of preoperative and postoperative CT scans, and comparison of postoperative (actual) and predicted skeletal movements. The visual superimposition of two models can be used for qualitative and quantitative comparisons. With the three-dimensional models and landmarks registered to a standard orientation, the software provides a potential tool for measuring cephalometric distances and angles. Finally, the program calculates the vector of the proposed skeletal movement and provides a prescrip-

tion for the location of the osteotomy and for the design of a distraction device to accomplish the movement (see Figure 19-16). Ultimately, the system will also incorporate accurate dental and surface (skin) data.[66,83]

CONCLUSION

This chapter discussed the clinical characteristics, diagnosis, and treatment of congenital TMJ anomalies. The important concept of progression of the deformity with time and growth was emphasized. The purpose of treatment in a growing child is to enhance growth potential in the mandible, to decrease or prevent secondary deformity in contiguous and contralateral facial skeletal structures, and to improve body image development.

REFERENCES

1. Kearns GJ, Padwa BL, Mulliken JB, Kaban LB: Progression of facial asymmetry in hemifacial microsomia, *Plast Reconstr Surg* 105:492-498, 2000.
2. Kaban LB, Mulliken JB, Murray JE: Three-dimensional approach to analysis and treatment of hemifacial microsomia, *Cleft Palate J* 18:90-99, 1981.
3. Murray JE, Kaban LB, Mulliken JB: Analysis and treatment of hemifacial microsomia, *Plast Reconstr Surg* 74:186-199, 1984.

4. Poswillo O: The pathogenesis of 1st and 2nd branchial arch syndrome, *J Oral Surg* 35:302, 1973.

5. Johnston MC, Bronsky PT: Animal models for human craniofacial malformations, *J Craniofac Genet Dev Biol* 11:277-291, 1991.

6. Kaban LB, Padwa BL, Mulliken JB: Surgical correction of mandibular hypoplasia in hemifacial microsomia: the case for treatment in early childhood, *J Oral Maxillofac Surg* 56:628-638, 1998.

7. Enlow OH: *Handbook of facial growth*, Philadelphia, 1975, WB Saunders.

8. Moss ML: Twenty years of functional cranial analysis, *Am J Orthod* 61:479-485, 1972.

9. Murray JE, Kaban LB, Mulliken JB, Evans CA: Analysis and treatment of hemifacial microsomia. In Caronni EP, editor: *Craniofacial surgery*, Boston, 1985, Little, Brown.

10. Pruzansky S: Not all dwarfed mandibles are alike, *Birth Defects* 1:120, 1969.

11. Mulliken JB, Kaban LB: Analysis and treatment of hemifacial microsomia, *Clin Plast Surg* 14(1):91-100, 1987.

12. Kaban LB, Moses ML, Mulliken JB: Correction of hemifacial microsomia in the growing child, *Cleft Palate J* 23(suppl 1):50-52, 1986.

13. Kaban LB, Moses ML, Mulliken JB: Surgical correction of hemifacial microsomia in the growing child, *Plast Reconstr Surg* 81:9-19, 1988.

14. Kaban LB, Mulliken JB, Murray JE: Facial growth after early correction of hemifacial microsomia. Abstract presented at the 68th Annual meeting of the American Association of Oral and Maxillofacial Surgeons, New Orleans, September 1986.

15. Moses MH, Kaban LB, Mulliken JB, et al: Facial growth after early correction of hemifacial microsomia. Abstract presented at the 64th Annual Meeting of the American Association of Plastic Surgeons, San Diego, May 1, 1985.

16. Vargervik K, Kaban LB: Management of hemifacial microsomia in the growing child. In Bell W, editor: *Modern practice in orthognathic and reconstructive surgery*, Philadelphia, 1991, WB Saunders.

17. Meurman Y: Congenital microtia and meatal atresia, *Arch Otolaryngol* 66:443, 1957.

18. Kaban LB, Evans C, Mulliken JB, et al: Analysis and treatment of hemifacial microsomia. In Shelton DW, Irby WB, editors: *Current advances in oral and maxillofacial surgery*: orthognathic surgery, ed 5, St Louis, 1986, CV Mosby.

19. Bennun RD, Mulliken JB, Kaban LB, Murray JE: Microtia: a microform of hemifacial microsomia, *Plast Reconstr Surg* 76:859-863, 1985.

20. Vento AR, LaBrie RA, Mulliken JB: OMENS classification of hemifacial microsomia, *Cleft Palate J* 28(1):68-76, 1989.

21. Mulliken JB, Ferraro NF, Vento AR: A retrospective analysis of growth of the constructed condyle-ramus in children with hemifacial microsomia, *Cleft Palate J* 26(4):312-317, 1989.

22. Horgan JE, Padwa BL, LaBrie RA, Mulliken JB: OMENS-plus: analysis of craniofacial and extracraniofacial anomalies in hemifacial microsomia, *Cleft Palate Craniofac J* 32:405-412, 1995.

23. Posnick J: Surgical correction of mandibular hypoplasia in hemifacial microsomia: a personal perspective, *J Oral Maxillofac Surg* 56:639-650, 1998.

24. Padwa BL, Kaiser MO, Kaban LB: Occlusal cant in the frontal plane as a reflection of facial asymmetry, *J Oral Maxillofac Surg* 55:811-816, 1997.

25. Troulis MJ, Everett P, Seldin EB, et al: Development of a three-dimensional treatment planning system based on computed tomographic data, *Int J Oral Maxillofac Surg* 31:349-357, 2002.

26. Gateno J, Teichgraeber JF, Aguilar E: Computer planning for distraction osteogenesis, *Plast Reconstr Surg* 105:873-882, 2000.

26a. Obwegeser HL: Correction of the skeletal anomalies of otomandibular dysostosis, *J Maxillofac Surg* 2:73-92, 1974.

27. Mulliken JB, Kaban LB, Evans CA, et al: Facial skeletal changes following hypertelorbitism correction, *Plast Reconstr Surg* 56:122, 1998.

28. Padwa BL, Mulliken JB, Maghen A, Kaban LB: Midfacial growth after costochondral graft construction of the mandibular ramus in hemifacial microsomia, *J Oral Maxillofac Surg* 56:122-127, 1998.

29. Polley JW, Figueroa AA, Liou EJW, et al: Longitudinal analysis of mandibular asymmetry in hemifacial microsomia, *Plast Reconstr Surg* 99:328, 1997.

30. Vargervik K, Ousterhout DK, Farias M: Factors affecting long-term results in hemifacial microsomia, *Cleft Palate J* 23(suppl 1):53, 1986.

31. Melsen B, Bjerregaard J, Bundgaard M: The effect of treatment with functional appliances on a pathologic growth pattern of the condyle, *Am J Orthod* 90:503, 1986.

32. Cohen MM: Variability versus "incidental findings" in the first and second branchial arch syndrome: unilateral variants with anophthalmia, *Birth Defects Orig Artic Ser* 7:103, 1971.

33. Harvold EP, Vargervik K, Chierici G: *Treatment of hemifacial microsomia*, New York, 1983, Alan R Liss.

34. Murray JE, Kaban LB, Mulliken JB: Analysis and treatment of hemifacial microsomia. In Caronni EP, editor: *Craniofacial surgery*, Boston, 1985, Little, Brown.

35. Kane AA, Lo IJ, Christensen GE, et al: Relationship between bone and muscles of mastication in hemifacial microsomia, *Plast Reconstr Surg* 99:990, 1997.

36. Tanzer RC: The total reconstruction of the auricle: the evolution of a plan of treatment, *Plast Reconstr Surg* 47:523, 1971.

37. Brent B: The correction of microtia with autogenous cartilage grafts: the classic deformity, *Plast Reconstr Surg* 66:1, 1980.

38. Brent B, Byrd HS: Secondary ear reconstruction with cartilage grafts covered by axial, random and free flaps of temporoparietal fascia, *Plast Reconstr Surg* 72:141, 1983.

39. Tulasne JF, Tessier PT: Results of the Tessier integral procedure for correction of Treacher Collins syndrome, *Cleft Palate J* 23(suppl 1):40-49, 1986.

40. Gorlin RJ, Pindborg J, Cohen MM: *Syndromes of the head and neck*, ed 2, New York, 1976, McGraw-Hill.

41. Poswillo D: The pathogenesis of the Treacher Collins syndrome (mandibulofacial dysostosis), *Br J Oral Surg* 13:1, 1975.

42. Cohen MM Jr: Malformations of the craniofacial region: evolutionary, embryonic, genetic, and clinical perspectives, *Am J Med Genet* 115:245-268, 2002.

43. Thomson A: Notice of several cases of malformation of the external ear, together with experiments on the state of hearing in such persons, *Month J Med Sci* 7:420, 1847.

44. Berry GA: Note on a congenital defect (coloboma) of the lower lid, *R Lond Ophthalmol Hosp Rep* 12:255, 1889.

45. Collins TE: Case with symmetrical congenital notches in the outer part of each lower lid and defective development of the malar bones, *Trans Ophthalmol Soc U K* 20:190, 1900.

46. Franchesetti A, Klein D: Mandibulofacial dysostosis: a new hereditary syndrome, *Acta Ophthalmol* 27:143, 1949.

47. Stovin JJ, Lyon JA, Clemmens RL: Mandibulofacial dysostosis, *Radiology* 74:225, 1960.

48. Kaban LB, Mulliken JB, Murray JE: Craniofacial deformity. In Welch KJ, editor: *Pediatric surgery*, Chicago, 1986, Year Book Medical Publishers.

49. Kaban LB: Congenital and acquired growth abnormalities of the temporomandibular joint. In Keith DA, editor: *Surgery of the temporomandibular joint*, Boston, 1988, Blackwell Scientific Publications.

50. Codivilla A: On the means of lengthening, in the lower limbs, the muscles and tissues which are shortened through deformity, *Am J Orthop Surg* 2:353, 1905.

51. Ilizarov GA: The tension-stress effect on the genesis and growth of tissues. Part I. The influence of stability of fixation and soft-tissue preservation, *Clin Orthop* 238:249, 1989.

52. Ilizarov GA: The tension-stress effect on the genesis and growth of tissues: Part II. The influence of the rate and frequency of distraction, *Clin Orthop* 239:263, 1989.

53. Ilizarov GA: The principles of the Ilizarov method, *Bull Hosp Jt Dis Orthop Inst* 48:1, 1988.

54. McCarthy J, Staffenberg DA, Wood RL, et al: Lengthening the human mandible by gradual distraction, *Plast Reconstr Surg* 89:1, 1992.

55. Snyder C, Levine GA, Swanson HM, Browne EZ: Mandibular lengthening by gradual distraction: preliminary report, *Plast Reconstr Surg* 51:506, 1973.

56. Micheli S, Miotti B: Lengthening of mandibular body by gradual surgical orthodontic distraction, *J Oral Surg* 35:187, 1977.

57. Costantino PD, Shybut G, Friedman CD, et al: Segmental mandibular regeneration by distraction osteogenesis: an experimental study, *Arch Otolaryngol Head Neck Surg* 116:535, 1990.

58. Klotch DW, Ganey TM, Slater-Haase A, Sasse J: Assessment of bone formation during osteogenesis: a canine model, *Otolaryngol Head Neck Surg* 112:291, 1995.

59. Perrott DH, Berger R, Vargervik K, Kaban LB: Use of a skeletal distraction device to widen the mandible: a case report, *J Oral Maxillofac Surg* 51:435, 1993.

60. Chin M, Toth B: Distraction osteogenesis in maxillofacial surgery using internal devices. Review of five cases, *J Oral Maxillofac Surg* 54:45, 1996.

61. Chin M, Toth B: Le Fort III advancement with gradual distraction using internal devices, *Plast Reconstr Surg* 100:819, 1997.

62. Monasterio FO, Molina F, Andrade L, et al: Simultaneous mandibular and maxillary distraction in hemifacial microsoma in adults: avoiding occlusal disasters, *Plast Reconstr Surg* 100:852, 1997.

63. Padwa BL, Kearns GJ, Todd R, et al: Simultaneous maxillary and mandibular distraction osteogenesis: a technique and case report, *Int J Oral Maxillofac Surg* 28:2, 1999.

64. Troulis MJ, Glowacki J, Perrott DH, Kaban LB: Effects of latency and rate one bone formation in a porcine mandibular distraction model, *J Oral Maxillofac Surg* 58(5):507-514, 2000.

65. Seldin EB, Troulis MJ, Kaban LB: Evaluation of a semiburied fixed-trajectory curvilinear distraction device in an animal model, *J Oral Maxillofac Surg* 57(12):1442-1446, 1999.

66. Troulis MJ, Everett P, Seldin EB, et al: Three-dimensional treatment planning system based on computed tomographic data, *Int J Oral Maxillofac Surg* 31:349-357, 2002.

67. Steinbacher DM, Kaban LB, Troulis MJ: Treatment of tracheostomy-dependent children with severe micrognathia, *J Oral Maxillofac Surg* August 2003 (in press).

68. Moore MH, Guzman-Stein G, Prodman TW, et al: Mandibular lengthening by distraction for airway obstruction in Treacher Collins syndrome, *J Craniofac Surg* 5:22, 1994.

69. Cohen SR: Early decannulation with bilateral mandibular distraction for tracheostomy-dependent patients (Discussion), *Plast Reconstr Surg* 103:58, 1999.

70. Denny AD, Talisman R, Hanson PR, Recinos RF: Mandibular distraction osteogenesis in very young patients to correct airway obstruction, *Plast Reconstr Surg* 108:302-311, 2001.

71. Morovic CG, Monasterio L: Distraction osteogenesis for obstructive apneas in patients with congenital craniofacial malformations, *Plast Reconstr Surg* 105:2324, 2000.

72. Sidman J, Sampson D, Templeton B: Distraction osteogenesis of the mandible for airway obstruction in children, *Laryngoscope* 111:1137-1146, 2001.

73. Williams JK, Maull D, Grayson BH, et al: Early decannulation with bilateral mandibular distraction for tracheostomy-dependent patients, *Plast Reconstr Surg* 103:48, 1999.

74. Cohen SR, Ross DA, Burstein FD, et al: Skeletal expansion combined with soft-tissue reduction on the treatment of obstructive sleep apnea in children: physiologic results, *Otolaryngol Head Neck Surg* 119:476-485, 1998.

75. Vannier MW, March JL, Warren JD: Three-dimensional CT reconstruction images for craniofacial surgical planning and evaluation, *Radiology* 150:179-184, 1984.

76. Levy RA, Edwards WT, Meyer JR, Rosenbaum AE: Facial trauma and 3-D reconstructive imaging: insufficiencies and correctives, *AJNR Am J Neuroradiol* 13:885, 1992.

77. Ayoub AF, Wray D, Moos KF, et al: Three-dimensional modeling for modern diagnosis and planning in maxillofacial surgery, *Int J Adult Orthod Orthognath Surg* 1:225, 1996.

78. Bill JS, Reuther JF, Dittmann, et al: Stereolithography in oral and maxillofacial operation planning, *Int J Oral Maxillofac Surg* 24:98, 1995.

79. Everett P, Seldin EB, Troulis M, et al: A 3-D system for planning and simulating minimally-invasive distraction osteogenesis of the facial skeleton. Proceedings MICCAI (Medical Image Computing and Computer-Assisted Intervention) 2000, Proceedings of the Third International Conference, Pittsburgh, Pa.

80. Gateno J: Accuracy of custom stereolithographic templates for the installation of an external multiplanar distractor, *J Oral Maxillofac Surg* 57:96, 1999.

81. Gateno J, Teichgraber JF, Aguilar E: Distraction osteogenesis: a new surgical technique for use with the multiplanar mandibular distractor, *Plast Reconstr Surg* 105:883-888, 2000.

82. Xia J, Ip HHS, Samman D, et al: Computer-assisted three-dimensional surgical planning and simulation: 3D virtual osteotomy, *Int J Oral Maxillofac Surg* 29:11-17, 2000.

83. Everett PC, Seldin EB, Troulis M, et al: A 3-D system for planning and simulating minimally invasive distraction osteogenesis of the facial skeleton. In Delp SL, DiGioia AM, Jaramaz B, editors: MICCAI 2000. Proceedings of the Third International Conference on Medical Image Computing and Computer-Assisted Intervention, Pittsburgh, Pa, October 2000. New York, 2000, Springer-Verlag, pp 1029-1039.

CHAPTER 20

Acquired Abnormalities of the Temporomandibular Joint

Leonard B. Kaban

Acquired temporomandibular joint (TMJ) diseases include primary (e.g., condylar hyperplasia) and secondary (e.g., posttraumatic) growth abnormalities, pathologic conditions of the TMJ (such as tumors, juvenile rheumatoid arthritis (JRA), infection, postradiation defects), and temporomandibular disorders and facial pain (see Chapter 18). This chapter is devoted to acquired anatomic and pathologic TMJ abnormalities.

CONDYLAR HYPERPLASIA
General Considerations

Condylar hyperplasia is the most common postnatal growth abnormality of the TMJ. It occurs more frequently in females than in males and it is caused by an abnormal hypermetabolic growth center in the affected condyle. The condition must be differentiated from mild hemifacial microsomia on the opposite side (i.e., condylar hypoplasia) and from a generalized asym-

metric growth pattern (mandibular hemihypertrophy) not accompanied by a localized hyperactive condylar region.[1-4]

Children with condylar hyperplasia typically are born with a symmetric jaw. They and their families recall the first sign of asymmetry during the onset of puberty. Asymmetric jaw growth progresses simultaneously with the rapid increase in overall body size. After a variable period, the abnormal growth center becomes quiescent and progression of the deformity ceases. This cycle of abnormal growth generally continues over several years. In approximately two thirds of patients who come to the surgeon or orthodontist for evaluation, the condition is stable, in the quiescent phase of condylar hyperplasia.[5] TMJ symptoms, such as noise in the joint or discomfort with function, are uncommon. Patients may exhibit limitation of motion, particularly an inability to translate, because the condylar head is disproportionately large in relation to the glenoid fossa. There are two growth patterns in this disorder:

1. *Vertical.* Excessive mandibular growth occurs in a predominantly vertical direction. The patients always exhibit increased vertical height of the ramus and often of the body. Intraorally, there is an open bite on the affected side (before the development of dental compensation); there is usually no crossbite on the unaffected side. As the abnormal ramus grows excessively, the chin point and dental midline become slightly deviated toward the normal side (Figures 20-1 to 20-5).

2. *Rotational.* In this pattern, there is not only a vertically long ramus on the affected side, but the mandibular body is convex and the chin point and dental midline are significantly deviated toward the normal side. Intraorally, there is a crossbite on the unaffected side. The clinical

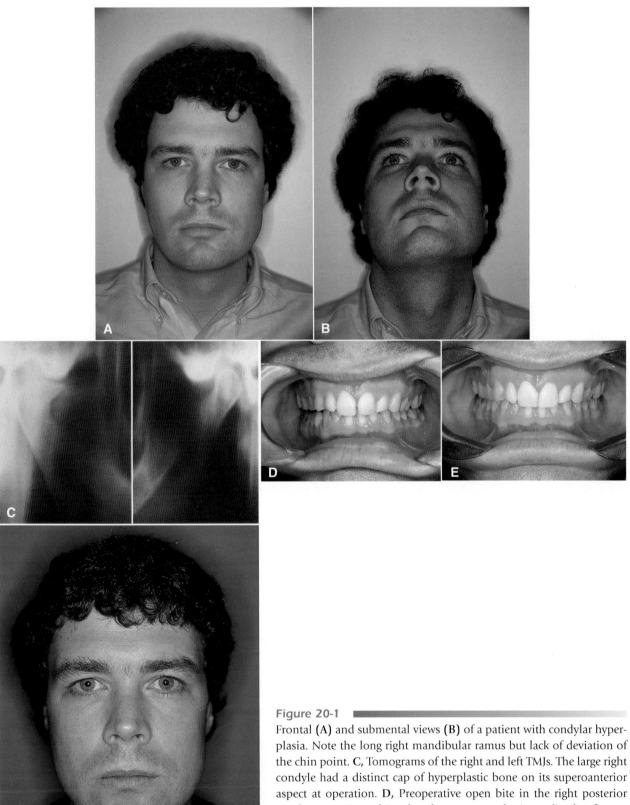

Figure 20-1

Frontal (**A**) and submental views (**B**) of a patient with condylar hyperplasia. Note the long right mandibular ramus but lack of deviation of the chin point. **C,** Tomograms of the right and left TMJs. The large right condyle had a distinct cap of hyperplastic bone on its superoanterior aspect at operation. **D,** Preoperative open bite in the right posterior quadrant. **E,** Open bite closed spontaneously, immediately after an abnormal condylar bone mass was excised. **F,** Facial symmetry is maintained 4 years postoperatively.

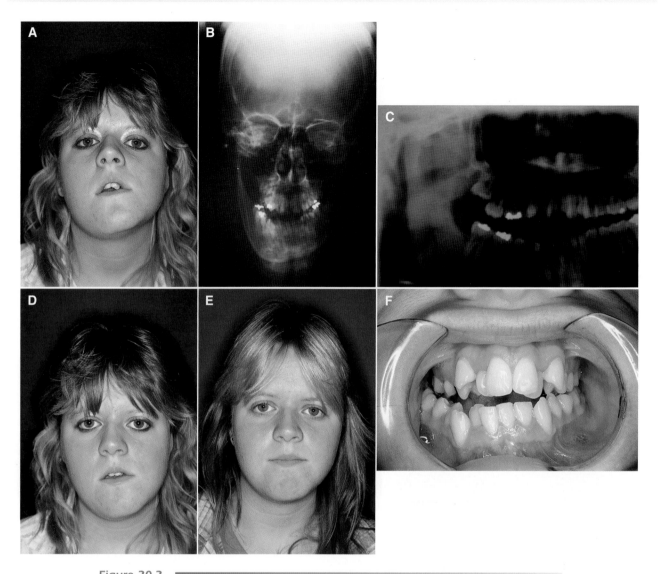

Figure 20-2

A, Submental view of a teenager with right condylar hyperplasia, vertical pattern. **B,** Antero-posterior cephalogram demonstrates vertical dysplasia of the mandible with a right posterior open bite. **C,** Panoramic radiograph shows long right condylar neck, open bite on the right side, and no deviation of midline. Preoperative (**D**) and 1 year postoperative (**E**) views. The patient had a high condylectomy as a growth-arresting procedure and an inferior border ostectomy. **F,** Intraoral view of the occlusion 1 year postoperatively. Note the spontaneous closure of the open bite after the condylectomy.

appearance of this group often resembles that of patients with end-stage hemifacial microsomia (Figures 20-6 to 20-8).

Diagnosis

History and Physical Examination. The diagnosis of condylar hyperplasia is made by the history of progressive mandibular asymmetry developing after birth.

While the asymmetry is most commonly noticed during or after the onset of puberty, it can be manifest between the ages of 4 and 7 years, when the mandible is also growing rapidly. Physical examination demonstrates one of the two patterns described (see Figures 20-1 to 20-9). In patients with the vertical pattern, there may be an occlusal cant downward on the affected side. This occurs, with time, as dental compensations (i.e., supraeruption of the teeth) result in spontaneous closure of the open bite.

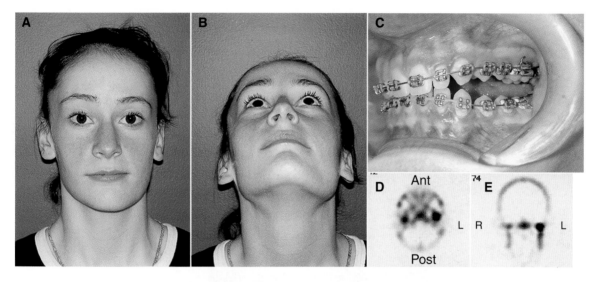

Figure 20-3 ▰

Uncompensated left condylar hyperplasia, vertical pattern. Frontal (**A**) and submental (**B**) views of a 15-year-old patient with an elongated left mandibular ramus indicative of condylar hyperplasia. **C,** Intraoral view shows the left posterior open bite before the development of dental compensations. **D,** SPECT scan showing the increased uptake of the left condyle. **E,** Similarly, the left condyle is hyperactive.

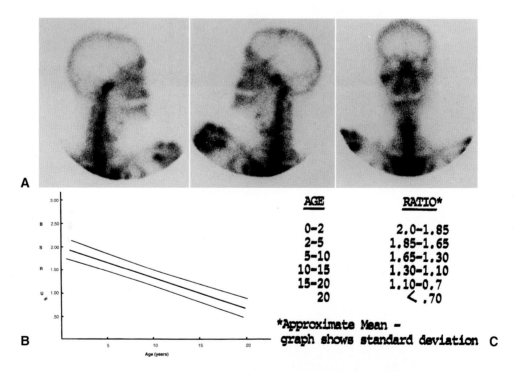

Figure 20-4 ▰

Skeletal scintigraphy. **A,** Computerized technetium scan of the right and left condylar, ramus, and body regions along with the fourth lumbar vertebra. The ratio of uptake of these regions to the fourth lumbar vertebra is calculated and compared with the normal standards (see text). In patients with active condylar hyperplasia, uptake in the abnormal condyle will be more than two standard deviations greater than normal, confirming the diagnosis. **B,** Standard curve of bone seeking radioisotope uptake (BSRU) and age in normal patients. **C,** Normal uptake ratios and age taken from standard curve. (**B** and **C** from Cisneros G, Kaban LB: *J Oral Maxillofac Surg* 42:513-520, 1985.)

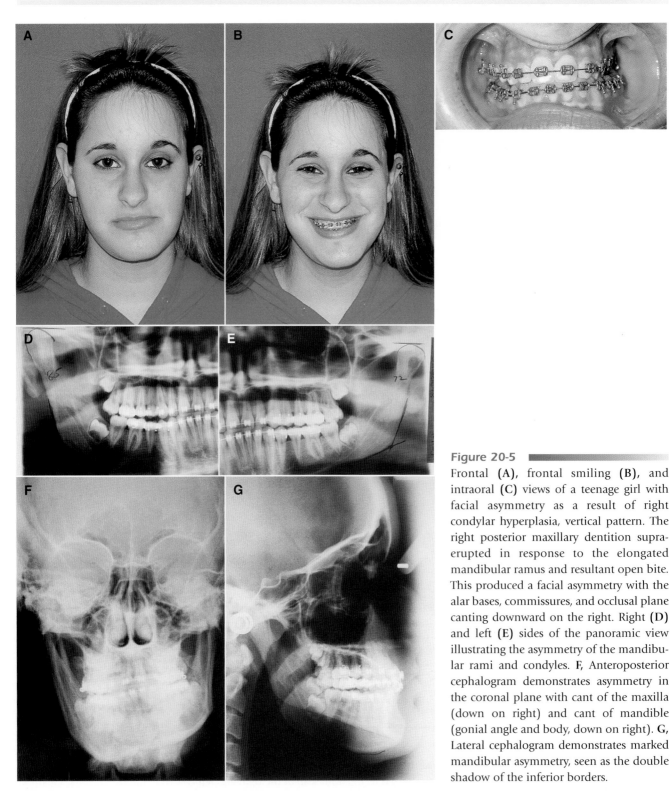

Figure 20-5

Frontal **(A)**, frontal smiling **(B)**, and intraoral **(C)** views of a teenage girl with facial asymmetry as a result of right condylar hyperplasia, vertical pattern. The right posterior maxillary dentition supra-erupted in response to the elongated mandibular ramus and resultant open bite. This produced a facial asymmetry with the alar bases, commissures, and occlusal plane canting downward on the right. Right **(D)** and left **(E)** sides of the panoramic view illustrating the asymmetry of the mandibular rami and condyles. **F,** Anteroposterior cephalogram demonstrates asymmetry in the coronal plane with cant of the maxilla (down on right) and cant of mandible (gonial angle and body, down on right). **G,** Lateral cephalogram demonstrates marked mandibular asymmetry, seen as the double shadow of the inferior borders.

Condylar hyperplasia is differentiated from mild hemifacial microsomia, on the opposite side, by the absence of ear anomalies, soft tissue contour deficiency, cranial nerve VII paresis, and palatal deviation with function (all manifestations of first and second branchial arch defects). Patients with condylar hyperplasia often have class III occlusion on the affected side and class I on the unaffected side, whereas those with hemifacial microsomia may have class II occlusion on both sides. In addition, the mandibular asymmetry of hemifacial microsomia is accompanied almost always by secondary abnormality in the midface. This is because the anomaly is present at birth and mandibular hypoplasia has a profound effect on vertical growth of the midface.

Imaging Studies. Panoramic and TMJ radiographs demonstrate asymmetry in the condylar head and neck regions. The condyle is larger, and the neck longer, on the affected side. The unaffected ramus-condyle unit is normal in morphology. Skeletal scintigraphy using ^{99m}Tc diphosphonate is a useful diagnostic tool.[3,4,6-11] Patients with condylar hyperplasia exhibit increased uptake in the affected condyle when compared with controls, whereas the uptake in the condyles of patients with hemifacial microsomia is reduced markedly[3,4] (Figure 20-4).

Skeletal scintigraphy has been used in medicine and surgery for many years.[12-15] The technique depends upon increased uptake of a radioactive substance in metabolically active (e.g., healing, growing, neo-

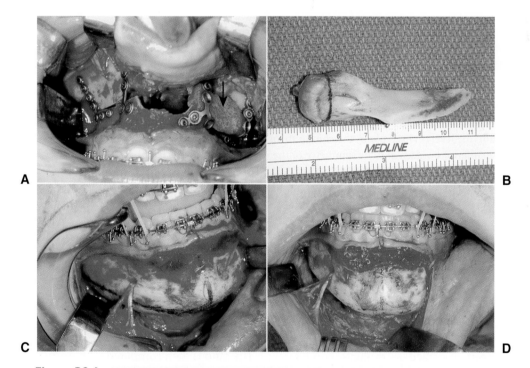

Figure 20-6

Intraoperative and postoperative views of teenager shown in Figure 20-4. **A,** Intraoperative view of Le Fort I osteotomy rigidly fixed. The right side was shortened and the left side slightly elongated and stabilized with a bone graft *(arrow)*. The center of rotation of the movement was determined by measurements to ensure the proper relationship of the upper anterior teeth to the upper lip. **B,** A right vertical ramus osteotomy was performed endoscopically, the segment removed, and the hyperplastic condylar head (marked in pencil) removed. The segment was replaced and rigidly fixed. The left side was treated with a sagittal split osteotomy, rigidly fixed. **C,** The inferior border ostectomy is marked. **D,** Mandibular body after the segment was removed (note the dissected mental nerve).

Continued

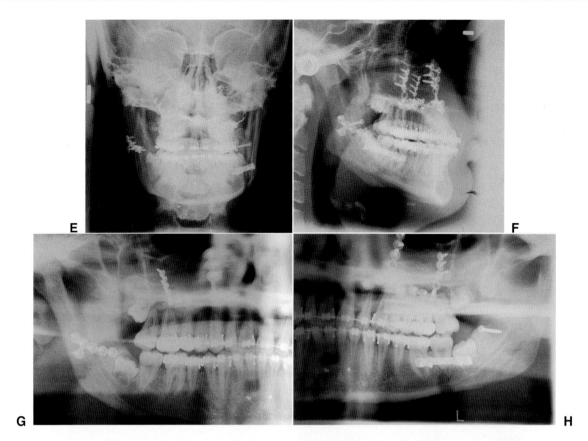

Figure 20-6—continued
Postoperative anteroposterior (**E**) and lateral (**F**) cephalograms and right (**G**) and left (**H**) panoramic views demonstrating correction of the asymmetry. Note the correction of the cant, the level occlusal plane, the chin in the midline, the correction of the double shadow of the inferior borders, and the symmetry of the right and left ramus lengths.

plastic) bone and decreased uptake in necrotic, devascularized, or otherwise hypometabolic bone. Both quantitative[5] and subjective bone scan evaluation techniques have been described to evaluate condylar hyperplasia.[10,16] Cisneros and Kaban developed normal standards of technetium-99m methylene diphosphonate (Tc 99m MDP) uptake in the condyle, ramus, and body regions of the mandible.[3,4] Comparison of Tc 99m MDP uptake with the normal standards by age has provided an objective method for diagnosis of condylar hyperplasia in patients with mandibular asymmetry (see Figure 20-4). A ratio of uptake of the condyle to the fourth lumbar vertebra (a standard bone for scanning purposes) is calculated by the following formula:

$$\text{Ratio of uptake} = \frac{\text{Uptake in condyle} - \text{Background counts}}{\text{Uptake in L4} - \text{Background counts}}$$

The ratio is then compared with normal standards by age (see Figure 20-4). Using this technique, it is possible to (1) differentiate the normal from the abnormal side of the mandible (Is the small side hypoplastic or the large side hyperplastic?), (2) determine the presence of an abnormal condylar growth center versus generalized asymmetric mandibular growth, and (3) differentiate between an actively progressive versus a stable growth abnormality.[3,4] Pogrel, Kaban, and others have also correlated increased uptake in the affected condyle with condylar hyperplasia using Tc 99m MDP uptake in single photon emission computed tomography (SPECT) scans[17] (Figure 20-4).

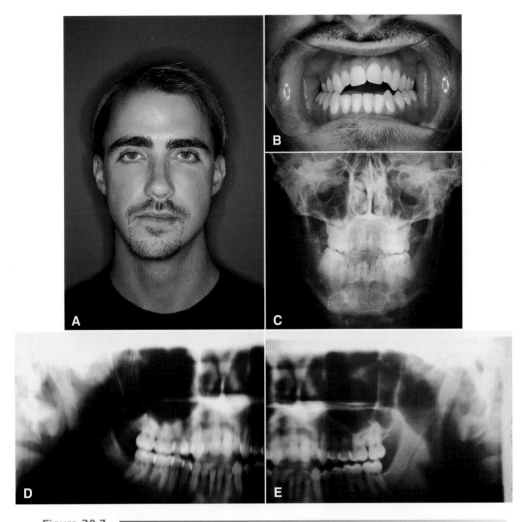

Figure 20-7

Condylar hyperplasia, rotational or horizontal pattern. **A,** Frontal view of a patient with progressive deviation of the chin (to the right), beginning in his mid-to-late teens. The deformity has been stable for the past 3 years. A growth-arresting procedure is not indicated in this case; the plan is to correct the end-stage anatomic deformity. **B,** Intraoral view demonstrates an open bite and crossbite, worse on the right. The mandibular dental midline is deviated to the right. **C,** Anteroposterior cephalogram demonstrates deviation of the chin to the right and mandibular asymmetry. Panoramic radiographs of the right **(D)** and left **(E)** rami show the increased size of the condyle and neck on the left side.

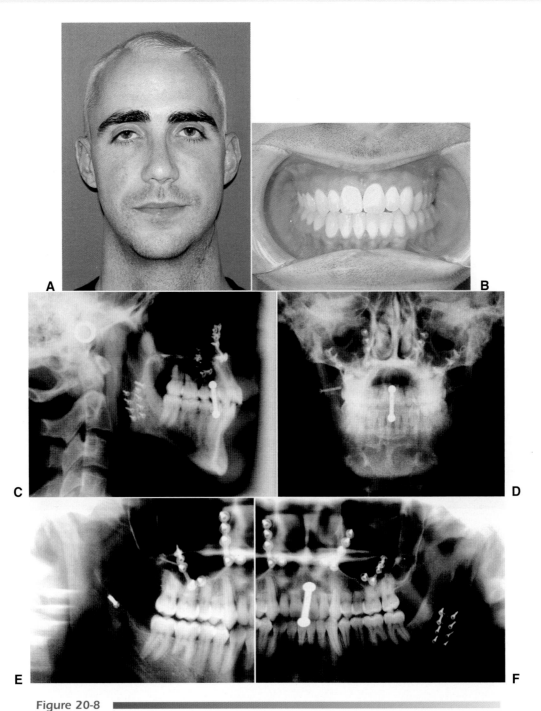

Figure 20-8

Same patient as in Figure 20-6, 2 years postoperatively. Frontal **(A)** and intraoral **(B)** views demonstrate correction of the facial and dental asymmetry, as well as the maxillary width deficiency. Anteroposterior **(C)** and lateral **(D)** cephalograms and right **(E)** and left **(F)** panoramic views demonstrate correction of the skeletal asymmetry by Le Fort I osteotomy of the maxilla, right sagittal split osteotomy, left endoscopic condylectomy, and vertical ramus osteotomy.

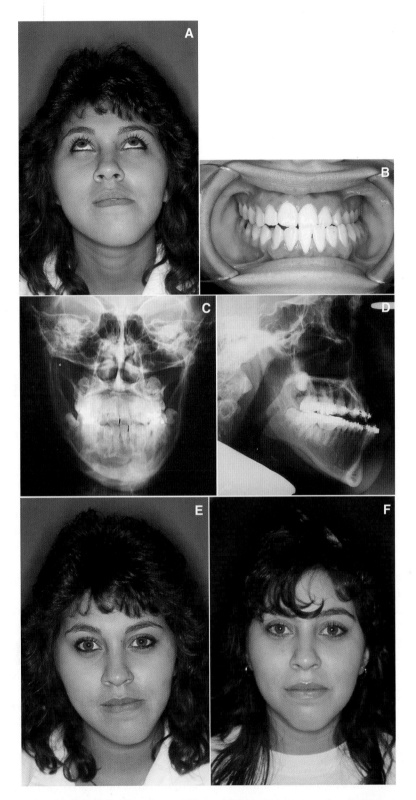

Figure 20-9

Stable right condylar hyperplasia, rotational pattern. Submental (A) and intraoral (B) photographs of a teenage patient with stable right condylar hyperplasia. Note the rotational pattern with deviation of the chin point and mandibular dental midline to the left, as well as a crossbite on the left. Bone scan revealed equal uptake in both condylar regions with normal values for her age. C, Anteroposterior cephalogram demonstrates convex shape of the right mandibular body and deviation of symphysis and mandibular dental midline to the left, consistent with right condylar hyperplasia. D, Preoperative lateral cephalogram with teeth decompensated and an anterior crossbite. Preoperative (E) and 1 year postoperative (F) frontal photographs demonstrate the symmetry achieved with bilateral mandibular osteotomies. A growth-arresting procedure was not necessary.

Treatment

To develop a treatment plan, the surgeon must make the correct diagnosis and determine whether abnormal condylar growth is progressive or stable. Patients in the active phase may be observed until the growth cycle is complete or may be offered a growth-arresting procedure (high condylectomy). This is most advantageous when carried out early in the cycle, before development of dental compensations, to prevent the need for bimaxillary orthognathic surgery (see Figures 20-1 to 20-3). Patients who have both active condylar hyperplasia and secondary deformities requiring correction will benefit from simultaneous high condylectomy and orthognathic surgery[18-20] (see Figures 20-5 and 20-6).

High condylectomy is performed through a standard preauricular incision; the hyperplastic condylar region is usually well demarcated and easily identified as a soft, marrow-like cap on the condylar head. This is excised (high condylectomy), leaving the normal condylar stump in place.

Troulis and Kaban[19] described a minimally invasive endoscopic technique for high condylectomy. A 1.5-cm submandibular incision is made to expose the mandible and create an optical cavity. The hyperplastic condylar head can be identified and the abnormal region removed (see Figures 20-5 and 20-6). Bimaxillary correction of the jaw asymmetry (if necessary) is then completed in the standard fashion using Le Fort I and mandibular osteotomies.

Patients with a clinically stable deformity, confirmed by a normal bone scan, are treated by orthodontic decompensation of the teeth and standard orthognathic surgical correction (see Figure 20-9). In these patients, high condylectomy is not performed unless there are TMJ symptoms such as decreased motion, pain, or marked deviation on opening because of mechanical interference by the large condylar head.

CONDYLAR RESORPTION OR CONDYLYSIS

Condylar resorption, or condylysis, is a curious acquired TMJ disorder that is manifested by progressive alteration of condylar shape and decrease in condylar mass or size. As a result, most patients exhibit a decrease in posterior face height, retrognathism, and progressive anterior open bite with clockwise rotation of the mandible. Although the cause is unknown, condylar resorption has been associated with rheumatoid arthritis, systemic lupus erythematosus, steroid use, trauma, neoplasia, orthodontic treatment, and orthognathic surgery.[21-32] In most cases, however, there is no identifiable precipitating event,[33] hence the term *idiopathic condylar resorption.* This condition is usually

bilateral and appears to have a predilection for females with an age range of 15 to 35 years. They often have preexisting TMJ dysfunction and a high mandibular plane angle.[31,32,34,35]

The management of condylar resorption remains controversial. Orthognathic surgical correction has been advocated,[28,36] but the reported results are satisfactory only if condylar resorption has ceased preoperatively and the condyles have stabilized. Bone scintigraphy of the mandibular condyles may be used to evaluate ongoing resorption.[3,6-11,17] Condylectomy and reconstruction with either autogenous materials (e.g., costochondral grafts) or alloplastic materials represent other treatment modalities. Crawford et al.[36] reviewed a group of seven patients with progressive condylar resorption who underwent orthognathic surgical procedures: five showed skeletal evidence of continued resorption and relapse postoperatively, and one showed further relapse after a second orthognathic surgical procedure. Merkx and Van Damme[37] treated eight patients who developed condylar resorption after sagittal split osteotomy. They noted unsatisfactory results in four patients after repeated orthognathic surgery, but more stable results in four patients treated by an occlusal appliance and other orthodontic or prosthodontic management. Arnett and Tamborello[38] reported six patients with progressive condylar resorption treated by orthognathic surgery; five had further resorption postoperatively. The one stable case was the only patient who had preoperative occlusal appliance therapy to stabilize the TMJ. A second orthognathic surgery group (eight patients) had TMJ stabilization with appliances and antiinflammatory medications *before* the operation; in seven of these patients the results were stable over the long term. They therefore advocated stabilization of the TMJs before the operation to prevent further resorption. Additionally, they suggested that compression of the condyle by operative positioning and fixation may result in resorption, particularly in susceptible females. Arnett and Tamborello[38] also suggest that maxillary orthognathic surgery alone should be considered for management of these patients, because there is no dissection of the mandibular soft tissues and there should be no adverse forces placed on the condyles with this procedure. Our data confirm that TMJ symptoms and muscle hyperactivity must be treated and stabilized before proceeding with any orthodontic treatment or orthognathic surgical correction in this group of teenagers.[31,39] The Massachusetts General Hospital protocol for management of teenagers with condylysis includes (1) documentation of the diagnosis by history of TMJ symptoms and progressive open bite, (2) documentation of progressive occlusal and condylar changes by evaluation of serial radiographs, photographs, and dental casts, (3) Tc 99m MDP quantitative bone scan to determine

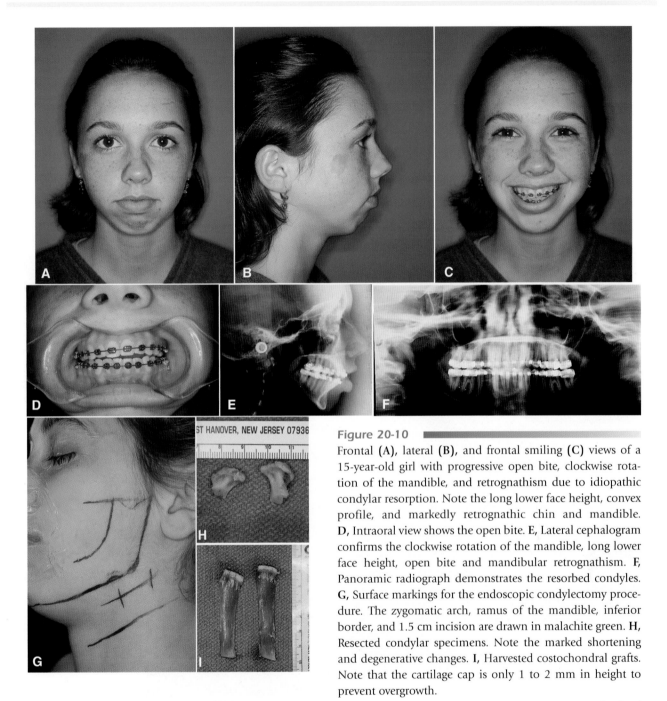

Figure 20-10

Frontal (**A**), lateral (**B**), and frontal smiling (**C**) views of a 15-year-old girl with progressive open bite, clockwise rotation of the mandible, and retrognathism due to idiopathic condylar resorption. Note the long lower face height, convex profile, and markedly retrognathic chin and mandible. **D,** Intraoral view shows the open bite. **E,** Lateral cephalogram confirms the clockwise rotation of the mandible, long lower face height, open bite and mandibular retrognathism. **F,** Panoramic radiograph demonstrates the resorbed condyles. **G,** Surface markings for the endoscopic condylectomy procedure. The zygomatic arch, ramus of the mandible, inferior border, and 1.5 cm incision are drawn in malachite green. **H,** Resected condylar specimens. Note the marked shortening and degenerative changes. **I,** Harvested costochondral grafts. Note that the cartilage cap is only 1 to 2 mm in height to prevent overgrowth.

Continued

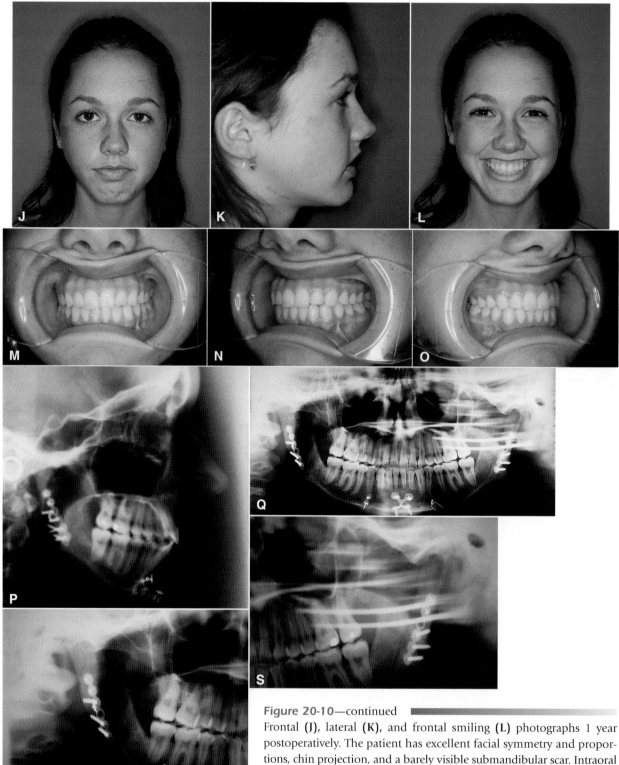

Figure 20-10—continued
Frontal (J), lateral (K), and frontal smiling (L) photographs 1 year postoperatively. The patient has excellent facial symmetry and proportions, chin projection, and a barely visible submandibular scar. Intraoral frontal (M) and right (N) and left (O) lateral views demonstrate the stable corrected occlusion. Lateral cephalogram (P) and panoramic radiograph (Q) of the patient 1 year postoperatively. Note the corrected open bite, the normal jaw relations, and the remodeling of the costochondral grafts, inferior border and genioplasty segment. Right (R) and left (S) close-up panoramic views show the remodeling of the grafts into what looks like a native condyle.

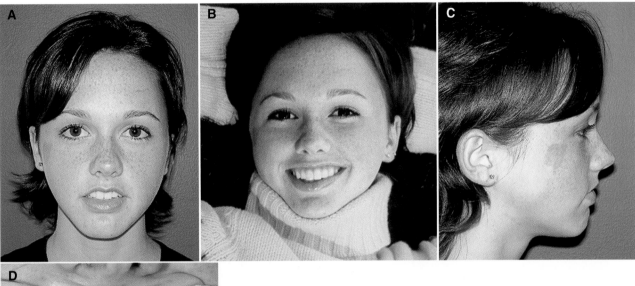

Figure 20-11

Same patient as in Figure 20-10, 4 years later. Frontal **(A)**, frontal smiling **(B)** (sent in by patient after graduation from high school), and lateral **(C)** views 4 years postoperatively. The result has been stable, with no changes in the skeleton or the occlusion. Note the barely visible scar. **D,** Intraoral view of the stable class I occlusion.

activity of the resorptive process, (4) management of TMJ symptoms by splint therapy, physical therapy, muscle relaxants, nonsteroidal antiinflammatory drugs, and other modalities as indicated, (5) longitudinal observation for at least 2 years to document response to treatment and stability of the condition, (6) orthognathic correction for stable patients with negative bone scan findings, and (7) condylectomy and costochondral graft reconstruction for patients with progressive condylar resorption and persistent TMJ symptoms or persistent positive bone scan results.

Huang, Pogrel, and Kaban[31] reported a series of 28 patients with progressive bilateral condylar resorption, of which 24 patients were treated by either orthognathic surgery (n = 18) or condylectomy and costochondral graft (n = 6). Only 56% (10 of 18) of patients treated by orthognathic surgical correction of the malocclusion remained asymptomatic postoperatively. The remainder had either continued condylar resorption (4 of 18) or TMJ symptoms (4 of 18). They predicted that the latter

group would also progress to skeletal relapse. In contrast, all patients (n = 6) treated with condylectomy and costochondral grafts remained stable and asymptomatic during the follow-up period. An additional six patients were treated in this manner by the senior author,[39] and all have remained asymptomatic with no skeletal or occlusal relapse.

The risk factors for relapse of condylar resorption after orthognathic surgery include difficulty controlling TMJ symptoms preoperatively, large magnitude of movements, and bimaxillary surgery.[31] Even patients who appear to have a period of clinical stability of TMJ dysfunction preoperatively exhibit a high risk of relapse after orthognathic surgery.

The results with condylectomy and costochondral graft reconstruction appear to be more favorable (Figures 20-10 and 20-11) than with orthognathic surgery. This is because condylectomy duplicates the natural end-point of idiopathic condylysis, i.e., resorption of the sigmoid notch.

ACQUIRED ABNORMALITIES OF MORPHOLOGY AND MOTION OF VARIOUS CAUSES

Trauma, radiation therapy, surgical excision of TMJ tumors, JRA, and infection may all result in mandibular deformity or mandibular hypomobility. Children with decreased mandibular motion, of any cause, often exhibit abnormal growth.

Trauma

Trauma to the chin, because of a fall, is a common occurrence in childhood. The spectrum of injuries ranges from abrasion or laceration of the skin to bilateral subcondylar and mandibular symphysis fractures. Cervical spine fractures occasionally are reported.[40] Unilateral or bilateral intracapsular or subcondylar fractures are the most common mandibular fractures in

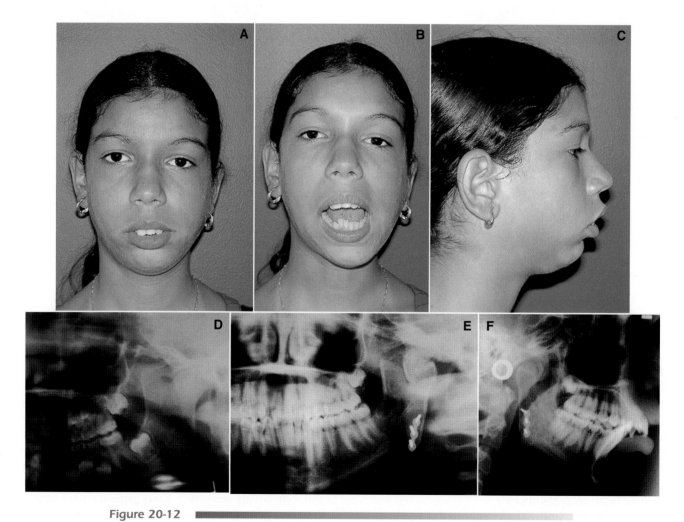

Figure 20-12

Frontal (**A**), frontal at maximum incisal opening (MIO) (**B**), and lateral (**C**) facial photographs of a 13-year-old girl with recurrent ankylosis of the left TMJ secondary to trauma sustained in a motor vehicle accident. **D,** Panoramic radiograph before the first operation demonstrates bony ankylosis of the left TMJ. **E,** Panoramic radiograph after the patient developed re-ankylosis. She had had a condylectomy and coronoidotomy at another institution. The TMJ was reconstructed with a costochondral graft. There was no soft tissue lining in the joint. **F,** Lateral cephalogram documenting the mandibular retrognathism.

Continued

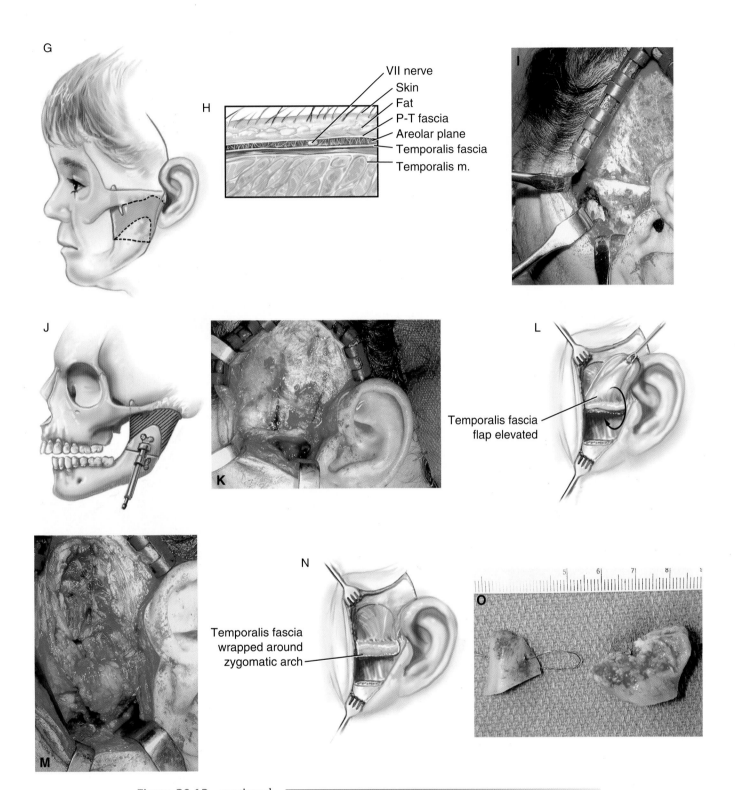

Figure 20-12—continued

G, The proposed preauricular incision with a coronal extension is shown in red. **H,** Diagram shows the anatomy in the temporal region (of the coronal extension). **I,** Intraoperative view after dissection was completed. A preauricular incision with a temporal extension was used. Note the bony ankylotic mass and the coronoid process with obliteration of the sigmoid notch. **J,** The standard ankylosis release was carried out: excision of the ankylotic mass and coronoidectomy (shaded areas). Instead of reconstructing the ramus with a costochondral graft, a horizontal osteotomy was made in the ramus to create a transport disk, and a Synthes (Paoli, PA) semiburied distraction device was placed. **K,** After excision of the ankylotic mass and coronoidectomy, the temporalis flap is drawn with malachite green. **L,** A partial-thickness muscle flap is elevated. **M,** Flap is dissected and rotated over the arch and sutured in place. **N,** The temporalis flap is wrapped around the zygomatic arch and sutured to the medial soft tissues (i.e., lines the glenoid fossa area). **O,** Speci-men: ankylotic mass and coronoid process.

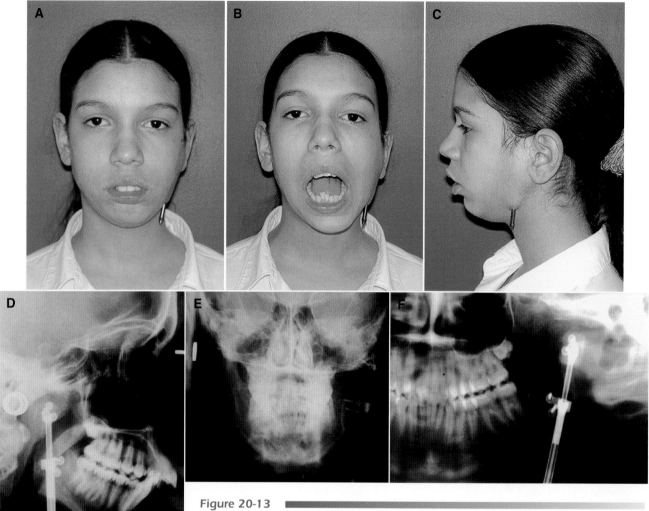

Figure 20-13

Same patient as in Figure 20-12 at end of distraction osteogenesis and end of treatment. Frontal (**A**), frontal opening (**B**), and lateral (**C**) photographs at end distraction. The patient was mobilized and she was started on physical therapy immediately post-operatively. She was comfortable because there was no donor site operation and no period of maxillomandibular fixation. Lateral (**D**) and anteroposterior (**E**) cephalograms and panoramic radiograph (**F**) at the end of DO demonstrating the lengthened mandibular ramus.

Continued

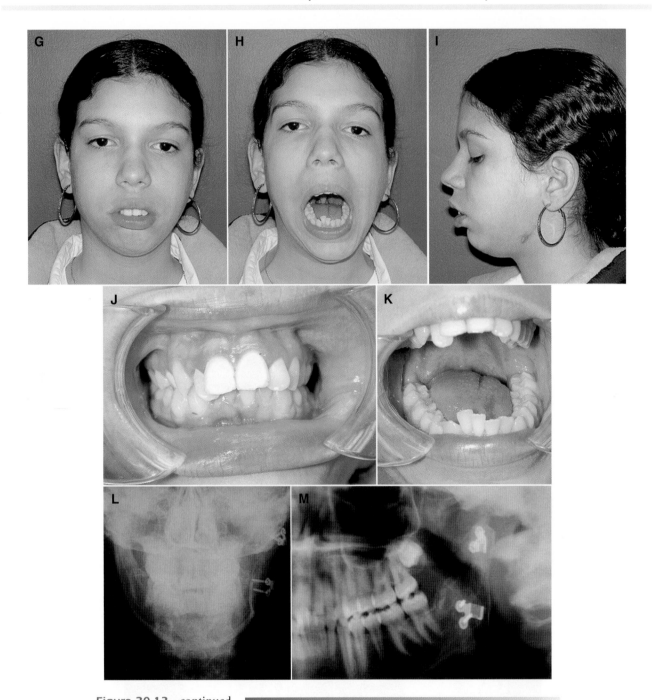

Figure 20-13—continued
Frontal (G), frontal opening (H), and lateral (I) photographs 1 year after completion of treatment. The patient maintained her TMJ motion and will begin presurgical orthodontic treatment to correct her preexisting malocclusion. Closed (J) and open (K) intraoral views, with the patient opening 39 mm at 1 year. Anteroposterior cephalogram (L) and panoramic radiograph (M) at 1 year. The ramus lengthening is demonstrated by the space between the retained footplates.

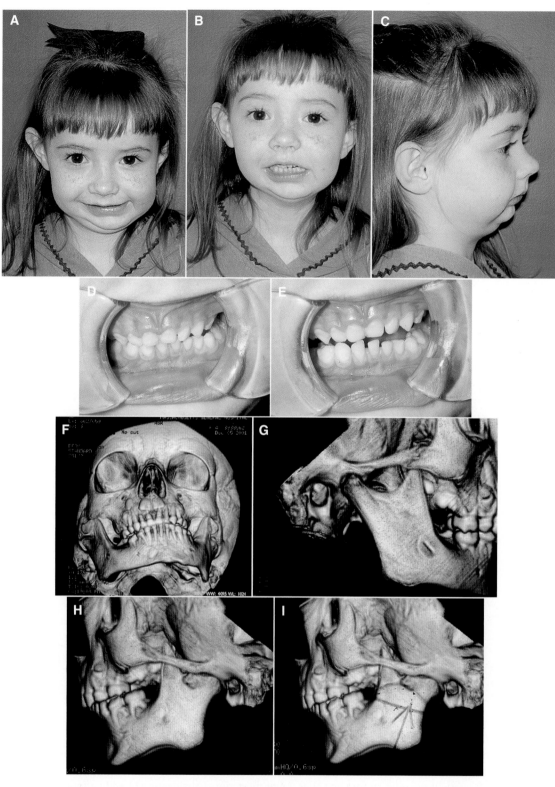

Figure 20-14

A 3-year old child with bony ankylosis of the left TMJ after a fall. Frontal **(A)**, frontal at maximum incisal opening (MIO) **(B)**, and lateral **(C)** facial photographs. The child is retrognathic and has an MIO of 1 mm. Closed **(D)** and open **(E)** intraoral views demonstrating the 1 mm MIO. **F,** Three-dimensional CT image documents the mandibular asymmetry and chin point deviation to the left. **G,** CT image of normal right mandible. **H,** CT image of left mandible illustrating the bony ankylosis of the TMJ, obliteration of the sigmoid notch with bone, and marked coronoid hyperplasia. **I,** CT image with proposed operative plan: excision of the ankylotic mass, coronoidectomy, distal osteotomy to create a transport disk and vector of movement of disk.

children. Diagnosis and management of these fractures is outlined in Chapter 25. In this section, we discuss the treatment of posttraumatic ankylosis.

The most common serious complication of a condylar fracture in a child is ankylosis. This usually occurs after closed reduction and prolonged immobilization of the jaw. Blood in the TMJ becomes organized, and a fibrous scar develops that subsequently becomes calcified and ossified (bony ankylosis). Lack of motion results in loss of the "functional matrix" of bone and muscle interaction. This leads to growth failure and a short ramus-condyle unit on the affected side. With

unilateral ankylosis, the patient develops a mandibular asymmetry (Figures 20-12 to 20-15). Patients with bilateral ankylosis develop retrognathia and open bite (Figures 20-16 to 20-18).

Treatment. The best treatment for posttraumatic ankylosis and the resultant growth abnormality is prevention.[41-43] However, for those patients who have developed ankylosis, surgical correction involves the following principles (see Figures 20-12 to 20-18): (1) aggressive, total excision of the ankylotic segment in the condylar-TMJ region, including removal of the medially displaced condylar fragment (see Figures 20-14 and

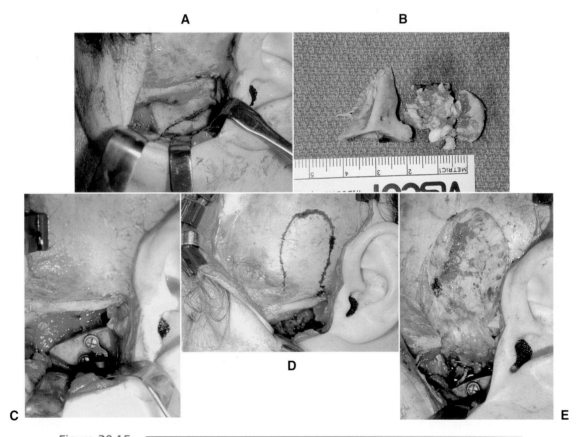

Figure 20-15

Intraoperative and end treatment views of child in Figure 20-14. **A,** After the dissection is completed, using a preauricular incision with a temporal extension, the zygomatic arch, ankylotic mass, and coronoid process are visible. **B,** The coronoid process and the mixed bony and cartilaginous ankylotic mass after excision. **C,** Intraoperative photograph shows the gap and the proximal footplate of the distraction device (Synthes, Paoli, PA). The temporalis flap is outlined (**D**) and rotated (**E**) over the zygomatic arch and sutured in place.

Continued

F   G

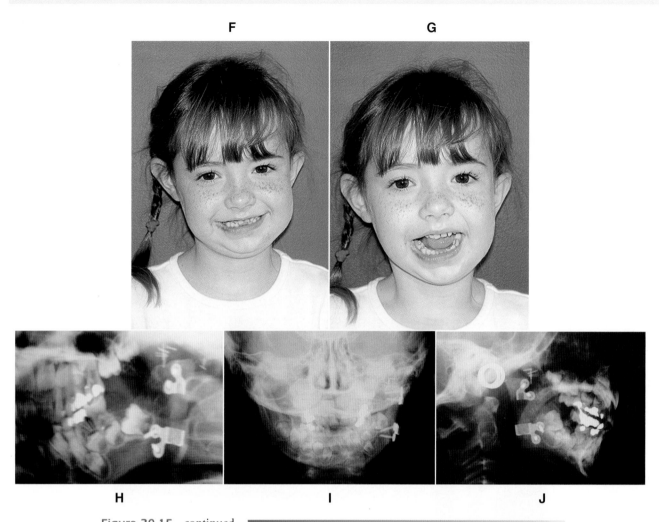

H   I   J

Figure 20-15—continued Frontal **(F)** and frontal opening **(G)** 1 year postoperatively. The child has excellent movement and function. The maximum opening is now limited only by the arc of motion determined by the steepness of the mandibular plane and the close distance between the chin and the trachea. Panoramic **(H)**, anteroposterior **(I)**, and lateral **(J)** cephalograms 1 year postoperatively demonstrating the mandibular lengthening, improved position of the chin, and retrognathic mandible.

20-15), (2) coronoidectomy on the affected side to eliminate the restrictive effect of the temporalis muscle, (3) lining of the joint with temporalis fascia or the native disk if it can be salvaged, (4) removal of the opposite coronoid if steps 1 to 3 do not result in enough motion to permit dislocation of the normal TMJ (approximately 35 to 50 mm of maximal incisal opening), (5) reconstruction of the ramus-condyle unit with costochondral graft and rigid fixation, (6) creation of an open bite on the affected side to permit settling of the bone graft; the open bite should be maintained with an orthodontic appliance for 3 to 6 months, (7) early mobilization with minimal intermaxillary fixation (no more than 10 days), and (8) aggressive physiotherapy. Simple, minimal excision of the ankylotic segment in childhood is not adequate treatment, because it does not address the ramus height asymmetry and the incidence of recurrent ankylosis is high.[44]

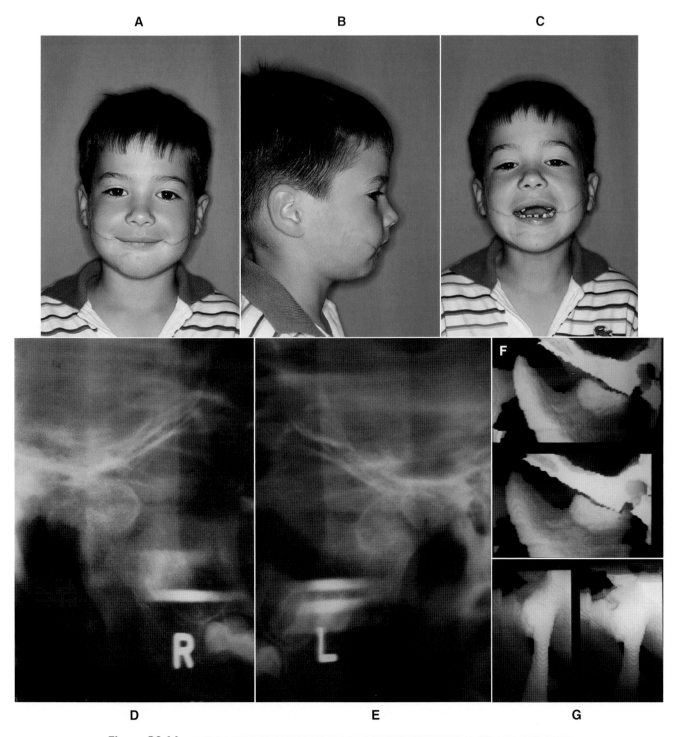

Figure 20-16

A 3-year old boy with bilateral bony ankylosis after a vehicular accident, which also produced bilateral lacerations of the commissures. Frontal **(A)**, lateral **(B)**, and frontal MIO **(C)** photographs. Note the maximal opening of 1 to 2 mm. Right **(D)** and left **(E)** panoramic views of the ankylotic masses of the TMJs. Right sagittal **(F)** and left coronal **(G)** CT scans. The right view shows the ankylosis and coronoid hyperplasia. The left view demonstrates the bony fusion of the condyle to the skull base.

Continued

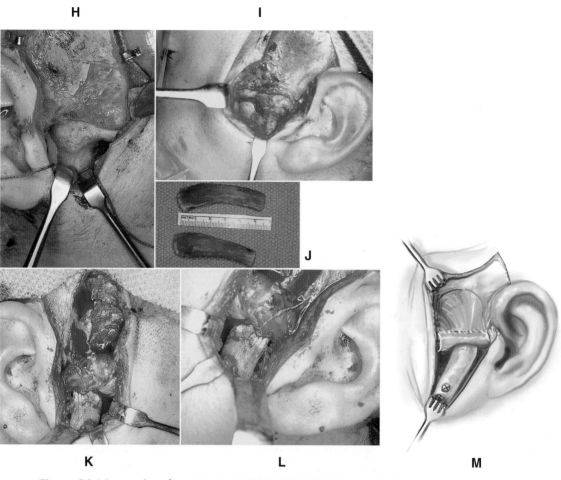

Figure 20-16—continued

Right **(H)** and left **(I)** TMJs exposed after the dissection was completed. On the right, the bony ankylotic mass is visible. On the left, both the mass and the coronoid process are demonstrated. **J.** Harvested costochondral grafts with 1 to 2 mm cartilaginous caps. Right **(K)** and left **(L)** TMJs after temporalis flaps have been sutured in place and the costochondral grafts secured. **M,** Diagram of left costochondral graft secured in place.

The protocol has been modified, when possible, by substituting ramus lengthening by distraction osteogenesis for reconstruction with costochondral grafts.[45,46] This has the advantage of eliminating the donor site operation and allowing immediate mobilization of the patient's TMJ(s). The surgical procedure is the same as described above except for the bony reconstruction of the ramus-condyle unit. After the jaw is mobilized and the lining created with a temporalis muscle–fascia flap

or the native disk (steps 1 to 4), the native mandibular stump is reshaped to make it narrow and rounded at the top. A corticotomy is created distally, leaving enough bone to serve as a transport disk. The distraction device is secured, the corticotomy completed, and mobility of the segment tested. The wound is then closed in layers. There is no need to create an open bite on the affected side, and the patient begins jaw motion exercises the night of the operation (see Figures 20-12 to 20-15).

Radiation Therapy

Therapeutic radiation to the mandible and TMJ region, in the growing child, produces a growth abnormality by its destruction of actively dividing cells and small blood vessels. Intimal hyperplasia produces narrowing of small vascular channels, which has a negative impact on bone metabolism and the capacity of bone to recover from injury. The magnitude of the growth defect is related to the amount of radiation and the age at which it was received.[47-49]

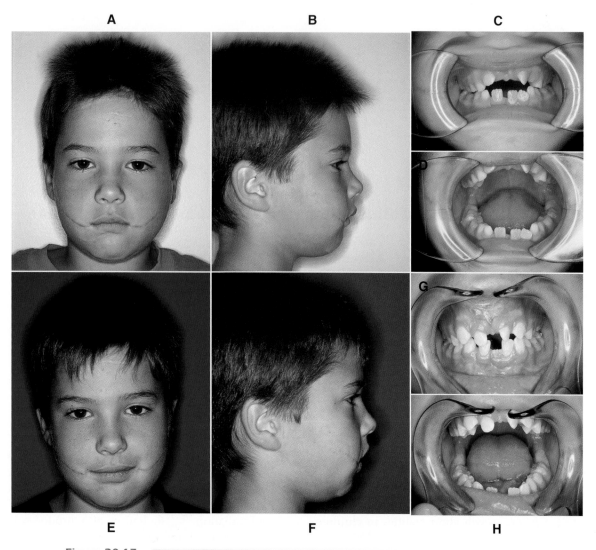

Figure 20-17

Same child as in Figure 20-16 1 and 2½ years postoperatively. Frontal (**A**) and lateral (**B**) facial photographs 1 year postoperatively. Intraoral closed (**C**) and open (**D**) views demonstrating completely normal MIO in the 40 mm range. Frontal (**E**) and lateral (**F**) facial photographs 2½ years postoperatively. Intraoral closed (**G**) and open (**H**) views demonstrating maintenance of the normal MIO.

Continued

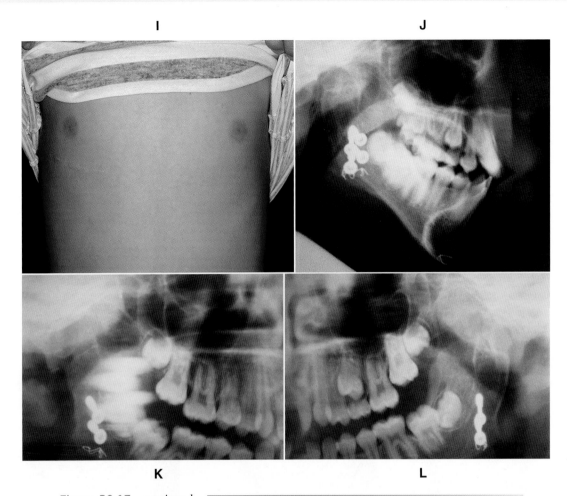

Figure 20-17—continued

I, The patient's chest 2 years postoperatively. The right inframammary incision is well healed. J, Lateral cephalogram demonstrates a stable occlusion without increase in overjet with time. Right (K) and left (L) panoramic views at 2½ years with remodeling of the costochondral grafts.

Although the data on mandibular radiation therapy are scarce, there have been studies on the effects of radiation on the spines of growing children. Neuhauser[48] reported that less than 1000 rads of radiation to the spine resulted in no growth abnormalities in children regardless of age. In contrast, more than 2000 rads always produced a growth disturbance. When the child received 1000 to 2000 rads, growth defects occurred in patients less than 2 years of age but not in those older than 2 years. Propert, Parker, and Kaplan[49] reported that children who received radiation before 6 years of age or during puberty (times of rapid and large amounts of growth) showed the greatest growth disturbances after

radiation therapy to the spine. Several studies have demonstrated in rodents inhibition of ossification, damage of the intermediate and hypertrophic zones of condylar cartilage, fibrosis, and marrow hypoplasia after TMJ irradiation.[50-52] Radiation also produces fibrosis, scarring, and induration of the surrounding soft tissues and muscles of mastication, resulting in decreased motion. This, in turn, contributes to abnormal mandibular growth. The resultant deformity is a very small mandible (Figures 20-19 and 20-20).

The soft tissue and bone abnormalities of the irradiated mandible are primarily vascular, become progressively worse, and are not treatable. Therefore, the

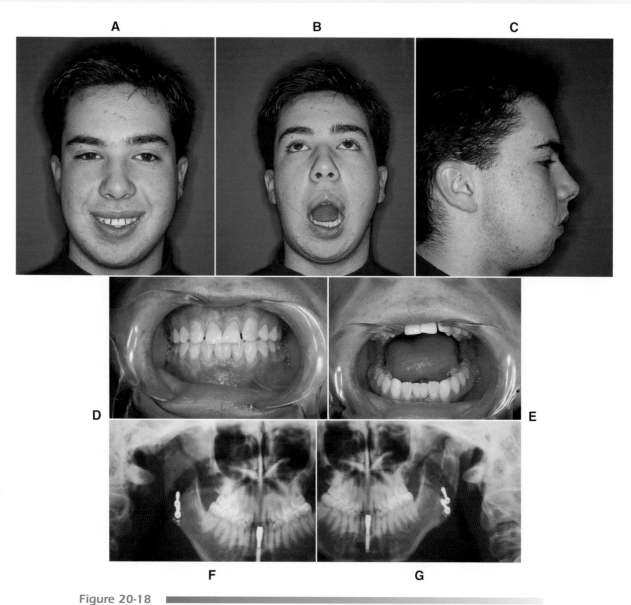

Figure 20-18

The same patient as in Figures 20-16 and 20-17, now 11 years postoperatively. Frontal **(A)**, frontal opening **(B)**, and lateral **(C)** facial views. Note maintenance of the normal MIO. The patient has a vertically long and retrusive chin and is planned for a genioplasty. Closed **(D)** and open **(E)** intraoral views. Right **(F)** and left **(G)** panoramic radiographs show remodeling of the costochondral grafts.

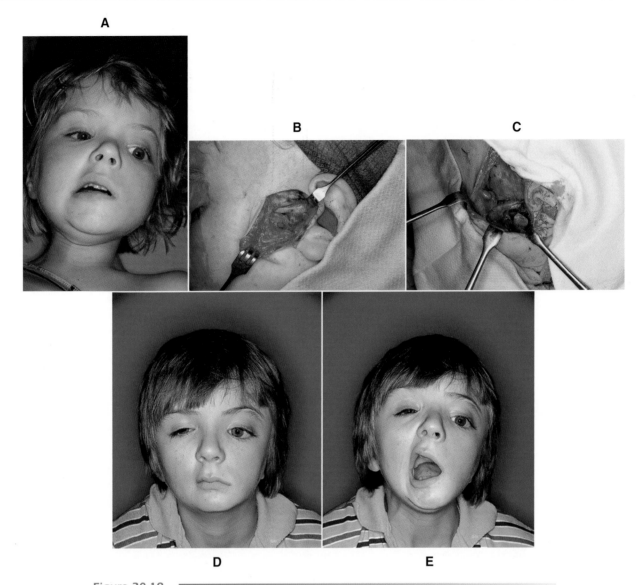

Figure 20-19

Child with left TMJ fibro-osseous ankylosis secondary to radiation therapy. **A,** Maximum opening before ankylosis release. **B,** Intraoperative view of ankylosed segment showing fibro-osseous fusion to the zygomatic arch. **C,** Costochondral graft in place. **D,** and **E,** Normal opening (3 cm) 1½ years postoperatively.

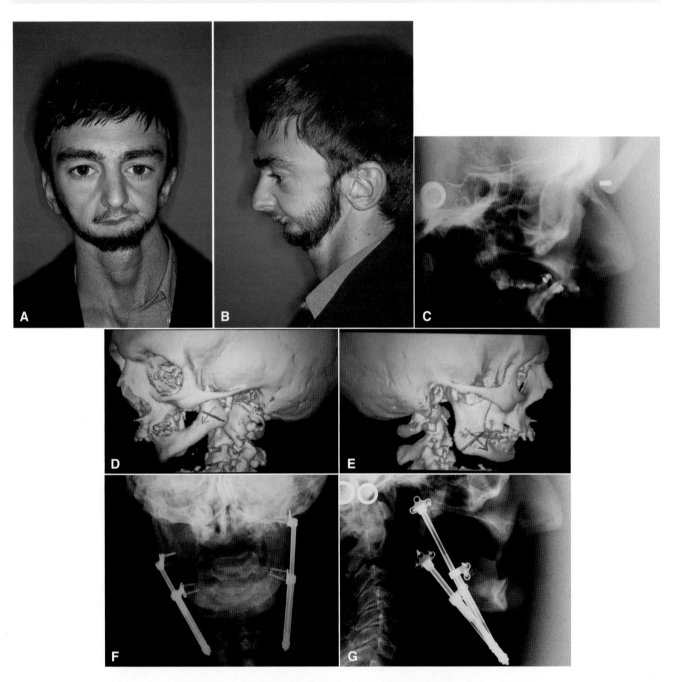

Figure 20-20

This patient received radiation therapy to the left ramus and TMJ region for an osteosarcoma at age 2½. He had limited motion and severe mandibular retrognathism. Frontal **(A)** and lateral **(B)** photographs showing the severe retrognathism and short lower face height. **C,** Lateral cephalogram documents the clinical findings. **D,** Left lateral 3D CT image demonstrates the markedly hypoplastic left ramus/condyle unit. The proposed osteotomy is diagrammed on the CT with the vector of movement. **E,** Right lateral 3D CT image with the osteotomy and vector of mandibular movement. Frontal **(F)** and lateral **(G)** cephalograms after removal of infected teeth and at the end of distraction. The jaw was advanced asymmetrically 30 mm on the left and 20 mm on the right.

Continued

results of operative correction of postradiation ankylosis and asymmetry are poor. Vascularized soft tissue or composite bone and soft tissue flaps may be required to achieve a satisfactory result. Asymmetry is treated by osteotomy or bone grafts, or both, with costochondral junction for the condylar head with a similarly poor prognosis. Encouraging results have been achieved with mandibular elongation by distraction osteogenesis in these irradiated patients.[53,54]

The patient illustrated in Figure 20-19 had ankylosis secondary to radiation therapy for histiocytosis, followed by osteomyelitis of the left mastoid and TMJ region. It should be pointed out that radiation would no longer be used for such a lesion in this location. The patient shown in Figure 20-20 received radiation treatment for an osteosarcoma of the mandibular ramus/ condyle unit at 2½ years of age. He developed a severe facial asymmetry and micrognathia as a result of this treatment.

Tumors of the Temporomandibular Joint

Tumors of the ramus of the mandible or TMJ region in children are rare, but when they occur, one must consider excision of the lesion and reconstruction to restore symmetric ramus length and function. Excision of jaw tumors in children is not accompanied by progressive growth abnormality if the TMJ and mandible are reconstructed[55] (see Chapter 15).

The primary TMJ neoplasms most frequently occurring in children are benign mesenchymal tumors, including giant cell lesions, myxomas, and fibro-osseous lesions.

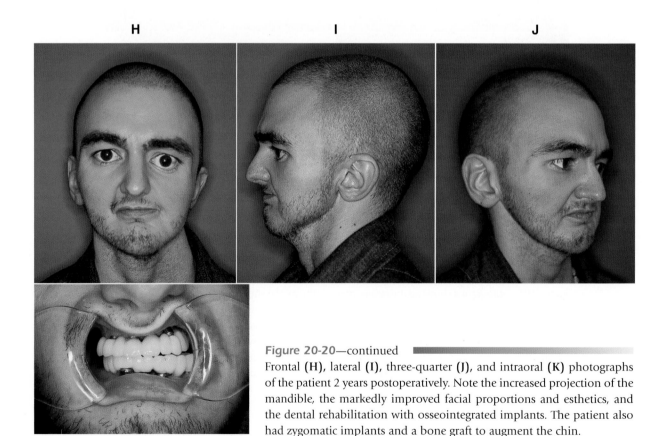

Figure 20-20—continued
Frontal (**H**), lateral (**I**), three-quarter (**J**), and intraoral (**K**) photographs of the patient 2 years postoperatively. Note the increased projection of the mandible, the markedly improved facial proportions and esthetics, and the dental rehabilitation with osseointegrated implants. The patient also had zygomatic implants and a bone graft to augment the chin.

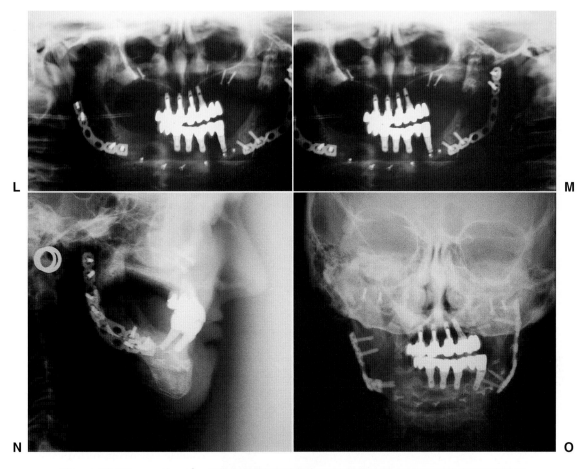

Figure 20-20—continued
Right (**L**) and left (**M**) panoramic views. **N** and **O**, Lateral cephalograms 2 years postoperatively. These radiographs document the stability of the result and the clinical findings. Note that the reconstruction plates for the mandible were used because the distraction devices were removed early because of lack of patient tolerance.

Giant cell and fibro-osseous lesions may occur in association with aneurysmal bone cysts, which are also common.[56] Finally, one must always consider eosinophilic granuloma (Langerhans cell histiocytosis) in a child with a localized, lytic bone lesion. The child usually has a history of a slow-growing, nonpainful mass and either a progressive decrease in jaw motion or a deviation of the mandible on opening. Plain radiographs and computed tomography scans reveal a radiolucent or mixed radiolucent and radiopaque lesion of the ramus and TMJ region. Management of the benign mesenchymal tumors of childhood is based on clinical behavior, radiographic appearance and, to some extent, histologic

diagnosis.[55] A detailed discussion of the diagnosis and management of primary jaw tumors in children is presented in Chapter 15. In this chapter, remarks are confined to excision of TMJ tumors and reconstruction.

The tumor is approached through a preauricular incision extended into the temporal fossa. A second submandibular incision sometimes is needed for exposure to do the resection and reconstruction. When the mandibular ramus is excised during childhood, ramus height must be restored by costochondral reconstruction as soon as possible. When this is done, normal facial growth can be expected (Figures 20-21 to 20-23). Reconstruction is carried out using the same principles

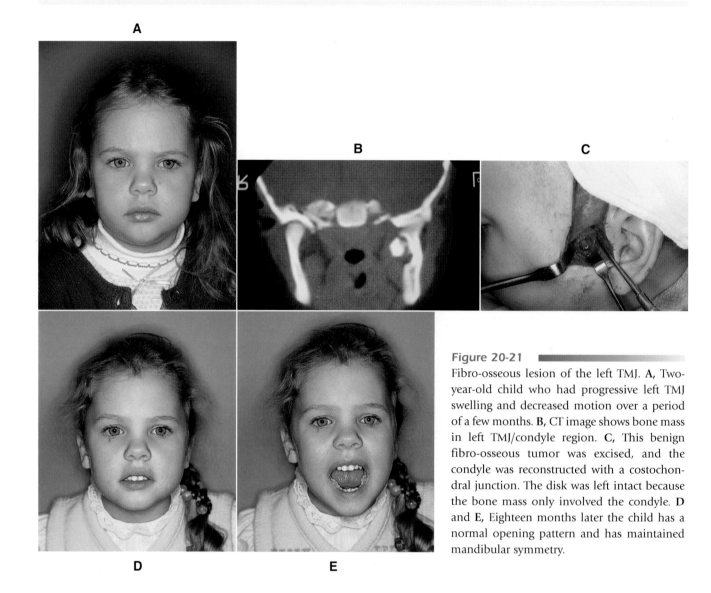

A

B

C

D

E

Figure 20-21

Fibro-osseous lesion of the left TMJ. **A,** Two-year-old child who had progressive left TMJ swelling and decreased motion over a period of a few months. **B,** CT image shows bone mass in left TMJ/condyle region. **C,** This benign fibro-osseous tumor was excised, and the condyle was reconstructed with a costochondral junction. The disk was left intact because the bone mass only involved the condyle. **D** and **E,** Eighteen months later the child has a normal opening pattern and has maintained mandibular symmetry.

described for costochondral grafts in previous sections. An open bite is created to permit settling of the graft postoperatively.

Osteomyelitis

Since the advent of antibiotics, chronic osteomyelitis is a rare cause of ankylosis of the mandible. However, when it does occur, it is usually associated with trauma, radiation, or contiguous spread of infection from an adjacent area of the maxillofacial skeleton. In contrast, in many developing countries, osteomyelitis still occurs because of hematogenous spread of distant infection. For the purposes of this discussion, we are interested specifically in the sequelae of osteomyelitis (Figure 20-24).

Osteomyelitis of the mandibular ramus and TMJ usually is accompanied by bony or fibrous ankylosis. Decreased motion leads to a progressive growth abnormality that resembles hemifacial microsomia. Management consists of control of infection by debridement and proper antibiotics. Once the patient is infection free, the ankylotic segment is excised, and the mandibular ramus and TMJ are reconstructed with a costochondral junction.

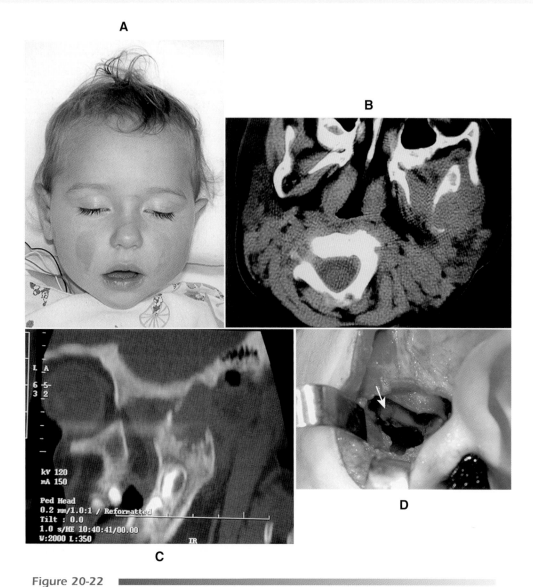

Figure 20-22

An infant with a lytic lesion of the left ramus and condyle. **A,** Frontal photograph shows slight fullness in left preauricular region. Axial **(B)** and sagittal **(C)** CT images demonstrate the lesion, with bony expansion and cortical thinning and perforation. **D,** At exploration, a frozen section revealed an eosinophilic granuloma. The lesion was enucleated, and this photograph shows the defect. Note that the intact disk is visible in the joint *(arrow)*.

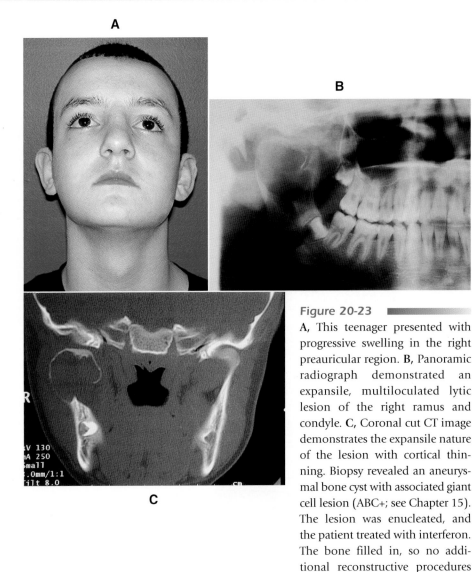

Figure 20-23

A, This teenager presented with progressive swelling in the right preauricular region. **B,** Panoramic radiograph demonstrated an expansile, multiloculated lytic lesion of the right ramus and condyle. **C,** Coronal cut CT image demonstrates the expansile nature of the lesion with cortical thinning. Biopsy revealed an aneurysmal bone cyst with associated giant cell lesion (ABC+; see Chapter 15). The lesion was enucleated, and the patient treated with interferon. The bone filled in, so no additional reconstructive procedures were planned.

Juvenile Rheumatoid Arthritis

JRA is a common chronic disease that affects approximately 200,000 children in the United States.[57,58] The incidence of TMJ involvement in this autoimmune disorder is not well documented. A prospective study at Children's Hospital in Boston has revealed that while only a small number of patients (1 in 37) have TMJ symptoms at the onset of JRA, about 50% (17 in 37) develop some (noise, pain, decreased motion) within the first 5 years after onset of the disease.[59] Most patients who develop symptoms also develop radiographic abnormalities: condylar and glenoid fossa erosions and decreased joint space. In a few patients, JRA results in mandibular growth deficiency on the basis of joint inflammation, condylar resorption, and decreased motion.

The characteristic deformity with unilateral TMJ involvement is mandibular asymmetry. Patients with

A   B   C

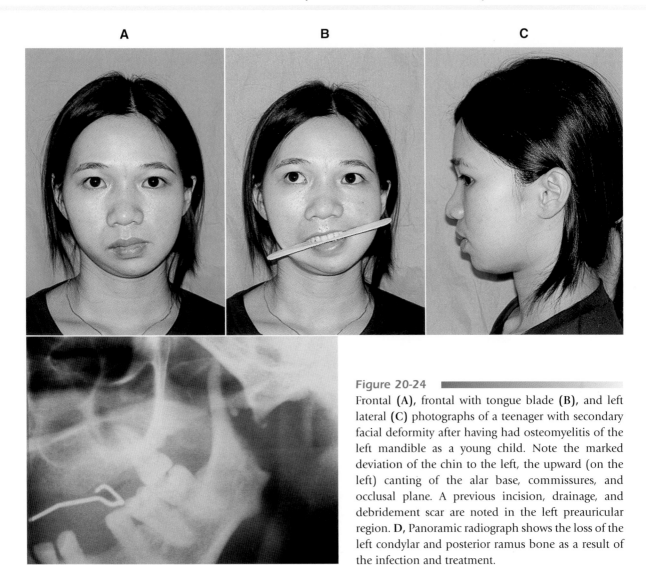

D

Figure 20-24

Frontal **(A)**, frontal with tongue blade **(B)**, and left lateral **(C)** photographs of a teenager with secondary facial deformity after having had osteomyelitis of the left mandible as a young child. Note the marked deviation of the chin to the left, the upward (on the left) canting of the alar base, commissures, and occlusal plane. A previous incision, drainage, and debridement scar are noted in the left preauricular region. **D**, Panoramic radiograph shows the loss of the left condylar and posterior ramus bone as a result of the infection and treatment.

bilateral TMJ involvement may develop retrognathia and open bite. Before the morphologic deformity can be treated, the inflammatory disease must be under control and adequate mandibular motion must be achieved. Rarely, because of pain and decreased motion, a condylectomy is performed, and the joint is reconstructed with a costochondral junction. If the primary disease is well controlled, the prognosis for long-term relief of pain and good motion is favorable. The malocclusion and dentofacial deformity are then treated by osteotomy and TMJ reconstruction, as dictated by skeletal configuration and severity of the defect. Figure 20-25 shows a teenage female with juvenile onset rheumatoid arthritis. She had severe pain and limitation of motion of the left TMJ. All other joints involved were under control with nonsteroidal antiinflammatory drugs.

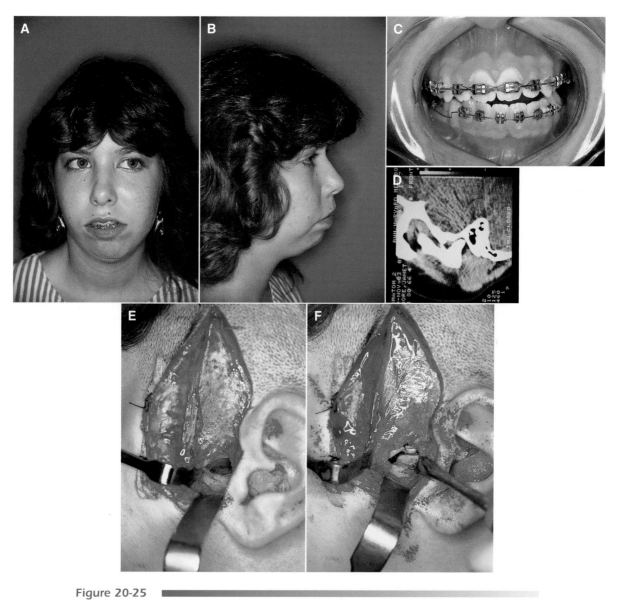

Figure 20-25

Juvenile rheumatoid arthritis. Frontal **(A)** and lateral **(B)** photographs demonstrate chin and mandibular dental midline deviated to the left, as well as mandibular retrognathism. **C,** Intraoral view shows the dental midline deviated to the left and an open bite. **D,** CT image documents decreased joint space and flattening of the condylar head, which was severely eroded at operation. **E** and **F,** Intraoperative views after the condyle was debrided and reconstructed with a costochondral graft. The roof of the glenoid fossa was lined with costal cartilage.

Continued

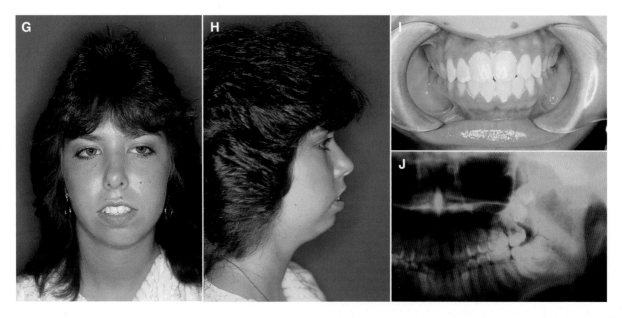

Figure 20-25—continued
Frontal (**G**), lateral (**H**), and intraoral (**I**) views 1½ years postoperatively. The mandible is symmetric, with the chin point corresponding to the facial midline. The mandibular dental midline is coincident with the maxillary dental midline, and the open bite is corrected. Patient has good jaw motion. **J,** Panoramic radiograph shows remodeling of the costochondral graft.

CONCLUSION

In this chapter, we discussed acquired growth abnormalities of the TMJ. Normal growth of the mandible depends upon the interaction of the neuromuscular complex with the bony mandible. The requirements for normal and symmetric mandibular growth are (1) TMJs located in symmetrically equivalent positions in relation to the skull base, (2) symmetric ramus height, (3) symmetric motion provided by the muscles of mastication, and (4) normal range of motion.

The goal of management is to restore the mandible and TMJ to a normal anatomic and functional state. The prognosis for normal growth in the long term is best for those patients who have isolated, acquired, skeletal defects. Those patients who have severe deformities involving the skeleton and soft tissues and those patients who have had radiation therapy have a less favorable prognosis.

REFERENCES

1. Hovell JH: Condylar hyperplasia, *Br J Oral Surg* 1:105, 1963.
2. Walker RJ: Condylar hyperplasia. In Bell WH, Proffit WR, White RB, editors: *Surgical correction of dentofacial deformities*, Philadelphia, 1980, WB Saunders.
3. Cisneros G, Kaban LB: Computerized skeletal scintigraphy for assessment of mandibular asymmetry, *J Oral Maxillofac Surg* 42:513-520, 1985.
4. Kaban LB, Treves ST: Skeletal scintigraphy for assessment of mandibular growth and asymmetry. In Treves ST, editor: *Pediatric nuclear medicine*, New York, 1985, Springer-Verlag.
5. Cisneros G, Kaban LB: Computerized skeletal scintigraphy for assessment of mandibular asymmetry, *J Oral Maxillofac Surg* 42:513-520, 1984.
6. Matteson SR, Proffit WR, Terry BC, et al: Bone scanning with 99m-technetium phosphate to assess condylar hyperplasia, *J Oral Maxillofac Surg* 60:356-367, 1985.
7. Gray RJ, Sloan P, Quayle AA, Carter DH: Histopathological and scintigraphic features of condylar hyperplasia, *Int J Oral Maxillofac Surg* 19:65-71, 1990.
8. Pogrel MA: Quantitative assessment of isotope activity in the temporomandibular joint regions as a means of assessing unilateral condylar hypertrophy, *J Oral Maxillofac Surg* 60:15-17, 1985.
9. Robinson PD, Harris K, Coghlan KC, Altman K: Bone scans and the timing of treatment for condylar hyperplasia, *Int J Oral Maxillofac Surg* 19:243-246, 1990.
10. Gray RJ, Horner K, Testa HJ, et al: Condylar hyperplasia: correlation of histological and scintigraphic features, *Dentomaxillofac Radiol* 23:103-107, 1994.
11. Harris SA, Quayle AA, Testa HJ: Radionuclide bone scanning in the diagnosis and management of condylar hyperplasia, *Nucl Med Commun* 5:373-380, 1984.

12. Silberstein EB, Saenger EL, Tofe AJ, et al: Imaging of bone metastases with 99m-Tc-Sn-EHDP (diphosphate), 18F and skeletal radiography, *Radiology* 107:551, 1973.

13. Barrett MB, Smith PHS: Bone imaging with 99Tc in polyphosphate: a comparison with 18F and skeletal radiography, *Br J Radiol* 17:387, 1974.

14. Stevenson JS, Bright RW, Dunson GL, et al: Technetium 99m phosphate bone imaging: a method for bone graft healing, *Radiology* 110:391, 1974.

15. Roser SM, Mena I: Diphosphonate dynamic imaging of experimental bone grafts and soft tissue injury, *Int J Oral Surg* 7:488, 1978.

16. Donoff RB, Jeffcoat MK, Kaplan ML: Use of miniaturized detector in facial bone scanning, *Int J Oral Surg* 7:482, 1978.

17. Pogrel MA, Kopf J, Dodson TB, et al: A comparison of single-photon emission computed tomography and planar imaging for quantitative skeletal scintigraphy of the mandibular condyle, *Oral Surg Oral Med Oral Pathol* 80:226-231, 1995.

18. Wolford LM, Mehra P, Reiche-Fischel O, et al: Efficacy of high condylectomy for management of condylar hyperplasia, *Am J Orthod Dentofacial Orthop* 121:136-150, 2002.

19. Troulis MJ, Kaban LB: Endoscopic approach the ramus/condyle unit: clinical applications, *J Oral Maxillofac Surg* 59:503-509, 2001.

20. Bertolami F, Bianchi B, DeRiu G, et al: Hemimandibular hyperplasia treated by early high condylectomy: a case report, *Int J Adult Orthodon Orthognath Surg* 16:227-234, 2001.

21. Ogus H: Rheumatoid arthritis of the temporomandibular joint, *Br J Oral Surg* 12:275, 1975.

22. Ogden GR: Complete resorption of the mandibular condyles in rheumatoid arthritis, *Br Dent J* 160:95, 1986.

23. Ramon Y, Samra H, Oberman M: Mandibular condylysis and apertognathia as presenting symptoms in progressive systemic sclerosis (scleroderma), *Oral Surg Oral Med Oral Pathol* 63:269, 1987.

24. Lanigan DT, Myall RW, West RA, et al: Condylysis in a patient with a mixed collagen vascular disease, *Oral Surg Oral Med Oral Pathol* 48:198, 1979.

25. Osial TA, Avakian A, Sassouni V, et al: Resorption of the mandibular condyles and coronoid processes in progressive systemic sclerosis (scleroderma), *Arthritis Rheum* 24:729, 1981.

26. Iizuka T, Lindqvist C, Hallikainen D, et al: Severe bone resorption and osteoarthrosis after miniplate fixation of high condylar fractures, *Oral Surg Oral Med Oral Pathol* 72:400, 1991.

27. Lindqvist C, Soderholm AL, Hallikainen D, et al: Erosion and heterotopic bone formation after alloplastic temporomandibular joint reconstruction, *J Oral Maxillofac Surg* 50:942, 1992.

28. Philips RM, Bell WH: Atrophy of mandibular condyles after sagittal ramus split osteotomy: report of case, *J Oral Surg* 36:45, 1978.

29. Sesenna E, Raffaini M: Bilateral condylar atrophy after combined osteotomy for correction of mandibular retrusion, *J Maxillofac Surg* 13:263, 1985.

30. Bouwman JPB, Kerstens HCJ, Tuinzing DB: Condylar resorption in orthognathic surgery, *Oral Surg Oral Med Oral Pathol* 78:138, 1994.

31. Huang YL, Pogrel MA, Kaban LB: Diagnosis and management of condylar resorption, *J Oral Maxillofac Surg* 55:114-119, 1997.

32. Wolford LM, Cardenas L: Idiopathic condylar resorption: diagnosis, treatment protocol and outcomes, *Am J Orthod Dentofac Orthop* 116:667-677, 1999.

33. Rabey GP: Bilateral mandibular condylysis—a morphanalytic diagnosis, *Br J Oral Surg* 15:121-134, 1997.

34. Moore KE, Gooris PJJ, Stoelinga PJW: The contributing role of condylar resorption to skeletal relapse following mandibular advancement surgery: report of five cases, *J Oral Maxillofac Surg* 49:448, 1991.

35. Kerstens HCJ, Tuinzing DB, Golding RP, et al: Condylar atrophy and osteoarthritis after bimaxillary surgery, *Oral Surg Oral Med Oral Pathol* 69:274, 1990.

36. Crawford JG, Stoelinga PJW, Blijdorp PA, et al: Stability after reoperation for progressive condylar resorption after orthognathic surgery: report of seven cases, *J Oral Maxillofac Surg* 52:460, 1994.

37. Merkx MAW, Van Damme PA: Condylar resorption after orthognathic surgery: evaluation of treatment in 8 patients, *J Craniomaxillofac Surg* 22:53, 1994.

38. Arnett GS, Tamorello JA: Progressive class II development: female idiopathic condylar resorption, *Oral Maxillofac Surg Clin North Am* 2:699, 1990.

39. Troulis MJ, Williams WB, Kaban LB: Endoscopic condylectomy and costochondral graft reconstruction of the ramus condyle unit, *J Oral Maxillofac Surg* 61 (suppl 1):63-64, 2003.

40. Bertolami CN, Kaban LB: Chin trauma: a clue to associated mandibular and cervical spine injury, *J Oral Maxillofac Surg* 53:122-126, 1982.

41. Kaban LB, Mulliken JB, Murray JE: Facial fractures in children: 109 fractures in 122 patients, *Plast Reconstr Surg* 59:15-20, 1977.

42. Mulliken JB, Kaban LB, Murray JE: Management of facial fractures in children, *Clin Plast Surg* 4:491-502, 1977.

43. James D: Maxillofacial injuries in children. In Rowe NL, Williams JL, editors: *Maxillofacial injuries*, London, 1985, Churchill Livingstone.

44. Munro I, Chen YR, Park BY: Simultaneous total correction of temporomandibular joint ankylosis and facial asymmetry, *Plast Reconstr Surg* 77:517-527, 1986.

45. Dean A, Alamillos F: Mandibular distraction in temporomandibular ankylosis, *Plast Reconstr Surg* 104:2021-2031, 1999.

46. Papageorge MB, Apostolidis C: Simultaneous mandibular distraction and arthroplasty in a patient with temporomandibular joint ankylosis and mandibular hypoplasia, *J Oral Maxillofac Surg* 57:328-333, 1999.

47. Shelton D: Late effects of condylar irradiation in a child: a review of the literature and report of a case, *J Oral Maxillofac Surg* 35:478-482, 1977.

48. Neuhauser EBD, Wittenborg MH, Berman CZ, Cohen J: Irradiation effects on the growing spine, *Radiology* 59:637, 1952.

49. Propert JC, Parker BR, Kaplan HS: Growth retardation in children after megavoltage irradiation of the spine, *Cancer* 32:634, 1972.

50. Burstone MS: The effect of x-irradiation on the development of the mandibular joint of the mouse, *J Dent Res* 29:358, 1950.

51. Furstman LL: Effect of x-irradiation on the mandibular condyle, *J Dent Res* 49:419, 1970.

52. Barr JS, Langley JR, Gall EA: The effect of roentgen irradiation on epiphyseal growth: experimental studies upon the albino rat, *Am J Roentgenol* 49:104, 1943.

53. Troulis MJ, Padwa B, Kaban LB: Distraction osteogenesis: past, present and future, *Facial Plast Surg* 14:205-215, 1998.

54. Gantous A, Phillips JH, Catton P, Holmberg D: Distraction osteogenesis in the irradiated canine mandible, *Plast Reconstr Surg* 93:164-168, 1994.

55. Chuong R, Kaban LB: Jaw tumors in children: a ten year experience, *J Oral Maxillofac Surg* 43:323-332, 1985.

56. Padwa B, Denhart B, Kaban LB: Aneurysmal bone cyst-plus, *J Oral Maxillofac Surg* 55:1144-1151, 1997.

57. Sinn DP: Mandibular deficiency secondary to juvenile rheumatoid arthritis. In Bell WH, Proffit WR, White RB, editors: *Surgical collection of dentofacial deformities*, Philadelphia, 1980, WB Saunders.

58. Turpin DL, West RA: Juvenile rheumatoid arthritis: a case report of surgical-orthodontic treatment, *Am J Orthod* 73:312-320, 1978.

59. Wilkes J, Hoch S, Kaban LB: TMJ disease in association with juvenile rheumatoid arthritis. Presented at the annual meeting of the International Association of Dental Research, Las Vegas, Nevada, March 1985.

CHAPTER 21

Orthognathic Surgery in the Growing Child

Bonnie L. Padwa

CHAPTER OUTLINE

Surgical correction of mandibular, maxillary, and midface deformities in the growing patient have been advocated by many clinical investigators. When treating children with craniofacial anomalies, the clinician is faced with the challenging dilemma of the fourth dimension, time. In general, surgical correction is reserved for patients who do not respond to orthopedic growth modification or for those whose deformities are too severe to camouflage by orthodontic tooth movement. When an operation is performed before complete skeletal maturation, growth with time, the fourth dimension, is introduced as a confounding variable and treatment outcomes may be less predictable.[1] On the other hand, in the severely deformed patient, early correction may be beneficial and should be considered.

Many of the goals of orthognathic surgery in children are similar to those in adults. These include improvement of masticatory function and facial appearance, enlargement of the upper airway in obstructive sleep apnea, and facilitation of occlusal correction beyond the range of orthodontic treatment. In the growing patient, procedures are performed more commonly to enlarge the upper airway in cases of syndromic and nonsyndromic micrognathia and to aid body image and psychosocial development.

This chapter focuses on correction of maxillofacial deformities in children, with particular attention to the effects of these procedures on facial growth and on long-term skeletal stability. Specific orthognathic surgical procedures are discussed when technical considerations vary because of age.[2,3]

FACIAL GROWTH CONSIDERATIONS

When planning orthognathic surgery in children, it is important to understand the timing and progression of craniofacial growth and development. For the purposes of this discussion, we focus on the relationship between growth dynamics and the ability to surgically correct a skeletal deformity. The orbit attains 90% of its final size by 7 years of age.[4] Nasal morphology and size reach the mature state in girls by 16 years of age. However, the nose continues to grow in boys up to and beyond 18 years.[5]

The mandible is the last facial bone to complete growth. Singh and Savara[6,7] found that anteroposterior maxillary growth is finished largely by the beginning of puberty and that any further growth is predominantly vertical. Transverse growth ends with eruption of the second permanent molars.[6] Growth in height of the maxilla is a result of bone apposition on the alveolar process in association with tooth eruption. Appositional growth at the sutural connections of the maxilla occurs in a cephalad direction toward the frontal and zygomatic bones. Growth in anteroposterior length of the maxilla occurs at the sutures of the palatine bones and by apposition at the maxillary tuberosities. The steepest slope of maxillary growth has been reported between ages 10 and 12 years for girls and 1 to 3 years later for boys. Buschang et al.[8] reported that maxillary growth does not exhibit the characteristic adolescent acceleration seen in the mandible.

The pattern of mandibular growth closely follows that of general body growth with an increase during puberty.[9] Length of the mandible in the sagittal plane and vertical alveolar height both exhibit a significant increase between ages 9 and 13 years in girls and 11 and 17 years in boys.[10] Mandibular growth in girls is usually complete by 17 years of age or 2½ to 3 years after the first menstrual period. In boys, it can continue until after age 20. Overall growth curves become flat between the ages of 16 and 18 years in girls and 17 to 19 years in boys.

There is considerable individual variation in facial growth.[11] Therefore, predictions from general databases are not necessarily helpful for the clinician trying to decide on the timing of orthognathic surgery in children.

TIMING OF ORTHOGNATHIC SURGERY

When planning orthognathic surgery in the growing child, the surgeon must consider the following questions: (1) Will the operation have a positive or an adverse effect on overall facial growth? (2) Will correction of a skeletal defect in one facial bone prevent or accentuate secondary deformity of ipsilateral and contralateral structures? (3) Is growth of the abnormal bone improved postoperatively (e.g., does early mandibular advancement improve the growth pattern of the hypoplastic jaw)? and (4) What is the expected stability of the correction? In adults, the stability of a maxillofacial surgical correction depends on the magnitude of the movement, soft tissue tolerance, adequacy of the fixation, and the occlusion.

In general, orthognathic surgery should be delayed until development is complete in patients with growth excess conditions (mandibular prognathism). However, surgical correction during growth is feasible with the expectation of favorable long-term outcomes in certain growth deficiency conditions.[1]

It appears that early orthognathic surgery has little inhibitory effect on facial growth. This would explain the relapse potential when the jaw is moved in the opposite direction of growth, such as mandibular setback in children with prognathism. Some authors have suggested that an early operation may beneficially alter remaining growth by changing the functional milieu and environment of the jaws and associated soft tissues.[12,13] Orthognathic surgery in young patients is safe. Precious et al.[12] retrospectively reported no cases of emergency release of intermaxillary fixation, infection, loss of teeth or bone, or nerve injury in adolescent patients (mean age, 13.9 years; range, 6 to 15 years).

Delaying an operation until maturation does minimize the risk of recurrence in growth excess conditions. However, this approach may not be pragmatic or desirable in specific patients. For example, in a boy with severe skeletal deformities, orthodontic management may be extended throughout high school and into college while awaiting correction. This is not always in the patient's best psychosocial and oral health interests.[1]

EVALUATION

The surgeon must consider the patient and family history when contemplating orthognathic surgery for children and adolescents. In young females, the onset of menses is a helpful guide. Most girls complete growth approximately 2½ to 3 years after menarche. The recent growth history and a change in shoe size may also indicate active general and facial growth. Facial morphology, size, and proportions, as well as occlusal relationships, are frequently consistent within a family. The "Hapsburg jaw" is a classic example of a familial tendency toward a prominent mandible. Similarly, mandibular hypoplasia may be a pattern found among family members. This information helps the surgeon and orthodontist predict growth and make rational treatment decisions.

Serial clinical examinations documented by photographs, cephalograms, hand-wrist films, and dental models are essential to document the rate and vector(s) of growth. Occasionally, computed tomography (CT) scans and skeletal scintigraphy with technetium 99-methylene diphosphonate (planar images or single photon emission computed tomography [SPECT] scans) are indicated to evaluate skeletal maturation.

Accurate diagnosis and careful treatment planning, taking growth into consideration, are critical to achieve a successful result in the pediatric patient undergoing orthognathic surgery. A frank discussion with the child and family regarding the indications, potential risks (particularly the potential need for additional operations), and expectations of the procedure is especially important.

MANDIBULAR RETROGNATHIA

General Considerations

Mild mandibular hypoplasia may be managed by orthodontic maneuvers that camouflage, rather than correct, the skeletal deformity. The success of orthodontic management depends on the extent of mandibular deficiency, amount of remaining maxillary and mandibular growth, patient cooperation, and the type of mechanics used. There are few reasons not to attempt these modalities before surgical correction in some patients, but there is little reason to continue these forms of management if the growth response is not favorable or if the mandibular deficiency is excessive.[1]

Mandibular deficiency is a commonly encountered facial skeletal condition that is amenable to surgical correction in children.[13-15] Precious and colleagues[12] reported that more than 69% of their growing patients who had early orthognathic surgery had class II jaw relations (mandibular hypoplasia). There have been several reports on the stability of mandibular advancement during childhood and its effects on growth.[14-16]

Freihofer[14] reported on a series of seven patients under the age of 17 years who had mandibular advancement by bilateral sagittal split osteotomy (BSSO). The mandible grew another 1.5 to 2 degrees postoperatively. Because this growth was in the same direction as the operative movement, it had no negative effect on the late clinical results. Wolford et al.[15] evaluated 12 actively growing children (age range, 8 to 16 years), a mean of 3.5 years after BSSO, with an average advancement of 5.4 mm. Using serial lateral cephalograms, they reported relapse of less than 5% of the movement. Postoperative growth occurred primarily in a vertical direction. These authors concluded that mandibular advancement can be performed safely and successfully in actively growing patients. Similarly, Snow et al.[16] reported a series of 12 growing patients who had BSSO. Mandibular growth continued postoperatively, and class I occlusion and good facial aesthetics were maintained throughout a 5-year follow-up period. Postoperative facial growth in these patients occurred in a vertical direction; the chin point did not advance. In contrast, Huang and Ross[17] reported on 22 patients who had mandibular advancement at a mean age of 14.1 years and who exhibited no clinically significant postoperative growth of the mandible.

Wolford et al.[18] differentiate between those patients who exhibit mandibular retrognathism with normal versus those with deficient mandibular growth rates. The former group is born with a small mandible or a mandible that is positioned posteriorly relative to the maxilla because of the location of the glenoid fossa. These children have normal and proportionate rates of maxillary and mandibular growth that is unaltered by orthognathic surgical correction. Harmonious postoperative maxillary and mandibular growth can be expected with a stable surgical result. In contrast, progressive worsening of mandibular retrusion and class II malocclusion occur in patients with an inherently deficient mandibular growth rate (e.g., posttraumatic growth deficiency, growth deficiency after radiation therapy, hemifacial microsomia, Treacher Collins syndrome). In these patients, recurrence may occur despite surgical correction of jaw position because of inherently deficient mandibular growth potential.

The consensus in the literature is that mandibular advancement in growing children can be performed safely and with no adverse effect on lower jaw development. It appears that many younger patients have further growth following mandibular advancement. However, most of this growth is expressed vertically and results in minimal forward movement in the dentition and pogonion. Therefore, early mandibular advancement in children with mandibular hypoplasia can be expected to provide a stable clinical result.

Technique

The technique of BSSO in growing patients is similar to that in adults. However, several anatomic differences must be considered. The second and third molar tooth buds and roots may be in close proximity to the vertical cut in the buccal cortex. It may be necessary to remove the third molar tooth bud, but every attempt should be made to maintain the second molar. The location of the vertical osteotomy may need to be changed to avoid these teeth.

The lingula is located more posteriorly and superiorly on the ramus in children than in adults. This may require extension of the medial cut of the osteotomy to the posterior border to give more surface area of contact.[3] In addition, there may be difficulty splitting the mandible because of its elasticity, thinness of the cortical bone, and relatively short posterior vertical mandibular body height.[18] During the mixed dentition, rigid internal fixation may not be possible because of the developing tooth buds (Figures 21-1 to 21-3).

Mandibular advancement may also be accomplished by distraction osteogenesis. This technique provides several advantages in a growing child. The operation is of smaller magnitude than BSSO and is easily accomplished in those 13 to 15 years of age. The corticotomy is made through the third molar tooth bud extraction socket, and the distraction device is placed. For standard orthognathic surgery cases, we use the Leibinger (Leibinger, L.P., Dallas, Tex.) intraoral semi-custom distraction device. This device is fashioned in the operating room by adjusting the length and the bends on the arms that attach to the footplates. The wounds are closed with chromic catgut suture, leaving the anterior arms and the turning mechanism exposed intraorally (Figure 21-4).

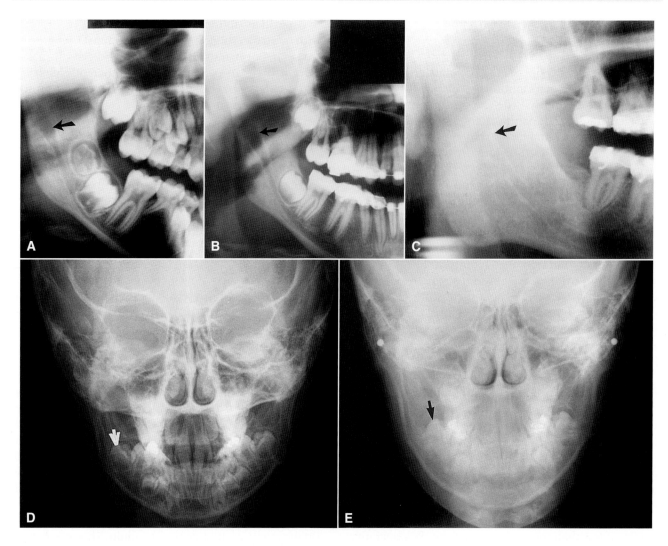

Figure 21-1

Panoramic radiograph of patients 8 years (**A**), 12 years (**B**), and 20 years (**C**) of age demonstrating the relationship of the mandibular foramen *(arrows)* to the posterior border of the mandible. Anteroposterior cephalograms of patients at age 7 years (**D**) and 12 years (**E**) demonstrating the position of the molar teeth in relation to the mandible and inferior alveolar canal.

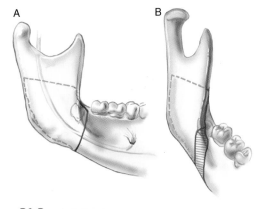

Figure 21-2

A and **B,** Sagittal split osteotomy (see text for details). Note that the medial cut extends to the posterior border of the ramus.

The distraction protocol used at the Massachusetts General Hospital and the Children's Hospital includes a latency period of 48 hours, distraction rhythm of one full turn twice a day, and a rate of 1 mm of advancement per day. If the child cannot tolerate the twice per day rhythm because of discomfort, we have the family do a half turn four times a day instead. The mandible is advanced to an overcorrected, edge-to-edge anterior occlusion, which is finalized during the postoperative orthodontic phase of treatment. The consolidation period is at least twice the number of days as distraction, and healing is confirmed by ultrasound. Specific details on distraction protocol, follow-up, and ultrasound evaluation of the healing wound are provided in Chapters 24 and 25.

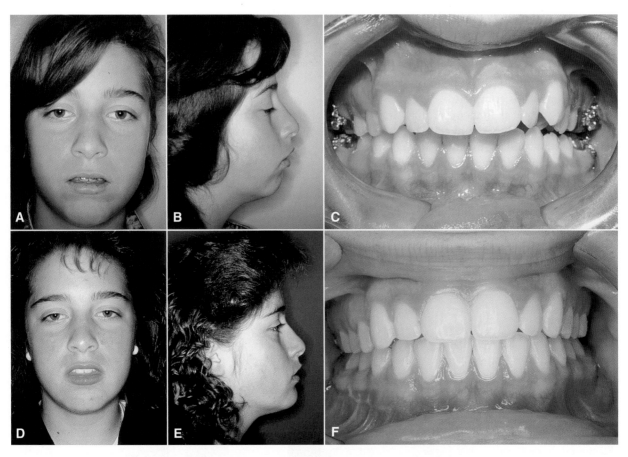

Figure 21-3
Preoperative frontal (**A**), lateral (**B**), and intraoral (**C**) photographs of a 12-year-old girl with mandibular retrognathia. Frontal (**D**), lateral (**E**), and intraoral (**F**) photographs 1 year after bilateral sagittal split osteotomies and completion of orthodontic treatment. The sagittal jaw relations remain stable.

MANDIBULAR PROGNATHISM
General Considerations

Mandibular prognathism is a growth excess condition, and latent postpubertal mandibular growth is seen commonly in patients with this disorder. Delaying an operation until growth is completed is prudent because it minimizes the risk of recurrent class III malocclusion. However, this is not always realistic. In cases of severe prognathism, patients may suffer from problems with psychosocial adjustment, teasing from other children, and speech and masticatory difficulties. In these children and adolescents, surgical correction is indicated before the completion of growth. The parents and child must be educated properly so they understand the benefits of early correction while also understanding the potential need for an additional operation if there is recurrence based on late growth.

Friehofer[14] found considerable occlusal relapse after mandibular setback in adolescent patients. He reported

a 26% reoperation rate for this group. Cook and Hinrichsen[22] had a similar experience and reported relapse in 5 of 34 patients undergoing mandibular set back. All five patients with significant relapse were less than 19 years of age at the time of correction. One of these patients required reoperation at the end of growth.

Wolford and colleagues[18] differentiate between normal and accelerated growth rates in children with mandibular hyperplasia. Those with normal growth maintain the same jaw relations over time. Mandibular growth is initiated from a forward position relative to the maxilla, or the mandible is disproportionately large at birth. In these patients, operative correction does not alter the rate of mandibular growth. Harmonious maxillary and mandibular growth continues postoperatively and a stable surgical correction can be expected. In contrast, patients with an accelerated mandibular growth rate exhibit progressive skeletal and occlusal disharmony and worsening class III jaw and dental relationships with time. This condition often develops during the pubertal growth spurt and may continue after corrective jaw surgery. In these cases, postoperative results are usually unstable and another operation often will be required after growth is complete.

A variety of technical maneuvers may improve the stability of early operative correction of mandibular prognathism. Mandibular osteotomy accompanied by a growth-arresting procedure (high condylectomy) or orthodontic forces (reverse pull head gear) may improve the long-term surgical outcome. Wolford and LeBlanc[20] reported favorable initial results in adolescents with mandibular prognathism who had mandibular setback and bilateral high condylectomies. The use of bimaxillary

surgery, before completion of growth, to treat mandibular prognathism has been proposed. This strategy has proved no more successful than single-jaw surgery.[1] Overcorrection of the occlusion may also be useful, but there is no way to determine the magnitude needed to account for postoperative growth.

It is difficult to determine accurately the cessation of growth in any individual child. A hand-wrist radiograph, serial cephalograms, recorded growth curves and, in special cases, technetium 99-m methylene diphosphonate bone scans are all useful modalities to help predict the appropriate time for an operation. In summary, early skeletal correction is appropriate for the indications noted above, with no danger of untoward effects on subsequent mandibular growth.

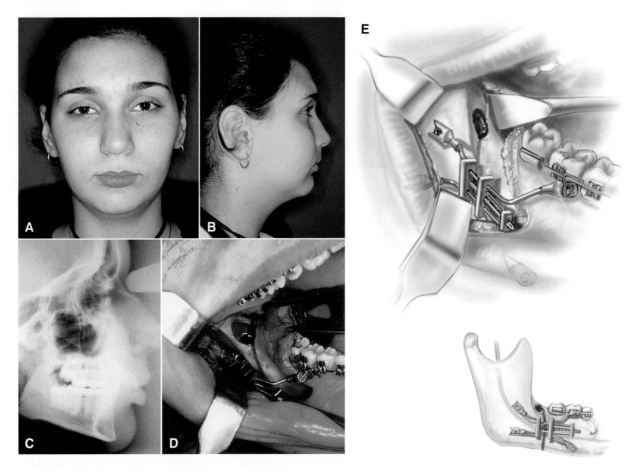

Figure 21-4

A 13-year-old girl with mandibular retrognathism and deep bite treated by distraction osteogenesis. Frontal **(A)** and lateral **(B)** photographs and lateral cephalogram **(C)** of the patient preoperatively in centric relation. Note the retrognathic mandible, approximately 10 mm of overjet, and deep bite. **D,** Intraoperative view of right mandible after third molar had been removed, corticotomy performed, and a Leibinger (Leibinger, L.P., Dallas, Tex.) semiburied distraction device had been fixed to the mandible and teeth. **E,** Diagrammatic representation of intraoperative view.

Continued

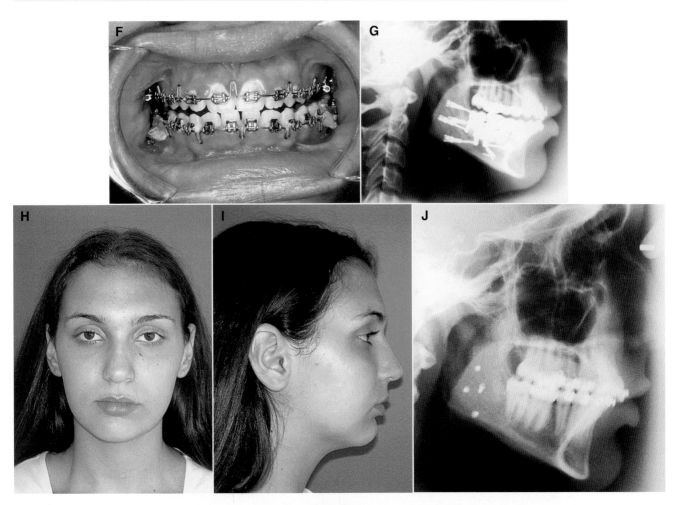

Figure 21-4—continued F, Intraoral view of occlusion at end of distraction. Note that the patient is overcorrected to an edge-to-edge bite. G, Lateral cephalogram at the same time point illustrates the overcorrection. Frontal (H) and lateral (I) photographs and lateral cephalogram (J) 1 year after treatment. Note orthognathic profile and increased lower face height with improved appearance.

Technique

Mandibular prognathism is corrected with a variety of surgical techniques, the most common being the bilateral sagittal split and vertical ramus osteotomies. The technical variations for performing a BSSO in the growing patient were discussed previously. The anatomic differences also apply to the vertical ramus osteotomy so that the cut is usually more posterior than that in an adult. Rigid fixation should be used to control the condylar position and minimize postoperative occlusal difficulties. In young patients, rigid fixation should be applied cautiously to avoid injury to developing teeth[18] (Figure 21-5). Troulis et al.[21] reported an endoscopic approach to the ramus condyle unit for vertical ramus osteotomy. This technique provides minimally invasive access and improved visibility while making the osteotomy and applying rigid internal fixation.

CHIN DEFORMITIES
General Considerations

Deformities of the anterior mandible occur in all three planes (vertical, horizontal, and sagittal), affecting the height, width, and anteroposterior dimensions of the chin. Surgical techniques to correct deformities include osseous recontouring and osteotomies to change the chin position. Both recontouring and osteotomies can be performed with or without bone grafts, bone substitutes, or alloplastic implants.[18] The operation should be chosen to address the patient's specific defect(s) and can be done on a young patient. Although the procedures have no significant effect on subsequent facial growth, the position of the maxilla and mandible may change with growth and influence the final outcome.

In young patients, the developing teeth and inferior alveolar (mental) nerve closely approximate the inferior

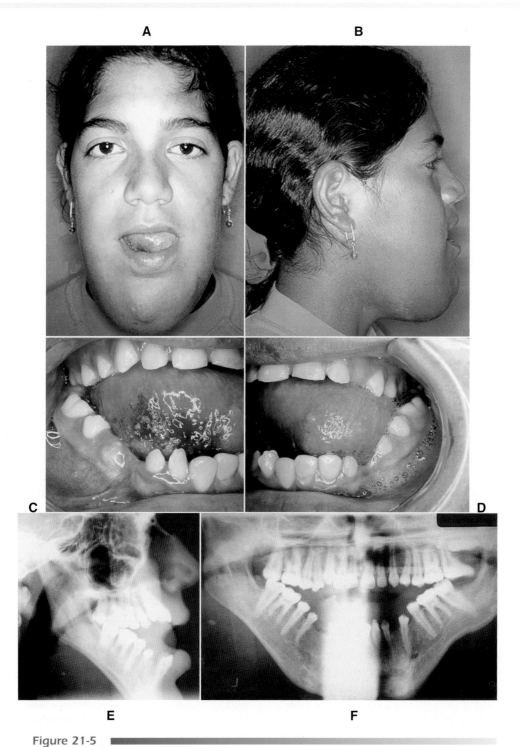

Figure 21-5

A to D, Frontal, lateral, and intraoral photographs of a 13-year-old girl with a large cervicofacial lymphatic malformation, associated mandibular prognathism, and extensive anterior open bite. E and F, Lateral cephalogram and Panorex show obtuse mandibular plane angle, overgrowth of mandibular body, and anterior open bite.

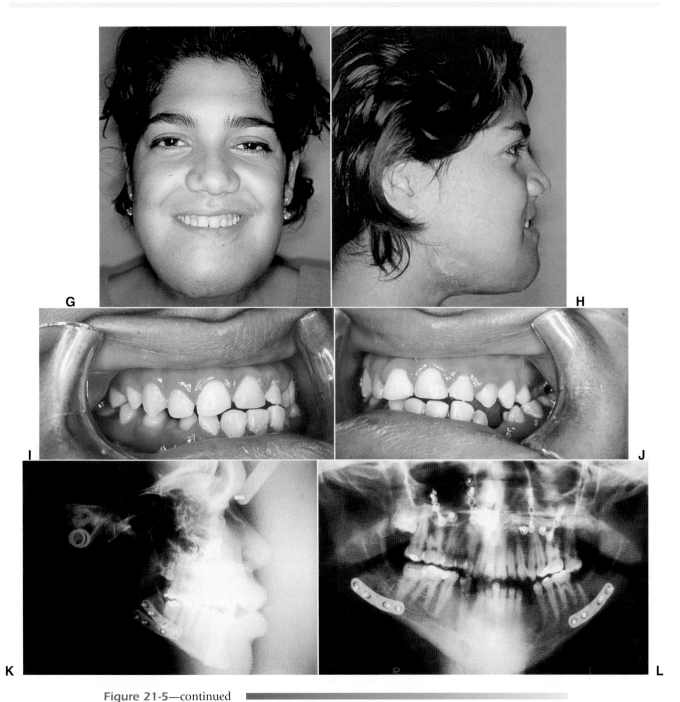

Figure 21-5—continued
G to **J,** Five years after Le Fort I osteotomy, bilateral mandibular body ostectomies, reduction genioplasty, and resection of submandibular lymphatic malformation, the open bite remains closed with improvement in mandibular prognathism. **K** and **L,** Postoperative lateral cephalogram and Panorex show a stable correction of the open bite and improved sagittal relations of the maxilla and mandible.

border of the mandible, placing these structures at risk during an osteotomy. Chin operations, therefore, should be delayed until the patient is 12 years or older so that dentoalveolar development is complete.[18] However, augmentation genioplasty with alloplastic implants can be performed at an earlier age provided the implant can be fixed to the bone without damaging the underlying structures.[18]

Technique

There are a variety of techniques for changing the position of the chin.[22] The sliding horizontal osteotomy can be tailored to treat the patient's specific deformity. The segment can be advanced to augment chin prominence, rotated to correct asymmetry, split to either widen or narrow the symphyseal region, and down-grafted to lengthen the lower face height with an interpositional bone graft. Alternatively, a step osteotomy can be performed to produce the same effect without the need of a bone graft harvested from another site. However, in children this osteotomy may not be possible because of the decreased distance between the inferior border and the mandibular teeth. Rigid fixation with plates and screws can be used in children, but careful attention must be paid to the position of tooth roots and tooth buds.

VERTICAL MAXILLARY HYPERPLASIA
General Considerations

Vertical growth of the maxilla ends after sagittal growth and is generally complete by 12 to 14 years of age. Several authors have addressed the issue of maxillary growth and its effect on skeletal and occlusal stability after Le Fort I osteotomy for correction of vertical maxillary excess.[23-27]

Washburn et al.[23] reported on 16 patients (mean age, 14 years; range, 10 to 16) who underwent repositioning of the maxilla for vertical maxillary excess and were followed for 36.7 months (range, 12 to 78 months). The patients had stable skeletal and occlusal relationships and acceptable esthetic outcomes. They speculated that the disproportionate growth characteristic (clockwise rotation of the mandible and increased mandibular plane angle) of vertical maxillary excess might be affected favorably by early operative intervention.

Proffit and colleagues[24] compared postoperative stability of patients less than 18 years of age at the time of surgery with those who were older. They found no difference in stability between the younger and older groups, and they concluded that the outcome of surgical repositioning of the maxilla during growth is as predictable as it is in adults.

Vig and Turvey[25] examined vertical maxillary growth in 20 subjects, 13.7 to 16.5 years of age, a mean of 3.3 years after surgical repositioning of the maxilla. They used wire osteosynthesis and maxillomandibular fixation in this group of patients. The vertical dimension of the maxilla increased postoperatively, with a statistically significant increase in the vertical position of the maxillary incisors and molars. The growth was primarily in the dentoalveolar segment. Despite this growth, the patients exhibited postoperative occlusal stability. They concluded that the clinical results and patient acceptance justified the early surgical approach.

Mogavero et al.[26] assessed the effects of superior repositioning of the maxilla on adolescent maxillary growth. Forty-eight patients had superior repositioning of the maxilla for correction of vertical maxillary excess: 23 with rigid and 25 with wire fixation. These patients were compared with closely matched unoperated controls. The mean age at operation was 14.5 years for the rigid and 14.6 for the wire fixation group. The follow-up was 1.9 years for the rigid and 2.3 for the wire group. In these patients, the maxilla was advanced and impacted an average of 2 mm in each direction. There were no statistically significant differences in vertical maxillary growth between the two surgical and control groups during the observation period. The authors concluded that Le Fort I osteotomy had little or no effect on vertical maxillary growth. Wolford,[27] on the other hand, observed that the most predictable results were obtained if the operation was performed after age 14 years in girls and age 16 in boys. He speculated that continued vertical growth might produce recurrence of vertical maxillary excess in patients operated on earlier.

Long-term clinical success after surgical correction of vertical maxillary excess, before complete maturation, depends on the mandibular response to continued vertical maxillary growth. If the mandibular ramus does not grow vertically with the maxilla, clockwise rotation of the mandible occurs and the patient begins to appear retrognathic. This is more likely to happen if the presurgical condition includes an anterior open bite. However, if vertical maxillary growth is matched by vertical growth of the mandibular ramus, the patient maintains an orthognathic profile and proper overbite.[1]

Mojdehi and colleagues[28] studied the mandibular growth response to superior maxillary repositioning by Le Fort I osteotomy in adolescents. Postoperatively they found no change in the vertical growth pattern, the mandible rotated backward, and there was no inhibition of mandibular growth. They concluded that early maxillary impaction does not normalize or inhibit the existing vertical growth pattern and that the mandible undergoes adaptive changes in response to maxillary repositioning.

Technique

Le Fort I osteotomy in growing patients should be delayed until after the eruption of the maxillary canines and second molars. This allows the surgeon to perform the appropriate osteotomy without damaging the teeth[3] (Figures 21-6 and 21-7). The technique does not differ from that in adults.

SECONDARY CLEFT LIP AND PALATE MAXILLARY HYPOPLASIA

Oronasal Fistula and Alveolar Cleft

The goals of operative closure of oronasal fistulas and bone grafting alveolar clefts are (1) to separate the oral and nasal cavities, (2) to stabilize and consolidate the maxilla with a bony union, (3) to provide adequate bone for the central incisor and canine teeth and to support the alar base, and (4) to provide adequate bone volume in the lateral incisor position to support a dental implant. Alveolar bone grafting in infancy has been associated with inhibition of midface growth, whereas patients treated after age 9 years show little growth inhibition. Therefore, the consensus is to close the oronasal fistula and bone graft the alveolar cleft with autogenous iliac bone marrow during the late mixed dentition (canine root one-half to two-thirds formed).

In patients with bilateral complete cleft lip and palate, the position of the premaxilla and its relation to the lip and nose must be evaluated. When the premaxilla is severely protrusive and inferiorly displaced, surgical premaxillary repositioning may be necessary during the mixed dentition or as part of a multiple segment Le Fort I osteotomy in teenagers (Figures 21-8 and 21-9). However, some authors report that the protrusive premaxilla becomes more retrusive by the time the child reaches the permanent dentition stage and therefore repositioning is never indicated.[29]

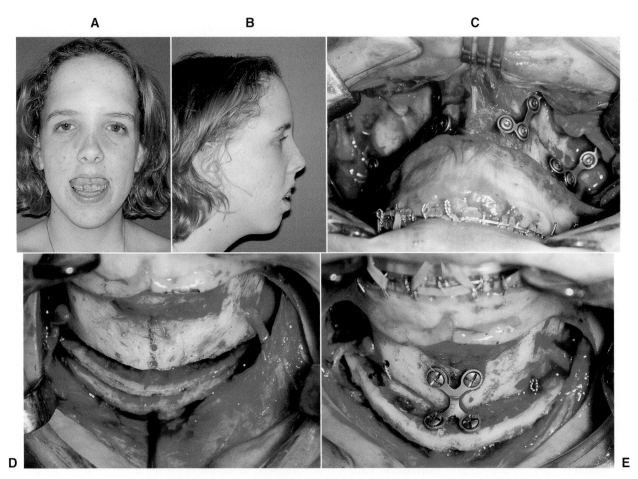

A   B   C

D   E

Figure 21-6
Frontal resting (**A**) and lateral (**B**) photographs of a teenager with vertical maxillary excess as part of Marfan syndrome. Note also the mandibular retrognathia. **C**, Intraoperative view of Le Fort I osteotomy with rigid internal fixation after 7 mm of impaction and shortening, advancement genioplasty (**D** and **E**) with removal of a wedge of bone.

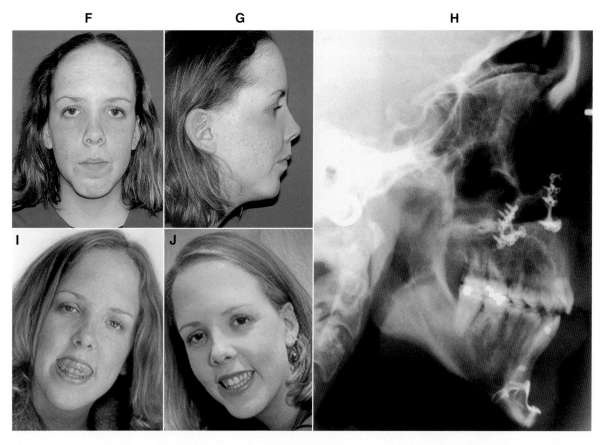

Figure 21-6—continued
Frontal (**F**) and lateral (**G**) photographs 1 year postoperatively. Note the improved esthetic result and much improved lip competence. **H**, Lateral cephalogram demonstrates some reopening of the bite because of dental tipping. Preoperative school photograph (**I**) and graduation photograph (**J**) 2 years postoperatively. Note the marked esthetic improvement in facial proportions and chin projection.

Premaxillary setback in infancy or early mixed dentition has been associated with a decrease in forward growth of the premaxilla and the development of midface retrusion.[30] On the other hand, Padwa and colleagues[31] found that a protrusive premaxilla can be repositioned after age 6 to 8 years without deleterious effects on midfacial growth (Figure 21-9).

Maxillary Hypoplasia

A significant number of patients with cleft lip and palate develop maxillary hypoplasia. This three-dimensional deficiency results in class III malocclusion (sagittal plane), narrowed arch (horizontal plane), inadequate tooth show, and overclosure of the mandible (vertical plane). Many factors contribute to poor maxillary growth in patients with clefts. Herber and Lehman[32] suggest that there is no intrinsic deficiency in these patients but that prior surgical procedures inhibit maxillary growth. Mechanical molding action of the muscles; tight, scarred tissues from earlier surgical repairs; and the presence of a pharyngeal flap may all contribute to deficient growth and development of the cleft maxilla.[33,34]

The reported incidence of maxillary hypoplasia in patients with clefts varies by author. Bardach et al.[35] noted only 4% of patients with clefts required orthognathic correction. Ross,[36] Rosenstein et al.,[37] Cohen et al.,[38] and DeLuke et al.,[39] reported that 22% to 26% of patients with clefts had dentofacial deformities requiring orthognathic correction. Le Fort I osteotomy to advance and inferiorly position the maxilla is more common in the later series. More aggressive management of dentoskeletal deformities rather than an absolute increase in incidence may explain this difference.[38]

Treatment of maxillary hypoplasia by the traditional orthognathic surgical approach necessitates delay until skeletal maturity. Freihofer[14] found unacceptable outcomes in 71% of patients who had Le Fort I osteotomy before 16 years of age and in 46% of those operated

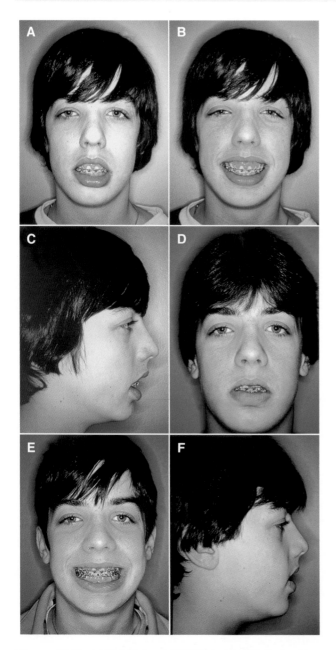

Figure 21-7

Frontal **(A)**, smiling **(B)**, and lateral **(C)** photographs of a 13-year-old boy with extreme maxillary excess. Frontal **(D)**, smiling **(E)**, and lateral **(F)** photographs 1 year after 10 mm maxillary impaction with turbinectomy, demonstrating improved facial proportions.

on between 16 and 17 years of age. Pseudorelapse, caused by continued mandibular growth after maxillary advancement, occurred in 75% of his patients. Transverse relapse occurred in 25% to 50% of patients, regardless of whether the maxillary arch was expanded before or at the time of advancement. In total, 55%

of these patients required reoperation. Therefore, Freihofer[14] recommended delaying Le Fort I osteotomy until eruption of the permanent dentition and completion of growth.

Some children with cleft lip and palate have severe midfacial hypoplasia that is apparent early in life. These patients may develop severe psychosocial problems and therefore would benefit from midface advancement before skeletal maturation. This can be accomplished by distraction osteogenesis. With a relatively minor procedure there can be dramatic improvement in facial morphology and dental relations at an early age.[40] As sagittal jaw discrepancy increases in adolescence, final presurgical orthodontics and Le Fort I osteotomy may be required. This may involve a smaller movement than if treatment had been delayed and the patient has had the benefits of the early correction (Figure 21-10).

In patients with clefts, scarred palatal soft tissues may resist maxillary advancement by conventional surgical techniques. However, incremental movement using distraction osteogenesis facilitates gradual advancement of the skeleton over large distances because the soft tissue can accommodate gradually.[41] Altuna et al.[42] applied and tested the principle of distraction osteogenesis on the maxillas of primates. This study and others showed that this technique could be applied successfully to the maxilla.[43,44]

Molina et al.[45] were the first to use distraction osteogenesis in patients with cleft lip and palate and maxillary hypoplasia. A Le Fort I osteotomy was made and an external reverse headgear with elastic traction was used to gradually advance the maxillary segment. Polley and Figueroa[40] used an external, adjustable, rigid distraction device placed at the time of Le Fort I osteotomy. Active distraction was started on the third or fourth postoperative day at a rate of 1 mm/day until the desired amount of maxillary movement (both vertical and horizontal) was achieved. The neutral fixation period was 2 to 3 weeks, and then the device was removed in the office. Night-time retention with a removable orthodontic face mask and elastic traction (12 to 16 oz) was used for 6 weeks postoperatively. Cohen[46] used a partially buried distraction device to distract the maxilla forward in patients with cleft lip and palate and maxillary hypoplasia.

Maxillary distraction osteogenesis can also be used in adolescent patients to overcome the scarred soft tissues, restriction of a pharyngeal flap, and soft tissue resistance to large movements. In these patients, the distraction device can be used to advance the maxilla and for retention. It may be more practical, in adolescent patients, to remove the device before complete consolidation and to secure the maxilla in its predetermined position with rigid internal fixation.[47] If a mandibular osteotomy for prognathism is required, it can be performed at this time.

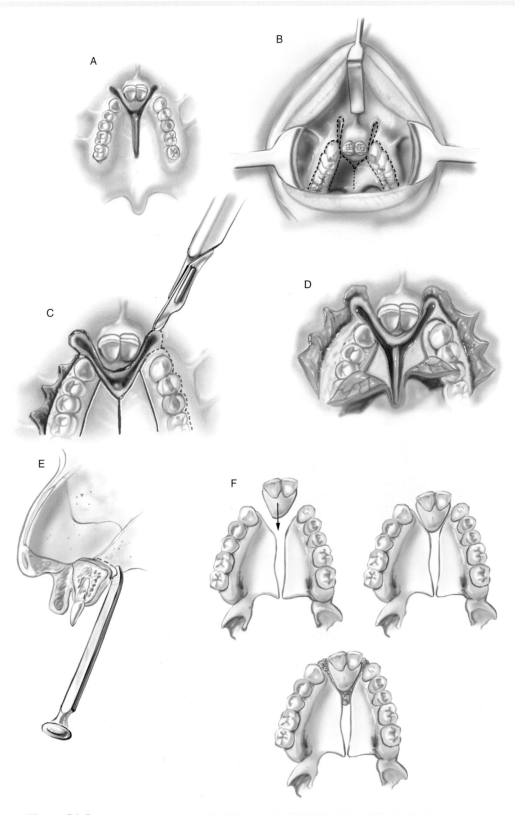

Figure 21-8 ▬▬▬▬▬▬
A, Occlusal view of a patient with bilateral cleft lip and palate with residual oronasal fistula.
B, Same view with incisions outlined. Note that the fistulas are incised around the entire
circumference. **C** and **D,** The fistulas are dissected, and the nasal lining is sutured. **E,** Osteotomy
of the premaxilla (if necessary; see Figure 21-9) is done from the palatal side, and the segment
is repositioned. **F,** Bone grafts are placed, and the oral side is then closed with advancement
flaps or buccal rotation flaps.

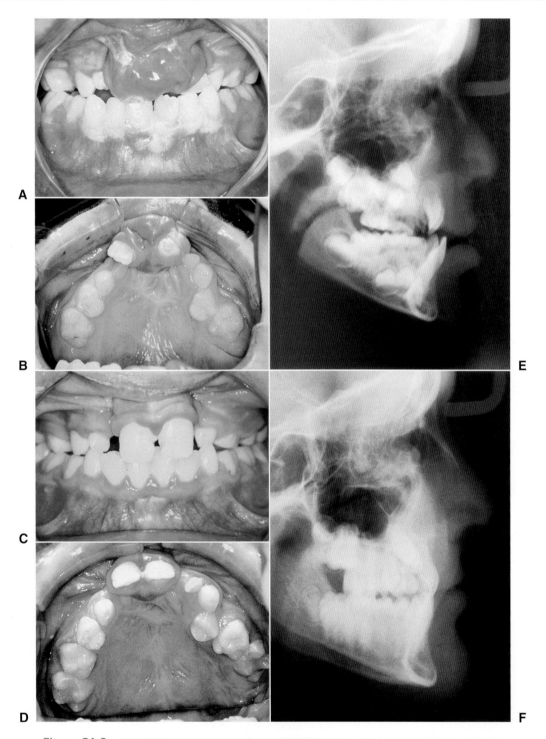

Figure 21-9

A 10-year-old boy with a repaired bilateral cleft lip and palate. **A** and **B,** Intraoral views demonstrate the anteriorly and inferiorly displaced premaxilla. **C,** Preoperative lateral cephalogram. **D** and **E,** Intraoral views after the premaxilla was superiorly repositioned, fistulas closed, and an iliac crest bone graft placed. The alignment of the premaxilla has improved. **F,** Postoperative lateral cephalogram 1 year after the procedure documents the improved position of the premaxilla.

When correction of maxillary deficiency at the Le Fort I level is indicated before cessation of growth, the operation should be delayed until the permanent canines and second molars have erupted. If a Le Fort I osteotomy is done before eruption of these teeth, the osteotomy should be placed at the highest level possible to minimize damage to the permanent dentition.

Absent Lateral Incisor

The incidence of an absent maxillary lateral incisor on the cleft side is 51.8%.[48] The incisor can be replaced by orthodontic closure of the space with forward move-ment of the canine into the lateral incisor position, or with a removable or fixed prosthesis. Orthodontic movement of the canine into the lateral incisor position can result in transverse maxillary deficiency and a poor esthetic result due to lack of symmetry with the noncleft side. Fabrication of a removable or fixed restoration to replace the lateral incisor may not be esthetically acceptable if there is a contour defect of the alveolar ridge. Additionally, fabrication of a fixed bridge requires preparation of healthy adjacent teeth. Closure of the lateral incisor space can also be accomplished with a multisegment Le Fort I osteotomy at the time of maxillary advancement (Figures 21-11 and 21-12).

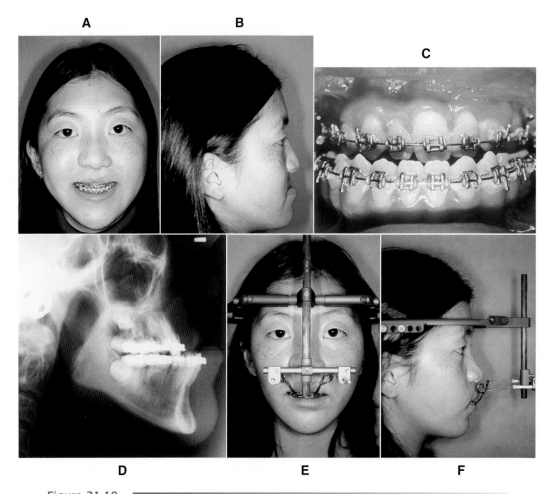

Figure 21-10

Frontal (A), lateral (B), and intraoral (C) photographs and lateral cephalogram (D) of a 13-year-old girl with left unilateral complete cleft lip and palate and severe maxillary hypoplasia who had lip and palate repair in infancy—pharyngeal flap at age 7 and palatal expansion and alveolar cleft grafting at age 10. Frontal (E) and lateral (F) photographs after Le Fort I osteotomy and placement of external distraction device. Distraction started on fifth postoperative day at a rate of 1 mm a day for 16 days. The device was removed in the office 5 weeks later.

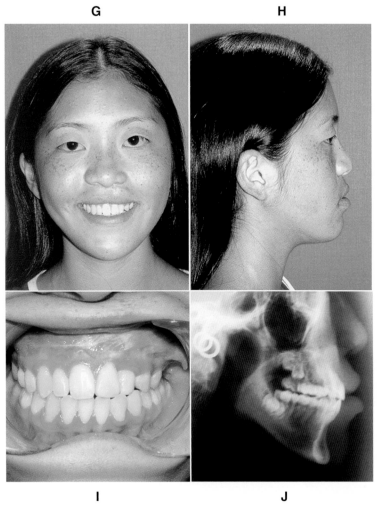

Figure 21-10—continued
Frontal (**G**), lateral (**H**), and intraoral (**I**) photographs 1 year later show improved esthetics, and the lateral cephalogram (**J**) demonstrates the stable correction.

Replacement of the lateral incisor with an osseointegrated implant is a desirable alternative approach. Verdi et al.[49] were the first to describe the successful use of an endosseous implant to restore the edentulous alveolar cleft region. Takahashi et al.[50] reported results of 21 implants placed in 19 previously bone-grafted alveolar clefts. There was sufficient bone in all but five patients who required a secondary bone graft. The overall survival rate for these implants was 90.5% during the follow-up period, ranging from 1 to 3 years.

Although the alveolar cleft may have been grafted previously, there may be inadequate bone for an implant and a supplemental bone graft may be necessary. Kearns et al.[51] studied the optimal timing of placement of endosseous implants in bone-grafted alveolar clefts. They found that the interval between bone graft and implant placement was important. The greater the interval beyond 4 months, the more likely that there would be inadequate bone volume to accept an implant. The optimal time for implant placement was 3 months after the bone graft (Figures 21-11 to 21-13).

Conclusion

As a general rule, skeletal correction, orthodontic intervention, and final prosthetic rehabilitation should be completed before soft tissue revisions and rhinoplasty are considered. Schendel and Delaire[52] performed nasal correction synchronously with labial revision and maxillary advancement. However, Marsh[53] suggests that definitive rhinoplasty should be deferred until 6 months after maxillary advancement. This allows the

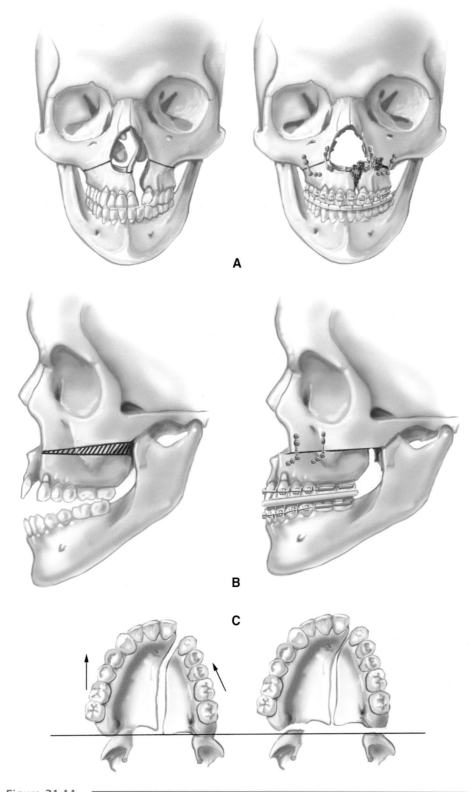

Figure 21-11

Frontal (**A**), lateral (**B**), and palatal (**C**) views of Le Fort I in two segments for advancement, anterior lengthening, and reduction of the dental gap with closure of the oronasal fistula and bone graft to the alveolar cleft.

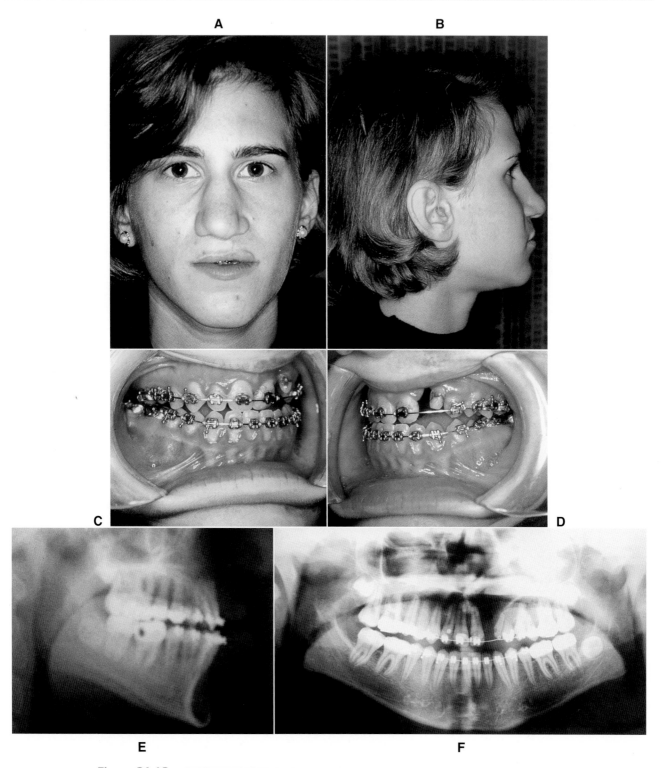

Figure 21-12
Frontal **(A)**, lateral **(B)**, and intraoral **(C and D)** photographs of a 16-year-old girl with a left unilateral complete cleft lip and palate. The lateral cephalogram **(E)** shows the retruded maxilla, and the panoramic radiograph **(F)** demonstrates the aveolar cleft. The space is significantly larger than a lateral incisor.

Continued

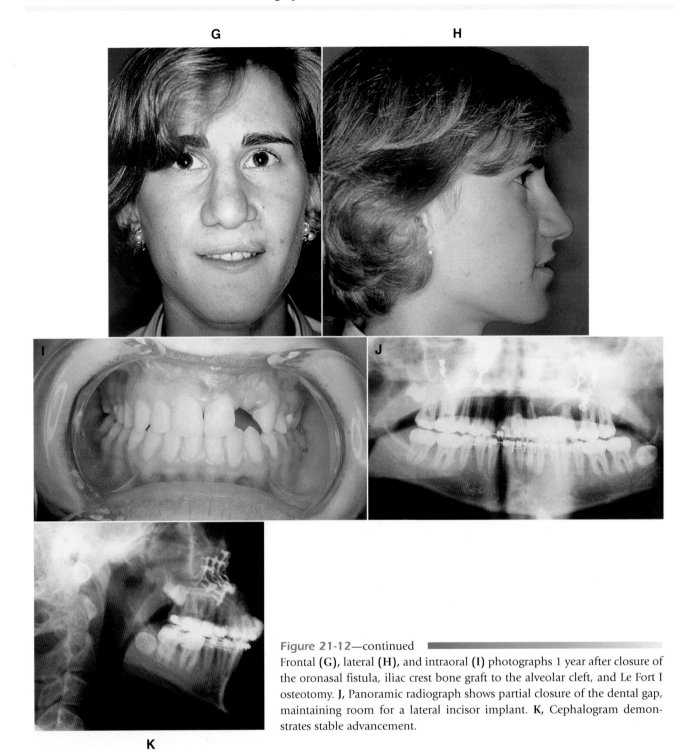

G

H

I

J

Figure 21-12—continued

Frontal (**G**), lateral (**H**), and intraoral (**I**) photographs 1 year after closure of the oronasal fistula, iliac crest bone graft to the alveolar cleft, and Le Fort I osteotomy. **J**, Panoramic radiograph shows partial closure of the dental gap, maintaining room for a lateral incisor implant. **K**, Cephalogram demonstrates stable advancement.

K

surgeon and patient to evaluate the changes in the nose and lip as a result of the dentoskeletal movement. Definitive nasolabial revision can then be planned accordingly.

Ferrario and colleagues[54] found that nasal growth in cleft patients was almost complete by the age of 13 in girls and several years later in boys. Genecov et al.[55] reported that soft tissue nasal growth continues in both sexes after skeletal growth has subsided, being relatively independent of the underlying hard tissue structures. Therefore, correction of the nasal deformity in patients with clefts should be deferred until after early maxillary advancement by either conventional surgery or distraction osteogenesis. Final nasal correction

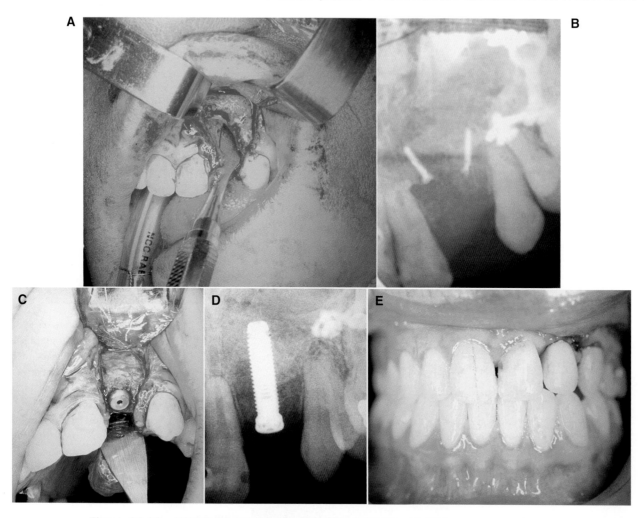

Figure 21-13

Same patient as shown in Figure 21-12, 2 years later. **A,** A bony defect is present in the previously grafted alveolar cleft. **B,** A supplemental bone graft from the chin was secured with screws. **C** and **D,** Three months later the screws were removed, and an implant was placed. **E,** Final occlusion with implant replacement of the maxillary incisor.

should also be delayed until after Le Fort I osteotomy in those patients undergoing maxillary advancement in late adolescence.

CRANIOSYNOSTOSIS
General Considerations

Patients with syndromic craniosynostosis have little downward and forward growth of the midface after the mixed dentition stage, and they develop relative mandibular prognathism.[56] The argument for early midface advancement is that a well-interdigitated occlusion is the key to stability and normal growth.[57] However, many researchers reported that after Le Fort III advancement in children there was little growth of the midface.[58,59] It appears that Le Fort III osteotomy in pediatric patients has neither adverse nor favorable

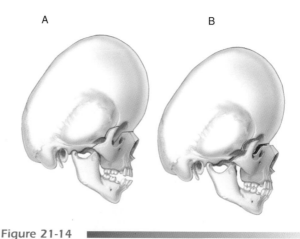

Figure 21-14

A, Diagram of subcranial Le Fort III osteotomy. **B,** After midface distraction bony callus forms in nasofrontal, lateral orbit, zygomatic arch, and between tuberosity and pterygoid plates.

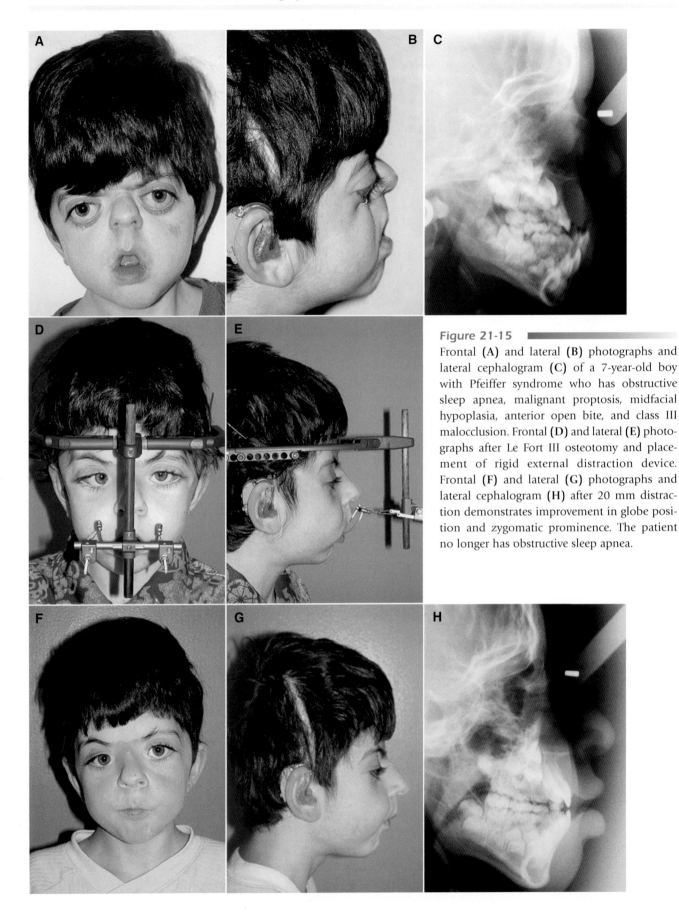

Figure 21-15

Frontal **(A)** and lateral **(B)** photographs and lateral cephalogram **(C)** of a 7-year-old boy with Pfeiffer syndrome who has obstructive sleep apnea, malignant proptosis, midfacial hypoplasia, anterior open bite, and class III malocclusion. Frontal **(D)** and lateral **(E)** photographs after Le Fort III osteotomy and placement of rigid external distraction device. Frontal **(F)** and lateral **(G)** photographs and lateral cephalogram **(H)** after 20 mm distraction demonstrates improvement in globe position and zygomatic prominence. The patient no longer has obstructive sleep apnea.

effects on midfacial growth and no adverse effects on mandibular growth.[60,61] If the midface deficiency is severe and the patient has malignant proptosis, obstructive sleep apnea, or significant psychosocial concerns a Le Fort III osteotomy may be done while the child is growing. The family must be informed that the patient may develop recurrent midface retrusion and class III occlusion as the mandible grows normally beyond the corrected midface. Additional surgical procedures including Le Fort III osteotomy, Le Fort I osteotomy, or mandibular setback might be required.

The technique of distraction osteogenesis has been applied to the midface with excellent results and has had a major impact on the treatment of children with syndromic craniosynostosis.[62,63] The technique is associated with less operative time, less morbidity (e.g., blood loss), and a shorter hospital stay when compared with conventional operative procedures. The magnitude of midface advancement that can be obtained with distraction has been reported to be three times greater than that with standard Le Fort III osteotomy.[63] Additionally, the postoperative stability and correction of respiratory disturbances is much improved with this technique. The final position of the midface should be set with the inferior orbital rim and malar complex in mind.

Because of the technical considerations noted above, surgeons have begun to use distraction to advance the midface in young children more frequently.[64,65] A conventional Le Fort III osteotomy performed early in life (deciduous dentition stage) is likely to be inadequate after the completion of facial skeletal growth. Recurrent class III occlusion is common in this setting.[66,67] Midface advancement with distraction osteogenesis may allow enough overcorrection so that the need for a repeat Le Fort III osteotomy in the teenage years is diminished. The Le Fort III distraction is performed to correct deficient growth in the upper midface and is not meant to correct dental arch discrepancies. Le Fort I osteotomy will likely be necessary to maximize occlusal relationships (Figures 21-14 and 21-15) at a later time.

Technique

The standard subcranial midface advancement is illustrated in Figure 21-12.

CONCLUSION

This chapter reviews the indications and techniques for facial skeletal correction in childhood, emphasizing the effects on facial growth. Since the first edition of this book, the techniques of rigid internal fixation and distraction osteogenesis have improved greatly the armamentarium of the surgeon for correction of skeletal

deficiencies during childhood. In the future, the concept of prevention of deformities and growth modification by nonsurgical techniques may further increase the possibilities for treatment of craniomaxillofacial skeletal anomalies.

REFERENCES

1. Turvey TA, Simmons K: Orthognathic surgery before completion of growth, *Oral Maxillofac Surg Clin North Am* 6:121, 1994.
2. Kaban LB: Surgical correction of the facial skeleton in childhood. In Kaban LB, editor: *Pediatric oral and maxillofacial surgery*, Philadelphia, 1990, WB Saunders.
3. Bell WH, Proffit WR, White RP: *Surgical correction of dentofacial deformities*, Philadelphia, 1980, WB Saunders.
4. Tessier P, Delaire J, Bittel J, et al: Consideration sur le development de l'orbite; ses incidences sur la croissance faciale, *Rev Stomat (Paris)* 66:27, 1965.
5. Meng HP, Goorhuis J, Kapila S, et al: Growth changes in the nasal profile from 7 to 18 years of age, *Am J Orthod Dentofacial Orthop* 94:317, 1988.
6. Singh IJ, Savara BS: Norm of size and annual increments of seven anatomical measures of maxillae in girls from three to sixteen years of age, *Angle Orthod* 36:312, 1966.
7. Savara BS, Singh IJ: Norms of size and annual increments of seven anatomical measures of maxillae in boys from three to sixteen years of age, *Angle Orthod* 38:104, 1968.
8. Buschang PH, Tanguay R, Turkewicz J, et al: Polynomial approach to craniofacial growth: description and comparison of adolescent males with normal occlusion and those with untreated class II malocclusion, *Am J Orthod Dentofacial Orthop* 90:437, 1986.
9. Green LF: Interrelationship among height, weight and chronological, dental and skeletal ages, *Angle Orthod* 31:189, 1961.
10. Knowles CC: Long-term results of mandibular osteotomy: an interim report on the treatment of young subjects, *Dent Pract Dent Rec* 20:318, 1970.
11. Moss ML: Vertical growth in the human face, *Am J Orthodont* 50:359, 1964.
12. Precious DS, McFadden LR, Fitch SJ: Orthognathic surgery for children: analysis of 88 consecutive cases, *Int J Oral Surg* 14:466, 1985.
13. Schendel SA, Wolford LM, Epker BN: Mandibular deficiency syndrome. III. Surgical advancement of the deficient mandible in growing children: treatment in twelve patients, *J Oral Surg* 45:364, 1978.
14. Freihofer HP: Results of osteotomies of the facial skeleton in adolescence, *J Maxillofac Surg* 5:267, 1977.
15. Wolford LM, Schendel SA, Epker BN: Surgical-orthodontic correction of mandibular deficiency in growing children: long-term treatment results, *J Maxillofac Surg* 7:61, 1979.
16. Snow M, Turvey TA, Waller D: Surgical mandibular advancement in adolescents: postsurgical growth related to stability, *Int J Adult Orthodon Orthognath Surg* 64:143, 1991.
17. Huang CS, Ross RB: Surgical advancement of the mandible in growing children, *Am J Orthod* 82:89, 1981.
18. Wolford LM, Spiro CK, Mehra P: Consideration for orthognathic surgery during growth. I. Mandibular deformities, *Am J Orthod Dentofacial Orthop* 119:95, 2001.
19. Thurmueller P, Troulis MJ, Rosenberg A, Kaban LB: Changes in the condyle and disk in response to distraction osteogenesis of the minipig mandible, *J Oral Maxillofac Surg* 60:1327, 2002.
20. Wolford LM, LeBlanc JP: Condylectomies to assist disproportionate class III mandibular growth. Presented at the 43rd meeting of the American Cleft Palate Association, Poster Session, New York City, 1986, p 27.

21. Troulis MJ, Kearns GJ, Perrott DH, Kaban LB: Extended genioplasty: long term cephalometric, morphometric and sensory results, *Int J Oral Maxillofac Surg* 29:167, 2000.

22. Cook RM, Hinrichsen G: The mandibular sagittal split osteotomy: a clinical and cephalometric review, *Trans Congr Int Assoc Oral Surg* 4:252, 1973.

23. Washburn MC, Schendel SA, Epker BN: Superior repositioning of the maxilla during growth, *J Oral Maxillofac Surg* 40:142, 1982.

24. Proffit WR, Phillips C, Tulloch JFC: Surgical versus orthodontic correction of skeletal class II malocclusion in adolescents: effects and indications, *Int J Adult Orthodon Orthognath Surg* 7:209, 1992.

25. Vig KWL, Turvey TA: Surgical correction of vertical maxillary excess during adolescence, *Int J Adult Orthodon Orthognath Surg* 4:119, 1989.

26. Mogavero FJ, Buschang PH, Wolford LM: Orthognathic surgery effects on maxillary growth in patients with vertical maxillary excess, *Am J Orthod Dentofacial Orthop* 111:288, 1997.

27. Wolford LM, Karras SC, Mehra P: Considerations for orthognathic surgery during growth, part 2: maxillary deformities, *Am J Orthod Dentofacial Orthop* 119:102, 2001.

28. Mojdehi M, Buschang PH, English JD, et al: Postsurgical growth changes in the mandible of adolescents with vertical maxillary excess growth patterns, *Am J Orthod Dentofacial Orthop* 119:106, 2001.

29. Vargervik K: Growth characteristics of the premaxilla and orthodontic treatment principles in bilateral *cleft lip and palate,* Cleft Palate J 20:289, 1983.

30. Friede H, Pruzansky S: Long-term effects of premaxillary setback on facial skeletal profile in complete bilateral cleft lip and palate, *Cleft Palate J* 22:97, 1985.

31. Padwa BL, Sonis A, Bagheri S, et al: Children with repaired bilateral cleft lip/palate: effect of age at premaxillary osteotomy on facial growth, *Plast Reconstr Surg* 104:1261, 1999.

32. Herber SC, Lehman JA: Orthognathic surgery in the cleft lip and palate patient, *Clin Plast Surg* 20:755, 1993.

33. Cheung LK, Samman N, Hui E, et al: The 3-dimensional stability of maxillary osteotomies in cleft palate patients with residual alveolar clefts, *Br J Oral Maxillofac Surg* 32:6-11, 1994.

34. Vig KWL, Turvey TA: Orthodontic-surgical interaction in the management of cleft lip and palate, *Clin Plast Surg* 12:735, 1985.

35. Bardach J, Morris H, Olin W, et al: Late results of multidisciplinary management of unilateral cleft lip and palate, *Ann Plast Surg* 12:235, 1984.

36. Ross RB: Treatment variables affecting facial growth in complete unilateral cleft lip and palate, *Cleft Palate J* 24:5, 1987.

37. Rosenstein S, Kernahan D, Dado D, et al: Orthognathic surgery in cleft patients treated by early bone grafting, *Plast Reconstr Surg* 87:835, 1991.

38. Cohen SR, Corrigan M, Wilmot J, et al: Cumulative operative procedures in patients aged 14 years and older with unilateral or bilateral cleft lip and palate, *Plast Reconstr Surg* 96:267, 1995.

39. DeLuke DM, Marchand A, Robles EC, et al: Facial growth and the need for orthognathic surgery after cleft palate repair: literature review and report of 28 cases, *J Oral Maxillofac Surg* 55:694, 1997.

40. Polley JW, Figueroa AA: Management of severe maxillary deficiency in childhood and adolescence through distraction osteogenesis with an external, adjustable, rigid distraction device, *J Craniofac Surg* 8:181, 1997.

41. Chin M, Toth BA: Distraction osteogenesis in maxillofacial surgery using internal devices: review of five cases, *J Oral Maxillofac Surg* 54:45, 1996.

42. Altuna G, Walker DA, Freeman E: Surgically assisted rapid orthodontic lengthening of the maxilla in primates—a pilot study, *Am J Ortho Dentofac Orthop* 107:531, 1995.

43. Rachmiel A, Potparic Z, Jackson IT: Midface advancement by gradual distraction, *Br J Plast Surg* 46:201, 1993.

44. Staffenberg DA, Wood RJ, McCarthy JG, et al: Midface distraction advancement in the canine without osteotomies, *Ann Plast Surg* 34:512, 1995.

45. Molina F, Ortiz Monasterio F: Maxillary distraction: three years of clinical experience. In Proceedings of the 65th Annual Scientific Meeting of the American Society of Plastic and Reconstructive Surgeons, Plastic Surgical Forum, Vol. XIX. 1996:54.

46. Cohen SR, Burstein FD, Stewart MB, et al: Maxillary-midface distraction in children with cleft lip and palate: a preliminary report, *Plast Reconstr Surg* 99:1421, 1997.

47. Wong GB, Padwa BL: Le Fort I soft tissue distraction: a hybrid technique, *J Craniofac Surg* 13:572, 2002.

48. Tsai TP, Huang CS, Huang CC, et al: Distribution patterns of primary and permanent dentition in children with unilateral complete cleft lip and palate, *Cleft Palate Craniofac J* 35:154, 1998.

49. Verdi F, Lanzi G, Cohen S, et al: Use of the Branemark implant in the cleft palate patient, *Cleft Palate Craniofac J* 28:301, 1991.

50. Takahashi T, Fukuda M, Yamaguchi T, et al: Use of endosseous implants for dental reconstruction of patients with grafted alveolar clefts, *J Oral Maxillofac Surg* 55:576, 1997.

51. Kearns G, Perrott DH, Sharma A, et al: Placement of endosseous implants in grafted alveolar clefts, *Cleft Palate Craniofac J* 34:520, 1997.

52. Schendel SA, Delaire J: Functional musculoskeletal correction of secondary unilateral cleft lip deformities: combined lip-nose correction and Le Fort I osteotomy, *J Maxillofac Surg* 9:108, 1981.

53. Marsh JL, Galic M: Maxillofacial osteotomies for patients with cleft lip and palate, *Clin Plast Surg* 16:803, 1989.

54. Ferrario VG, Sforza C, Poggio CE, et al: Three-dimensional study of growth and development of the nose, *Cleft Palate Craniofac J* 34:309, 1997.

55. Genecov JS, Sinclair PM, Dechow PC: Development of the nose and soft tissue profile, *Angle Orthod* 60:191, 1990.

56. Kreiborg S, Aduss H: Pre- and postsurgical facial growth in patients with Crouzon's and Apert's syndromes, *Cleft Palate J* 23(Suppl 1):78, 1986.

57. Munro IR: The effect of total maxillary advancement on facial growth, *Plast Reconstr Surg* 62:751, 1978.

58. Bachmayer DI, Ross RB, Munro IR: Maxillary growth following Le Fort III advancement surgery in Crouzon, Apert, and Pfeiffer syndromes, *Am J Orthod Dentofacial Orthop* 90:420, 1986.

59. Carthy JG, LaTrenta GS, Breitbart AS, et al: The Le Fort III advancement osteotomy in the child under 7 years of age, *Plast Reconstr Surg* 86:633, 1990.

60. Bu BH, Kaban LB, Vargevik K: Effect of Le Fort III osteotomy on mandibular growth in patients with Crouzon and Apert syndromes, *J Oral Maxillofac Surg* 47:666-671, 1989.

61. Kaban LB, West B, Conover M, et al: Midface position after Le Fort III advancement, *Plast Reconstr Surg* 73:758, 1984.

62. Cedars MG, Linch DL, Chin M, et al: Advancement of the midface using distraction techniques, *Plast Reconstr Surg* 103:429, 1999.

63. Fearon JA: The Le Fort III osteotomy: to distract or not distract? *Plast Reconstr Surg* 107:1091, 2001.

64. Toth BA, Kim JW, Chin M, et al: Distraction osteogenesis and its application to the midface and bony orbit in craniosynostosis syndromes, *J Craniofac Surg* 9:100, 1998.

65. Swennen G, Schliephake H, Dempf R, et al: Craniofacial distraction osteogenesis: a review of the literature: part 1: clinical studies, *Int J Oral Maxillofac Surg* 30:89, 2001.

66. Kaban LB, Conover M, Mulliken JB: Midface position after Le Fort III advancement: a long-term follow-up study, *Cleft Palate J* 23(Suppl 1):75, 1986.

67. Ousterhout DK, Vargervik K, Clark S: Stability of the maxilla after Le Fort III advancement in craniosynostosis syndromes, *Cleft Palate J* 23(Suppl 1):91, 1986.

CHAPTER 22

Microtia and Ear Reconstruction in Children

Roland D. Eavey

The coexistence of jaw and ear malformations is well recognized in patients who have first and second pharyngeal arch syndromes such as Treacher Collins and hemifacial microsomia. Perhaps less appreciated is the rather high incidence of a spectrum of mandibular anomalies in patients who come to the pediatrician and auricular surgeon with "isolated" microtia.[1] It is important that the association between ear and jaw anomalies and the full range of first and second pharyngeal arch deformities be understood. Because congenital mandibular anomalies generally worsen progressively with time, early treatment may prevent progression to more severe end-stage deformities.

Conversely, the oral and maxillofacial surgeon will immediately comprehend the visible external auricular malformation but might not appreciate the advances in auricular and auditory reconstruction available to these patients. In this chapter, we provide an overview of contemporary auricular correction techniques. Because these conditions are rare and the anomalies complex, surgeons attempting these corrections should have the appropriate experience and training. Ideally, the jaw and ear reconstructive surgeons should evaluate each patient in a multidisciplinary clinic so that a coordinated plan for all the patient's anomalies and associated problems can be developed efficiently.

GENERAL CONSIDERATIONS

The ear is an obvious esthetic unit of the face and functions to provide hearing and equilibrium. The ear, which develops embryologically in three parts, includes multiple tissue types: skin, fat, bone, cartilage, nerve, blood vessels, and mucous membrane.[2-7] The *external ear* is formed by ectoderm and mesoderm. It includes the external auditory meatus, tympanic membrane, and auricle and functions to collect sound.[7] The *middle* ear is formed by endoderm and includes the eustachian tube and ossicles and serves to transmit sound.[7] The *internal* ear is formed predominately of ectoderm and includes the membranous labyrinth, cochlea, organ of Corti, and the semicircular canals. The internal ear structures convert sound waves into nerve impulses and maintain equilibrium.

The auricle, which forms by the third fetal month, is the product of maturation and coalition of six hillocks originating from the mandibular (first) and hyoid (second) arches. The tragus forms from the first pharyngeal (mandibular) arch. The second (hyoid) arch produces the other five hillocks that go on to form the remainder of the auricle (Figure 22-1). The branchial groove between the two arches invaginates to produce the external auditory canal.[8] The external ear is initially located in the lower neck and ascends (as the mandible develops) to the side of the head and the level of the eyes.[7]

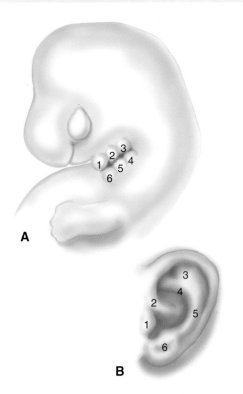

Figure 22-1
Embryologic development of the auricle. **A,** The six hillocks that coalesce to form the ear. **B,** The auricle with its derivative hillocks labeled.

A wide spectrum of auricular malformations can occur due to the involvement of multiple tissue types and the complex embryologic development of the ear. The mildest deformity is a malpositioned (low-set)[7,9] ear of normal shape. In the most severe deformities, there is no morphologically recognizable external ear and the external auditory canal, meatus, and tragus are absent. Commonly, with microtia (literally, little ear) there is an amorphous rudimentary cartilaginous mass superiorly and a lobule-like tissue mass inferiorly. Anotia (congenital absence of the external ear) also occurs and generally is associated with a low-lying hairline. Less common is stenosis or atresia of the external auditory canal in the presence of a well-developed auricle.[10] Of significance, in patients with an associated mandibular malformation, is that the relative position of the external ear may change significantly when jaw reconstruction has been completed.

Syndromic and nonsyndromic microtia have an estimated incidence of 1 in 10,000 live births (in metropolitan Atlanta).[9] The incidence is higher in other geographic locations,[11-16] when a child is born to a diabetic mother,[17,18] or when a child is exposed to varicella in utero.[19] A variable familial pattern has been noted[9,18,20-24] and there is an increased incidence of isolated microtia in subsequent siblings.[20-24] Monozygotic or dizygotic twins do not neces-

sarily both develop microtia, suggesting that the genetic or intrauterine environment is not solely responsible.[25] Genetic animal models are being developed and exist in nature.[26-30]

The most common form of microtia occurs in isolation. However, specific syndromes have been associated with microtia and atresia. Treacher Collins syndrome, a result of a mutation in the gene *TCOF1*,[31] is associated with bilateral microtia, whereas unilateral microtia is more common in hemifacial microsomia. In a prospective clinical study of 100 consecutive patients with "microtia," 40 were determined to have unrecognized hemifacial microsomia.[1] Other deformities or syndromes that have been associated with auricular anomalies (although less commonly) include hypertelorbitism, cervical fistula and nodules, mixed or conductive hearing loss, thickened earlobes, incudostapedial abnormalities, the lacrimoauriculodentodigital syndrome, micrognathia, and deafness.[32,33] Trisomies 13-15, 18, and 22 have been reported with microtia as one of multiple anomalies.[34-36] Antenatal detection of microtia by ultrasonography is now possible.[37]

Currently, three possible mechanisms for microtia have been proposed. A mouse model, reported by David Poswillo, demonstrates similar malformations caused by rupture of the stapedial artery during development.[38,39] A second model, failure of neural crest migration, has been implicated in the pathogenesis of microtia. This hypothesis is strengthened circumstantially by the known teratogenic effect of maternal ingestion of vitamin A on the second pharyngeal arch.[40] In animal models (mice), the second pharyngeal arch does not develop when migration of the neural crest is retarded by vitamin A.[5] This selectivity of vitamin A toxicity produces microtia but spares the tragus, which is a first arch derivative (Figure 22-2). However, the tragus is affected in most cases of microtia, so this theory has infrequent applicability. Furthermore, the unilateral nature of most cases is not consistent with the neural crest migration theory.

The third theory is that auricular malformation may occur due to intrauterine deformation (pressure phenomenon).[41] In support of this is the finding that auricular malformations may occur in association with limb malformations caused by abnormal intrauterine position or amniotic bands.

Classification systems to grade the degree of severity of auricular malformations have been reported. For example, Meurmann[42] described a grade I deformity as mild hypoplasia and mild cupping with all structures present. Grade II is manifested by absence of the external auditory canal and variable hypoplasia of the concha. Grade III consists of an absent auricle, with an anteriorly and inferiorly displaced lobule.[42] Other subjective grading systems have also been reported but are of little practical use beyond communication between physicians. Analysis of the specific anatomic features is more impor-

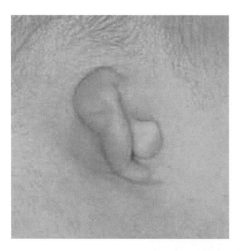

Figure 22-2

Vitamin A teratogenicity. Note the presence of a tragus, which usually is absent in microtia. (From Eavey RD, Cheney ML: Reconstruction of the auricle. In Nadol JB, Schuknecht HF: *Surgery of the ear and temporal bone*, New York, 1993, Raven.)

tant for decisions concerning management and auricular construction and reconstruction.

EVALUATION AND CARE OF THE PATIENT BEFORE SURGICAL CORRECTION

Infancy

An auricular malformation is immediately and easily recognizable at birth. The obvious and deforming nature of the anomaly, its rarity and, consequently, the understandable lack of experience on the part of the nurses and pediatricians often make for a stressful situation for the parents and family. Therefore, parents should be offered counseling by an experienced auricular surgeon for reassurance and advice on the sequence of management and future repair.[43] After the initial concern about the esthetics of the auricle, parental attention then focuses on hearing. A thorough brain stem–evoked response audiometric test should be performed as soon after birth as possible. Even in patients with unilateral microtia, the hearing must be evaluated. Although the contralateral normal-appearing ear has normal hearing (10-15 dB), in most cases, this must be demonstrated. The abnormal ear usually exhibits conductive hearing at 60 dB or more, and there may be associated sensorineural loss.[44]

With any significant conductive hearing loss, a bone-conduction aid should be considered because hearing is crucial to the development of normal speech and language.[44] The aid can be fixed by a headband or with double-sided tape. When the ear canal is present, a standard air-conduction hearing aid can be used.[8]

The infant should also be evaluated for other associated congenital malformations. Commonly associated abnormalities include mandibular hypoplasia, epibulbar dermoids, eyelid malformations, coloboma, cleft palate, facial nerve malfunction, vertebral body abnormalities, and renal and cardiac anomalies. Hemifacial microsomia and Treacher Collins syndrome should be ruled out (see Chapter 18).

Early Childhood

In children with isolated microtia, the anatomy and mucosal lining of the nasopharynx along the eustachian tube to the middle ear and mastoid region is present as in unaffected patients. Therefore, these patients have the same risk for otitis media and its associated complications as children with normal ears.[45] However, the risk associated with effusion in the normal ear is serious because the patient might then develop bilateral hearing loss. Therefore, antibiotics should be prescribed for suspected acute otitis media, even without otoscopic confirmation. Persistent effusion with substantial conductive loss on the normal side requires tube placement.[43,44]

Another concern with infants who have small or deformed ear canals is the development of an acquired cholesteatoma. Although visualization can be difficult, otorrhea, a tiny polyp in the small canal, or even mastoiditis may be the first signs of cholesteatoma.[9]

Physical Examination

Auricular Position. When viewed from the side (i.e., lateral view), the abnormal ear is smaller in vertical height than the contralateral ear. Normally, the most cephalad portion of the ear lies approximately at the level of the lateral brow. In the normally oriented auricle, an imaginary line drawn from the most superior portion of the helix through the lobule is roughly parallel with the dorsum of the nose. The microtic ear is caudad to this level, and a microtic ear exhibits a more vertical axis of orientation than a normal auricle (Figure 22-3). In the frontal view, the lobule is 3 to 5 mm higher on the microtic side, the superior portion of the auricle is lower, and there is no tragal prominence.[9]

Cartilaginous Appendage. In microtia, there may be considerable variation in the appearance of the cartilaginous appendage (external ear cartilaginous framework). In patients with mild deformities, the superior cartilaginous portion of the auricle may allow otoplasty-type techniques for reconstruction without adding new tissue.[46] In severe microtia, the volume of cartilaginous remnant determines the quantity and quality of overlying soft tissue coverage. The amount of available soft tissue coverage is critical, especially when the planned corrective

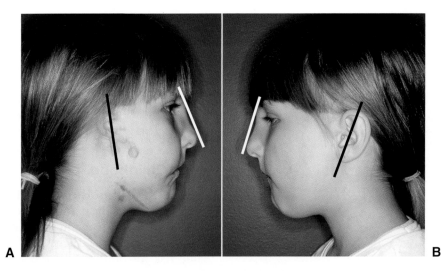

Figure 22-3

Lateral views of 6-year-old child with right microtia. The abnormal ear **(A)** is smaller in vertical height, is caudal, and has a more vertical axis of rotation as compared with the orientation of the normal ear **(B)**. When an imaginary line is drawn from the most superior part of the helix and through the lobule, in the normal ear the line lies roughly parallel to the dorsum of the nose.

procedure includes a rib cartilage graft.[61] The contour of the overlying soft tissue is also important. When the skin is smooth, it can be adapted better to the underlying cartilaginous framework. Skin with deep convolutions is difficult to adapt. Auricular features that are present and well formed should be incorporated into the reconstruction when possible.

Lobular Remnant. Even in the most severe malformations, a lobular remnant is usually present but abnormally positioned (superiorly and anteriorly) (Figure 22-3). The remnant should be rotated posteriorly and inferiorly. Placement of the lobule in a position similar to that of the opposite ear helps to achieve symmetry between the sides. Additionally, this lobule-like tissue is usually adequate to place an earring, which helps to improve the eventual aesthetic result.[8]

Hairless Zone Around the Auricle. In most patients with microtia, a hairless cutaneous rim exists above the ear. With anotia, the hairline can be extremely low. The hairless zone is important during the first stage of reconstruction because the superior portion of the cartilaginous framework, of necessity, will reside under hair-bearing skin. After ear construction, the patient will require permanent hair removal to achieve a reasonable esthetic result. This may be accomplished by excision of the hair-bearing skin and placement of a split-thickness skin graft or by laser treatment.

Skin Tags. Skin tags are frequently present. These tags should not, as a rule, be removed during infancy.[9]

Their removal should be delayed to avoid vascular compromise of the overlying skin. Also, tags are three-dimensional anatomic entities that occasionally can be used by the reconstructive surgeon.[62]

Presence of a Meatus, Canal, and Tympanic Membrane. In severe microtia, the meatus and canal are usually absent. When the canal is present, the potential for hearing preservation is enhanced.[47] However, the presence of a canal, especially if narrow, makes the patient susceptible to secondary cholesteatoma. Also, the position of auricular reconstruction may be compromised in these instances because the fixed canal (which may be low) cannot be moved. Finally, to minimize soft tissue scarring, the otologic surgeon must not reconstruct a canal stenosis until after the external ear has been repaired. It is important that the otologic and auricular surgeons (if not the same surgeon) work as a team to stage appropriately the entire reconstruction.

The presence of a tympanic membrane is very beneficial because there is an increased chance that clinical hearing may be achieved and otoscopic monitoring is possible.[45]

Contralateral Ear. The contralateral ear must be evaluated carefully for appearance and function (hearing) before the reconstruction. Usually, minor otologic anomalies are present and must be noted. In addition, the normal contralateral ear serves as the model for reconstruction and associated otoplasty techniques are often necessary to enhance the overall symmetry.[8]

RECONSTRUCTIVE CONSIDERATIONS

Patient and Family Preparation

Surgical correction of the severely microtic ear requires several staged procedures. The child and the parents must be prepared for multiple, sequential operations, and they should be apprised of the potential risks and benefits of this elective undertaking. The parents, with or without professional counseling help, must make the decision as to whether the child is appropriately prepared for and able to cope with multiple procedures (see Chapter 3).

A decision must be made as to whether surgical reconstruction of the middle ear for hearing will be attempted. Auricular reconstruction should precede aural atresia correction because surgical procedures to improve hearing produce considerable scarring which limits the amount of usable skin. In patients with unilateral microtia, the abnormal external appendage is perceived to be a severe congenital malformation, whereas the hearing deficit usually can be overcome with aids. These patients usually have normal speech and language development with the normal-hearing contralateral ear.

Finally, it is important that major surgical decisions be developed in a collaborative way, with all involved surgeons (especially the otologic and auricular) having the appropriate input. In patients with a malformed mandible or midface or both, surgical reconstruction should also be coordinated with the maxillofacial surgeon. In select cases, the jaw and auricular surgeries can be performed simultaneously (see Chapter 19).

Timing. Timing of surgical reconstruction of the auricle is important. When the ear is only mildly to moderately deformed, correction can be performed during early childhood (below the age of 5 to 6 years). This is especially true if the corrective procedures include only removal of extraneous tags or otoplasty techniques. However, with most microtia cases, correction of the deformity requires costal cartilage harvest. In these patients, the operation should be delayed until approximately the age of 6 years to allow for growth and development and adequate quantity of cartilage.

Techniques

Camouflage. In some cases, the parents choose to avoid an operation(s) and to camouflage the deformity with hair growth to conceal the appendage. They may choose this option because intervening medical problems increase the risk of an operation, because they feel the child can adjust to the deformity with camouflage, or because the child is not psychologically prepared to undergo an operation at the time. The parents should be counseled and should be made aware of the possibility of doing the correction at a later date.

Molding. The potential for nonoperative correction of a slightly malformed and pliable auricle in newborns by application of tape has been reported.[48] This noninvasive measure has had questionable benefit but may be of some use in rare cases when carried out during the first few days after birth.

Osseointegrated Implants. This technique, popularized in Europe, involves a prosthetic auricle anchored by osseointegrated titanium implants.[49] The technique must be applied at a somewhat older age to allow the skull cortex to become sufficiently thick to anchor the implants. Advantages include fewer operations with less morbidity, a fine "arm's length" result if the prosthesis is well made, and no donor site morbidity. Disadvantages include a prosthesis that requires daily hygiene, an unsightly appearance when the prosthesis is not in place, an abnormal feel when the prosthesis is touched, the need for a lifetime of both summer and winter prosthetic replacements, as well as the permanent loss by amputation of the original microtic ear. A prosthetic ear, however, does provide fine back-up technique if the auricular area has, for example, been altered irretrievably by trauma, previous unsuccessful surgery, or possibly regional burns.

Use of Contralateral Cartilage and Skin. Use of the contralateral cartilage and skin to reconstruct the affected auricle has been advocated by Davis.[46] This technique is applicable for unilateral cases that are amenable to correction with the small amount of ear conchal cartilage and postauricular skin obtainable without producing an unacceptable deformity of the normal ear. These moderately malformed ears should be about 50% of the width and 75% of the vertical height of the contralateral side. Such an auricle typically has a missing or diminutive tragus, no conchal bowl, a reasonable but shortened helix, a minimal to nonexistent antihelix, a near-normal lobule, and a small postauricular sulcus. Each ear must be custom crafted. The final enhanced result is accomplished in one or two stages with minimal morbidity and no visible donor scars. This technique, when successful, usually provides an ear of symmetric width and projection and visible convolutions; the overall vertical height is approximately 80% to 85% of the normal ear. The touch of the ear is obviously normal because the donor materials are autogenous auricular elastic cartilage and skin (Figure 22-4). Such soft tissue reconstructive surgery is much more demanding than classic rib reconstruction and should not be undertaken by an inexperienced microtia surgeon.

Rib Construction

The "workhorse" technique for reconstruction of a typical severe microtia uses costal cartilage and was developed creatively by Tanzer[50] and subsequently has been modi-

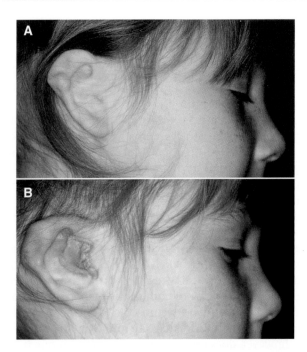

Figure 22-4

A moderate ear deformity has been corrected in a single stage from contralateral ear postauricular skin and cartilage, with no visible scars elsewhere on the body. **A,** Preoperative view. **B,** Postoperative view. Note enhanced size and contours.

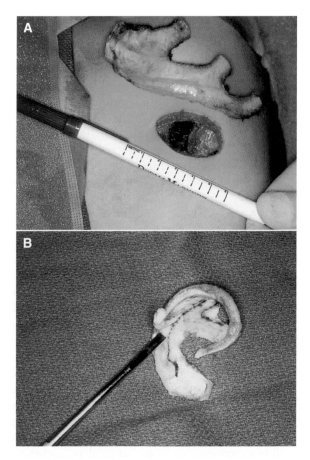

Figure 22-5

Ear reconstruction using rib. **A,** Rib harvest. **B,** Creation of rib framework. (**A** from Eavey RD, Ryan DP: *Arch Otolaryngol Head Neck Surg* 122:617-620, 1996.)

fied.[51-55] Reconstruction traditionally is performed at age 6 years or older for two reasons: (1) the ear usually achieves adult size by age 6 years and hence the constructed ear can be crafted to its final required size without taking into account further growth, and (2) by this age, the child is usually large enough to allow the harvest of an adequate amount of cartilage to make an appropriately sized ear framework.

The staged operation starts with rib harvest. The rib is carved and reconfigured into the shape of an auricle (Figure 22-5). The rib framework is then implanted into a skin envelope on the side of the head where the ear should be located. In patients with severe hemifacial microsomia undergoing simultaneous or sequential jaw distraction or reconstruction, ear placement must be considered relative to the eventual jaw appearance and position rather than the current size and location (Figure 22-6). In a subsequent operation, the lobule can be created from the fleshy portion of the malformed ear or, on occasion, created from cartilage. A functional postauricular sulcus is designed by separating the rib framework from the side of the head and placing skin grafts (Figure 22-7). Tragal construction can be done as a separate stage or in conjunction with one of the earlier stage procedures.

Reconstructive Middle Ear Surgery

Once the auricle has been created, repair of the external auditory canal and middle ear can be considered. If anatomically possible, the procedure can be done between phases of auricular reconstruction or after auricular reconstruction is completed.[44,56]

Atresia surgery usually is more formidable than conventional middle ear and mastoid surgery. However, with adequate anatomy, an external auditory canal can be drilled and an eardrum placed. The ossicles, although malformed, usually do function as a mobile assembly to conduct sound. The facial nerve will be positioned abnormally and in theory could be damaged. Although initial attention is focused on the actual atresia operation, potentially more significant issues may result from postoperative problems. Despite skin grafting, in some patients the new external auditory canal will become stenosed completely during the early postoperative period (weeks). Even if the canal is patent, sometimes the hear-

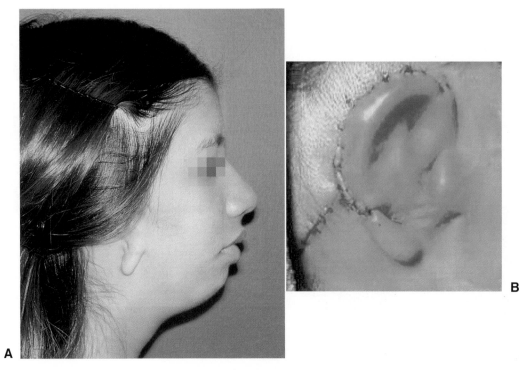

Figure 22-6

A, Preoperative lateral view of a patient with microtia who will undergo a simultaneous mandibular and auricular reconstruction (see also Figure 18-6). **B,** Lateral intraoperative view after the third stage, at which a postauricular sulcus was created. Note the auricular contours, which were created at the first operation (when the rib ear framework was carved), as well as the lobule, which was originally the small microtic ear rotated to a more natural location at the second stage.

ing result may be less than optimal or may decline again after a year. The patient will require periodic otologic visits for canal evaluation and possible cerumen debridement.

Most patients with aural atresia are not optimal candidates for an operation based on computed tomography (CT) imaging results. When the condition is unilateral, the contralateral hearing by default, although suboptimal, is adequate to permit development of speech and normal function. Therefore, in unilateral cases, an operation generally is reserved for patients with CT results indicating a high likelihood of improvement. When the condition is bilateral, aural atresia correction is indicated more strongly.

Yeakley and Jahrsdoerfer[57] have developed a 10-point surgical rating on high-resolution CT scans. The scale is based on the presence of key structures: stapes, open oval window, greater than 3 mm of middle ear space, course of the facial nerve, malleus–incus complex, mastoid pneumatization, round window, and appear-ance of the external ear. Patients with a presurgical score of less than or equal to 5 are not considered surgical candidates because the risks are greater than the potential benefits.

Tissue Engineering

Through the science of tissue engineering, creating a new ear from a patient's own tissue may one day be possible. Initially, only the xenograft model of "the mouse with the ear on its back" existed. In this model, cells are cultured in vitro and then allowed to mature in vivo, but in another species (i.e., an immunoincompetent mouse or rat).[58] Major advances have led to the robust production of healthy autogenous auricular cartilage created in vitro in immunocompetent animals.[59,60] Assuming this technique becomes reality, fewer staged reconstructive procedures should be necessary, patients should experience less morbidity, and the finished ear should have a more natural feel.[9,61-63]

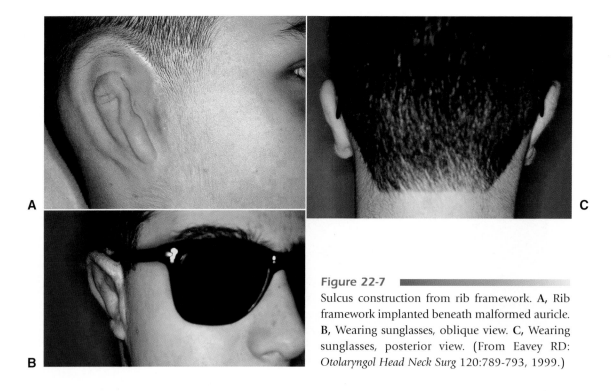

Figure 22-7

Sulcus construction from rib framework. **A,** Rib framework implanted beneath malformed auricle. **B,** Wearing sunglasses, oblique view. **C,** Wearing sunglasses, posterior view. (From Eavey RD: *Otolaryngol Head Neck Surg* 120:789-793, 1999.)

CONCLUSION

Microtia frequently is associated with mandibular malformations. Both oral and maxillofacial and ear surgeons should be aware of these associations to facilitate a multidisciplinary approach to these patients.

ACKNOWLEDGMENTS

Betty Treanor provided expert assistance to families with microtia and expert word processing help for this chapter. Drs. Maria Troulis and Leonard Kaban are valued colleagues who have taught me much about mandibular malformation and reconstruction. Our patients are a constant source of inspiration.

REFERENCES

1. Troulis MJ et al, unpublished data.
2. Schuknecht H: *Pathology of the ear*, Cambridge, MA, 1974, Harvard University Press, pp 184-186.
3. Wolff D, Bellucci RJ, Eggston A: *Surgical and microscopic anatomy of the temporal bone*, New York, 1971, Hafner, pp 1-26.
4. Pearson A: *The development of the ear: a manual prepared for the use of graduates in medicine*, Rochester, MN, 1967, American Academy of Ophthalmology and Otolaryngology.
5. Anson BJ, Donaldson JA: *Surgical anatomy of the temporal bone*, Philadelphia, 1981, WB Saunders, pp 23-31.
6. Jarvis BL, Johnston MC, Sulik KK: Congenital malformations of the external, middle, and inner ear produced by isotretinoin exposure in mouse embryos, *Otolaryngol Head Neck Surg* 102:391-401, 1990.
7. Sadler TW: *Langman's medical embryology*, ed 5, Baltimore, 1985, Williams & Wilkins.
8. Eavey R, Cheney M: Reconstruction of congenital auricular malformation. In Nadol J, Schuknecht H, editors: *Surgery of the ear and temporal bone*, New York, 1993, Lippincott, Williams & Wilkins.
9. Kamil SH, Aminuddin BS, Bonassar LJ, et al: Tissue-engineered human auricular cartilage demonstrates euploidy by flow cytometry, *Tissue Eng* 8:85-92, 2002.
10. Grundfast KM, Camilan F: External auditory canal stenosis and partial atresia with associated anomalies, *Ann Otol Rhinol Laryngol* 95:505-509, 1986.
11. Castilla EE, Lopez-Camelo JS, Campana H: Altitude as a risk factor for congenital anomalies, *Am J Med Genet* 86:9-14, 1999.
12. Harris J, Kaleen B, Robert E: The epidemiology of anotia and microtia, *J Med Genet* 33:809-813, 1996.
13. Lopez-Camelo JS, Oriolio IM: Heterogeneous rates for birth defects in Latin America: hints on causality, *Genet Epidemiol* 13:469-481, 1996.
14. Nelson SM, Berry RI: Ear disease and hearing loss among Navajo children—a mass survey, *Laryngoscope* 94:316-323, 1984.
15. Castilla EE, Orioli IM: Prevalence rates of microtia in South America, *Int J Epidemiol* 15:364-368, 1986.
16. Aase JM: Microtia—clinical observations, *Birth Defects* 16:289-297, 1980.
17. Ewart-Toland A, Yankowitz J, Winder A, et al: Oculoauriculovertebral abnormalities in children of diabetic mothers, *Am J Med Genet* 90:303-309, 2000.
18. Mastroiacovo P, Corchia C, Botto LD, Let al: Epidemiology of genetics and microtia-anotia: a registry based study on over one million births, *J Med Genetics* 32:453-457, 1995.
19. Jones KL, Johnson KA, Chambers CD: Offspring of women infected with varicella during pregnancy: a prospective study, *Teratology* 49:29-32, 1994.

20. Cremers C: Meatal atresia and hearing loss: Autosomal dominant and autosomal recessive inheritance, *Int J Pediatr Otorhinolaryngol* 8:211-213, 1985.

21. Kessler L: Observation of an over six generations simple dominant inheritance of microtia of the first degree, *HNO* 15:113-116, 1967.

22. Ostavik KH, Medbo S, Mair IW: Right-sided microtia and conductive hearing loss with variable expressivity in three generations, *Clin Genet* 38:117-120, 1990.

23. Gupta A, Patton MA: Familial microtia with meatal atresia and conductive deafness in five generations, *Am J Med Genetics* 59:238-241, 1995.

24. Llano-Rivas I, Gonzalez-del Angel A, del Castillo V, et al: Microtia: a clinical and genetic study at the National Institute of Pediatrics in Mexico City, *Arch Med Res* 30:120-124, 1999.

25. Neal GS, Hawkins GD: Left microtia in one monozygotic twin. A case report, *J Reprod Med* 37:375-377, 1992.

26. Naora H, Kimura M, Otani H, et al: Transgenic mouse model of hemifacial microsomia: cloning and characterization of insertional mutation region on chromosome 10, *Genomics* 3:515-519, 1994.

27. Cousley R, Naora H, Yokoyama M, et al: Validity of the hfm transgenic mouse as a model for hemifacial microsomia, *Cleft Palate Craniofac J* 39:81-92, 2002.

28. Kaur S, Singh G, Stock JL, et al: Dominant mutation of the murine *Hox-2.2* gene results in developmental abnormalities, *J Exp Zool* 264:323-326, 1992.

29. Bleyl DW: Microtia in a Wistar rat, *Z Versuchstierkd* 25:285-286, 1983.

30. Basrur PK, Yadav BR: Genetic diseases of sheep and goats, *Vet Clin North Am Food Anim Pract* 6:779-802, 1990.

31. Isaac C, Marsh KL, Paznekas WA, et al: Characterization of the nucleolar gene product, treacle, in Treacher Collins syndrome, *Mol Biol Cell* 11:3061-3071, 2000.

32. Konigsmark BW, Gorlin RJ: *Genetic and metabolic deafness*, Philadelphia, 1976, WB Saunders, pp 49-73.

33. Melnick M, Myrianthopoulos NC: *External ear malformations: epidemiology, genetics, and natural history*, vol 15. The National Foundation March of Dimes Birth Defects. Original article series. New York, 1979, Alan R Liss, pp 122-123.

34. Saito R, Fujimoto A, Fujita A, et al: Temporal bone histopathology of atresia auris congenita with chromosome aberration, *Acta Otolaryngol Suppl* 393:96-104, 1983.

35. Verloes A, Seret N, Bernier N, et al: Branchial arch anomalies in trisomy 18, *Ann Genet* 34:22-24, 1991.

36. Bacino CA, Schreck R, Fischel-Ghodsiam N, et al: Clinical and molecular studies in full trisomy 22: further delineation of the phenotype and review of the literature, *Am J Med Genet* 56:359-365, 1995.

37. Shih JC, Shyn MK, Lee CN, et al: Antenatal depiction of the fetal ear with three-dimensional ultrasonography, *Obstet Gynecol* 91:500-505, 1998.

38. Poswillo D: The pathogenesis of the first and second branchial arch syndrome, *Oral Surg* 35:302-328, 1973.

39. Phelps PO, Poswillo D, Lloyd GAS: The ear deformities in mandibulofacial dysostosis (Treacher Collins syndrome), *Clin Otolaryngol* 6:15-28, 1981.

40. Lammer EJ, Chen DJ, Hoar RM, et al: Retinoic acid embryopathy, *N Engl J Med* 313:837-841, 1985.

41. Jones KL, editor: *Smith's recognizable patterns of malformation*, ed 4. Philadelphia, 1988, WB Saunders, p 634.

42. Meurman Y: Congenital microtia and meatal atresia, *Arch Otolaryngol* 66:443, 1957.

43. Eavey RD: Management strategies for congenital ear malformations, *Pediatr Clin North Am* 36:1521-1534, 1989.

44. Eavey RD: Microtia and significant auricular malformation: 92 pediatric patients, *Arch Otolaryngol Head Neck Surg* 121:557-562, 1995.

45. Zalzal GH: Acute mastoiditis complicated by sigmoid sinus thrombosis in congenital aural atresia, *Int J Pediatr Otorhinolaryngol* 14:31-39, 1987.

46. Davis J, editor: *Otoplasty: aesthetic and reconstruction techniques*, New York, 1997, Thieme-Verlag.

47. Koutakis SE, Helidonis E, Jahrsdoefer RA: Microtia grade as an indicator of middle ear development in aural atresia, *Arch Otolaryngol Head Neck Surg* 121:885-886, 1995.

48. Muraoka M, Nakai Y, Sasaki T, et al: Tape attachment therapy for correction of congenital malformations of the auricle: clinical and experimental studies, *Laryngoscope* 95:167-176, 1985.

49. Tjellstrom A: Osseointegrated implants for replacement of absent or defective ears, *Clin Plast Surg* 62:355-366, 1940.

50. Tanzer RC: Total reconstruction of the external ear, *Plast Reconstr Surg* 23:1-15, 1959.

51. Brent B: The correction of microtia with autogenous cartilage grafts. I. The classic deformity, *Plast Reconstr Surg* 66:1-12, 1980.

52. Nagata S: New method of total reconstruction of the auricle for microtia, *Plast Reconstr Surg* 92:187-200, 1993.

53. Eavey RD: Surgical repair of the auricle for microtia. In Bluestone CD, Stool SE, editors: *Atlas of pediatric otolaryngology*, Philadelphia, 1994, WB Saunders.

54. Eavey RD, Ryan DP: Refinements in microtia surgery, *Arch Otolaryngol Head Neck Surg* 122:617-620, 1996.

55. Eavey RD: Microtia repair: creation of a functional postauricular sulcus, *Otolaryngol Head Neck Surg* 120:789-793, 1999.

56. Schuknecht HF: Congenital aural atresia, *Laryngoscope* 99:908-917, 1989.

57. Yeakley JW, Jahrsdoerfer RA: CT evaluation of congenital aural atresia: what the radiologist and surgeon need to know, *J Comput Assist Tomogr* 20(5):724-731, 1996.

58. Haisch A, Klaring S, Groger A, et al: A tissue-engineering model for the manufacture of auricular-shaped cartilage implants, *Eur Arch Otorhinolaryngol* 259(6):316-321, 2002.

59. Saim AB, Cao Y, Weng Y, et al: Engineering autogenous cartilage in the shape of a helix using an injectable hydrogel scaffold, *Laryngoscope* 110(10 Pt 1):1694-1697, 2000.

60. Kamil SH, Kojima K, Vacanti MP, et al: In vitro tissue engineering to generate a human-sized auricle and nasal tip, *Laryngoscope* 113(1):90-94, 2003.

61. Arevalo-Silva CA, Cao Y, Vacanti M, et al: Influence of growth factors on tissue engineered pediatric elastic cartilage, *Arch Otolaryngol Head Neck Surg* 126:1234-1238, 2000.

62. Arevalo-Silva CA, Eavey RD, Cao Y, et al: Internal support of tissue-engineered cartilage, *Arch Otolaryngol Head Neck Surg* 126:1448-1452, 2000.

63. Arevalo-Silva CA, Cao Y, Weng Y, et al: The effect of fibroblast growth factor and transforming growth factor-ß on porcine chondrocytes and tissue-engineered elastic cartilage, *Tissue Eng* 7:81-88, 2001.

CHAPTER 23

Sequential Management of the Child with Cleft Lip and Palate

Bonnie L. Padwa and John B. Mulliken

CHAPTER OUTLINE

Cleft lip and palate (CLP) is the most common craniofacial anomaly, with an overall incidence of 1 in 750 live births. Although localized to a small anatomic area, the cleft deformity requires specialized care by many disciplines. It is a three-dimensional anomaly, involving soft and skeletal tissue, that changes in the fourth dimension with growth and function. In this chapter we present the protocols for sequential management of the child with cleft lip and palate at the Children's Hospital, Boston. Since the techniques of repair are covered extensively in the literature, we focus here on the principles of management.

The etiology of nonsyndromic CLP is multifactorial and heterogeneous; both genetic and environmental factors have been implicated. Using pedigree and linkage analysis, several investigators have identified putative genes for CLP. Melnick et al.[1] and Marazita et al.[2] proposed that most cases of CLP result from a single dominant gene with low penetrance. Chung and coworkers[3] have identified a single recessive gene. Recently, with the use of DNA fragments (restriction fragment length polymorphisms [RFLPs]), several genes have been identified in patients with CLP, including those for the gene products transforming growth factor α (TGFα), epidermal growth factor (EGF), retinoic acid receptor α (RARα), cytochrome p450, nicotinamide adenine dinucleotide (NADH) dehydrogenase, and the sonic hedgehog gene *(SHH)*.[4-7] TGFα and EFG are both in the epidermal growth factor family; they direct the contact, fusion, and merging of facial prominences. Both RARα and *SHH* regulate the expression of homeobox *(Hox)* genes during embryonic patterning and neural crest cell migration.

Lynch and Kimberling[8] reported an increase in inheritance when a family member has a CLP. Once a couple has a child with a CLP, the risk of having a second child affected increases 40-fold, becoming approximately 4%, and the risk for a third child is 10%. In a study by Mitchell and Risch,[9] multivariate analysis was used to determine whether sex of the proband, sibling sex, and severity of the proband's defect or family history were the best predictors of recurrence risk among siblings of individuals with nonsyndromic cleft lip with or without cleft palate. Recurrence risks in siblings were not significantly related to the sex of the proband. However, severity of the proband's deformity, graded by the extent of the labial defect (incomplete versus complete, as well as unilateral versus bilateral), was found to be a significant predictor of sibling recurrence, whereas involvement of the secondary palate in the proband was not. A positive family history of clefting (i.e., at least one affected first-degree relative in addition to the proband) and the sex of the sibling were also found to correlate with risk of recurrence. After adjusting for the effects of family history, the risk to siblings of probands with bilateral labial cleft is twice the risk to siblings of probands with unilateral defects (odds ratio [OR] = 2.00; 95% confidence interval [CI] 1.25 - 3.19). A positive family history of clefting increases the risk to siblings by greater than fourfold (OR = 4.49; 95% CI 2.74 - 7.35), after adjusting for the severity of the proband's labial cleft.

There are wide ethnic and racial variations in the occurrence of CLP. It occurs more commonly in Asians (2.1 in 1000) than it does in whites (1.0 in 1000) and those of African descent (0.41 in 1000).[8]

Nonsyndromic cleft lip and palate is composed of two separate genetic entities: cleft lip and palate (CLP) and isolated cleft palate (CP). The distribution of orofacial clefts is 25% cleft lip alone, 50% CLP, and 25% isolated CP. CLP occurs more commonly and with greater severity in males than in females. The left:right:bilateral ratio for labial clefting is 6:3:1.[10] Approximately 10% to 20% of patients with CLP have associated anomalies, usually (central nervous system, cardiac, musculoskeletal) as part of a known syndrome (e.g., van der Woude's syndrome). CLP is twice as common as isolated CP. Isolated CP occurs in 1 in 2000 births. In contrast to CLP, there is no racial predilection in isolated CP and it is more common in females. Additionally, 20% to 70% of these patients have associated anomalies, Stickler syndrome being the most common, often appearing as Robin sequence.[11]

In 1993 the American Cleft Palate-Craniofacial Association (ACPA) proposed parameters of care designed to help standardize the treatment of patients with CLP and CP.[12] The objectives were to advocate for the concept of interdisciplinary care and to encourage the use of treatment protocols that emphasize thoughtful timing of interventions (operations, speech therapy, dental and psychosocial treatment) to coincide with the child's physical, cognitive, dental, and psychosocial development. The goals of the cleft team are to carry out periodic assessments, to make suggestions about the timing and sequencing of care to ensure long-term benefits, and to minimize revisions, complications, and costs.

Cleft centers around the world have interpreted these goals differently and, as such, there are a variety of treatment protocols for the management of these infants, children, and adolescents. This chapter outlines the approach to the care of cleft patients at Children's Hospital, Boston, that has evolved during the past 40 years by the faculty of the Cleft Palate Clinic and Craniofacial Center.

PRENATAL DIAGNOSIS AND COUNSELING

Intrauterine diagnosis of orofacial clefts is possible by ultrasonography, but the sensitivity is technician dependent. Complete clefts (CLP) are seen easily at 16 weeks' gestation; however, incomplete clefts are seen more readily at 27 weeks. Palatal clefts are difficult to visualize by prenatal ultrasonography.[13] Currently, between 14% and 25% of cleft lip, with or without CP, is detected antenatally.[14] About 12% of presumably isolated clefts will be one feature in a broader pattern of malformations.

As ultrasonography becomes more widely used in pregnancy and imaging technology improves, CLP will be identified more commonly during prenatal life. In efforts to meet the needs for information regarding cause and management, pregnant women and their partners are referred increasingly to cleft and craniofacial treatment centers. Information regarding the extent of the defect and the presence or absence of associated abnormalities is usually incomplete.

Prenatal diagnosis of CLP is occurring more commonly during both routine screening and with high-resolution ultrasonography. The family or obstetrician may request prenatal consultation with a surgeon. Matthews et al.[15] surveyed all families referred to the cleft program with a prenatal diagnosis of cleft between 1990 and 1994. Of 80 newborn referrals, 13 had a prenatal diagnosis. These children had a higher incidence of bilateral cleft than the average population (53.8% versus 28.7%, p < 0.03, chi square test). No isolated CPs were identified. Nine families were available for follow-up. Of note, only one third of the families felt that they had been given adequate information about clefts by their obstetrician or ultrasonographer.[16]

Parents should meet with the appropriate members of the cleft team in order to receive information needed to make informed decisions based on professional advice and realistic data. The ultimate decision regarding outcome and management, including termination, belongs to the prospective parents. Clinicians have their own thoughts; however, their responsibility is to help the couple make their own decisions based upon their personal religious, moral, and cultural values.[17]

INFANCY
General Considerations

Patients with CLP require interdisciplinary care from a team of providers including a geneticist, plastic surgeon, oral and maxillofacial surgeon, otolaryngologist, dentist, orthodontist, speech therapist, audiologist, psychologist, social worker, and nurse. The role of each specialist depends on the age of the patient.

During the first days of the infant's life, it is critical that both parents learn the proper technique for feeding the child. Infants with a palatal cleft cannot generate the negative intraoral pressure needed to suck from a bottle. They frequently tire before their caloric requirements are met, leading to failure to thrive. The nurse on the team, or another feeding specialist, must instruct the parents in the use of a special feeding device for the infant. We prefer the Haberman nipple, which delivers milk under slight pressure, more posteriorly in the oropharynx.

Because of the abnormal insertion of the levator veli palatine and tensor veli palatine, children with palatal clefts have difficulty ventilating the eustachian tubes. This results in the accumulation of fluid in the middle ear and repeated episodes of otitis media. Ear infections must be treated promptly with antibiotics, or scarring of the tympanic membrane will result in hearing loss. If the child has frequent ear infections, fluid collection, and abnormal audiologic study findings, myringotomy tubes are placed at the time of palatal repair.

Dentofacial Orthopedics

In unilateral complete cleft lip and palate (UCCLP) or bilateral complete cleft lip and palate (BCCLP) with a protruding premaxilla, labial repair is often completed with tension on the closure. Although dehiscence is unlikely, tension is more likely to cause a heavy and wide scar and distortion of the prolabium and nose. The best scar occurs following closure during infancy; therefore, it is imperative to provide a favorable environment for primary nasolabial repair. This is the basis for preoperative dentofacial alignment.

Orthopedic appliances bring the dentoalveolar segments together, facilitating a tension-free labial repair that requires less undermining of tissues. In addition, alveolar approximation forms the skeletal platform for correction of the nasal deformity and permits gingivoperiosteoplasty (GPP); alveolar closure eliminates an oronasal fistula. When this technique is used, alveolar bone formation may obviate the need for bone grafting in the mixed dentition.[18] There is one report suggesting that dentofacial orthopedics may play a role in minimizing the number of nasolabial revisions in children with repaired unilateral complete cleft lip.[19]

There is a long-standing controversy over active versus passive dentofacial orthopedics. We believe an active device gives better alignment of the alveolus and labial elements. An alginate model of the maxilla is taken in the office and the appliance fabricated within the first few weeks of life. The device is placed soon afterward while the child is under general anesthesia.

Activating the appliance over the ensuing weeks aligns the arches. The appliance is removed at the time of labial repair and replaced with a passive appliance to maintain the alveolar position.

Management of the Cleft Lip and Nasal Deformity

The primary focus of repair of cleft lip has always been the labial closure. However, during the past 30 years, surgeons have paid more attention to the nasal deformity. Because of successful dentofacial orthopedics, many centers repair the unilateral complete cleft lip and the nasal deformity in a single stage. However, in our center a preliminary lip-nasal adhesion is done after dentofacial orthopedics and before definitive repair of the unilateral cleft lip. Reasons for this two-stage repair are that it (1) minimizes tension, (2) increases the bulk of the orbicularis oris muscle to construct the philtral ridge, (3) increases the vertical dimension of labial elements, particularly on the medial side, and (4) gives the surgeon two chances to correct the position of the lower lateral cartilage.[20]

Timing of Nasolabial Repair

Labial repair is traditionally carried out when the child is approximately 10 weeks of age, weighs 10 pounds, and has a serum hemoglobin value of 10 mg/ml. However, there is no scientific basis for these guidelines. It is important to wait until the period of postnatal anemia has corrected (after 1 month). The child should be gaining weight and growing before undergoing nasolabial repair (Figures 23-1 and 23-2).

For unilateral incomplete cleft lip (the cleft extends part way up the cutaneous lip and there may or may not be a cleft of the alveolus and secondary palate), nasolabial repair is done at 3 to 5 months of age, along with alveolar closure as needed. For UCCLP, dentofacial orthopedics is done before lip-nasal adhesion and GPP at 3 to 4 months; more definitive nasolabial repair is undertaken at 5 to 6 months. However, in the rare variant of unilateral complete cleft lip and alveolus with an intact secondary palate (about 10% of patients), an earlier lip adhesion is done at 1 month of age; at least 2½ to 3 months later the definitive repair is completed with GPP.

For the uncommon bilateral symmetric incomplete cleft lip, nasolabial repair is done at 3 to 4 months of age, along with alveolar closure if needed. In the most common variant, BCCLP, dentofacial orthopedics begins at 1 to 2 months of age followed by synchronous (one-stage) repair of the primary palate (nose, lips, and alve-

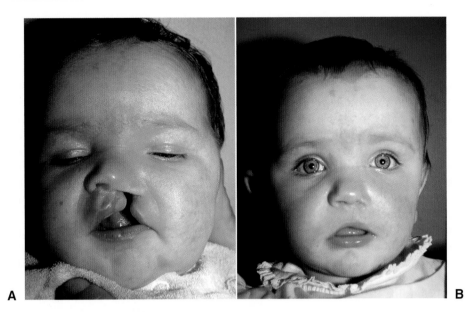

Figure 23-1

A, An infant with a left unilateral complete cleft lip and palate. **B,** Following labial adhesion, formal nasolabial repair, and palatal closure. Note the hypoplastic left alar lobule.

olus).[21-23] However, in the asymmetric variant (complete or incomplete), dentofacial orthopedics is done on the complete side followed by lip-nasal adhesion and GPP. The surgical field is now level, and synchronous nasolabial repair is done just as in BCCLP. If a child is brought in for treatment after 8 to 10 months of age, dentofacial orthopedics is not possible because the premaxilla is no longer moveable. In these children a bilateral nasolabial repair is done with a premaxillary osteotomy and positioning. However, if the child is close to 1 year or older, speech is paramount and, therefore, the bilateral CP is closed with premaxillary positioning and the nasolabial repair is done as a second stage.

Techniques of Nasolabial Repair

In the early 1950s, Millard[24] realized that the popular triangular flap technique often aligned the peak of the cupid's bow in its normal position but violated the natural lines of the philtral column and dimple. Rather than merely rotating the lower third of the central lip, he conceptualized the high release and subsequent rotation of the whole medial lip segment, thereby returning it to its normal position. The lateral lip segment was then prepared and advanced to meet the leading edge of the rotated medial lip segment. Through the years, Millard and others have added various refinements to his initial technique. Today most surgeons, in closure of unilateral cleft lip, follow Millard's rotation-advancement principle, although every surgeon has personal technical variations (Figure 23-2).

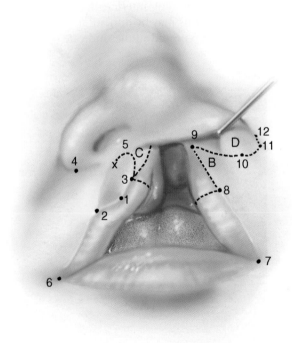

Figure 23-2

Diagrammatic representation of the rotation advancement principle of unilateral complete cleft lip repair. Note the inferior rotation of the medial segment and advancement of the lateral segment. (From Millard DR, ed: *Cleft craft: The evolution of its surgery,* vol I, *The unilateral deformity,* Boston, 1976, Little, Brown.)

The techniques used to repair a bilateral cleft lip derive from those used for the unilateral counterpart. Although there are some common elements in the repair of the unilateral and bilateral cleft lip, the bilateral repair has special challenges that make it more difficult; it cannot be thought of as just a double form (mirror image) of a unilateral repair (Figure 23-3). The results for bilateral cleft lip repair have never been as good as those for the unilateral form. Over the past decade, the following principles that guide the surgeon's hand in closing bilateral cleft lip have been established: (1) maintain symmetry, (2) design the prolabium of proper size and shape, (3) ensure primary muscular continuity, (4) construct the median tubercle from lateral labial elements, and (5) perform primary construction of the columella and nasal tip.[21-23] The fifth principle has resulted in a major improvement in the appearance of children with bilateral cleft lip.

Management of the Cleft Palate

A child with either an unrepaired or an inadequately repaired palate who reaches the age of speech development requires an operation to achieve velopharyngeal competence. Otherwise, the child develops compensatory articulation patterns that interfere with intelligibility. These compensations may be difficult to eliminate once established. Most reported studies indicate that children

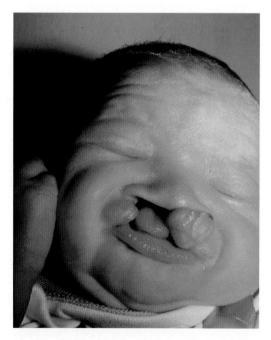

Figure 23-3

A newborn with bilateral complete cleft lip and palate. Note severe angulation of the premaxillary segment.

without hearing impairment or cognitive delays have significantly fewer compensatory articulation and abnormal speech patterns when the palate is repaired before 2 years of age.

The objective of palatal closure is to construct a functional mechanism for velopharyngeal competence. Separation of the oral and nasal cavities is also believed to improve ventilation of the middle ear by proper orientation of the velar muscles. The fundamental principle of palatal closure is to release the abnormal attachments from the posterior edge of the hard palate and retroposition the muscle bundles in a transverse axis (intravelar veloplasty).

At Boston's Children's Hospital palatal closure is done at 8 to 10 months of age; the standard technique is two-flap palatoplasty with levator retropositioning and vomerine flap(s) if needed (Figure 23-4). Myringotomy tubes are placed during the same period of anesthesia, as is usually necessary.

Some CLP centers follow a protocol that involves a two-stage palatoplasty. In an attempt to avoid detrimental effects of palate repair on maxillary growth, algorithms were developed to delay palate closure, allowing facial growth to proceed. Often these protocols involved obturation of the hard palate with a prosthetic appliance, with or without early repair of the soft palate. Patients treated with such protocols have been reported to have good facial growth. However, they have had significant speech problems that are difficult to correct.[25] There have been many additional reports to confirm that early CP repair (before 1 year) results in improved speech when compared with later repair.[26-29] Based on this information, early palatal repair is recommended, but the effects on maxillary growth should be taken into consideration and monitored.

EARLY CHILDHOOD
Speech

Speech and language assessment begins at age 1½ to 2 years to detect abnormalities in articulation and resonance. Even the most experienced surgeons, using a variety of techniques, will have patients (an average of 10% to 15%) who develop velopharyngeal incompetence after palatoplasty.[27,30,31] Perceptual evaluation by an experienced speech and language pathologist focuses on standardized testing of speech and ratings of oronasal resonance. Specifically, weak production of plosive and fricative consonants, visible nasal emission during consonant production, compensatory articulation errors, and hypernasal resonance are identified (see Chapter 5).

When our speech pathologist detects an abnormal speech mechanism by subjective clinical examination, dynamic anatomic information during function is obtained by videofluoroscopy or nasopharyngoscopy or

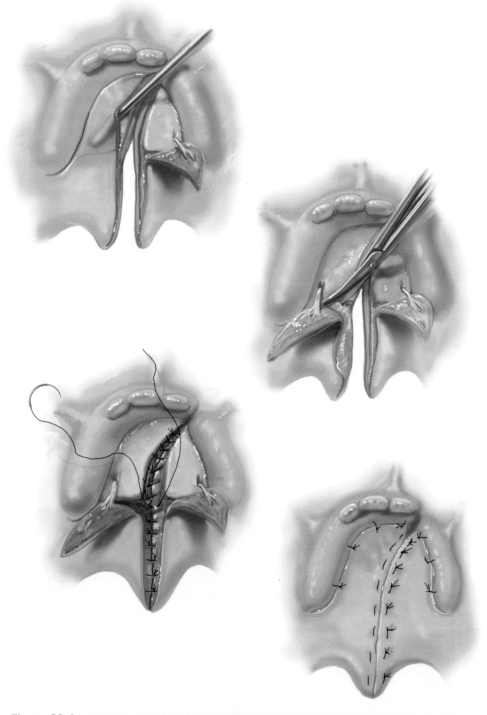

Figure 23-4
Diagrammatic representation of the sequence of the Bardach two flap palatoplasty. (From Posnick J: *Craniofacial and maxillofacial surgery in children and young adults,* Philadelphia, 2000, WB Saunders.)

both. These studies demonstrate the magnitude and direction of movement of the velum, motion of the pharyngeal walls, position of contact (or lack of contact) between velum and pharyngeal walls during speech, and the size and orientation of the residual velopharyngeal gap.

The two most common procedures for correction of velopharyngeal insufficiency are the pharyngeal flap and the sphincter pharyngoplasty. In our center the gold standard is the superiorly based pharyngeal flap, designed on the basis of location and extent of lateral pharyngeal wall motion. The raw undersurface of the flap is lined with tissue from the nasal side of the soft palate to prevent contracture and narrowing of the flap. The donor site on the posterior pharyngeal wall is closed, if possible, to minimize bleeding and postoperative pharyngeal pain. Depending on the size of the flap, most patients exhibit some degree of transient airway obstruction during the postoperative period.

Dental

Children with CLP have a number of dental problems, including abnormal eruption patterns, supernumerary teeth, missing teeth, hypoplastic enamel, and dental and skeletal malocclusion. It is important for these patients to have an evaluation by a dentist, as early as age 3 years, to establish a baseline examination and to familiarize the patient with the dental environment.

Nasolabial Revisions

Nasolabial revisions are considered before age 3 years, before facial image develops and before the child has a memory of operations. The residual deformities for the unilateral form can be separated into those involving the lip and those involving the nose. Nasal stigmata include slumping of the lower lateral cartilage, lateral vestibular webbing, and laterally displaced alar base. The labial problems are a weakness of the median tubercle and relative fullness of the free margin of the lateral labial element and sometimes a vertically short lip. Usually these residual asymmetries can be corrected (Figure 23-5).

Often the asymmetry of the nose is more noticeable than the residual labial deformity. The lower lateral cartilage can be resuspended, the vestibular web can be effaced, and the alar base can be repositioned to be symmetric with the opposite side. The contour of the free margin of the lip is corrected by either resection of redundant mucosa and submucosa and sometimes the addition of a submucosal or dermal graft to the median tubercle. A tiny unilimb Z-plasty just at the vermilion cutaneous junction is used to lengthen the lip. Correction of the nasal deformity is the most common revision with repaired unilateral complete cleft lip.[19]

In our center the revision rate for children with bilateral cleft lip is less than that for unilateral cleft lip.[32] The procedures include resuspension of the mucosa in the anterior gingivolabial sulcus, autogenous graft to

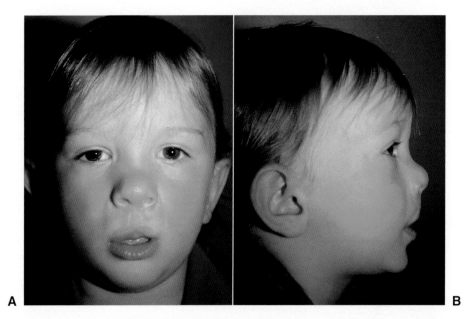

Figure 23-5 ▬▬▬▬▬▬▬▬▬▬▬▬▬▬▬▬▬▬▬

A, The patient shown in Figure 23-3 with BCCLP at age 4 years after synchronous nasolabial repair and palatal closure. **B,** Note the obtuse nasolabial angle and acceptable midfacial position.

the median tubercle, and narrowing of the interalar dimension. Our patients do not require secondary columellar lengthening (Figures 23-6 and 23-7).

LATE CHILDHOOD
Phase I Orthodontics

The cleft patient in the mixed dentition often exhibits asymmetric maxillary constriction (the minor segment is collapsed) with anterior crossbite and poor dental alignment. Malformed, missing, or supernumerary teeth are obvious. The goals of treatment are to reposition the maxillary segments, to create proper arch form and width, and to prepare the cleft site for alveolar bone grafting and for later orthodontics.

Phase I orthodontic treatment begins with placement of a differential expansion appliance to increase the transverse dimension of the anterior (canine region) more than that of the posterior (first molar region) maxilla. Also during this phase, exfoliating deciduous and supernumerary teeth in the cleft region are removed, and orthodontic manipulation of the maxillary incisor to move the crown away from the cleft is done if it can be completed without placing the apex of the root into the alveolar cleft. These maneuvers improve the success rate of the alveolar bone graft.

Phase I orthodontic treatment is started early enough to complete alignment and expansion before eruption of the canine tooth on the cleft side. It the treatment is completed too early, it may be difficult to maintain the expansion and alignment until the patient is ready for alveolar bone grafting. The bone graft is placed when the maxillary canine root is one-half to two-thirds formed (age 8 to 12 years). This provides bony and periodontal support without adversely affecting midfacial growth. However, if there is a viable lateral incisor, the graft can be placed when the root of this tooth is one-half to two-thirds formed (age 5 to 7 years).

Alveolar Bone Grafting

Preoperative expansion of the maxillary segments allows better access to the alveolar recipient site, permits nasal floor closure, and maintains the arches in their proper positions. Alveolar bone grafting provides bony support of teeth adjacent to the cleft, helps to stabilize the maxillary segments, allows closure of the oronasal fistula, enhances the aesthetic appearance of the alveolus, gives support to the alar base of the nose, and provides bone for a titanium implant.

Cancellous bone is used for alveolar grafting because the particles transfer living osteoblasts and the architecture promotes more rapid vascularization than cortical or corticocancellous block grafts. Particulate marrow remodels quickly and permits eruption of the teeth. Cancellous graft can be harvested from the ilium, calvaria, tibia, or mandible. We prefer ilium, because an adequate amount of bone can be harvested from this site. The bone should be placed within the cleft from the piriform aperture to the level of the alveolar crest.

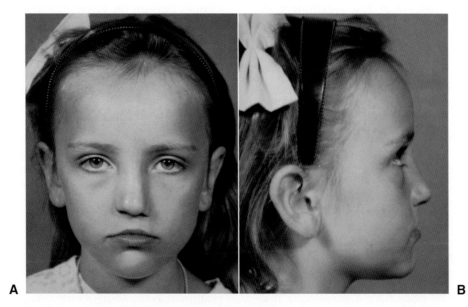

A   **B**

Figure 23-6

A, The patient shown in Figure 23-1 with UCCLP at age 9 years. Labial height and nasal contour are maintained. **B,** Midfacial retrusion is more evident.

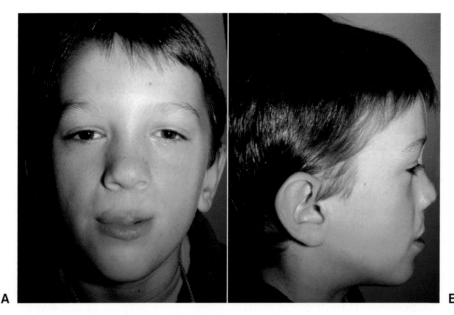

Figure 23-7

A and B, The patient shown in Figures 23-3 and 23-5 at age 11 years. Interalar distance is close to the inter-medial canthal distance. Midfacial retrusion is obvious; the nasolabial angle has narrowed.

Each donor site has inherent risks and complications that are common to all (bleeding, infection, etc.) and also those that are site specific (gait disturbance, paresthesia, and so forth.) (see Chapter 9). In addition to an adequate graft, there must be sufficient soft tissue available to cover the bone in a watertight pocket between nasal and oral linings. Gingival mucoperiosteal flaps are used for oral closure over an alveolar bone graft, because they are well vascularized, are in close proximity to the cleft, and can be mobilized to provide a tension-free closure. The gingival flap also provides attached gingiva for dental eruption through the cleft site.

Dental eruption through the alveolar graft occurs in most patients. Our results are similar to those reported in the literature. Cohen and colleagues[33] reported that 95% of canines erupted and did not require surgical exposure. Van der Walk[34] found spontaneous eruption of the canine in 77% of patients, and 20% required either bony or soft tissue uncovering. Similarly, da Silva Filho et al.[35] reported that 72% of patients had eruption of the maxillary canine after alveolar cleft grafting, and 6% required orthodontic traction for eruption.

Premaxillary Positioning

Despite successful labiopalatal repair, children with bilateral complete CLP often have a persistently malpositioned premaxilla. The premaxilla is sometimes protruded, lingually rotated, and vertically elongated in infants with repaired bilateral cleft lip and palate. There are two indications for surgical repositioning. First, premaxillary osteotomy may be necessary to facilitate revision of the nasolabial soft tissues.[36] Second, there is often a need for premaxillary positioning in combination with secondary bone grafting. The goals of premaxillary repositioning are (1) to align and stabilize the dental arch, (2) to improve inclination and vertical position of the incisors, and (3) to permit eruption of canines through the bone graft. The premaxilla is stabilized with an acrylic splint and secured to orthodontically bonded maxillary teeth.

The timing of premaxillary osteotomy in patients with repaired bilateral complete cleft lip and palate is controversial. Primary osteotomy and stabilization of the premaxilla (i.e., at the time of labial repair) is rarely necessary because of success with presurgical dentofacial orthopedics. Osteotomy of the premaxilla, in combination with secondary bone grafting, is often necessary. We do not hesitate to reposition the premaxilla, because Padwa and colleagues[37] found that a protrusive premaxilla can be positioned after age 6 to 8 years without deleterious effects on midfacial growth.

ADOLESCENCE
Phase II Orthodontics

Treatment in the adult dentition requires a well thought out, comprehensive plan that involves input from all practitioners (plastic surgeon, oral and maxillofacial surgeon, orthodontist, and prosthodontist) involved in the patient's care. This interdisciplinary approach helps avoid mistakes and misunderstandings during the last stage of treatment.

The final phase of orthodontia begins in the permanent dentition and is coordinated to end with the completion of skeletal growth. If there is uncertainty as to how the mandible will grow, orthodontic manipulation should be delayed until growth is completed. The orthodontic plan is determined by whether the final treatment will include orthodontics alone or in combination with an operation. This strategy should be settled before treatment is initiated. The orthodontic plan should provide the optimal dental aesthetics while minimizing the need for prosthetic replacement of teeth.

Operative Correction of Maxillary Hypoplasia

A number of patients with CLP develop maxillary hypoplasia. Ross,[38] Rosenstein et al.,[39] Cohen et al.,[40] and DeLuke et al.[41] reported a 22% to 26% incidence of CLP patients requiring an orthognathic procedure for maxillary deficiency. However, the need for maxillary advancement is a subjective assessment not judged by standardized criteria. Hence, the incidence of orthognathic correction of the cleft maxilla can vary depending on the criteria applied. In our center we favor operative correction over orthodontic compensation.

The maxilla is hypoplastic in all three planes, resulting in class III malocclusion (sagittal plane), narrow arch (horizontal plane), and inadequate dental show and overclosure of the mandible (vertical plane). This hypoplasia extends from the dentition to the infraorbital rims. A lack of understanding of the three-dimensional nature of the cleft maxillary deformity can result in inappropriate treatment. A patient with a vertically short maxilla and relative mandibular prognathism is best treated by maxillary advancement in the sagittal plane, with disimpaction and elongation in the vertical plane. This allows clockwise rotation of the mandible and will likely obviate the need for mandibular setback (Figures 23-8 and 23-9).

Although advancement of the maxillary dentoalveolar unit does improve the posture of the upper lip and nasal tip projection, Le Fort I advancement does not change the superior aspect of the middle third of the face.[42] We favor malar augmentation with implants in the infraorbital region extending to the zygomatic arch, which can be placed at the time of the Le Fort procedure to improve the projection of the upper midface. Variations on the Le Fort II osteotomy have been proposed for some patients with midfacial retrusion. Cleft patients with retrusion of the nose, infraorbital rims, and malar eminences are candidates for these procedures and occasionally for a Le Fort III osteotomy.

Before the introduction of maxillary advancement by distraction osteogenesis, results were unpredictable in patients who required a major maxillary movement. Mandibular setback was often necessary, even with a normally positioned mandible, if the sagittal discrepancy was greater than 10 to 15 mm.[43] However, this bimaxillary strategy often compromised the long-term aesthetic outcome, because the maxilla was inadequately advanced and lengthened. Incremental movement of the maxilla using distraction osteogenesis permits gradual advancement over a large distance, because the scarred soft tissues of the palate or pharyngeal flap can accommodate to this incremental expansion. We use Le Fort I distraction osteogenesis in patients with clefts who have a pharyngeal flap and who need large maxillary advancement (>10 mm).

Modification of the maxillary osteotomy may be necessary in patients with oronasal fistulas and alveolar clefts, unilateral deformities, paranasal hypoplasia, and maxillary-zygomatic hypoplasia. If the greater maxillary segment is in good position but the lesser segment is medially and posteriorly displaced, a segmental osteotomy can be incorporated with the Le Fort I osteotomy to correct the position of the minor segment.[43] Posnick and Tompson[44] reported correction of maxillary hypoplasia with concomitant residual fistulas, alveolar defects, and cleft dental gaps in one procedure. The major and minor segments are moved differentially to correct the maxillary hypoplasia, close the cleft dental gap and fistula, and graft the alveolar cleft. This procedure offers an alternative when the fistula has not been closed and the alveolar cleft has not been bone grafted during the mixed dentition.

Velopharyngeal Incompetence after Maxillary Advancement

The velopharyngeal mechanism of cleft patients can fail after maxillary advancement. Maxillary advancement moves the soft palate away from the posterior pharyngeal wall and thus can have an effect on speech by increasing the patency of the nasal airway, changing the occlusion, and altering velopharyngeal function.[42] Unfortunately, it is not always possible to predict which cleft patients will develop velopharyngeal incompetence after Le Fort I advancement. There is some evidence to suggest that the incidence of velopharyngeal insufficiency following Le Fort I osteotomy correlates with preoperative velopharyngeal function and the amount of maxillary movement. David et al.[45] reported deterioration in velopharyngeal competence with maxillary advancement of more than 10 mm. Sader et al.[46] found that maxillary advancement up to 7 mm is possible without loss of velopharyngeal function. However, Watzke et al.[47] reported no relationship between the

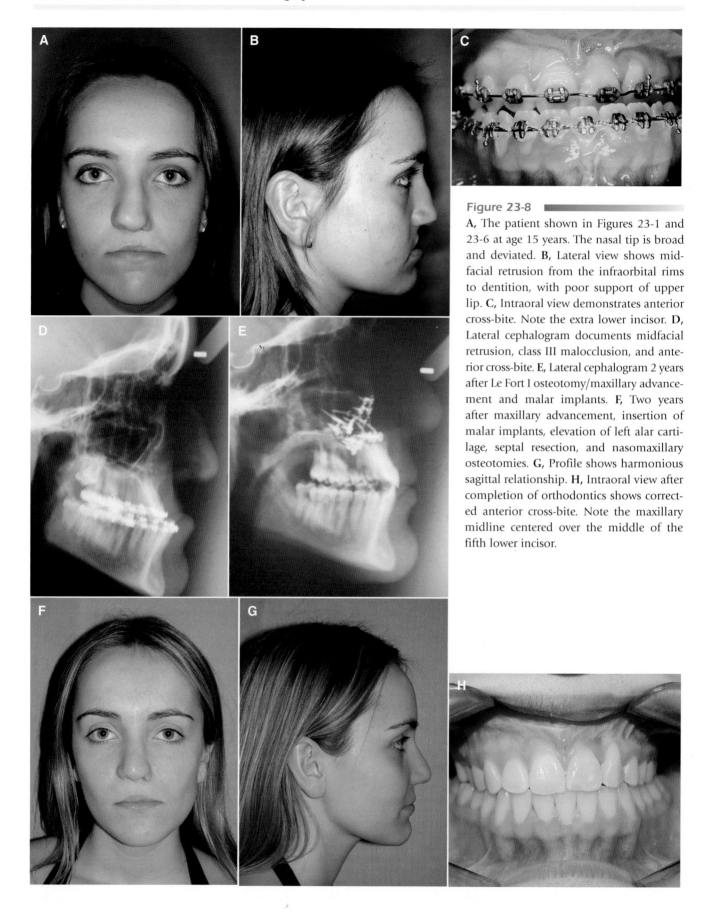

Figure 23-8

A, The patient shown in Figures 23-1 and 23-6 at age 15 years. The nasal tip is broad and deviated. **B,** Lateral view shows midfacial retrusion from the infraorbital rims to dentition, with poor support of upper lip. **C,** Intraoral view demonstrates anterior cross-bite. Note the extra lower incisor. **D,** Lateral cephalogram documents midfacial retrusion, class III malocclusion, and anterior cross-bite. **E,** Lateral cephalogram 2 years after Le Fort I osteotomy/maxillary advancement and malar implants. **F,** Two years after maxillary advancement, insertion of malar implants, elevation of left alar cartilage, septal resection, and nasomaxillary osteotomies. **G,** Profile shows harmonious sagittal relationship. **H,** Intraoral view after completion of orthodontics shows corrected anterior cross-bite. Note the maxillary midline centered over the middle of the fifth lower incisor.

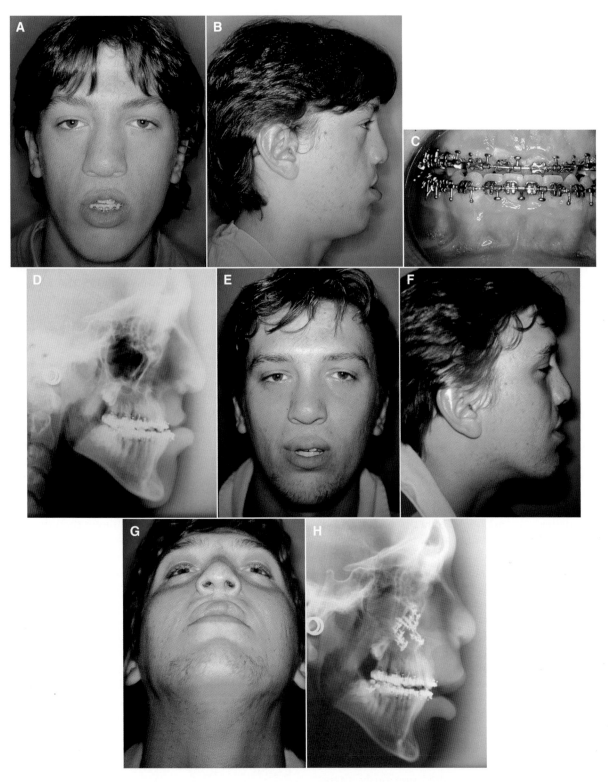

Figure 23-9

A, The patient shown in Figures 23-3, 23-5, and 23-7 at age 17. The nasal pyramid has widened. **B,** Lateral view shows midfacial retrusion, flattened nasal tip, poorly supported upper lip, and lower lip ectropion. **C,** Intraoral photograph shows anterior cross bite and class III occlusion. **D,** Lateral cephalogram documents midfacial retrusion, class III malocclusion, and anterior cross bite. **E and F,** Five years after maxillary advancement and malar augmentation and 1 year after nasomaxillary osteotomies to narrow the pyramid, septal resection, cartilage strut graft to nasal tip, and submucosal graft from lower tip to median tubercle. Note normal nasolabial angle and improved upper/lower lip harmony. **G,** Normal ratio of columellar length–to–nasal tip protrusion. **H,** Lateral cephalogram 1 year after Le Fort I maxillary advancement and malar augmentation.

amount of maxillary advancement and velopharyngeal function. The risk of velopharyngeal insufficiency following maxillary distraction is similar to the 16% to 23% risk observed with standard Le Fort I osteotomy.[48]

In our center, all patients with CLP undergoing Le Fort I osteotomy have a baseline preoperative speech assessment, which includes a subjective clinical evaluation by a speech therapist and nasopharyngoscopy to assess soft palate and lateral pharyngeal wall movement. In patients with borderline or gross velopharyngeal insufficiency, videofluoroscopy is done. Patients are reevaluated 3 to 6 months postoperatively by the speech therapist, and further studies are obtained if necessary. If a patient develops velopharyngeal insufficiency, a superiorly based pharyngeal flap can be placed 6 to 12 months after Le Fort I osteotomy.

Replacement of Absent Maxillary Lateral Incisor

Patients with repaired CLP often have a hypoplastic or absent maxillary lateral incisor on the cleft side. There are a variety of ways to substitute for the missing incisor, and the treatment choice should be an integral part of the overall plan. The correction is determined by each patient's particular arch form, dentition, and occlusion. Orthodontic closure of the space with anterior movement of the canine into the position of the lateral incisor is an option but can result in transverse maxillary deficiency and poor aesthetics because of a lack of symmetry with the noncleft side. Fabrication of a removable or fixed restoration to replace the lateral incisor may be aesthetically acceptable, especially if there is a defect in the alveolar ridge. However, if the bone graft is inadequate and there is a persistent alveolar cleft without bony union of the maxilla, there can be micromotion across a fixed restoration, leading to failure of the prosthesis. Additionally, if there is an associated oronasal fistula, oral hygiene is often poor, further compromising the long-term viability of the fixed restoration.

Replacement of the lateral incisor with an osseointegrated implant is an increasingly popular approach. As with implant placement at any site, there must be adequate volume and quality of bone. Although the alveolar cleft may have been grafted previously, there may be insufficient bone in this area for an implant, and a supplemental bone graft may be necessary. Kearns et al.[49] found that the interval between bone graft and implant is important. The greater the interval beyond 4 months, the more likely it was that there would be inadequate bony volume to accept an implant. The bone-grafted alveolar cleft can be augmented with additional graft and an implant placed 3 months later.

Final Revisions

As a general rule, orthodontic intervention, skeletal correction, and prosthetic habilitation are completed before soft tissue nasolabial revision and rhinoplasty are considered. These final surgical procedures should be deferred until at least 6 months after maxillary advancement. This allows for an appreciation of the changes in the nose and lip secondary to the dentoskeletal movement. Surgical advancement of the maxilla is accompanied by changes in the overlying soft tissue. Therefore, to achieve an acceptable aesthetic result, one must consider the soft tissues and their response to skeletal correction. The soft tissue response to skeletal movements is difficult to predict in both the cleft and non-cleft individual.[50] The repaired cleft lip may be thinner and less flexible, and the lower lip often is everted and hypertrophied in appearance.[51] Freihofer[52,53] studied the effects on soft tissue after movement of the maxilla on the nasal and labial profile in both cleft and noncleft patients and he found no difference in the response. In the cleft patient, the average advancement ratio of the nasal tip to maxilla was 2:7 and to the nasal base was 4:7. The upper labial profile advanced an average of 50% of the advancement of the maxillary dental arch. They also showed a pattern of decreasing ratios from *subnasale* to *labrale superius,* the opposite of what is seen in noncleft individuals. Ewing and Ross[50] reported ratios for soft tissue movement per unit advancement of the maxilla. The lip to hard tissue response was 0.6:1, which was larger than that reported in other studies. In addition, maxillary advancement greater than 4 mm produced a corresponding thinning of the upper lip, which was unrelated to the original lip thickness. After the first year, soft tissue changes were insignificant.

Six to twelve months after maxillary advancement, formal rhinoplasty, which can include nasomaxillary osteotomies, septal resection, final adjustment of the alar cartilages, and narrowing interalar width, can be done in combination with labial mucosal adjustment based on dental show. A pharyngeal flap can be done if maxillary advancement caused velopharyngeal insufficiency.

CONCLUSION

The successful habilitation of a child born with cleft lip and palate requires close cooperation among the many specialists on a high-volume team. A coordinated approach is preferred to help the child achieve ideal speech, occlusion, facial appearance, and self-esteem. Poor outcomes are related to nonexistent protocols, fragmented care, lack of periodic assessment, and low patient volume.[54,55] Unnecessary, unproductive, and unproved interventions should be avoided because they exhaust the patient, family, and healthcare system, produce unfulfilled expectations, and introduce secondary deformities. Providing the patient with the ability to pursue and achieve personal success in life without particular regard to the original cleft deformity is the ultimate goal.

REFERENCES

1. Melnick M, Bixler D, Fogh-Andersen P, Connelly PM: Cleft lip +/- palate: an overview of the literature and an analysis of Danish cases born between 1941-1968, *Am J Med Genet* 6:83-87, 1980.
2. Marazita ML, Spence MA, Melnick M: Major gene determination of liability to cleft lip with or without cleft palate: a multiracial review, *J Craniofac Genet Dev Biol* 2(suppl):89-97, 1986.
3. Chung CS, Bixler D, Watanabe T, et al: Segregation analysis of cleft lip with or without cleft palate: a comparison of Danish and Japanese data, *Am J Hum Genet* 39:603-611, 1986.
4. Abbott BD, Pratt RM: Retinoid and EFG alter embryonic mouse palatal epithelial and mesenchymal cell differentiation in organ culture, *J Craniofac Genet Dev Biol* 7:219-240, 1987.
5. Shaw D, Ray A, Marazita M, Field L: Further evidence of a relationship between the retinoic acid receptor alpha locus and non-syndromic cleft lip with or without cleft palate (CL+/–P), *Am J Hum Genet* 53:1156-1157, 1993.
6. Rosvold EA, Gasser DL, Rhodes M, Buetow KH: Association of detoxification enzyme polymorphisms with cleft lip and palate (abstract), *Am J Hum Genet* 55(suppl):A48, 1994.
7. Orioli IM, Vieira AR, Castilla EE, et al: Mutational analysis of the sonic hedgehog gene in 220 newborns with oral clefts in a South American (ECLAMC) population, *Am J Med Genet* 108:12-15, 2002.
8. Lynch HT, Kimberling WJ: Genetic counseling in cleft lip and cleft palate, *Plast Reconstr Surg* 68(5):800-815, 1981.
9. Mitchell LE, Risch N: Correlates of genetic risk for non-syndromic cleft lip with or without cleft palate, *Clin Genet* 43:255-260, 1993.
10. Wilson MEAC: A ten-year survey of cleft lip and cleft palate in South West region, *Br J Plast Surg* 25:224-228, 1972.
11. Rollnick BR, Pruzansky S: Genetic services at a center for craniofacial anomalies, *Cleft Palate J* 18(4):304-313, 1981.
12. Parameters for evaluation and treatment of patients with cleft lip/palate or other craniofacial anomalies, American Cleft Palate-Craniofacial Association, March, 1993, *Cleft Palate Craniofac J* 30(suppl):S1-16, 1993.
13. Benacerraf BR, Mulliken JB: Fetal cleft lip and palate: sonographic diagnosis and postnatal outcome, *Plast Reconstr Surg* 92:1045-1051, 1993.
14. Jones MC: Prenatal diagnosis of cleft lip and palate: detection rates, accuracy of ultrasonography, associated anomalies, and strategies for counseling, *Cleft Palate Craniofac J* 39:169-173, 2002.
15. Matthews MS, Cohen M, Viglione M, Brown AS: Prenatal counseling for cleft lip and palate, *Plast Reconstr Surg* 101(1):1-5, 1998.
16. Mulliken JB, Benacerraf BR: Prenatal diagnosis of cleft lip: what the sonologist needs to tell the surgeon, *J Ultrasound Med* 20: 1159-1164, 2001.
17. Saal HM: Prenatal diagnosis: when the clinician disagrees with the patient's decision, *Cleft Palate Craniofac J* 39:174-178, 2002.
18. Pfeifer TM, Grayson BH, Cutting CB: Nasoalveolar molding and gingivoperiosteoplasty versus alveolar bone graft: an outcome analysis of costs in the treatment of unilateral cleft alveolus, *Cleft Palate Craniofac J* 39:26-29, 2002.
19. Mulliken JB, Martinez-Perez D: The principle of rotation advancement for repair of unilateral complete cleft lip and nasal deformity: technical variations and analysis of results, *Plast Reconstr Surg* 104(5):1247-1260, 1999.
20. Vander Woude DL, Mulliken JB: Effect of lip adhesion on labial height in two-stage repair of unilateral complete cleft lip, *Plast Reconstr Surg* 100:567-572, 1997.
21. Mulliken JB: Principles and techniques of bilateral complete cleft lip repair, *Plast Reconstr Surg* 75:477z
22. Mulliken JB: Bilateral complete cleft lip and nasal deformity: an anthropometric analysis of staged to synchronous repair, *Plast Reconstr Surg* 96(1):9-23, 1995.
23. Mulliken JB: Primary repair of bilateral cleft lip and nasal deformity, *Plast Reconstr Surg* 108(1):181-194, 2001.
24. Millard RD: *Cleft craft: the evolution of its surgery. I. The unilateral deformity,* Boston, 1976, Little, Brown and Company.
25. Bardach J, Morris HL, Olin WH: Late results of primary veloplasty: the Marburg project, *Plast Reconstr Surg* 73(2):207-218, 1984.
26. Dorf DS, Curtin JW: Early cleft palate repair and speech outcome, *Plast Reconstr Surg* 70(1):74-81, 1982.
27. Marrinan EM, LaBrie RA, Mulliken JB: Velopharyngeal function in nonsyndromic cleft palate: relevance of surgical technique, age at repair, and cleft type, *Cleft Palate Craniofac J* 35:95-100, 1998.
28. Rohrich RJ, Rowsell AR, Johns DF, et al: Timing of hard palate closure: a critical long-term analysis, *Plast Reconstr Surg* 98(2): 236-246, 1996.
29. Ysunza A, Pamplona C, Mendoza M, et al: Speech outcome and maxillary growth in patients with unilateral complete cleft lip/palate operated on at 6 versus 12 months of age, *Plast Reconstr Surg* 102(3):675-679, 1998.
30. Kirschner RE, Wang P, Jawad AF: Cleft-palate repair by modified Furlow double-opposing Z-plasty, *Plast Reconstr Surg* 104(7): 1998-2010, 1999.
31. Vedung S: Pharyngeal flaps after one- and two-stage repair of the cleft palate: a 25-year review of 520 patients, *Cleft Palate Craniofac J* 32(3):206-215, 1995.
32. Mulliken JB, Wu JK, Padwa BL: Repair of bilateral cleft lip: review, revisions, and reflections, *J Craniofac Surg* Sept 2003 (in press).
33. Cohen M, Polley JW, Figueroa AA: Secondary (intermediate) alveolar bone grafting, *Clin Plast Surg* 20(4):691-705, 1993.
34. van der Wal KG, van der Meulen BD: Eruption of canines through alveolar bone grafts in cleft lip and palate, *Nederlands Tijdschrift voor Tandheelkunde* 108(10):401-403, 2001.
35. da Silva Filho OG, Teles SG, Ozawa TO, et al: Secondary bone graft and eruption of the permanent canine in patients with alveolar clefts: literature review and case report, *Angle Orthod* 70(2):174-178, 2000.
36. Heidbuchel KLWM, Kuijpers-Jagtman AM, Freihofer HPM: An orthodontic and cephalometric study on the results of the combined surgical-orthodontic approach of the protruded premaxilla in bilateral clefts, *J Craniomaxillofac Surg* 21:60-66, 1993.
37. Padwa BL, Sonis A, Bagheri S, et al: Children with repaired bilateral cleft lip/palate: effect of age at premaxillary osteotomy on facial growth, *Plast Reconstr Surg* 104:1261, 1999.
38. Ross RB: Treatment variables affecting facial growth in complete unilateral cleft lip and palate: part 6. Techniques of palate repair, *Cleft Palate J* 24(1):64-77, 1987.
39. Rosenstein S, Kernahan D, Dado D, et al: Orthognathic surgery in cleft patients treated by early bone grafting, *Plast Reconstr Surg* 87(5):835-839, 1991.
40. Cohen SR, Corrigan M, Wilmot J, et al: Cumulative operative procedures in patients aged 14 years and older with unilateral or bilateral cleft lip and palate, *Plast Reconstr Surg* 96(2):267-271, 1995.
41. DeLuke DM, Marchand A, Robeles EC, et al: Facial growth and the need for orthognathic surgery after cleft palate repair: literature review and report of 28 cases, *J Oral Maxillofac Surg* 55(7):694-697, 1997.
42. Marsh JL, Galic M: Maxillofacial osteotomies for patients with cleft lip and palate, *Clin Plast Surg* 16(4):803-814, 1989.

43. Herber SC, Lehman JA: Orthognathic surgery in the cleft lip and palate patient, *Clin Plast Surg* 20(4):755-768, 1993.

44. Posnick JC, Tompson B: Cleft-orthognathic surgery: complications and long-term results, *Plast Reconstr Surg* 96:255-266, 1995.

45. David DJ, Sells RK, Maegawa J: The effects of maxillary osteotomy on speech in cleft lip and palate patients. In Transactions of the VIIIth International Congress of Cleft Palate and Related Craniofacial Anomalies, Singapore, 1997, pp 655-659.

46. Sader R, Hess U, Zeilhofer HF, et al: Maxillary advancement and velopharyngeal closure in cleft patients. In Transactions of the VIIIth International Congress of Cleft Palate and Related Craniofacial Anomalies, Singapore, 1997, pp 651-654.

47. Watzke I, Turvey TA, Warren DW, et al: Alterations in velopharyngeal function after maxillary advancement in cleft palate patients, *J Oral Maxillofac Surg* 48(7):685-689, 1990.

48. Guyette TW, Polley JW, Figueroa A, et al: Changes in speech following maxillary distraction osteogenesis, *Cleft Palate Craniofac J* 38(3):199-205, 2001.

49. Kearns G, Perrott DH, Sharma A, et al.: Placement of endosseous implants in grafted alveolar clefts, *Cleft Palate Craniofac J* 34(6):520-525, 1997.

50. Ewing M, Ross RB: Soft tissue response to orthognathic surgery in persons with unilateral cleft lip and palate, *Cleft Palate Craniofac J* 30:320-327, 1993.

51. Pensler JM, Mulliken JB: The cleft lip-lower lip deformity, *Plast Reconstr Surg* 82:602-608, 1988.

52. Freihofer HP: The lip profile after correction of retromaxillism in cleft and non-cleft patients, *J Maxillofac Surg* 4:136-141, 1976.

53. Freihofer HP: Changes in nasal profile after maxillary advancement in cleft and non-cleft patients, *J Maxillofac Surg* 5:20-27, 1977.

54. Bearn D, Mildinhall S, Murphy T: Cleft lip and palate care in the United Kingdom—the Clinical Standards Advisory Group (CSAG) Study. Part 4: outcome comparisons, training, and conclusions, *Cleft Palate Craniofac J* 38(1):38-43, 2001.

55. Shaw WC, Dahl E, Asher-McDade C: A six-center international study of treatment outcome in patients with clefts of the lip and palate: part 5. General discussion and conclusions, *Cleft Palate Craniofac J* 29(5):413-418, 1992.

CHAPTER 24

Facial Trauma I: Midfacial Fractures

Arnulf Baumann, Maria J. Troulis, and Leonard B. Kaban

CHAPTER OUTLINE

Facial fractures are less common in children than in adults, and pediatric midfacial fractures, which include nasal, zygomatic, orbital, and Le Fort injuries, are especially rare.[1] Overall, these fractures account for approximately 5% of all facial fractures, but the reported incidence ranges from 1.5% to 15%, depending on the demographics of the study and the types of injuries included.[1] In children younger than 12 years, midfacial fractures make up from 1.5% to 8% of all facial fractures treated in trauma centers.[2-8] In children younger than 5 years, the reported incidence is even lower: 1.0% to 1.5% of all facial fractures. This number has remained unchanged during the last four decades.[1,5,9-12] Kaban et al., evaluating children only,[10] reported 80 midfacial fractures (nasal, zygomaticomaxillary, and orbit) in 109 patients who sustained 122 facial injuries during a 10-year period. In a follow-up study, with an additional 9 years of data, 184 of 262 facial fractures were in the midface.[13,14]

Iida et al.[8] reported a series of 26 facial fractures in a group of children less than 10 years of age. Two of the fractures were in the midface and the rest in the mandible. In contrast, Iida found 80 isolated midfacial fractures and 291 mandible fractures in a series of children from ages 10 to 19 years.

The major causes of midfacial fractures, in order of frequency, are motor vehicle accidents, sports-related injuries, and falls.[1,15,16] The increased popularity of multispeed bicycles, dirt bikes, and off-road vehicles (e.g., snowmobiles, go-carts) in the hands of untrained and unprotected children and adolescents has contributed to an increasing number of maxillofacial injuries in these groups. Sports trauma is another source of pediatric facial fractures. Proper helmets, mouth protectors, and face guards are still not mandatory, or rules are not enforced, in many youth hockey and football leagues. Educational programs are needed to better inform parents, teachers, and coaches of the importance of preventing facial injuries. The most common pediatric midfacial fractures (in order of frequency) are nasal, orbital, zygomaticomaxillary, and Le Fort fractures.[1] Reliable epidemiologic data on nasal fractures are not readily available, because most of these cases are treated on an outpatient basis and, therefore, not entered in hospital databases.

The low incidence of midfacial fractures in children may be explained by the elasticity of the child's facial bones, the retrusive position of the maxilla, nose, and infraorbital rims, and the anatomic protection afforded by the prominent calvaria (Figure 24-1). In addition, young children lead relatively protected lives and their activities are closely supervised. During the first 5 years of life, the cranium enlarges in parallel with rapid growth of the brain; the forehead is prominent.[17] The maxillary and ethmoid sinuses are not fully developed and the

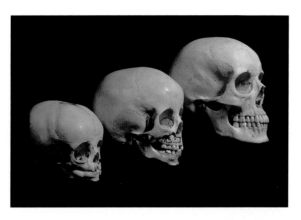

Figure 24-1

Left to right, Infant, mixed dentition, and adult human skulls illustrate the proportions and relative prominence of the skull, midface, and mandible at the three stages of development. (From Mulliken JB, Kaban LB, Murray JE: *Clin Plast Surg* 4: 491-502, 1977.)

midface is vertically short.[18] These factors result in a high skull-to-face ratio, with more exposure of the frontal bone, brain, and orbits and with the lower facial bones relatively protected. Messinger et al.[19] reviewed a series of 23 patients, with a mean age of 3.3 years, who sustained facial fractures. All 23 children had fronto-orbital fractures involving the orbital roof. Associated fractures in the lower maxillofacial skeleton occurred in only seven of these young patients. Later in childhood and in adolescence, development of the maxillary and other paranasal sinuses and downward and forward growth of the midface result in a shift of fractures to involve more often the zygomatic complex and the Le Fort levels of the midface.[20]

GENERAL CLINICAL MANAGEMENT

Although the incidence of pediatric facial trauma has not changed dramatically over time, there have been significant advances in diagnostic and treatment techniques. Plain facial radiographs (Waters', posteroanterior and lateral skull, and submental vertex views) traditionally were used to evaluate midfacial fractures. These radiographs had significant limitations in the pediatric age group. Positioning the child, lack of the child's ability to remain motionless, a short midface with undeveloped sinuses, and multiple tooth buds in the area often obscured fracture lines.[21,22] For these reasons, computed tomography (CT) has replaced these studies for the diagnosis of fractures in pediatric patients.

The metabolic management of pediatric trauma patients has also changed. Maintenance of normal fluid and electrolyte balance is critical in children, and our understanding of their cardiovascular physiology and fluid and electrolyte balance has advanced significantly.[21] Currently, standard metabolic management formulas based on age and weight are readily available for the surgeon to use (see Chapter 8).

The surgeon also must be cognizant of associated injuries, especially in a child who has been involved in a high-speed motor vehicle accident. Posnick et al.[12] reported that 33% of the patients who had sustained maxillofacial trauma also had concurrent injuries (head 42%, extremities 24%, eye 22%, thorax 10%, and abdomen 2%). Kaban, Mulliken, and Murray documented similar findings, with approximately 20% of patients having associated injuries (head 11%, extremities 4.5%, eye 1.8%, abdomen 0.9%, and cervical spine 0.9%).[10,21]

Airway management has also changed over the past few decades. Traditionally, tracheotomy was used to protect a child's airway after a midfacial fracture.[23,24] The trend then moved to short-term endotracheal intubation.[12,24,25] With the advent of fiberoptic intubation and rigid internal fixation (less maxillomandibular fixation), pediatric trauma patients seldom remain intubated for any significant period (see Chapter 8).

Finally, a major advance in the treatment of pediatric midfacial fractures has been the increasingly common use of rigid internal fixation. The entire midfacial skeleton can be exposed with the use of maxillary vestibular, subciliary, and supratarsal fold incisions. Additional exposure is achieved with a coronal incision and craniofacial dissection. Fractures can then be reduced and immobilized with miniplates or microplates.[21,26] Before the advent of rigid internal fixation, stabilization was managed with maxillomandibular fixation, with or without wire osteosynthesis and craniofacial suspension. Maxillomandibular fixation may lead to significant difficulties in airway management and nutrition limitations in children. Upper airway obstruction is common in children because they are particularly sensitive to even mild airway swelling, secretions, or other stimulation.

NASAL FRACTURES

Nasal fractures are the most common midfacial skeletal injury in the pediatric population.[1,10] This is not surprising, because the nose is a prominent skeletal structure and the nasal bones are fragile.[27] Kaban found that 41% (107 of 262 facial fractures) of children sustained a nasal fracture.[13,14] Anderson reported that 54% (75 of 139) of children had nasal fractures.[28] These fractures often are excluded from retrospective studies, because the patients are likely to be treated and discharged in the emergency room, a doctor's office, or an ambulatory surgery center. Therefore, they may not be entered in the hospital database, which usually includes only inpatients. In addition, a nasal fracture may be missed because the nose is not well developed and crepitus on palpation often is absent.[10]

Diagnosis

A thorough history is especially important, because a nasal fracture may be missed on physical examination if the child is uncooperative and difficult to examine.[11,17] The type of blow and its force and direction provide clues as to the likelihood of bony injury. The family's assessment of the appearance and of the child's ability to breathe through the nose are also critical (Figure 24-2). Clinical findings suggestive of a nasal fracture may include ecchymosis, overlying skin lacerations, swelling, epistaxis, septal hematoma, or intranasal lacerations. Palpable bony irregularities may be appreciated although difficult to detect because of a lack of cooperation and the usual absence of crepitus in children.[1,10] Although intramembranous ossification begins during the third month of fetal life, the resilient nasal bones in pediatric patients usually do not comminute. A lateral blow to the nose displaces the nasal bone medially, and the opposite nasal bone may override the frontal process of the maxilla. A blow from the front may fracture both nasal bones transversely, or the bones may separate in the midline, a so-called open book fracture.[10,24,29]

Intranasal examination should be carried out with a speculum to rule out septal deviation or hematoma. Septal hematoma requires early drainage to avoid resorption of the cartilage and subsequent saddle nose deformity. One septal hematoma was documented in the 107 nasal fractures reviewed by Kaban.[24]

Radiographs may be helpful for documentation of the injury, but the diagnosis should be made on the basis of the history and physical examination. A lateral nasal projection and Waters' view at 30 to 45 degrees are sufficient in most cases (Figure 24-3). Nasal fractures may be noted on CT scans of the trauma patient with multiple facial injuries.

Treatment

When indicated, an operation is performed after the swelling resolves.[11,17] Closed reduction should be performed very early (within a week), because fractures in children heal rapidly and mobility may be reduced significantly after 7 days.[10] In teenagers, nasal reduction may be accomplished with sedation and local anesthesia (lidocaine 0.5% with epinephrine 1:200,000

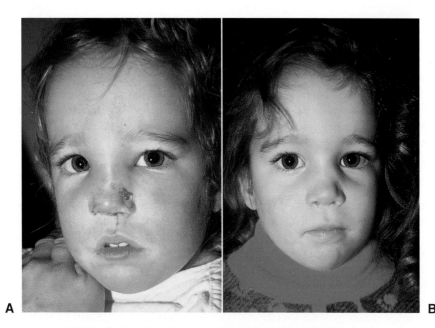

A   **B**

Figure 24-2

A, A 4-year-old girl with a nasal fracture. Physical findings may be subtle in children. The nasal bones are elastic, and the nasal bridge may not be fully developed. There is often no crepitation on palpation. The nasal bridge is widened, as illustrated in this patient. **B,** After closed reduction, intranasal pack, and splint. (Courtesy Dr. John B. Mulliken.)

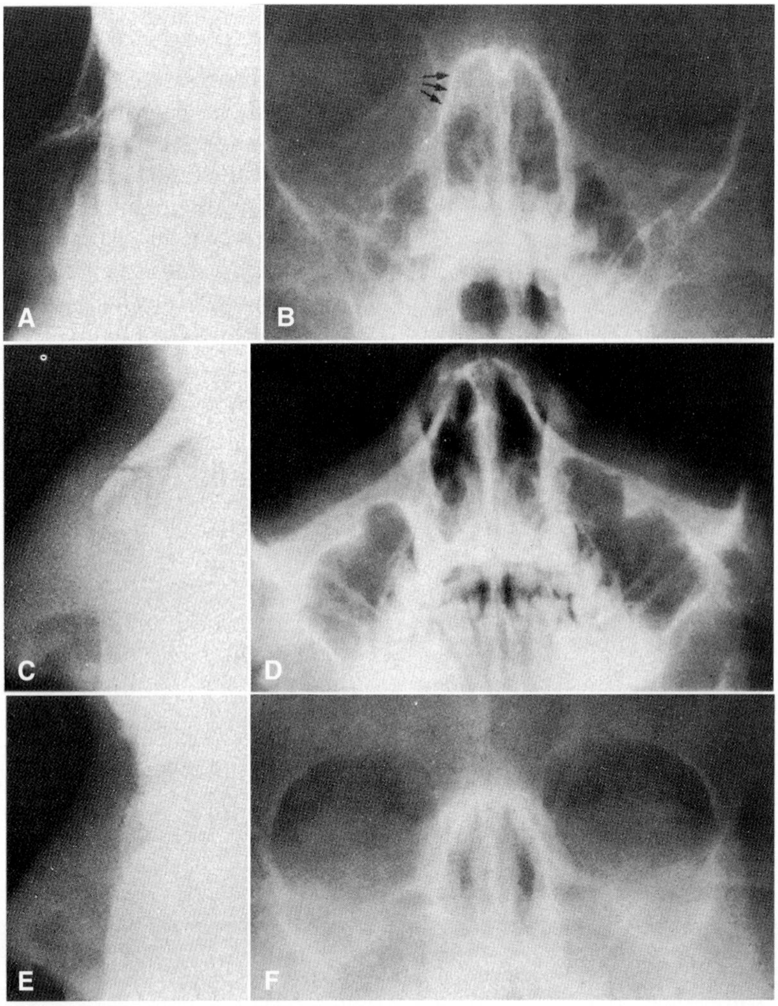

Figure 24-3

A, Child with "normal" lateral nasal x-ray; B, Waters' view shows depression of right nasal bone; C, transverse fracture of nose on lateral x-ray; D, Waters' view demonstrates angulation of right nasal bone; E, depressed nasal dorsum on lateral view with F, "normal" Waters' view. (From Mulliken JB, Kaban LB, Murray JE: *Clin Plast Surg* 4:491-502, 1977.)

for nerve block and infiltration, and intranasal topical cocaine 5%). In younger patients, general anesthesia is required.

The use of topical cocaine is important, not only as an anesthetic but also for vasoconstriction. It prevents reuptake of norepinephrine by adrenergic nerve endings.[30] Cocaine should be used for this reason even if nasal reduction is to be carried out under general anesthesia.

The nasal bones are elevated and reduced with an Ash forceps, Kelly clamp, or Rowe elevator. The purpose of treatment is to realign the nasal bones and straighten the septum. Intranasal packing and a splint are used to stabilize the reduction and provide hemostasis. The splint is made to cover the nose only. The forward projecting frontal bone in children causes a splint to ride off the

nose if it is secured to the forehead[11] (Figure 24-4). A septal hematoma must be drained on an emergent basis to avoid resorption of the cartilage, which causes the associated saddle nose deformity.[1]

Mustoe et al.[31] obtained follow-up data, by a telephone interview, on 30 of 107 children with nasal fractures. The average age at the time of injury was 8.6 years (range = 3 to 12) and the mean follow-up was 9 years. Therefore, the mean age at the time of reevaluation was 17.6 years, with most of the children having completed growth. All of the patients had their nasal injuries treated by closed reduction (as described above). Of 30 patients, 8 reported difficulty breathing, but only 3 required a submucous resection (2 of the 3 had an esthetic rhinoplasty). None of the 30 patients

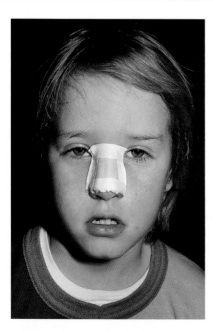

Figure 24-4
Proper nasal splint for a child (as described in text). (From Mulliken JB, Kaban LB, Murray JE: *Clin Plast Surg* 4:491-502, 1977.)

reported an underbite or midfacial hypoplasia. The conclusion was that closed reduction of a nasal fracture during childhood is not associated with later midfacial growth deficiency (Figure 24-5) or growth inhibition. Other authors have similarly reported a low incidence of midfacial growth deficiency in patients who sustained a nasal fracture in childhood.[32-34] The most frequent long-term complication of such an injury is a compromised airway caused by deviation and thickening of the septum or widening of the dorsum.[10,14]

ZYGOMATIC COMPLEX FRACTURES
Diagnosis

Zygomatic fractures are common in children. The four zygomatic suture lines do not ossify until the seventh decade in many patients.[35] The frontozygomatic and zygomaticotemporal sutures are particularly weak and susceptible to disruption.[29] In the Kaban et al.[10,13] retrospective study, there were 51 zygomatic fractures, of which two thirds involved the zygomatic-maxillary complex and one third involved the zygomatic arch alone.

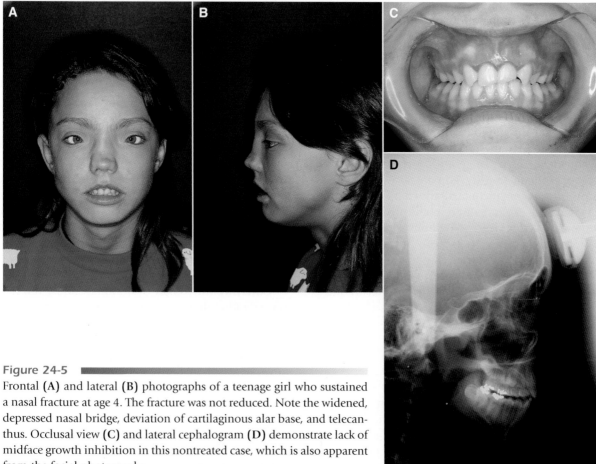

Figure 24-5
Frontal (**A**) and lateral (**B**) photographs of a teenage girl who sustained a nasal fracture at age 4. The fracture was not reduced. Note the widened, depressed nasal bridge, deviation of cartilaginous alar base, and telecanthus. Occlusal view (**C**) and lateral cephalogram (**D**) demonstrate lack of midface growth inhibition in this nontreated case, which is also apparent from the facial photographs.

There is a history of a blow to the cheek, usually with a fist or a blunt object. Zygomatic complex or arch fractures on the left side commonly are produced by a "right-handed" assailant. Physical examination may reveal a combination or all of the following: periorbital edema, ecchymosis and hematoma, conjunctival hemorrhage, antimongoloid slant of the lateral canthus, enophthalmos, palpable step deformities, and paresthesia in the distribution of the second division of the trigeminal nerve (Figures 24-6 to 24-8). There may be extraocular muscle dysfunction, secondary to injury or entrapment, resulting in limitation of upward gaze. This may be due to edema or hematoma in the orbital soft tissue, entrapment of orbital fat, and inferior rectus or inferior oblique muscles.[36] Palpation reveals tenderness and a diastasis at the frontozygomatic suture and tenderness and depression at the infraorbital rim and zygomatic arch. The cheek is flat, and there may be limitation of mandibular movement by impingement of the medially displaced arch on the coronoid process. Because of potential injury to the globe and the difficulty of performing a good ophthalmologic examination of injured children, an ophthalmologist should be consulted for all children with a zygomatic complex fracture.

Minimally displaced zygomatic fractures may be masked in young children by their subcutaneous fat and because poor cooperation immediately after the acute injury makes examination difficult. Asymmetry becomes evident with time, when the swelling goes down and some of the fat on the injured side atrophies (see Figure 24-8).

In the case of a zygomatic arch fracture, swelling, pain, and limitation of mandibular motion may be the only symptoms. The infraorbital nerve is not involved, hence there is no paresthesia. There is usually a palpable depression in the arch. There are no abnormalities of the orbit or globe in a pure zygomatic arch injury.

Historically, zygomaticomaxillary complex fractures and isolated arch fractures were confirmed by Waters' and submental vertex view radiographs. However, these radiographic techniques have been replaced by CT imaging because of the speed (especially with "light speed" scanners), superior clarity, and more accurate diagnostic information provided by this technique.[1] In addition, the positioning is easier for a child (see Figure 24-6).

Treatment

Zygomatic complex fractures with clinically significant displacement are treated by open reduction and rigid internal fixation.[26] The principles of fracture management in children do not differ from those in adults, but developing permanent dentition must be taken into consideration in children below age of 12 years. Treatment should be carried out 5 to 7 days after the injury, after the swelling has resolved but before the fracture consolidates. The frontozygomatic region is explored through an upper eyelid (supratarsal fold) incision[37] (Figure 24-9). This approach allows clear visualization of the suture, access for elevation of the zygoma, and room for placement of a miniplate. In children, most of these fractures are stable with one plate, perhaps because of the short distance (short lever arm) from the frontozygomatic suture to the infraorbital rim.[11] An intraoral buccal sulcus incision may be used, but in children less than 6 years of age, maxillary tooth buds are at risk during rigid fixation (even with microplates).[24,26] The infraorbital rim can be approached via an infraciliary incision, using a "stepped" dissection that results in less scarring and a low incidence of ectropion. The transconjunctival incision also provides sufficient access to the infraorbital rim for fixation. If a comminuted zygomatic arch fracture is associated with a displaced zygomatic complex fracture, the coronal incision may be combined with intraoral and infraciliary or transconjunctival incisions to give full exposure for exploration, reduction with internal fixation, and bone grafting when required. Resorbable plate systems may offer an alternative to titanium plates and screws in the pediatric trauma population.[38-40] The resorbable systems eliminate the need to remove plates and screws for fear of future problems or interference with growth.

Reduction of a zygomatic arch fracture can be done by the Gillies incision and elevation or an intraoral incision and elevation. Zygomatic arch fractures are usually stable after reduction.[10,41]

Kaban found that 31% (16 of 51) of patients with zygomaticomaxillary complex (ZMC) fractures had nondisplaced injuries requiring no intervention.[14] The remaining 35 children were treated by open reduction with either intraosseous wire fixation or a Caldwell-Luc approach to place a supporting pack in the maxillary sinus. There were no acute postoperative complications in these patients. However, three patients had long-term neurologic complaints: persistent paresthesia in the second division of the fifth cranial nerve (n = 2) and persistent third nerve palsy (n = 1).

Currently, microplate or miniplate and screw fixation is used rather than wire osteosynthesis when performing open reduction of zygomatic complex fractures in children (see Figure 24-6). Unfortunately, there are no reported long-term outcome studies of rigid internal fixation in a large series of pediatric patients with zygomatic fractures. Such studies are difficult to conduct because of the small number of patients and the loss of follow-up due to mobility of the population. Long-term data, however, are needed so that the aesthetic results, the effects on growth across the sutures, and the need to remove plates can be assessed.

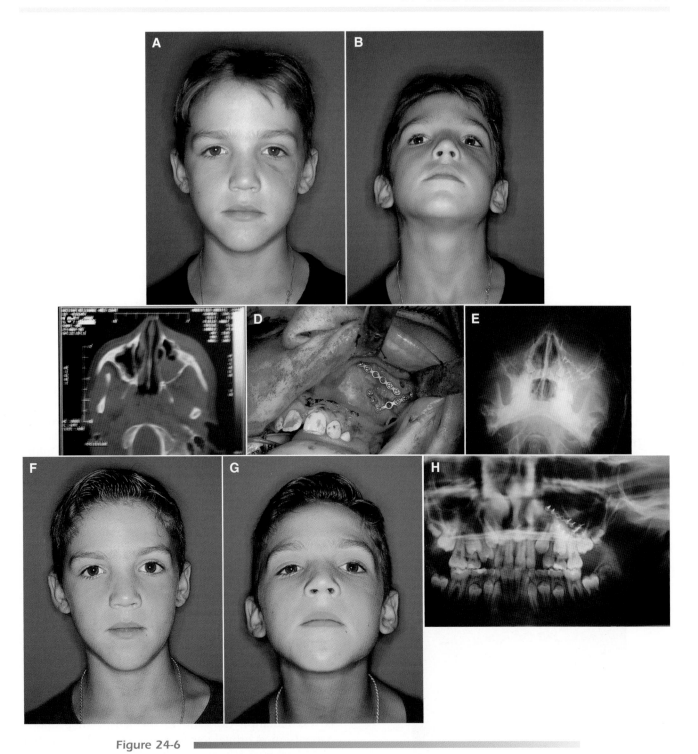

Figure 24-6

A young boy who sustained a blow to the left cheek. Frontal **(A)** and submental **(B)** photographs illustrate the typical findings of a zygomatic complex fracture: periorbital ecchymosis (mild in this case), antimongoloid slant of the lateral canthus, and depression of the cheek. Submental view better illustrates the marked left cheek depression. **C,** CT image shows a fracture at the anterior maxillary wall and a fluid-filled antrum. **D,** Intraoperative image shows the access via the intraoral, vestibular incision and the good reduction (achieved in this case with a Carroll-Gerard screw) and rigid internal fixation achieved using 2.0-mm plates (Synthes Maxillofacial, Paoli, PA). **E,** Postoperative submental vertex view confirms the proper reduction and symmetry. **F** and **G,** Good symmetry 1 year postoperatively. **H,** Panoramic radiograph 1 year postoperatively.

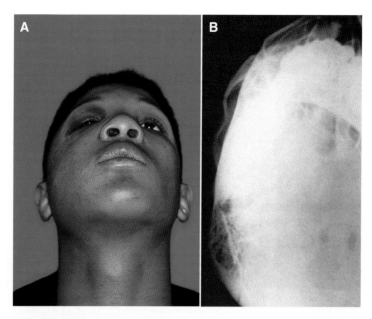

Figure 24-7

A, A teenage boy with a fracture of the right zygoma and zygomatic arch. **B**, Submental vertex radiograph demonstrates the depressed zygomatic arch fracture.

ORBITAL AND BLOWOUT FRACTURES
Diagnosis

The first description of posttraumatic enophthalmos was published in 1889 by Lang.[42] He concluded that the physical findings were secondary to fracture of the

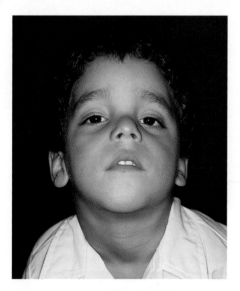

Figure 24-8

This 8-year-old child sustained a blow to the left cheek 1 month previously. He had a black eye and a swollen face. Waters' view radiograph was negative. He came to our clinic complaining of facial asymmetry. Physical examination revealed a depressed left zygoma and antimongoloid slant of the lateral canthus.

"orbital walls." Today, enophthalmos is attributed to a combination of herniation and atrophy of orbital fat, and increased orbital volume.[10,43] The source of injury may be a direct frontal blow to the orbit with a round object such as a baseball, tennis ball, doorknob, or fist. Physical examination may reveal periorbital ecchymosis, edema, and hematoma, as well as enophthalmos. Documentation of infraorbital nerve paresthesia and extraocular muscle dysfunction may be difficult in a pediatric patient (Figure 24-10). The child may refuse to move the eye because of pain, and a forced duction test is usually not possible in an awake child. Sedation or general anesthesia or both often are required to make the diagnosis of entrapment. All these children should be examined by an ophthalmologist.

A fine-cut (1-mm) CT scan, with three-dimensional reconstruction, should be obtained for the best anatomic delineation of the injury. The helical CT scan is desirable in children, because it reduces imaging time and there is less radiation exposure to the lens.[44] In pediatric patients, most orbital fractures involve the floor (20 out of 22 fractures), whereas in adults both the orbital floor and medial wall often are fractured.[45,46] In addition, most pediatric orbital floor fractures are located medial to the infraorbital nerve, and soft tissue is incarcerated in this region. The surgeon should be aware that soft tissue may be entrapped, even with an apparently small or subtle fracture.

Radiologic findings may be minimal because of the elasticity of the orbital floor. Tissue herniation into the maxillary sinus (tear drop sign) may not be evident because

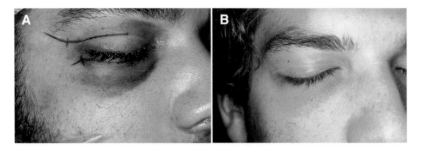

Figure 24-9

A, Supratarsal fold and infraciliary incisions for reduction of zygomatic fracture. **B,** Patient 3 months postoperatively, after supratarsal approach.

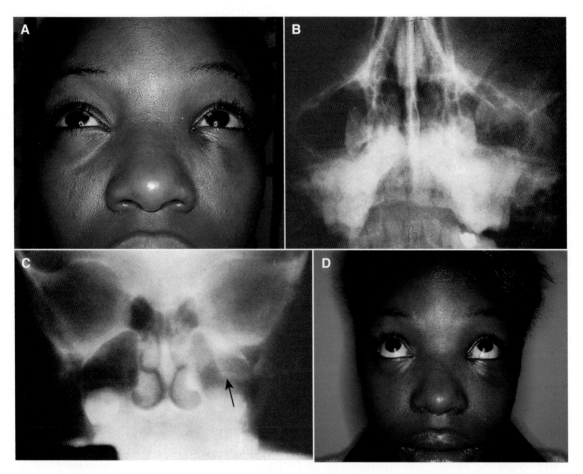

Figure 24-10

A, Frontal photograph of a 10-year-old girl with a left orbital blow-out fracture. Because of pain, the patient could not cooperate for testing of extraocular muscle function. A forced duction test under anesthesia revealed limitation of upward motion of the left globe. **B,** Waters' view radiograph demonstrates a cloudy antrum on the left side. A mucus-retention cyst is present on the right. **C,** Anteroposterior tomogram demonstrates orbital contents herniated into the left maxillary sinus *(arrow)* more clearly than on the Waters' view. **D,** Postoperative photograph shows full upward movement of the left globe.

of overlap of the fractured segment called a *trapdoor fracture*.[47] This is common in pediatric patients. When a child has diplopia and restriction of vertical gaze and little or no clinical evidence of soft tissue trauma (e.g., edema, ecchymosis), this fracture is referred to as *white-eyed blowout*.[48]

Many children can have significant nausea and vomiting after a blow to the eye. Nausea and vomiting may be a vagally mediated response to pain or other sensory feedback associated with extraocular muscle traction. This oculocardiac reflex consists of the triad of bradycardia, nausea, and syncope.[49]

Treatment

Pediatric patients demonstrating restriction and pain with ocular motion but who exhibit minimal signs of ocular trauma and minimal bone displacement (i.e., a trapdoor fracture or a white-eyed blowout), should be operated as soon as possible (within 24 to 48 hours).[50] Delay in surgical intervention may result in ischemic necrosis of the entrapped tissue.[49] In addition, early intervention may prevent fibrosis, thereby enhancing muscle recovery. Release of the soft tissue (fat, extraocular muscle) is the most important goal of the operation and allows for the return of ocular motility.[51]

Orbital fractures with a large orbital floor defect, without restriction in eye motility, can be explored in 5 to 7 days (when edema subsides). In the case of a large defect or a severely comminuted fracture, the orbital floor is reconstructed using either an alloplastic implant or an autologous bone graft. These fractures usually are found in adolescents and are treated in a manner similar to that used in adults. The primary goal is to prevent enophthalmos (Figure 24-11).

The infraorbital rim and orbital floor are approached through infraciliary or transconjunctival incisions. In a pure blowout fracture, the transconjunctival incision is recommended.[10,14,51-53] When there is a trapdoor fracture, it has been recommended to gently tease the entrapped tissue out of the fracture site using blunt dissection.[45] Alternatively, it is possible to create an osteotomy of the orbital floor, medial to the infraorbital nerve. This facilitates repositioning the orbital soft tissue with less dissection and manipulation, thereby avoiding further injury to the orbital contents. Endoscopic visualization of orbital floor fractures may be a useful tool in children and adolescents after the maxillary sinus is developed. Endoscopy is indicated to visualize areas difficult to access (posterior orbit) and to confirm complete repositioning of the entrapped soft tissue. Furthermore, when implants or bone grafts are used, endoscopic confirmation of the posterior extent of the implant or graft is useful[54] (Figure 24-12).

Of the 184 midfacial fractures reported by Kaban, 21 were blowout fractures.[13,14] Of the 21 patients, 17 underwent orbital floor exploration for enophthalmos, a large orbital floor defect, or significant limitation of upward gaze. Nine patients had orbital floor reconstruction with a Silastic implant, and eight patients had reduction with no implant. No late complications were reported in the nine patients who had Silastic implants, and none of the implants was removed in 1 to 8 years of follow-up.[10,11] There have been more recent reports recommending the use of Gelfilm or Medpor for orbital wall reconstruction in pediatric patients.[45] The use of autogenous bone grafts from the skull has also been recommended.[51] The choice of material often is made on the basis of the size and location of the orbital floor defect.

LE FORT FRACTURES
Diagnosis

Le Fort fractures are the least commonly reported midfacial injuries in children. The child's midface is protected by the prominent calvaria. There are no good data on the incidence of Le Fort fractures in those children who die as a result of craniocerebral and other injuries in high-speed motor vehicle accidents. In Rowe's series of midfacial fractures in children, 40% had skull fractures and 14% had cerebrospinal fluid rhinorrhea.[4,7] Perhaps with better restraints and more compliance, children will survive life-threatening injuries and receive treatment for associated midfacial fractures. The reported incidence may then rise to coincide with the true incidence.

Six Le Fort II and four Le Fort III fractures out of a total of 210 pediatric facial fractures were reported by Reil and Kranz.[55] Kaban et al.[10] reported no Le Fort fractures in a series of 122 pediatric facial fractures over a 10-year period. During the follow-up study (an additional 9 years), an additional 140 pediatric midfacial fractures were reported, of which only five were Le Fort fractures (all Le Fort III). Three of the five Le Fort fractures (60%) were the result of motor vehicle accidents. Iida et al.[8] reported only two Le Fort fractures in the age group from 0 to 9 years during a period between 1981 and 1996.

Physical examination may reveal all or a combination of the following: bilateral periorbital ecchymosis and edema, conjunctival hemorrhage, traumatic telecanthus, and elongation of the middle third of the face (Figures 24-13 and 24-14). The fractures are commonly comminuted in the nasoethmoidal region and may be split in the midline[1,14] (see Figure 24-14). In the Le Fort I fracture, the maxilla is mobile, but the nose and zygomas are stable. In the Le Fort II injury, the central segment of the midface (i.e., maxilla and nose) is mobile. Movement is palpable at the infraorbital rims and the nasofrontal suture. Le Fort III fractures exhibit mobility at the fron-

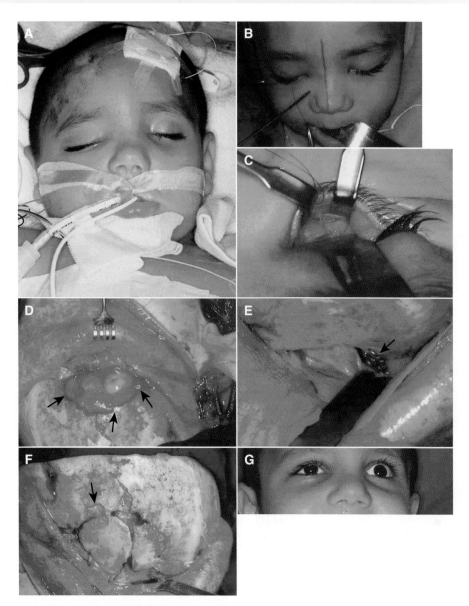

Figure 24-11

A, This 3-year-old boy came to the emergency room intubated after falling four stories. The child suffered naso-ethmoidal-orbital and anterior frontal sinus fractures. **B,** Intraoperative photograph shows the hypertelorism. **C,** Intraoperative view of the transconjunctival incision. The soft tissue was freed from the trapdoor fracture. No graft was required. **D,** Intraoperative view of the frontal sinus fractures *(arrows)*. **E,** The nasal fracture was reduced and fixed using a miniplate *(arrow)*. **F,** The sinus fracture was reduced and stabilized using a resorbable plate *(arrow)*. **G,** Postoperative result. A slight enophthalmos persists, although it is greatly improved and will be repaired in the future.

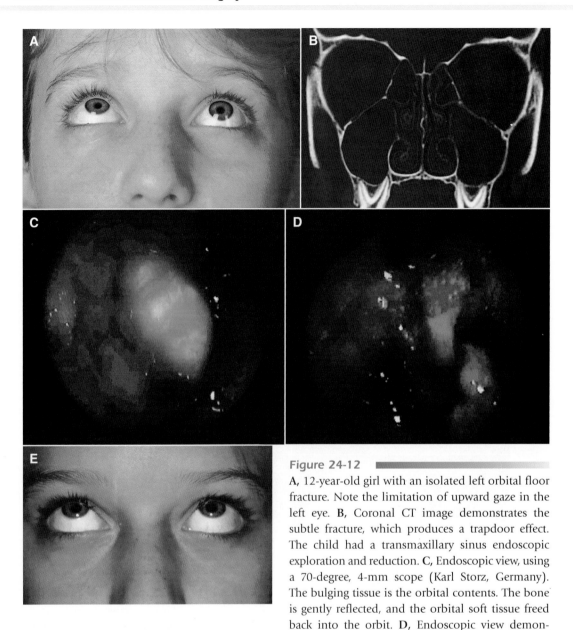

Figure 24-12

A, 12-year-old girl with an isolated left orbital floor fracture. Note the limitation of upward gaze in the left eye. **B,** Coronal CT image demonstrates the subtle fracture, which produces a trapdoor effect. The child had a transmaxillary sinus endoscopic exploration and reduction. **C,** Endoscopic view, using a 70-degree, 4-mm scope (Karl Storz, Germany). The bulging tissue is the orbital contents. The bone is gently reflected, and the orbital soft tissue freed back into the orbit. **D,** Endoscopic view demonstrates that the bone has been reduced. No plating or grafting is required. **E,** Postoperative photograph. Both eyes demonstrate good upward gaze.

tozygomatic and the nasofrontal sutures. With nasoethmoidal injuries, there may be crepitus over the nose and forehead. Often there is an associated malocclusion, but this may be difficult to judge in the pediatric patient because of dentoalveolar injuries and poor cooperation. Waters' view radiographs are not particularly helpful because swelling, lack of full development of the sinuses, overlapping structures, and multiple tooth buds in the maxilla mask the fractures. Fine-cut (1-mm) CT scan with three-dimensional reconstruction is the diagnostic imaging tool of choice for these fractures (see Figures 24-13 and 24-14).

Treatment

The principles of midfacial fracture treatment in pediatric patients are similar to those in adults. However, one has to consider the developing permanent dentition in children below the age of 12 years. This makes it difficult to stabilize the alveolar portion of the fracture by plates and screws. Because clinical union occurs much more rapidly in children, prolonged periods of immobilization are not necessary.

Le Fort I fractures in children less than age 6 rarely require surgical intervention and when they do, closed reduction with maxillomandibular fixation (usually with

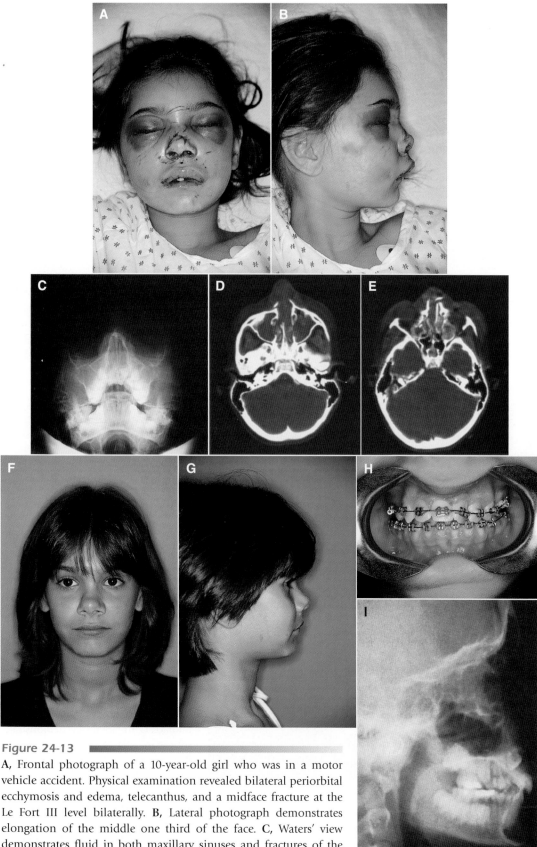

Figure 24-13

A, Frontal photograph of a 10-year-old girl who was in a motor vehicle accident. Physical examination revealed bilateral periorbital ecchymosis and edema, telecanthus, and a midface fracture at the Le Fort III level bilaterally. **B,** Lateral photograph demonstrates elongation of the middle one third of the face. **C,** Waters' view demonstrates fluid in both maxillary sinuses and fractures of the infraorbital rims. The specific fractures are difficult to delineate. **D** and **E,** Axial CT scans show the depressed midface, nasal fractures, and comminuted ethmoid complex. Frontal **(F)** and lateral **(G)** photographs, occlusal view **(H),** and lateral cephalogram **(I)** demonstrate normal facial appearance and midface development 3 years postoperatively.

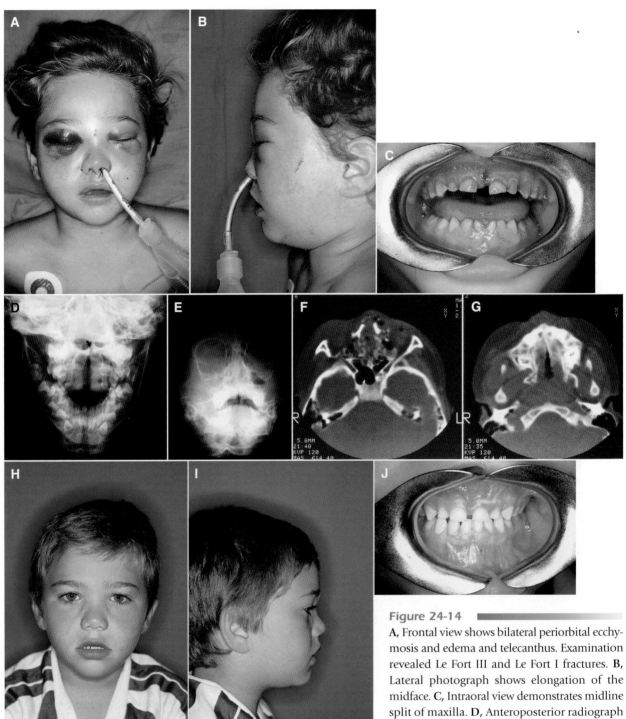

Figure 24-14

A, Frontal view shows bilateral periorbital ecchymosis and edema and telecanthus. Examination revealed Le Fort III and Le Fort I fractures. **B,** Lateral photograph shows elongation of the midface. **C,** Intraoral view demonstrates midline split of maxilla. **D,** Anteroposterior radiograph shows a midline fracture of maxilla, extending from the alveolar ridge into the nasal floor. **E,** Waters' view illustrates fluid in both maxillary sinuses, and the medial wall of orbit displaced on the patient's left. **F** and **G,** CT images show depressed midface, nasoethmoid fractures, and midline split of palate. **H,** One year postoperatively, the midface proportions are restored, and the telecanthus is corrected. Note the dacryocystorhinostomy incisions. **I,** Lateral photograph showing midface projection. **J,** Occlusion.

Stout wires) can be used. Suspension on the zygomatic arches or superior region of the piriform apertures can be used. At this age, plates and screws, even monocortical, cannot be applied safely to the tooth-bearing portion of the maxilla without damaging the tooth buds. It is also important to remember that the zygomatic arch is thin and the bone soft in this age group. Excessive tightening of wires can pull through the bone.

Le Fort II and III fractures are treated by open reduction and rigid internal fixation. The fractured bony segments are positioned properly, thereby restoring the facial skeleton and reestablishing the occlusion. Low-profile miniplates and microplates are recommended.[26] In Kaban's long-term follow-up study of the five Le Fort III fractures, one patient (see Figure 24-14) required bilateral dacryocystorhinostomies within 1 year after open reduction.[14] There were no other complications. One patient, followed to completion of growth, showed no midfacial retrusion (see Figure 24-13). The other four patients followed for at least 2 years have shown no tendency toward midfacial hypoplasia. It appears that midfacial fractures without tissue loss (particularly nasal septal cartilage damage), and with adequate reduction, do not result in midfacial growth inhibition. Schultz and Meilman[17] also reported no growth impairment in patients with midfacial fractures. However, they found that children with severe orbital and nasoethmoidal injuries often had residual local deformity. Posnick et al.[12] found no short-term growth abnormalities in children treated with rigid fixation of midfacial fractures. Schliephake et al.[56] also found no midfacial retrusion after midfacial fracture treatment in children.

CONCLUSION

The incidence of midfacial fractures in children is low because of the anatomic protection afforded by the prominent calvaria. Careful history, physical examination, and CT imaging provide the basis for the diagnosis of these injuries. Only minimally displaced fractures should be considered for observation alone. Early intervention should be considered when there are functional disturbances. Standard principles of rigid internal fixation can be also applied to pediatric patients, but not indiscriminately. The surgeon must be aware of the developing permanent dentition and growth of the young patient. Plates should not traverse a suture, because they may inhibit growth. The removal of plates and screws remains controversial in both adults and children.[57,58] Long-term follow-up studies are needed in the pediatric age group—especially in the areas of rigid fixation, biodegradable rigid fixation, and long-term stability of midfacial fractures—to better document the effects these injuries and the proposed treatments on growth and long-term function.

REFERENCES

1. Chuang SK, Dodson TB: Evaluation and management of pediatric midface injuries, *OMS Knowledge Update* 3:37-46, 2001.
2. Panagopoulos AP: Management of fractures of the jaws in children, *J Int Coll Surg* 8:806-811, 1957.
3. Hagan EH, Huelke OF: An analysis of 319 case reports of mandibular fractures, *J Oral Surg* 19:93, 1961.
4. Rowe NL, Killey HC: *Fractures of the facial skeleton*, ed 2. Baltimore, 1968, Williams & Wilkins, pp 173, 425.
5. Rowe NL: Fractures of the jaws in children, *J Oral Surg* 27:497-507, 1969.
6. VanHoof RF, Merkx CA, Stekelenburg EC: Different patterns of facial fractures in four European countries, *Int J Oral Maxillofac Surg* 6:3-11, 1977.
7. James O: Maxillofacial injuries in children. In Rowe NL, Williams JL: *Maxillofacial injuries*, London, 1985, Churchill Livingstone, pp 538-558.
8. Iida S, Kogo M, Sugiura T, et al: Retrospective analysis of 1502 patients with facial fractures, *Int J Oral Maxillofac Surg* 30:286-290, 2001.
9. MacLennan WO: Fractures of the mandible in children under age 6, *Br J Plast Surg* 9:125, 1956.
10. Kaban LB, Mulliken JB, Murray JE: Facial fractures in children: an analysis of 122 fractures in 109 patients, *Plast Reconstr Surg* 59:15-20, 1977.
11. Mulliken JB, Kaban LB, Murray JE: Management of facial fractures in children, *Clin Plast Surg* 4:491-502, 1977.
12. Posnick JC, Wells M, Pron G: Pediatric facial fractures: evolving patterns of treatment, *J Oral Maxillofac Surg* 51:836-844, 1993.
13. Kaban LB: Symposium on pediatric maxillofacial trauma: midfacial fractures in children. Presented at the 67th Annual Meeting of the American Association of Oral and Maxillofacial Surgeons, Washington, DC, October 3-7, 1985.
14. Kaban LB: Facial trauma I. Midface fractures. In Kaban LB, editor: *Pediatric oral & maxillofacial surgery*, Philadelphia, 1990, Saunders, pp 209-232.
15. Iizuka T, Thorén H, Annino DJ, et al: Midfacial fractures in pediatric patients. Frequency, characteristics and causes, *Arch Otolaryngol Head Neck Surg* 121:1366-1371, 1995.
16. Shelness A, Charles S: Children as passengers in automobiles: the neglected minority on the nation's highways, *Pediatrics* 56:271, 1975.
17. Schultz RC, Meilman J: Facial fractures in children. In Goldwyn RM: *Long-term results in plastic and reconstructive surgery*, Boston, 1980, Little Brown, pp 458-480.
18. Enlow DH: *Facial growth*, ed 3. Philadelphia, 1990, Saunders.
19. Messinger A, Radkowski MA, Greenwald MJ, Pensler JM: Orbital roof fractures in the pediatric population, *Plast Reconstr Surg* 84:213-216, 1989.
20. Posnick JC: Craniomaxillofacial fractures in children. In Kaban LB, editor: Oral and maxillofacial surgery in children and adolescents, *Oral Maxillofac Surg Clin North Am* 6(1):169-185, 1994.
21. Kaban LB: Diagnosis and treatment of fractures of the facial bones in children 1943-1993, *J Oral Maxillofac Surg* 51:722-729, 1993.
22. Holland AJ, Broome C, Steinberg A, Cass DT: Facial fracture in children, *Pediatr Emerg Care* 17:157-160, 2001.
23. Beatrous WP: Tracheostomy (tracheotomy): its expanded indications and its present status. Based on an analysis of 1000 consecutive operations and a review of the recent literature, *Laryngoscope* 78:3-55, 1968.
24. Kaban LB, Longaker MT: Ancillary surgical procedures. In Kaban LB, editor: *Pediatric oral & maxillofacial surgery*, Philadelphia, 1990, Saunders, pp 45-61.
25. Line WS Jr, Hawkins DB, Kahlstrom EJ, et al: Tracheostomy in infants and young children: the changing perspective 1970-1985, *Laryngoscope* 96:510-515, 1986.

26. Beirne OR, Myall RW: Rigid internal fixation in children. In Kaban LB, editor: Oral and maxillofacial surgery in children and adolescents, *Oral Maxillofac Surg Clin North Am* 6(1):153-167, 1994.

27. Nahum AM: The biomechanics of maxillofacial trauma, *Clin Plast Surg* 2:59-64, 1975.

28. Anderson PJ: Fractures of the facial skeleton in children, *Injury* 26:47-50, 1995.

29. Converse JM: Facial injuries in children. In Kazanjian VH, Converse JM: *The surgical treatment of facial injuries*, Baltimore, 1974, Williams and Wilkins, p 378.

30. Goodman LS, Gilman A: *The pharmacological basis of therapeutics*, ed 5. New York, 1975, Macmillan, p 387.

31. Mustoe TA, Kaban LB, Mulliken JB: Nasal fractures in children, *Br J Plast Surg* 10:135-138, 1987.

32. Fry H: Nasal skeletal trauma and the interlocked stresses of the nasal septal cartilage, *Br J Plast Surg* 20:146, 1961.

33. Winters HP: Isolated fractures of the nasal bones, *Arch Chir Neerl* 19:159, 1967.

34. Mayell MJ: Nasal fractures: their occurrence, management and some late results, *J R Coll Surg Edinb* 18:31, 1973.

35. Kokich V: Age changes in the human fronto-zygomatic suture from 20-95 years, *Am J Orthod* 69:411, 1976.

36. Koornneff L: Orbital septa: anatomy and function, *Ophthalmology* 86:876-880, 1979.

37. Chuong R, Kaban LB: Fractures of the zygomatic complex, *J Oral Maxillofac Surg* 44:283-288, 1986.

38. Eppley BL, Prevel CD, Sadove AM, Sarver D: Resorbable bone fixation: its potential role in craniomaxillofacial trauma, *J Craniomaxillofac Trauma* 2:56-60, 1996.

39. Triana RJ Jr, Shockley WW: Pediatric zygomatico-orbital complex fractures: the use of resorbable plating systems. A case report, *J Craniomaxillofac Trauma* 4:32-36, 1996.

40. Imola MJ, Hamlar DD, Shao W, et al: Resorbable plate fixation in pediatric craniofacial surgery: long term outcome, *Arch Facial Plast Surg* 3:79-90, 2001.

41. Pozatek ZW, Kaban LB, Guralnick WC: Fractures of the zygomatic complex: an evaluation of surgical management with special emphasis on the eyebrow approach, *J Oral Surg* 31:141-148, 1973.

42. Lang W: Traumatic enophthalmos with retention of perfect acuity of vision, *Trans Ophth Soc U K* 9:43, 1889.

43. Smith B, Regan WF: Blowout fracture of the orbit, *Am J Ophthalmol* 44:733-739, 1957.

44. Lakits A, Prokesch R, Schholda C, Bankier A: Orbital helical computed tomography in the diagnosis and management of eye trauma, *Ophthalmology* 106:2330-2335, 1999.

45. Bansagi ZC, Meyer DR: Internal orbital fractures in pediatric age group, characterization and management, *Ophthalmology* 107:829-836, 2000.

46. Burm JS, Chung CH, Oh SJ: Pure orbital blowout fracture: new concepts and importance of medial orbital blowout fracture, *Plast Reconstr Surg* 103:1839-1849, 1999.

47. Soll DB, Polley BJ: Trapdoor variety of blowout fracture of the orbital floor, *Am J Ophthalmol* 60:269-272, 1965.

48. Jordan DR, Allen LH, White J, et al: Intervention within days for some orbital floor fractures: the white-eyed blowout, *Ophthal Plast Reconstr Surg*14:379-390, 1998.

49. Sires BS, Stanley RB Jr, Levine LM: Oculocardiac reflex caused by orbital floor trapdoor fracture: an indication for urgent repair, *Arch Ophthalmol* 116:955-956, 1998.

50. Chandler DB, Rubin PAD: Development in the understanding and management of pediatric orbital fractures, *Int Ophthalmol Clin* 41(4):87-104, 2001.

51. Grant JH, Patrinely JR, Weiss AH, et al: Trapdoor fracture of the orbit in a pediatric population, *Plast Reconstr Surg* 109:482-495, 2002.

52. Ellis E III, Zide MF: *Surgical approaches to the facial skeleton*, Williams & Wilkins, 1995, Baltimore, pp 7-62.

53. Baumann A, Ewers R: Use of the preseptal transconjunctival approach in orbit reconstructive surgery, *J Oral Maxillofac Surg* 59:287-291, 2001.

54. Chen CT, Chen YR: Endoscopically assisted repair of orbital floor fractures, *Plast Reconstr Surg* 108:2011-2018, 2001.

55. Reil B, Kranz S: Traumatology of the maxillo-facial region in childhood, *J Maxillofac Surg* 4:197, 1976.

56. Schliephake H, Berten JL, Neukam FW, et al: Growth disorders following fractures of the midface in children, *Dtsch Zahnarztl Z* 45:819-822, 1990.

57. Bhatt V, Langford RJ: Removal of miniplates in maxillofacial surgery: University Hospital Birmingham experience, *J Oral Maxillofac Surg* 61:553-556, 2003.

58. Bartlett SP, DeLozier JB III: Controversies in the management of pediatric facial fractures, *Clin Plast Surg* 19(1):245-258, 1992.

Facial Trauma II: Dentoalveolar Injuries and Mandibular Fractures

Arnulf Baumann, Maria J. Troulis, and Leonard B. Kaban

CHAPTER OUTLINE

Mandibular fractures are the most common (56%) facial skeletal injury in hospitalized pediatric trauma patients.[1,2] Boys are affected twice as frequently as girls.[2,3] Dentoalveolar injuries are a more frequent facial injury (60%) in children (especially under the age of 5) but rarely require hospitalization.[2] For this reason, hospital databases do not include dentoalveolar trauma, because the child usually is treated by a dentist or oral maxillofacial surgeon in an office setting. Understanding of dentoalveolar and mandibular injuries is important because of the potential complications related to tooth eruption, alveolar development, occlusion, and facial growth.

A fall from a bicycle, steps, or climbing apparatus is the most common cause of mandibular or dentoalveolar trauma.[2] In 61.4% of bicycle-related injuries, children under the age of 15 years suffered some type of oral or maxillofacial injury.[4] Most of the oral or maxillofacial injuries were facial abrasions, cuts, and lacerations (50.3%), followed by oral soft tissue injuries (30.9%), dentoalveolar trauma (9.7%), and mandibular, nasal, and zygomatic fractures (9.1%). Over one half of these children were wearing bicycle helmets, which do not protect the face and jaw. Following falls, blunt trauma from an object (baseball bat, hockey puck) and motor vehicle accidents are the most common causes of mandibular and dentoalveolar injuries.[2,5-8] Although child abuse is a rare cause of maxillofacial trauma,[9-11] it should be considered in the patient who suffers repeated or recurrent injury. In most states, the clinician is legally obligated to report cases of suspected child battering to the authorities.[12-14]

Comprehensive physical evaluation is especially important because of the high incidence of associated injuries. In 1977, Kaban et al.[5] reported that 22 of 29 patients (75.8%) with mandibular fractures had additional injuries, including other facial fractures, extremity fractures, skull fractures, craniocerebral injuries, and cervical spine fractures. Patients who fall off a bicycle and sustain trauma to the chin and dentoalveolar structures should be evaluated thoroughly for cervical spine fracture. The coincidence of cervical spine injury (usually the upper cervical spine) (Figure 25-1) with mandibular fractures is well documented.[15-17] Lewis et al.[18] found that 9.6% of 982 patients with cervical spine injuries had facial fractures. Patients under 2 years of age are considered at high risk for cervical spine injury with other "isolated" face or head injuries. Because they cannot always relate that they have neck pain, their cervical spines must be evaluated using radiographs.[19]

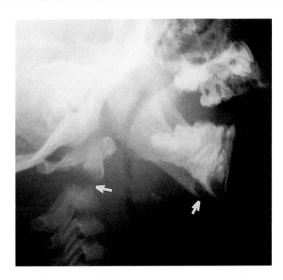

Figure 25-1

Lateral skull radiograph of a 3-year-old girl who sustained bilateral subcondylar and parasymphysis *(right arrow)* fractures of the mandible. There is a concomitant fracture dislocation of the odontoid process *(left arrow)* of the second cervical vertebra. Although the jaw is not closed (pain prevented full range of motion), the severe retrognathism and the open bite can be appreciated.

DENTAL TRAUMA AND DENTOALVEOLAR INJURIES

General Considerations

Dentoalveolar injuries may be quite dramatic, causing parents to panic and the child to cry uncontrollably, with blood, tooth, and soft tissue debris in the mouth. The most common location is the anterior maxilla, followed by the anterior mandible. Children with protrusive maxillary teeth are particularly at risk for repeated dentoalveolar trauma.[20,21] Frequently, the lips and alveolar soft tissues are injured also. When there is isolated trauma to the teeth and alveolus, the child's overall physical condition is usually normal. However, damage to the teeth and alveolar structures may occur in association with severe maxillofacial or multiple system injuries, which should not be overlooked.[6]

Intrusion and avulsion of teeth are common dentoalveolar injuries in young children.[22] Approximately one fourth of intrusion injuries will affect the developing tooth bud, resulting in enamel hypoplasia.[23] Epidemiologic studies reveal that one out of two children will sustain some sort of a dental injury (crown fracture being the most common), usually between the ages of 8 and 12.[22] Furthermore, dental trauma in children and adolescents has increased during the last 20 years.[24]

When a tooth is avulsed, the periodontal fibers and the neurovascular bundle at the root apex are severed. There may be concomitant damage to the socket and root. The prognosis of an avulsed tooth is largely dependent on the status of the cells of the periodontal ligament at the time of reimplantation.[25-28] If the periodontal ligament is intact, the consequences of tooth avulsion are usually minimal.[26,29] In contrast, when the cells are damaged, a severe inflammatory response over a large area of the root surface develops. This results in either ankylosis[30,31] or root resorption.[32] The tooth can also be lost due to a combination of an inflammatory response of the necrotic pulp and bacterial contamination.[33] Therefore, treatment strategies that decrease inflammation and contamination must be considered. For these reasons, handling and transportation of avulsed teeth by the parents will influence the outcome. When there is an isolated dentoalveolar injury, the parents usually telephone for advice. If so, they should be directed to retrieve the tooth and store it in an appropriate medium such as milk or the patient's saliva.[29]

Diagnosis

The force and nature of the traumatic event are determined from the account of a parent, the child, or any other witness. General physical examination is carried out and the child's condition is stabilized as necessary. Maxillofacial examination reveals missing, chipped, and mobile teeth, damaged or missing restorations or crowns, and other loose debris (e.g., glass, pebbles, dirt), as well as soft tissue injuries (Figures 25-2 and 25-3). The clinical examination should include a vitality test. If teeth or restorations are missing, their location must be determined. If this is not possible, a chest radiograph should be obtained to rule out aspiration (Figure 25-4). If not localized in the chest, then an abdominal radiograph should also be obtained.

Radiographs are necessary to document dental and alveolar fractures. In addition, root fragments remaining in the socket or between the alveolus and overlying soft tissue must be localized. A panoramic radiograph is most helpful but should be supplemented by periapical and occlusal radiographs. Periapical radiographs are used to determine dental fractures and may also localize radiopaque foreign bodies and teeth lodged in the surrounding soft tissues, most commonly the lips. Computed tomography scans may be helpful in severe dentoalveolar fractures.[34]

Andreasen and Andreasen described a classification of traumatic dental injuries based on the specific structures involved.[20] The following is a summary of this system:

1. Hard dental tissues and pulp:
    a. Fractures of the crown: enamel alone; enamel and dentin; enamel, dentin, and pulp (complicated crown fracture)

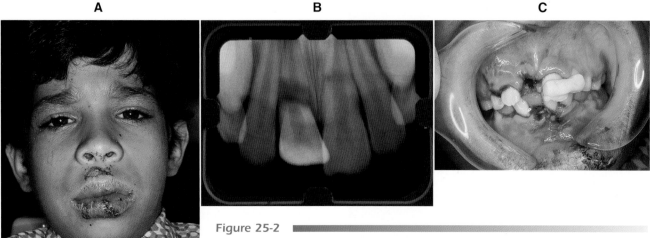

Figure 25-2

Dentoalveolar injuries. **A,** This patient sustained blunt trauma to the perioral region in a fight. The lower lip laceration has been sutured. **B,** Periapical radiograph shows that the upper left central incisor was partially avulsed and was repositioned. The right central incisor has a fracture of the cervical one third of the root and was extracted. **C,** Acid-etched splint stabilizing the central to the left lateral incisor, which was not injured.

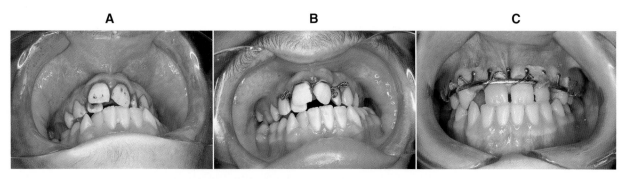

Figure 25-3

A, Occlusal photograph of patient with partially avulsed and loosened upper central incisors. **B,** The teeth were intruded and repositioned and were stabilized with Stout wiring from canine to canine. **C,** Another case, showing an arch bar immobilizing the partially avulsed maxillary central incisors and a fractured right lateral incisor. An arch bar was used from premolar to premolar to provide more stability than dental wires.

    b. Fractures of crown and root: enamel, dentin, cementum without pulpal exposure; enamel, dentin, cementum with pulpal exposure
    c. Root fracture: dentin, cementum, and pulp
2. Periodontal tissues: concussion without loosening, loosening without displacement (subluxation), loosening with partial displacement (extrusive or lateral luxation), complete avulsion, retained root
3. Alveolar bone: fractures of the alveolus, with or without comminution

Treatment

Guidelines for the management of traumatic dental injuries have been published by the International Association of Dental Traumatology for primary teeth and permanent teeth.[35-39] Significant changes in treatment of dental injuries have occurred during the last decade (based on increased knowledge of the biology of dental healing and retrospective studies). Treatment protocols have been developed for both primary and permanent dentitions.

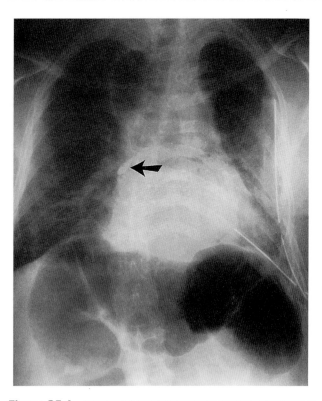

Figure 25-4
Chest radiograph shows premolar tooth *(arrow)* aspirated into right mainstem bronchus.

Treatment of dentoalveolar injuries of the *primary dentition* are based on the child's cooperation and life expectancy of the affected primary tooth.[22] Dental crown fractures involving the enamel usually require no treatment during the acute phase, unless the patient is bothered by sharp edges rubbing against the soft tissue. In these cases, the crown is smoothed with a bur. Complicated crown fractures with pulp exposure may be treated by partial pulpotomy if the apex is open in the young primary incisor. Pulpotomy with formocresol and zinc oxide eugenol is done if the normal physiologic resorption process has not started. Treatment of root fractures depends on the level of the injury. The mobile coronal fragment should be extracted in a tooth with either a crown-root or root fracture. However, root fragments that are not well visualized should not be removed if this is likely to damage underlying permanent tooth buds. For primary teeth that suffer periodontal injuries such as concussion or subluxation, only symptomatic relief and observation are recommended. Intruded teeth can be allowed to erupt spontaneously. In a retrospective study of 172 intruded teeth, most of them reerupted and survived with no complications (follow-up of 36 months).[40] However, after intrusion of a primary tooth, the developing permanent tooth may be affected, resulting in enamel abnormalities.[23] Extruded primary teeth should be extracted. Avulsed primary teeth should not be implanted because of the potential damage to the underlying permanent tooth bud. Alveolar fractures, although rare in this age group, should be repositioned and splinted to the adjacent teeth for 3 to 4 weeks.

Dentoalveolar injuries in the *permanent dentition* have psychological consequences for both the child and parents. It is important to make an effort to save traumatized teeth and dental segments.[17,35-39] Dental crown fractures involving the enamel usually require no acute treatment unless the patient is bothered by sharp edges, which can be smoothed down. Dental fractures extending into the dentin usually are treated with a temporary glass-ionomer cement or a permanent restoration using a bonding agent and composite resin. Fractures into the pulp require calcium hydroxide pulp capping or partial pulpotomy in an immature tooth or pulpectomy in a mature tooth, depending on the size of pulpal exposure.[35-39] Definitive endodontic treatment is carried out, depending on the tooth's vitality and level of root development.[41] In cases of crown and root fractures, in which the coronal fragment is attached to the gingiva and mobile, the coronal fragment should be stabilized with an acid etch–resin splint to adjacent teeth for 3 weeks. When there is a subgingival fracture, the site may be exposed by gingivectomy or surgical extrusion. If root formation is complete, root canal treatment is indicated.

Root fractures occur rarely, accounting for 0.5% to 7% of all dental trauma cases.[42] The treatment recommendations for root fractures have changed recently. Since the 1970s, rigid splinting was applied to bridge the fractured tooth for 2 to 3 months to allow for hard tissue bridging between the fragments.[20] However, a recent retrospective study showed that splinted teeth were associated with less hard tissue healing than teeth that were not splinted.[43] Endodontic treatment should be started if there is no vitality or if clinical signs of periodontitis and radiolucency appear.[44] In a recent study, teeth with a transverse fracture at the cervical third of the root were lost in 44% of the cases, but in only 8% of oblique fractures at the apical portion were the teeth lost.[45] Splinting had no influence on the tooth's survival in this study.[45] Therefore, teeth with a closed apex and transverse fracture above the middle third of the root should be extracted. In these cases, the lost teeth can be replaced with implants. When an implant is to be placed in the future, the root can be treated with calcium hydroxide and maintained so it preserves the alveolar bone.[46]

Subluxated or contused permanent teeth that are mobile, but not displaced, should be treated with a flexible splint for 7 to 10 days.[35-39] Intruded teeth should be allowed to erupt spontaneously. When root formation is complete, prophylactic extirpation of the pulp should be done 1 to 3 weeks after the injury. Loose and partially avulsed teeth (extruded teeth) are repositioned and stabilized with a splint for up to 3 weeks.

Avulsed teeth should be implanted as soon as possible. The extraoral time should be less than 60 minutes to avoid resorption.[28] If the root is contaminated, it is cleaned with saline solution. Before replantation, the blood clot should be removed from the socket. The socket walls should be examined and, if necessary, repositioned gently, and the tooth replanted slowly with slight digital pressure or by having the patient bite gently on a cotton roll. A permanent tooth with an open apex should be placed in a doxycycline solution (1 mg/20 ml saline) before it is replaced. Permanent teeth with a closed apex, which are to be replanted after an extraoral time of less than 60 minutes, should be immersed in a 2.4% sodium fluoride solution with a pH 5.5 for a minimum of 5 minutes to remove remaining periodontal ligament.[35-39] This procedure decreases the inflammatory response. If the extraoral time of a tooth with an open apex is greater than 60 minutes, the chance of revascularization is poor.[29,35-39] However, as stated earlier, virtually no tooth should be turned down for replantation. It is possible to achieve success occasionally, even with teeth that have been out of the oral environment for a long period (Figure 25-5). If the tooth is replanted, endodontic treatment should be initiated as early as possible. After replantation of the teeth, systemic antibiotics are administered (doxycycline 2 per day for 7 days or penicillin V 500 mg 4 times per day for 7 days or according to the patient's age and weight). Tetanus booster should also be considered. Replanted teeth should be followed clinically and radiographically for ankylosis or external or internal root resorption. Immature teeth are treated endodontically at the first sign of root resorption or pulp necrosis.

Dentoalveolar fractures are reduced and immobilized with arch bars or dental splints for 3 to 4 weeks (Figure 25-6). There are a variety of techniques to stabilize luxated and avulsed teeth with a splint. A wire-composite splint, bracket splint, resin splint, or titanium splint can be applied to the adjacent teeth (one firm tooth) using acid-etched composite. These splints maintain physiologic tooth mobility, which is important for periodontal healing.[47,48] In children with dentoalveolar injuries in whom a dry field cannot be maintained, an arch bar can be used. The duration of splinting dentoalveolar injuries is summarized in Table 25-1.

Commonly associated with dentoalveolar injuries are intraoral soft tissue injuries. Caregivers should be instructed about good oral hygiene in order to promote soft tissue healing. Soft diet for 2 weeks is indicated, and teeth should be brushed with a soft toothbrush after

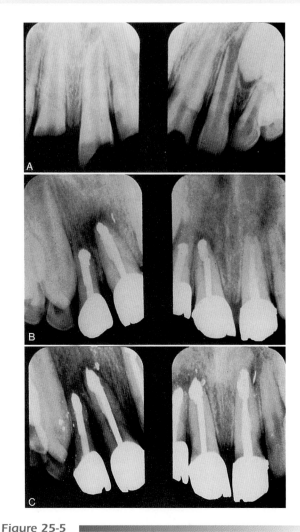

Figure 25-5

Replanted teeth. **A,** Periapical radiographs immediately after replantation of upper right and left central and right lateral incisors. These teeth were out of the mouth and in the dirt for several hours before replantation. The parents insisted that an attempt be made to save the teeth. **B,** Six months after replantation. Endodontic therapy was completed approximately 6 weeks after the acute injury, when the teeth were stable. **C,** Two years after apicoectomy and retrograde amalgams and 3 years after replantation. The teeth are stable, the periapical areas are filling in with bone, and there is no root resorption.

each meal. Topical use of chlorhexidine mouthrinse (0.1%) twice a day for 1 to 2 weeks may be advisable.[35-39] With significant soft tissue injuries, systemic antibiotics should also be prescribed.

MANDIBULAR FRACTURES
General Considerations

In adults, approximately 60% of mandibular fractures occur in the third molar, angle, or subcondylar regions (i.e., in the anatomically thinnest portion of the

A   B   C

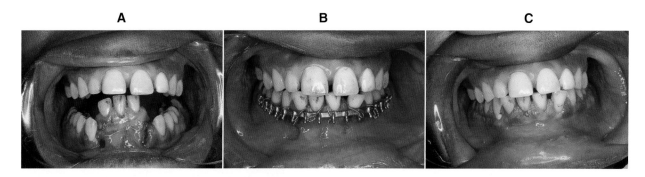

Figure 25-6

A, Intraoral photograph of a teenager who suffered a dentoalveolar fracture of the anterior mandible. **B,** An arch bar was placed to stabilize the segment. **C,** Occlusion after removal of the arch bar.

mandible). Specifically, approximately one third of fractures involve the condylar region, 20% to 30% the body, and 10% the symphysis.[17]

In children, condylar, subcondylar, and angle fractures account for 80% of the mandibular fractures.[17] Symphysis and parasymphysis fractures (15% to 20%) are more common than in adults, while body fractures occur only rarely.[10,49] In pediatric patients, the condylar region (36% to 50%) is affected most commonly.[2,5,17,50,51] In 2002, Iida[2] reported that in a series of eight children (ages 0 to 5 years) with facial fractures, six involved the condyle. With increasing age, the location of the mandibular fractures changes, and in adolescents the mandibular angle is fractured most commonly.[5,52]

Management of mandibular fractures in children differs somewhat from that in adults because of anatomic variation, rapidity of healing, degree of patient cooperation, and the potential for changes in mandibular growth. The treatment choice of fractures in the pediatric mandible depends on the age and the state of tooth development. The child's mandible is filled with teeth in various stages of development, and this has to be considered when deciding on a closed reduction with intermaxillary fixation versus open reduction with rigid internal fixation.

Diagnosis

The history of a mandibular fracture usually includes a fall or a blunt injury to the chin (Figures 25-7 and 25-8). There is often an accompanying laceration or abrasion. If there is a history of discomfort in the neck, a soft cervical collar should be placed immediately and cervical spine radiographs obtained before any further manipulation of the patient.[19,53] The child may have pain in one or both temporomandibular joints, indicating injury to the joint in the form of hemarthrosis or fracture. Often, the patient or parents complain that the "bite is off." It is imperative to determine how the occlusion is different:

1. Is there an anterior open bite?
2. Is the jaw more retruded?
3. Is the bite deviated to one side?

Retrognathism and open bite are indicative of bilateral subcondylar fractures. Unilateral subcondylar fractures usually result in an ipsilateral premature occlusion with crossbite or a contralateral lateral open bite.

Examination usually reveals a limitation of opening because of pain and muscle spasm. With unilateral subcondylar fractures, the jaw deviates toward the fracture on opening due to the unopposed action of the lateral pterygoid muscle on the normal condyle. There is often a prematurity or crossbite on the affected side and contralateral open bite (see Figure 25-8). If there are bilateral subcondylar fractures, the patient often has retrognathia and anterior open bite due to the resultant short rami and the depressor action of the suprahyoid muscles. Fractures in the tooth-bearing area are best demonstrated by

TABLE 25-1 Duration of Splinting in Dentoalveolar Injuries and Dental Trauma	
Type of Injury	**Time**
Subluxation	Optional splint for 7 to 10 days
Avulsed tooth	7 to 10 days
Extrusion	3 weeks
Lateral luxation	3 weeks; if radiograph shows marginal bone break, then additional 3 to 4 weeks
Crown/root fracture	3 weeks
Root fracture	3 to 4 weeks
Dentoalveolar fracture	3 to 4 weeks

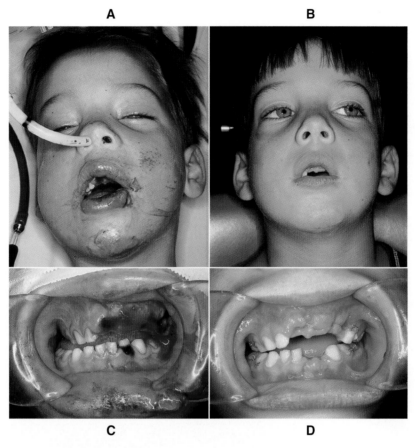

Figure 25-7

A, Frontal photograph illustrates a typical pediatric injury in this 6-year-old patient. He fell off a bicycle while riding downhill at high speed. Note the chin and lower lip laceration. The patient has decreased mandibular motion and pain in the temporomandibular joints bilaterally on opening. **B,** The same patient several weeks later after being released from fixation. The laceration is healed and the chin is in the midline. **C,** Intraoral photograph shows multiple missing teeth, blood around the lower left lateral incisor, and ecchymosis and hematoma in the buccal sulcus. There were a left parasymphysis and bilateral subcondylar fractures. **D,** Intraorally, the Ivy loops are still in place for use with training elastics. The occlusion is normal, and the opening pattern is midline, without deviation.

bimanual palpation, because there is often mobility across the fracture site. Frequently there is a hematoma in the buccal sulcus and ecchymosis in the floor of mouth in the area of fracture (Figure 25-9). The patient may have paresthesia or anesthesia in the distribution of the inferior alveolar nerve, although this is often difficult to assess in children.

The most useful radiographic study is the panoramic radiograph, which demonstrates the temporomandibular joints, ramus, angle, body, and symphysis of the mandible in one film (Figure 25-10). A mandibular occlusal radiograph helps document symphyseal fractures (Figures 25-11 and 25-12). A Towne's view shows the position and deviation of the condyles in the antero-

posterior plane (Figure 25-13). When a panoramic radiograph is not possible because of the lack of equipment or poor patient cooperation, a standard mandibular series is obtained: right and left lateral oblique, posteroanterior, and Towne's views (see Figure 25-13). In order to properly document a fracture, or lack thereof, films in two different planes must be obtained (see Figure 25-9). Computed tomography scans may be useful in children who cannot cooperate[55] but some fractures are missed unless a three-dimensional reconstruction is obtained. Three-dimensional computed tomography scans are also very important in documenting the position of the proximal segment in patients with condylar or subcondylar fractures.

A

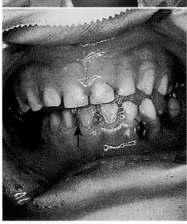

B

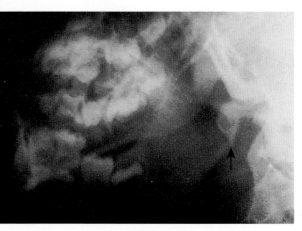

C

Figure 25-8 ▪▬▬▬▬▬

A, This 4-year-old child sustained trauma to the chin as a result of a fall from a porch. **B,** Intraorally, she had a crossbite on the left side, the mandibular dental midline deviated to the left, and the occlusion was premature on the left. She had a left subcondylar and a right parasymphysis fracture (separation between right central and lateral incisors). There was ecchymosis and hematoma in the mucosa over the symphysis. **C,** Lateral oblique radiograph demonstrates a left subcondylar fracture *(arrow)*.

Treatment

The management of mandibular fractures in children differs somewhat from that in adults, mainly because of the concern for possible disruption of normal growth. The main sites of growth are the condylar cartilage, the posterior border of the ramus, and the alveolar ridge. These areas of bone deposition account grossly for increases in the height, length, and width of the mandible. Bone fragments in children may become partially united as early as 4 days, and fractures become difficult to reduce by day 7. For this reason, treatment should be carried out as soon after the injury as possible.[5,7,50] Growth abnormalities may result from fracture dislocation of the condyle (effectively creating a short ramus and eliminating the "functional matrix" of lateral pterygoid function), trismus, or ankylosis.

In children, the mandibular cortex is thin and less dense than in adults, so care must be taken to avoid pulling a wire through the mandible.[1] The presence of tooth buds throughout the body of the mandible must be considered when doing an open reduction. Trauma to developing tooth buds and partially erupted teeth may occur when placing intraosseous wires or plates and screws for internal rigid fixation. This may result in failure of eruption of permanent teeth and a narrow atrophic alveolar ridge (Figure 25-14). However, failure of eruption of the teeth is not a common complication of open reduction with internal rigid fixation. Koenig et al.[56] found that 82% of the tooth buds in the fracture line of the mandible erupted normally, regardless if the method of treatment was open reduction with rigid fixation or closed reduction and maxillomandibular fixation. The shape and shortness of deciduous crowns may make the placement of circumdental wires and arch bars slightly more difficult in children. However, the narrow cervix of the tooth in relation to the crown and root provides better retention for wires (i.e., Stout wires or Ivy loops) (see Figure 25-9).

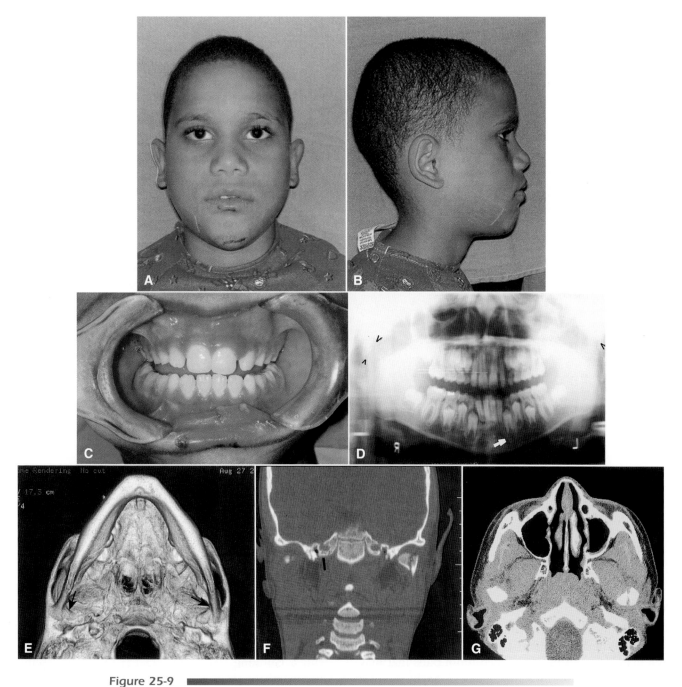

Figure 25-9

Frontal **(A)** and lateral **(B)** photographs of 10-year-old boy who fell, hitting his chin. **C,** Intraoral photograph shows a bilateral open bite. Examination revealed a lingual hematoma and mobility across the mandibular midline, as well as bilateral preauricular pain. **D,** Panoramic radiograph shows a left parasymphyseal fracture *(white arrow)* and raised suspicion about subcondylar fractures *(black arrowheads)*. **E,** The 3D CT image does not show the parasymphyseal fracture and shows some "unclear definition" of the medial aspects of both condyles *(arrows)*. Coronal **(F)** and axial CT **(G)** images clearly show the sagittally oriented high condylar fracture (intracapsular).

Continued

H

I

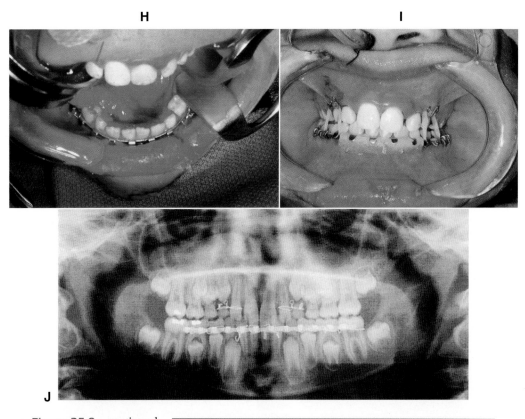

J

Figure 25-9—continued
H, Intraoperative photograph shows the lingual hematoma. **I,** Intraoperative photograph demonstrates immobilization and occlusion. **J,** Immediate postoperative Panorex. This child was treated with an acrylated arch bar, Ivy loops, guiding elastics, and opening exercises. It is important to reestablish function early to prevent ankylosis.

SPECIFIC MANDIBULAR FRACTURES
Body and Symphysis

The majority of body and symphysis fractures in children are nondisplaced, perhaps because of the elasticity of the mandible and the embedded tooth buds that may hold fragments together "like glue."[7,10] Slight occlusal discrepancies resulting from lack of a perfect reduction usually resolve spontaneously as the permanent teeth erupt and the bone undergoes remodeling with function. Nondisplaced body and symphysis fractures without malocclusion are treated by close observation (once or twice per week), blenderized diet, and avoidance of physical activities. If a body or symphysis fracture is displaced, closed reduction and immobilization is performed. The exact method of immobilization depends on the child's chronologic age and the stage of dental development.[10] In children under 2 years of age, the deciduous dentition may not be fully erupted and root development may be incomplete. In the mixed denti-

tion stage, only the 6-year molars may be adequate for circumdental wires. If possible, arch bars are placed, and the jaw is immobilized with elastics (see Figure 25-9). If the teeth are inadequate, the fracture site is immobilized with a Gunning (see Figure 25-12) or lingual splint. Intermaxillary fixation is used if the fracture is not immobilized adequately by the splint (i.e., if it is at the posterior region of the body beyond where the splint can be extended). In these cases, an impression is obtained (usually under general anesthesia), and the splint is constructed. If other injuries are being treated during the same anesthetic period, the splint should be inserted; otherwise a separate anesthetic is required. The fracture is reduced and the appliance fixed in place with circummandibular wires: one wire on either side of the fracture and an additional two wires to add stability to the splint. If intermaxillary fixation is also required, wires can be placed from the circummandibular wires to wires at the piriform rim or zygoma (care should be

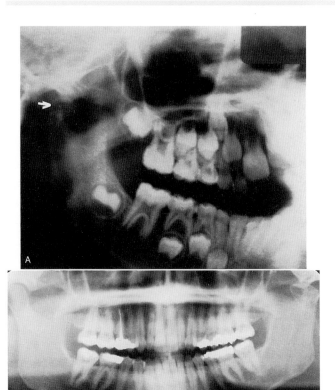

Figure 25-10
A, Panoramic radiograph showing a high right subcondylar fracture *(arrow)* with the condylar segment partially dislocated. **B,** Adult patient 22 years after left subcondylar fracture. Note the short ramus and remodeled condyle anterior to the glenoid fossa.

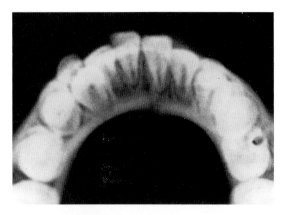

Figure 25-11
Occlusal radiograph illustrating a minimally displaced midline symphysis fracture.

taken not to saw through the zygoma or piriform rim when tightening the wires). The splint is left in place for 3 weeks. A general anesthetic usually is required to remove the appliance; the patient should be given prophylactic penicillin or clindamycin before the procedure. Alternatively, if possible, a monocortical microplate at the inferior border of the mandible can be placed. This is often easier and more efficient[57] (Figure 25-15).

Angle

Fractures at the angle (i.e., proximal to the tooth-bearing area) are not immobilized adequately by a mandibular splint alone; closed reduction and intermaxillary fixation for 3 weeks are required. If the dentition is inade-

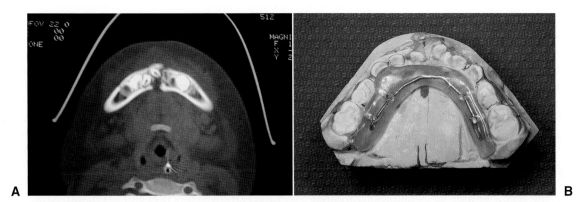

Figure 25-12
A, Axial CT image demonstrates symphyseal fracture. **B,** A lingual splint was used to treat the fracture. The splint can be wired to the teeth (preferably) or stabilized with circummandibular wires.

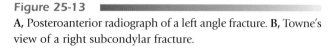

Figure 25-13
A, Posteroanterior radiograph of a left angle fracture. **B,** Towne's view of a right subcondylar fracture.

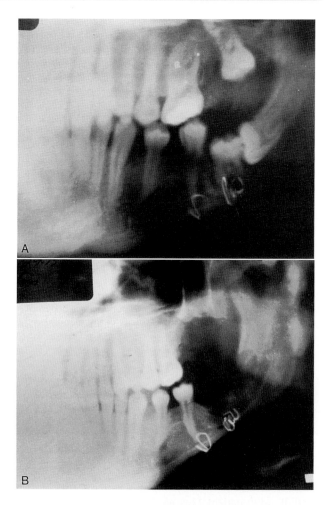

Figure 25-14
A, Intraosseous wiring of a posterior body fracture in a young child resulted in failure of eruption of the first molar and second premolar. **B,** After extraction to treat recurrent infection, the lack of development of the alveolar ridge is obvious.

quate, immobilization is achieved with Gunning splints on the maxilla and mandible. In these cases, it is important to avoid sawing through the bone when the wire is tightened. When performing an open reduction in children under the age of 5, it is possible to injure tooth buds near the angle when placing an intraosseous wire[17] or a plate and screws.

Condyle

Trauma to the chin producing temporomandibular joint injury is a frequent occurrence in childhood. The impact drives the mandibular condyle posterosuperiorly in the joint, against the skull base. The resultant injury may range from a capsular tear, to hemarthrosis, to a

fracture of the condylar head or neck. Occasionally, there is a crush injury to the condylar head producing a comminuted fracture. Pediatric fractures in the condylar region demonstrate the greatest potential for growth disturbance. Children less than 3 years of age with trauma to the condyle are at high risk for ankylosis.[1] Inadequate treatment or overtreatment may lead to growth retardation or growth excess, while excessive immobilization may result in mandibular hypomobility.[58] The two critical goals of treatment in these patients are (1) preservation of function and (2) maintenance of normal ramus height. When these are achieved, normal growth usually occurs.

Condylar fractures usually are classified by (1) location, i.e., intracapsular (condylar) or extracapsular (sub-

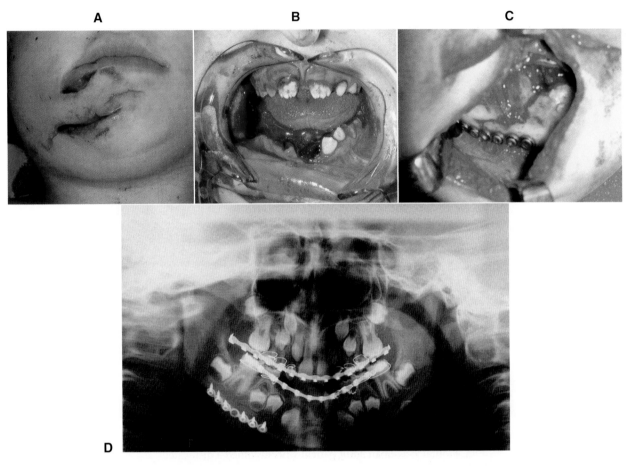

Figure 25-15
Frontal (**A**) and occlusal (**B**) photographs of a 7-year-old girl who fell off of a horse, suffering multiple lacerations and severe dentoalveolar trauma, including multiple dental avulsions. **C,** She also had a right mandibular fracture that was reduced and rigidly fixed at the inferior border with a 2.0 plate via a right chin laceration. **D,** Postoperative panoramic radiograph shows the rigid fixation of the mandibular fracture. The arch bars were used for stabilization of the dentoalveolar segments. (Courtesy Dr. Meredith August.)

condylar); (2) unilateral or bilateral; and (3) relationship of the proximal fragment to the glenoid fossa and the mandible. The fractures may be (a) nondisplaced, (b) displaced in fossa (referred to as *medial* and *lateral override depending*), or (c) dislocated, meaning the proximal head is out of fossa.[59] However, the location and degree of displacement of condylar fractures in *children in the primary and mixed dentition stage* are not useful variables for developing a treatment plan.[1] Rather, the amount of interincisal opening, dental age (primary, mixed, or permanent dentition), occlusion, and level of pain must be assessed carefully. If these are normal, treatment should consist of close observation and a blenderized diet.[1] For children, a better classification for

treatment planning would be based on the child's dental stage (i.e., primary, mixed, or permanent dentition).

Open reduction with internal rigid fixation rarely is indicated for pediatric condylar and subcondylar fractures, unless the displaced fragment produces a mechanical obstruction.[1,5,58-63] The overwhelming majority of condylar fractures in children can be treated adequately in a nonsurgical manner (observation, exercises, maxillo-mandibular fixation, training elastics, bite-opening splints)[5,50,58,62-71] (see Figure 25-9). Nonoperative management is overwhelmingly popular, because there are minimal complications and the outcomes are good with adults and children alike[59] (Figures 25-16 and 25-17).

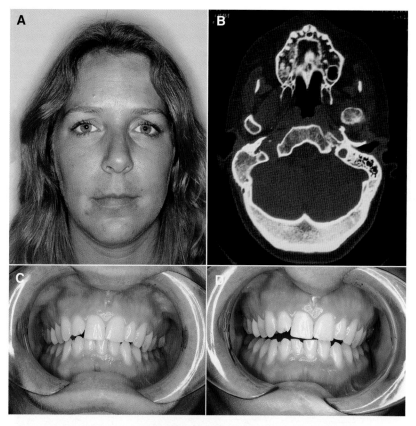

Figure 25-16

A, Frontal view of an adult patient who sustained a dislocated left subcondylar fracture 1 year previously. The left mandible is shorter than the right, and she deviates to the left on opening. **B,** Axial CT image demonstrates the dislocated condyle. **C,** Intraorally, maximum intercuspation is achieved with a habitual slide to the right and forward. **D,** In centric relation, she is premature on the left with an open bite on the right. This correlates with the short ramus on the left side.

In children with intracapsular condylar fractures or crush injuries (including hemarthrosis), there is a significant potential for ankylosis and growth disturbance.[17] Children less than 3 years of age with intracapsular fractures or crush injuries are at an increased risk for ankylosis.[1] They should be started early on mandibular exercises and jaw stretching to decrease the risk of this complication.[1] For older children, muscle relaxants and analgesics, as well as jaw stretching exercises, help to achieve normal function.

In children in the *primary and mixed dentition stage* with unilateral subcondylar fractures, analgesics and a blenderized diet for 5 to 7 days is usually adequate treatment. Minor malocclusions will correct spontaneously during this period. Deviation on opening is treated with midline opening exercises[72] (Figure 25-18).

If there is significant pain and severe malocclusion, a short period of immobilization for 7 to 10 days (with or without a bite-opening splint) is indicated. This treatment can be followed with training elastics as necessary.

In children in the *primary and mixed dentition stage* with bilateral subcondylar fractures, a relatively normal opening and stable occlusion may be present. In these cases analgesics and a blenderized diet for 7 to 10 days followed by soft diet for 2 weeks may be adequate (Figure 25-19). Minor malocclusions will correct spontaneously during growth. However, bilateral subcondylar fractures, especially if associated with dislocation, often produce an open-bite malocclusion because of the resultant short ramus and action of the suprahyoid muscles. In these cases, the jaw should be immobilized for 7 to 10 days (Figure 25-20). When fixation is released,

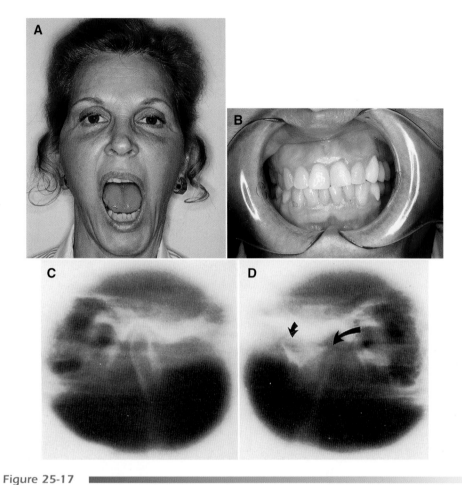

Figure 25-17

A, A patient opens with marked deviation to the left, 22 years after a left subcondylar fracture. **B,** Her occlusion is normal. **C,** Despite remodeling and partial growth of a new condyle *(large arrow)*, the ramus is short on the left side. When the condyle stump is dislocated *(small arrow)*, the mandibular ramus often remains short on the fractured side despite an attempt at regrowth of a condyle.

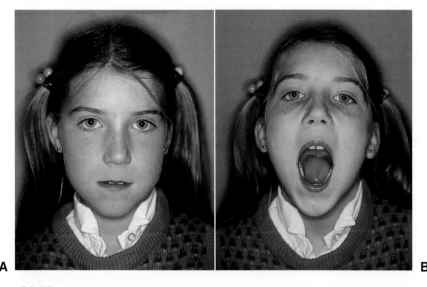

Figure 25-18

Frontal photographs at rest **(A)** and maximum jaw opening **(B)** document normal function in this child who had a unilateral subcondylar fracture treated without immobilization 6 months previously.

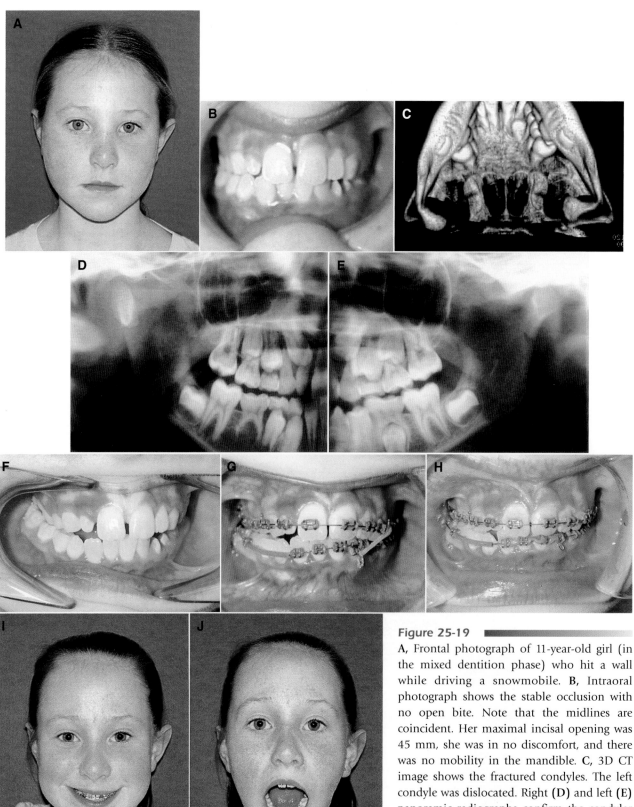

Figure 25-19

A, Frontal photograph of 11-year-old girl (in the mixed dentition phase) who hit a wall while driving a snowmobile. **B,** Intraoral photograph shows the stable occlusion with no open bite. Note that the midlines are coincident. Her maximal incisal opening was 45 mm, she was in no discomfort, and there was no mobility in the mandible. **C,** 3D CT image shows the fractured condyles. The left condyle was dislocated. Right **(D)** and left **(E)** panoramic radiographs confirm the condylar fractures. **F,** Intraoral photograph 2 weeks later shows the development of a right lateral crossbite. **G,** She was treated with one guiding elastic for 4 weeks. **H,** Her midlines remain coincident; she has no lateral slide and has resumed normal orthodontia. **I,** Frontal photograph shows good facial symmetry. **J,** Maximal incisal opening remains normal.

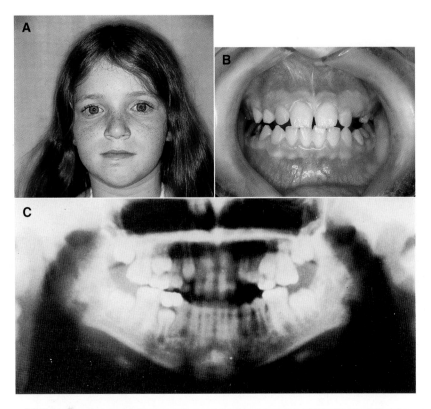

Figure 25-20
A, Frontal photograph of a 9-year-old girl who at age 7 suffered bilateral subcondylar fractures. She was treated with maxillomandibular fixation. Photograph shows facial symmetry.
B, Occlusal view demonstrates that the maxillary and mandibular dental midlines coincide.
C, Panoramic radiograph shows remodeling of the condyles.

the patient is placed in guiding elastics for another 7 to 10 days. If, after this period, a malocclusion persists, open reduction should be considered.

Children in the *permanent dentition stage* with unilateral or bilateral condylar fractures, especially if the fracture is dislocated, and who have persistent malocclusion after a course of intermaxillary fixation (7 to 10 days), should be considered for an open reduction to restore ramus length and to prevent progressive deformity (Figure 25-21). Restoration of normal symmetric jaw function provides the best chance for normal growth.[17,73] In older children there is less capacity for the bone to adapt and remodel, and the ramus height may not be regained.[66,67] Retrospective studies in adults show that the outcome of open reduction may be superior to that of nonsurgical therapy.[67,74-76] Furthermore, minimally invasive endoscopic approaches for subcondylar fractures may make surgeons less averse to open reduction and rigid fixation of condylar fractures.[74,77,78]

MANDIBULAR FRACTURES AND GROWTH ABNORMALITIES

Decreased vertical height of the mandibular body and alveolus may occur after a fracture of the horizontal ramus of the mandible if teeth are lost as a result of the injury or if hardware through tooth buds prevent dental eruption. Contour defects may result from severely comminuted and compound fractures in which the bone undergoes resorption during the remodeling process. In general, however, fractures of the mandibular body, per se, present little risk for long-term growth abnormalities.

Unilateral and bilateral condylar fractures, however, may result in mandibular asymmetry in the former and mandibular retrognathism and open bite in the latter. Much has been written about pediatric condylar fractures and facial growth. Most studies suggest that growth abnormality is rare and when it occurs it is often mild.[60-62,65,69] Leake et al.[72] demonstrated no growth abnormalities in 13 children with unilateral and 8 chil-

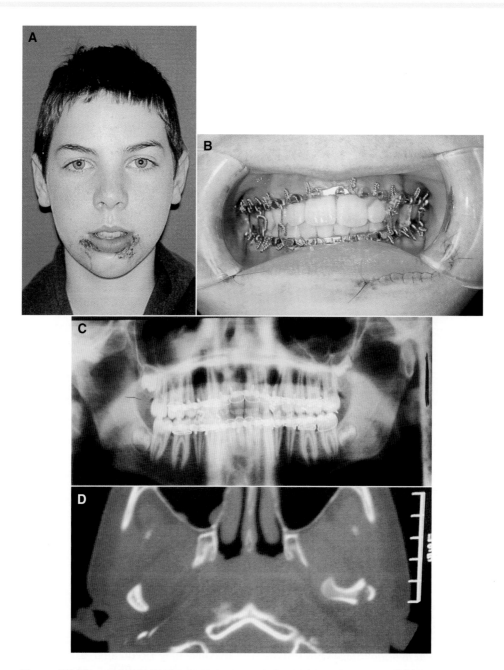

Figure 25-21

A, Frontal photograph of 15-year-old boy who suffered a left subcondylar fracture while snowboarding. **B,** He was treated with a 7-day course of maxillomandibular fixation. On attempt to remove the wire fixation he had a severe contralateral open bite and severe pain (requiring replacement of the wires). He was referred to our clinic. **C,** Panorex shows the rotated left condylar fragment. **D,** CT image confirms that the fragment is dislocated out of the fossa.

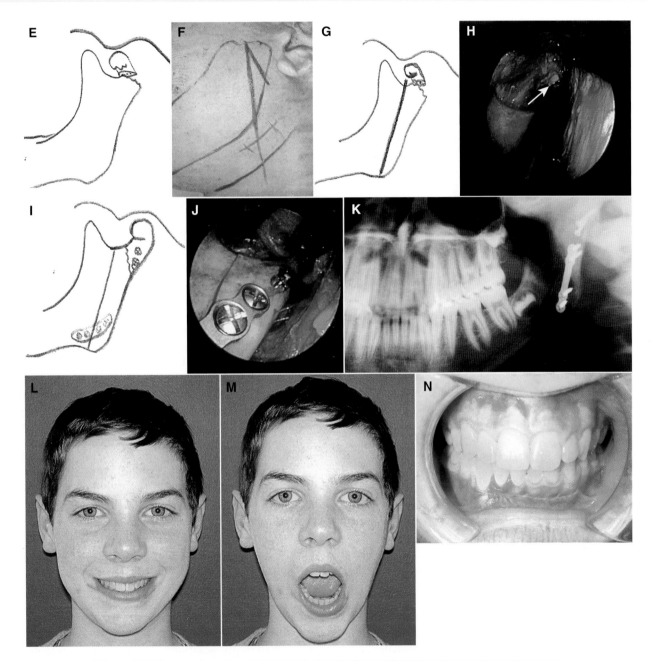

Figure 25-21—continued
E, Schematic of anticipated fracture. **F,** Photograph of the left side of the face. Intraoperatively, the mandibular landmarks, anticipated area of the fracture, and the proposed 1.5-cm incision are outlined in Malachite green. Schematic **(G)** and endoscopic **(H)** views of the distal mandible and the condylar stump, now easily accessed after a vertical ramus osteotomy was performed *(arrow* shows disc). Schematic **(I)** and endoscopic **(J)** views showing the condylar stump well reduced and fixed with two 2.0 screws; the proximal ramus is now fixed to the mandible with a 2.0 plate. **K,** The postoperative Panorex shows the proper alignment of the ramus/condyle unit. **L** and **M,** Frontal postoperative photographs show good symmetry and good interincisal opening. **N,** Intraoral postoperative photograph.

dren with bilateral subcondylar fractures treated with analgesics, liquid diet, and guiding elastics or exercises when necessary. Kaban et al.,[5] from the same institution, noted 1 patient out of a total of 39 patients with mandibular or subcondylar fractures who developed slight mandibular asymmetry after a subcondylar fracture. MacLennan found late facial growth deformities in patients who sustained intracapsular crush injuries prior to age 2.5.[60,64] Two studies by Walker[79] and Boyne,[80] involving monkeys, demonstrated that condylar fractures undergo remodeling with little growth abnormality after the injury.

Lund[58] carried out a prospective study of 38 growing patients with subcondylar fractures to determine what effect these injuries had on mandibular growth and to determine to what extent the condyle remodeled after fracture. This is the only significant prospective study of facial growth after condylar injury, and the material is of great interest to all surgeons who treat these injuries.

The 38 patients were from 4 to 17 years of age (32 patients were 12 years old or less and 6 were between 13 and 17). There were 11 bilateral fractures and 27 unilateral. Most patients (35 of 38) were treated by observation alone or in combination with intermaxillary fixation. Three patients had operative treatment: open reduction and fixation with K-rod (n = 1) and condylectomy (n = 2).

When trying to understand mandibular growth patterns after condylar fracture, it is important to realize that, as a result of the injury, the fractured side of the ramus is shorter than the unaffected side. In Lund's study, mandibular growth after condylar fracture was, in general, *greater* on the fractured than on the nonfractured side. The fractured ramus, which is initially shorter, has a greater incremental growth rate, so that a possible disproportion between the two sides is reduced with time. This was most evident when measuring the distance from the chin point to the condyle. Lund defined three types of mandibular growth in these patients:

1. Compensatory growth without overgrowth.
   The fractured side grows more than the normal side, but in the end it remains somewhat shorter than normal (13 of 27 patients, 48%). The clinical facial asymmetry becomes less evident.
2. Compensatory growth with overgrowth.
   The fractured side grows longer than the normal side (8 of 27 patients, 30%).
3. Dysplastic growth. The fractured side grows less than or at an equal rate to the normal side so that the difference in length between the two is accentuated with time.

The patients who demonstrated compensatory growth with overgrowth most commonly had only a small difference in ramus length immediately after injury. In other words, if the initial disproportion between the

fractured and nonfractured side was small, the patient had a greater chance of developing compensatory growth with overgrowth. Compensatory growth occurred in two patterns, similar to that seen in developmental condylar hyperplasia. In the predominantly vertical pattern, there is increased vertical length of the ramus with no deviation of the chin point. In the rotational pattern, there is an increased anteroposterior length of the mandible and progressive deviation of the chin point to the nonfractured side. Compensatory growth occurred only in those patients still growing at the time of injury. In summary, most patients who sustain condylar fractures (78%) show compensatory growth on the affected side and do not develop significant mandibular asymmetry. Dysplastic growth (i.e., progressive asymmetry with deviation of the chin toward the fractured side) developed in 22% of patients.

Most studies of growth after a condylar fracture have been retrospective and have started a considerable time after the primary injury.[5,50, 60, 61,63-65] If a mandibular asymmetry is noted, it is then attributed to decreased mandibular growth on the fractured side. The primary shortening of the mandible as a result of the injury is not considered. However, based on Lund's prospective observations beginning soon after the injury, most of these cases represent compensatory growth without overgrowth.

Lund also investigated the question of condylar remodeling after fracture. He defined two groups: (1) incomplete remodeling, in which the condyle was irregular or displacement remained at the fracture site and (2) complete remodeling. Complete remodeling occurred in 37 of 49 condyles and incomplete in 12 of 49. Patients with displaced condylar fractures (i.e., proximal fragment out of the fossa) had a greater chance of incomplete remodeling. Successful remodeling was also related to biologic age, occurring more frequently in the youngest patients. The difference between the remodeling in younger patients when compared with postpubertal adolescents was highly significant (p < 0.001).

Serial radiographs demonstrated that remodeling consisted of a combination of resorption and apposition. The process began at the time of injury and continued for a period of 5 to 49 months (mean = 23). When remodeling occurred successfully in displaced fractures, it consisted of resorption of the proximal condylar stump and outgrowth of a bony process on the ramus resembling a normal condyle. Other authors,[62,65,80] using serial radiographs, have also demonstrated partial resorption and remodeling of the condylar region after fracture. Norholt and Strobl found results similar to those of Lund in 1974.[66,67] They also found an age dependency on the amount of remodeling that occurred, that there was more complete remodeling (to a more radiologically normal-appearing condyle) in the younger age groups. However, function was normal in all age groups.

CONCLUSION

Dentoalveolar injuries and mandibular fractures in children occur most commonly as a result of a fall from a bicycle, steps, or climbing apparatus. Children with protrusive maxillary anterior teeth are particularly at risk for dentoalveolar injuries. These injuries are classified by the structures involved and depth of the injury: crown (enamel, dentin, pulp), root (cementum, dentin, pulp), and alveolus. This determines the treatment and ultimate prognosis of the injury.

Mandibular fractures in children most commonly occur in the condylar region, followed by the symphysis and angle. The fractures tend to be minimally displaced, and in the majority of cases, they can be treated without an operation, with a short period of immobilization. Significantly displaced mandibular fractures (especially in children in the permanent dentition stage) are reduced and immobilized using rigid internal fixation according the principles that are used in adults.

Fractures in the condylar region usually are treated using nonoperative therapies, especially in children in the primary and mixed dentition stages. In most children, the fracture heals and the condyle is remodeled with successful anatomic and functional results.

REFERENCES

1. Dodson TB: Mandibular fractures in children, *OMS Knowledge Update* 1(part II):95-107, 1995.
2. Iida S, Matsuya T: Pediatric maxillofacial fractures: their aetiological characters and fracture patterns, *J Craniomaxillofac Surg* 30:237-241, 2002.
3. Posnick JC, Wells M, Pron G: Pediatric facial fractures: evolving patterns of treatment, *J Oral Maxillofac Surg* 51:836-844, 1993.
4. Aceton CH, Nixon JW, Clark RC: Bicycle riding and oral/maxillofacial trauma in young children, *Med J Aust* 165:249-251, 1996.
5. Kaban LB, Mulliken JB, Murray JE: Facial fractures in children: an analysis of 122 fractures in 109 patients, *Plast Reconstr Surg* 59:15-20, 1977.
6. Kaban LB: Symposium on pediatric maxillofacial trauma: midface fractures in children. Presented at the 67th Annual Meeting of the American Association of Oral and Maxillofacial Surgeons, Washington, DC, October 2-7, 1985.
7. Mulliken JB, Kaban LB, Murray JE: Management of facial fractures in children, *Clin Plast Surg* 4:491-502, 1977.
8. Fortunato MA, Fielding AF, Guernsey LH: Facial bone fractures in children, *Oral Surg* 53:225-230, 1982.
9. Sowray JH: Localised injuries of the teeth and alveolar process. In Rowe NL, Williams J: *Maxillofacial injuries*, Edinburgh, 1985, Churchill Livingstone, pp 214-231.
10. James D: Maxillofacial injuries in children. In Rowe NL, Williams J: *Maxillofacial injuries*, Edinburgh, 1985, Churchill Livingstone, pp 538-559.
11. Tate RJ: Facial injuries associated with the battered child syndrome, *Br J Oral Surg* 9:41, 1971.
12. Schwartz S, Woolridge E, Stege D: Oral manifestations and legal aspects of child abuse, *J Am Dent Assoc* 95:586-591, 1977.
13. Laskin DM: The recognition of child abuse, *J Oral Surg* 36:349, 1978.
14. Needleman HL: Orofacial trauma in child abuse: types, prevalence, management and the dental profession's involvement, *Pediatr Dent* 8:71-80, 1986.
15. Bertolami CN, Kaban LB: Chin trauma: a clue to associated mandibular and cervical spine injury, *Oral Surg* 53:122-126, 1982.
16. Walker DG, Harrigan WF, Rowe NL: Clinical pathology conference on facial trauma: a panel discussion, *J Oral Surg* 27:575-585, 1969.
17. Kaban LB: Facial trauma II. Dentoalveolar injuries and mandibular fractures. In Kaban LB, editor: *Pediatric oral & maxillofacial surgery*, Philadelphia, 1990, WB Saunders, pp 233-260.
18. Lewis VL, Manson PN, Morgan RF, et al: Facial injuries associated with cervical fractures: recognition, patterns and management, *J Trauma* 25:90-93, 1985.
19. Laham JL, Cotcamp DH, Gibbons PA, et al: Isolated head injuries versus multiple trauma in pediatric patients: do the same indications for cervical spine evaluation apply? *Pediatr Neurosurg* 21:221-226, 1994.
20. Andreasen JO, Andreasen FM: Classification, etiology and epidemiology. In *Textbook and color atlas of traumatic injuries of the teeth*, ed 3, Copenhagen, 1994, Munksgaard, pp 151-180.
21. Lewis TE: Incidence of fractured anterior teeth as related to their protrusion, *Angle Orthod* 29:128-131, 1959.
22. Flores MT: Traumatic injuries in the primary dentition, *Dent Traumatol* 18:287-298, 2002.
23. von Arx T: Developmental disturbances of permanent teeth following trauma to the primary dentition, *Aust Dent J* 38:1-10, 1993.
24. Robertson A, Noren JG: Knowledge-based system for structured examination, diagnosis and therapy in treatment of traumatised teeth, *Dent Traumatol* 17:5-9, 2001.
25. Andreasen JO, Borum MK, Jacobsen HL, Andreasen FM: Replantation of teeth. I. Radiographic and clinical study of 110 human teeth replanted after accidental loss, *Acta Odontol Scand* 24:263-286, 1966.
26. Andreasen JO, Kristersson L: The effect of limited drying or removal of the periodontal ligament: periodontal healing after replantation of mature permanent incisors in monkeys, *Acta Odontol Scand* 39:1-13, 1981.
27. Andreasen JO, Borum MK, Jacobsen HL, Andreasen FM: Replantation of 400 avulsed permanent incisors. 4. Factors related to periodontal ligament healing, *Endod Dent Traumatol* 11:76-89, 1995.
28. Donaldson M, Kinirons MJ: Factors affecting the time of onset of resorption in avulsed and replanted incisor teeth in children, *Dent Traumatol* 17:201-205, 2001.
29. Trope M: Clinical management of the avulsed tooth: present strategies and future directions, *Dent Traumatol* 18:1-11, 2002.
30. Andreasen JO: Analysis of pathogenesis and topography of replacement root resorption (ankylosis) after replantation of mature permanent incisors in monkeys, *Swed Dent J* 4:231-240, 1980.
31. Hellsing E, Alatli-Kut I, Hammarström L: Experimentally induced dentoalveolar ankylosis in rats, *Int Endod J* 26:93-98, 1993.
32. Andersson L, Bodin I, Sorensen S: Progression of root resorption following replantation of human teeth after extended extraoral storage, *Endod Dent Traumatol* 5:38-47, 1989.
33. Tronstad L: Root resorption etiology, terminology and clinical manifestations, *Endod Dent Traumatol* 4:241-252, 1988.
34. Gahleitner A, Watzek G, Imhof H: Dental CT: imaging technique, anatomy, and pathologic condition of the jaws, *Eur Radiol* 13:366-376, 2003.

35. Flores MT, Andreasen JO, Bakland LK: Guidelines for evaluation and management of traumatic dental injuries, *Dent Traumatol* 17:1-4, 2001.

36. Flores MT, Andreasen JO, Bakland LK: Guidelines for evaluation and management of traumatic dental injuries, *Dent Traumatol* 17:49-52, 2001.

37. Flores MT, Andreasen JO, Bakland LK: Guidelines for evaluation and management of traumatic dental injuries, *Dent Traumatol* 17:97-102, 2001.

38. Flores MT, Andreasen JO, Bakland LK: Guidelines for evaluation and management of traumatic dental injuries, *Dent Traumatol* 17:145-148, 2001.

39. Flores MT, Andreasen JO, Bakland LK: Guidelines for evaluation and management of traumatic dental injuries, *Dent Traumatol* 17:193-196, 2001.

40. Holan G, Ram D: Sequelae and prognosis of intruded primary incisors: a retrospective study, *Pediatr Dent* 21:242-247, 1999.

41. Cvek M: Endodontic treatment of traumatized teeth. In Andreasen JO: *Traumatic injuries of the teeth*, Copenhagen, 1981, Munksgaard, pp 330-335.

42. Andreasen JO: Etiology and pathogenesis of traumatic dental injuries. A clinical study of 1298 cases, *Scand J Dent Res* 78:329-342, 1970.

43. Cvek M, Andreasen JO, Borum MK: Healing of 208 intraalveolar root fractures in patients aged 7-17 years, *Dent Traumatol* 17:53-62, 2001.

44. Barnett F: The role of endodontics in the treatment of luxated permanent teeth, *Dent Traumatol* 18:47-56, 2002.

45. Cvek M, Mejare I, Andreasen JO: Healing and prognosis of teeth with intra-alveolar fractures involving the cervical part of the root, *Dent Traumatol* 18:57-65, 2002.

46. Rodd HD, Davidson LE, Livesey S, Cooke ME: Survival of intentionally retained permanent incisor roots following crown root fractures in children, *Dent Traumatol* 18:92-97, 2002.

47. von Arx, T, Filippi A, Lussi A: Comparison of a new dental trauma splint device (TTS) with three commonly used splinting techniques, *Dent Traumatol* 17:266-274, 2001.

48. Ebeleseder KA, Glockner K, Pertl C, Städtler P: Splints made of wire and composite: an investigation of lateral tooth mobility, *Endod Dent Traumatol* 11:288-293, 1995.

49. Lehman JA, Saddawi ND: Fractures of the mandible in children, *J Trauma* 16:773, 1976.

50. Schultz RC, Meilman J: Facial fractures in children. In Goldwyn RM: *Long-term results in plastic and reconstructive surgery*, Boston, 1980, Little Brown, pp 458-480.

51. Cossio IP, Galvez EF, Perez GJL, et al: Mandibular fractures in children. A retrospective study of 99 fractures in 59 patients, *Int J Oral Maxillofac Surg* 23:329-331, 1994.

52. Thoren H, Iizuka T, Hallikainen D, Lindqvist C: Different patterns of mandibular fractures in children. An analysis of 220 fractures in 157 patients, *J Craniomaxillofac Surg* 20:292-296, 1992.

53. Bertolami CN, Kaban LB: Chin trauma: a clue to associated mandibular and cervical spine injury, *Oral Surg* 53:122-126, 1982.

54. Reference deleted in proofs.

55. Chacon GE, Dawson KH, Myall RW, Beirne OR: A comparative study of 2 imaging techniques for the diagnosis of condylar fractures in children, *Oral Maxillofac Surg* 61:668-672, 2003.

56. Koenig WR, Olsson AB, Pensler JM: The fate of developing teeth in facial trauma: tooth buds in the line of mandibular fractures in children, *Ann Plast Surg* 32:503-505, 1994.

57. Davison SP, Clifton MS, Davison MN, et al: Pediatric mandibular fractures: a free hand technique, *Arch Facial Plast Surg* 3:185-189, 2001.

58. Lund K: Mandibular growth and remodelling processes after condylar fracture: a longitudinal roentgencephalometric study, *Acta Odontol Scand* 32(suppl):3-117, 1974.

59. Sorel B: Mandibular condylar fractures, *OMS Knowledge Update* 3:47-62, 2001.

60. MacLennan WD: Consideration of 180 cases of typical fractures of the mandibular condylar process, *Br J Plast Surg* 5:122-128, 1952.

61. Thomson AG, Farmer AW, Lindsay WK: Condylar neck fractures of the mandible in children, *Plast Reconstr Surg* 34:452-463, 1964.

62. Gilhuus-Moe O: *Fractures of the mandibular condyle in the growth period*, Oslo, 1969, Universitetsforlaget, pp 28-44, 77-80, 117.

63. Leake DJ, Doykos J, Habal MB, et al: Long-term follow-up of fractures of the mandibular condyle in children, *Plast Reconstr Surg* 47:127-131, 1971.

64. MacLennan WD, Simpson W: Treatment of fractured mandibular condylar process in children, *Brit J Plast Surg* 18:423-427, 1965.

65. MacGregor AB, Fordyce GL: The treatment of fracture of the neck of the mandibular condyle, *Brit Dent J* 102:351-357, 1957.

66. Strobl H, Emshoff R, Rothler G: Conservative treatment of unilateral condylar fractures in children: a long-term clinical and radiologic follow-up of 55 patients, *Int J Oral Maxillofac Surg* 28:95-98, 1999.

67. Norholt SE, Krishnan V, Sindet-Pedersen S, Jensen I: Pediatric condylar fractures: a long-term follow-up study of 55 patients, *J Oral Maxillofac Surg* 51:1302-1310, 1993.

68. Thoren H, Hallikainen D, Iizuka T, Lindqvist C: Condylar process fractures in children: a follow-up study of fractures with total dislocation of the condyle from the glenoid fossa, *J Oral Maxillofac Surg* 59:768-773, 2001.

69. Hovinga J, Boering G, Stegenga B: Long-term results of nonsurgical management of condylar fractures in children, *Int J Oral Maxillofac Surg* 28:429-440, 1999.

70. Guven O, Keskin A: Remodelling following condylar fractures in children, *J Craniomaxillofac Surg* 29:232-237, 2001.

71. Dahlstrom L, Kahnberg KE, Lindahl L: 15 years follow-up on condylar fractures, *Int J Oral Maxillofac Surg* 18:18-23, 1989.

72. Leake DJ, Doykos L, Habal MB, et al: Long-term follow-up of fractures of the mandibular condyle in children, *Plast Reconstr Surg* 47:127-131, 1971.

73. Demianczuk AN, Verchere C, Phillips JH: The effect on facial growth of pediatric mandibular fractures, *J Craniofac Surg* 10:323-328, 1999.

74. Lee C, Mueller RV, Lee K, Mathes SJ: Endoscopic subcondylar fracture repair: functional, aesthetic, and radiographic outcomes, *Plast Reconstr Surg* 102:1434-1443, 1998.

75. Eckelt U: Condylar neck fractures, *Mund Kiefer Gesichtschir* 4(suppl 1):S110-S117, 2000.

76. Ellis E III, Simon P, Throckmorton GS: Occlusal results after open or closed treatment of fractures of the mandibular condylar process, *J Oral Maxillofac Surg* 58:260-268, 2000.

77. Troulis MJ, Kaban LB: Endoscopic approach to the ramus/condyle unit: clinical applications, *J Oral Maxillofac Surg* 59:503-509, 2001.

78. Schmelzeisen R, Lauer G, Wichmann U: Endoscope-assisted fixation of condylar fractures of the mandible, *Mund Kiefer Gesichtschir* 2(suppl):S168-S170, 1998.

79. Walker RV: Traumatic mandibular condylar fracture dislocations, *Am J Surg* 100:850-863, 1960.

80. Boyne PJ: Osseous repair and mandibular growth after subcondylar fractures, *J Oral Surg* 25:300-309, 1967.

Index

Page numbers followed by *f*, *t*, and *b*
indicate figures, tables, and boxed material,
respectively.